Functional Neurorehabilitation Through the Life Span

Functional Neurorehabilitation Through the Life Span

Dolores B. Bertoti MS, PT

Associate Professor and Dean
Alvernia College
Reading, PA
Pediatric Clinical Specialist,
Certified by the American Board
of Physical Therapy Specialists, 1993–2003

F. A. DAVIS • Philadelphia

F. A. Davis Company
1915 Arch Street
Philadelphia, PA 19103
www.fadavis.com

Printed in the United States of America

Last digit indicates print number: 10 9 8 7 6 5 4 3 2 1

Acquisitions Editor: Margaret Biblis
Developmental Editor: Peg Waltner
Cover Designer: The Creative Group

As new scientific information becomes available through basic and clinical research, recommended treatments and drug therapies undergo changes. The author(s) and publisher have done everything possible to make this book accurate, up to date, and in accord with accepted standards at the time of publication. The author(s), editors, and publisher are not responsible for errors or omissions or for consequences from application of the book, and make no warranty, expressed or implied, in regard to the contents of the book. Any practice described in this book should be applied by the reader in accordance with professional standards of care used in regard to the unique circumstances that may apply in each situation. The reader is advised always to check product information (package inserts) for changes and new information regarding dose and contraindications before administering any drug. Caution is especially urged when using new or infrequently ordered drugs.

Library of Congress Cataloging-in-Publication Data

Bertoti, Dolores.
   Functional neurorehabilitation through the life span / Dolores
Bertoti.
         p. ; cm.
Includes index.
   ISBN 0–8036–1107–2
   1. Nervous system—Diseases—Patients—Rehabilitation. 2.   Physical
therapy. 3.   Occupational therapy.
   [DNLM: 1.   Nervous System Diseases—rehabilitation—Case Report. 2.
Occupational Therapy—methods—Case Report. 3.   Physical Therapy
Techniques—methods—Case Report. WL 300 B547c 2003] I. Title.
   RC350.4.B476 2003
616.8′043—dc21
                                                                       2003048504

Dedication

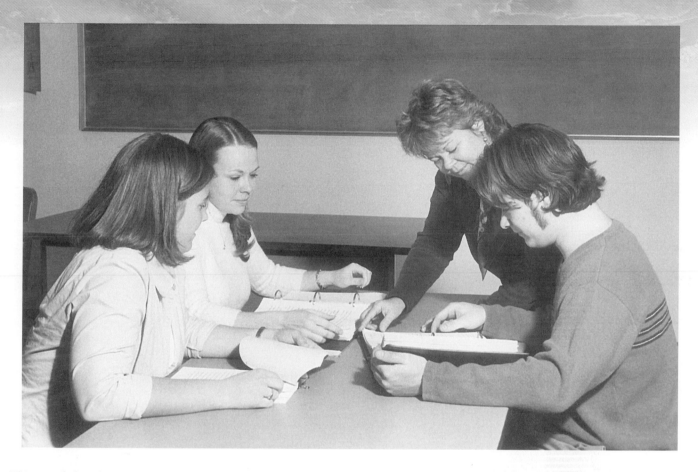

This work has been written in honor of all the patients and their families that have blessed me with their faith, unconditional love of each other, and courage. This work is devoted to all students, the clinicians of tomorrow, to whom I wish the joy of spending their professional days steeped in the continual pursuit of knowledge, relentless inquiry, deep caring, and the wisdom of gratefully knowing that you always receive twice as much as you give. You have all touched me forever and given me more blessings than I can ever count.

Preface

This book is the culmination of twenty-eight years of clinical practice, clinical inquiry, reading, writing, and teaching. I count my work as among one of my life's greatest blessings. I still love what I do as much as I did during my first clinical experience as a young volunteer, then as a student, therapist, and now teacher. How fortunate I am to awaken every day being able to do what I love!

This book literally has been in my head for about the past decade. As a board certified clinical specialist within the physical therapy profession and an educator in both physical therapy and occupational therapy programs, every day I see the symbiosis that must exist between clinical practice and advances in that profession's knowledge base. Informed clinical practice and ongoing scientific advances are equal catalysts for dedicated professionals who attempt to bring the best and most current insights to the practice arena for the benefit of the patient/client. Actually, the most exciting feature about the rehabilitation field *is* the dynamic, evolving nature of the field. As knowledge in the basic sciences increases, there will be a natural evolution of therapeutic approaches as practitioners develop their expertise in applying this new neuroscience knowledge to patient care. Concurrently, experienced practitioners will demand innovative answers and new ideas from the basic scientists to further develop the evolution of practice insights that occur in the science of clinical application. This text, as with others, will need ongoing revision as knowledge emerges and as clinicians and applied researchers strive for effectiveness, evidence, and measurable outcomes in clinical application.

The purpose of this text is to provide an integrated approach to basic neuroscience and applied neurorehabilitation, presented with practical applications illustrating the functional implications of neurological damage. This book attempts to answer one main question often posed by entry-level practitioners in the fields of occupational therapy and physical therapy as they initially encounter individuals with movement impairments and subsequent functional limitations caused by neurological disorders:

Do not tell me only what is going on with the patient/ client, but more importantly, what can I do to improve that person's function, where do I start, and how do I try to ensure that my intervention is really meaningful to that individual?

This text attempts to present the essentials of neuroscience and movement control and to provide practical applications by offering solutions to commonly encountered clinical dilemmas affecting an individual's ability to move effectively and efficiently as he or she attempts to function the best that he or she can under his or her unique given circumstances. This text presents a practical and therefore unique perspective to well-established and emergent rehabilitation practice. There really is no totally new information but rather unusual and fresh combinations of materials that have been presented elsewhere. What *is* new and original is the lens through which the same material is viewed, the lens of an educator and a problem-solving, experienced clinician.

Becoming a master clinician is possible only because of the teaching and insight gained from many of the professions' great masters. Although I reference the works of many authors throughout the text, it is imperative that I note, with deep humility, the guidance and knowledge already available from so many of our professions' leaders. Leaders and authors like Anne Shumway-Cook, Marjorie Woollacott, Susan O'Sullivan, Thomas Schmitz, Catherine Trombly, Janet Carr, Roberta Shepherd, Rona Alexander, Regi Boehme, Barbara Cupps, Lois Bly, Suzanne Campbell, Jane Case-Smith, Susan Duff, Susan Miller Porr, Ellen Berger Rainville, Darcy Umphred, Susan Ryerson, Kathryn Levit, Donna Cech, Suzanne "Tink" Martin, Mary Kessler, Laurie Lundy-Ekman, Jane Styer-Acevedo, Ann VanSant, Pamela Duncan, Faye Horak, Joan Valvans, Toby Long, Susan Herdman, Helen Cohen, Jacqueline Perry, Chuck Leonard, Katherine Ratliffe, Carol Oatis, and Becky Craik have all contributed great works from which our students and patients can benefit. I certainly have learned a great deal from all these talented leaders in the rehabilitation profession. I have built upon the work of these authors and acknowledge the contributions they have made to our professional body of knowledge. As cited throughout this text, I have attempted to reframe much of the information from the writings from these leaders into a consolidated, practical approach to life span intervention. This text attempts to present "best practice" insights, made clinically meaningful and easily applicable to patient care. This text is different in that it attempts to be extremely practical, focused on functional but personally meaningful outcomes, and approaches an understanding of the individual presenting for intervention at *any* stage throughout the life span.

As a physical therapist, I always have respected and relied on the professional expertise of my colleagues in the occupational therapy profession. I am honored to have been joined by the author of the *Occupational Therapy Guide to Practice*, Penelope Moyers, Ed.D. OTR/L, FAOTA, as a coauthor of Chapter 1. This introductory chapter portrays with intention the importance of both collegial teamwork and respect for professional autonomy. I also am honored to have the contributions of Catherine Emery, MS, OTR/L, BCN and Doré Blanchet, MS, OTR/L in Chapters 8 and 9 respectively. These talented occupational therapists are among the faculty at Alvernia College, and I am delighted to work side by side with them. Kate (Catherine Emery) is board certified in neurological occupational therapy and Doré Blanchet is a pediatric occupational therapist, with sensory integration certification.

This book is intended for use by educators and clinicians within physical therapy and occupational therapy. Although both professions are complementary, they are different and separate. The client, however, is *one whole* individual who often presents with multiple needs. The different and uniquely valuable insights of both professions reflect the separate roles of the rehabilitation team, all of whom are focused on maximizing an effective interaction between the person, the activity, and the environment, thereby facilitating an "enabling" rather than a "disabling" process. Occupational therapy and physical therapy professionals are locked arm in arm with helping their patients/clients strive for the overarching goal of improved function. The differences and unique skills characteristic of each discipline support the need for a close working relationship to thoroughly solve the problems of functioning in a way that might not be achieved by one discipline. Celebrating differences as well as similarities creates unending opportunities for professional growth. Ultimately, the patient clearly benefits from this collegial relationship. I have enjoyed creating this text and sincerely hope that it finds a place among its partners as the professions of physical therapy and occupational therapy continue to evolve and refine.

Acknowledgments

My husband, Willy, and our son, Christopher, encouraged me for years to "just write a book," challenging me to describe for new and aspiring clinicians the knowledge and insight I had gathered over years of practice, clinical study, writing, and teaching. They cheered me on during every aspect of this project, when "just write a book" translated into month after month of hard work. Christopher, our college-aged son, and his friends read many pieces of the text and the workbook, reminding me to keep my writing student-friendly and giving me great ideas. "The book" lived with all of us, earning a loved place in the midst of our family and home life. It was exciting for all of us. Thanks to both of you for all of your faith in me. I love you both beyond words.

Family is a wonderful support. My mother, son, nephew, brother, and husband all modeled for me in some of the photographs. How many authors are fortunate enough to have a talented brother willing to do the original artwork to help bring a dream into being? My brother, Timothy Brough, gave the gift of his love and talent, providing me, and now countless students of the future, with beautiful, original illustrations. He was able to listen to my description of what needed to be drawn and capture the essence of that information with an ingenious balance of clarity and detail. He is absolutely incredible. Thank you, Tim.

The artwork and photography for this book became possible because of the hard work and love of a great deal of people. Reggie Wickham, a world-class photographer, came to Alvernia College and photographed, with sensitivity and talent, the therapists and assistants working with clients or models. Therapists from among the faculty at Alvernia or the staff of Easter Seal of Berks County demonstrated their talent in an effort to share that talent with the clinicians and patients of tomorrow. The adults and children who participated in the photograph sessions humbled all of us with their enthusiasm and gifts of time and self. I am honored to know you. Out of respect for the privacy of these many wonderful individuals and their families who came forward to help create this text, the names and data in the cases of this text *do not match* the person in the photo. Rather, the data was created from clinical experience and the case was construed for educational purposes. Again, I humbly thank all who helped in this effort. You are a gift to me and now to countless others.

Alvernia College, where I am an Associate Professor and currently an Academic Dean, supported this effort every step of the way and in countless small and large measures. The assistance was palpable from every level, from the Board, Administration, faculty, staff, and students, contributing everything from a sabbatical for the bulk of the writing, to the use of the facilities for the photo sessions and the support of technology, bibliographical support, and the assistance of a very special student worker, Stacey Puzaskas. The college administration gave me tangible moral support for which I will be forever grateful. Their pride and belief in me sustained my motivation and energy.

The professionals at and associated with F. A Davis Company are phenomenal. Margaret Biblis is without doubt a professional of tremendous class. She has the wonderful ability to move an author through a total project, from the exciting birth of an idea, through its somewhat uncertain incubation, during the tiring middle phases, over the last hurdles when energy is low, and finally celebrating with everyone the team effort necessary to bring an idea to fruition. The greatest surprise gift came through the friendship I gained by working with my energetic and highly motivating developmental editor, Peg Waltner. Her knowledge, organizational abilities, honesty, and strength became a real support beam to me throughout the seemingly endless months of writing and revision. She was an honest, insightful coach to me throughout the months of writing, revision, and finalizing this text for production. Peg, you are the best!

In closing, I humbly thank my Dad who always believed that I could do anything I set my mind to, and God from Whom all blessings come and Who keeps me centered. They were both with me every step of the way.

Contributors

Doré Blanchet, MS, OTR/L
Assistant Professor
Alvernia College
Reading, PA

Catherine Emery, MS, OTR/L, BCN
Assistant Professor and Associate Dean
Alvernia College
Reading, PA

Penelope A. Moyers, Ed.D., OTR, FAOTA
Professor and Dean
University of Indianapolis
Indianapolis, IN

About the Author

Dolores Brough Bertoti is a 1975 graduate of Temple University with a BS in Physical Therapy, later earning an advanced Masters in Physical Therapy from the same university in 1984. She earned certification as a Pediatric Clinical Specialist in 1993 from the American Board of Physical Therapy Specialties, subsequently serving the board as an appointed member of the Specialization Academy of Content Experts (SACE), Pediatric Specialty Council as an item writer from 1997 to 1999. Dolores has been a physical therapist for 28 years, authoring eighteen publications in the areas of applied neurorehabilitation, pediatric clinical practice, electrotherapy, and clinical research. Her publications include case reports, clinical research, review articles, a home study course, text chapters, and now, a text and companion workbook. Her most recent publications include: Bertoti, D. B. (2002). Clinical practice: Pediatric physical therapy. In R. Scott, *Foundations of physical therapy*. New York: McGraw-Hill; Bertoti, D. B. (2002). Electrical stimulation: A reflection on current clinical practices. Research and Engineering Society of North America. *Assistive Technology, 12,* 21–32; Bertoti, D. B. (2000). *Cerebral palsy: Lifespan management.* Orthopaedic Section Home Study Course, Orthopaedic Interventions for the Pediatric Patient. American Physical Therapy Association; Stanger, M., & Bertoti D. B. (Eds.). (1997). An Overview of Electrical Stimulation for the Pediatric Population. *Pediatric Physical Therapy, 9* (special issue); and Bertoti, D. B. et al. (1997). Percutaneous intramuscular electrical stimulation as an intervention choice for children with cerebral palsy. *Pediatric Physical Therapy, 9,* 123–127. Active in clinical inquiry and scholarly writing, Dolores has been recognized as recipient of the following awards: American Physical Therapy Association Jack Walker Award for Excellence in Clinical Research (1989), Nominee American Physical Therapy Association Pediatric Research Award (1991), and the American Business Club National Therapist of the Year (1990).

Her clinical practice is hallmarked by several noteworthy, pioneering accomplishments. In 1977, Dolores founded the first early intervention program of the Easter Seal Society of Berks County, emphasizing her commitment to education for parents of children with challenges. She then participated in a statewide training program through Albright College, training therapists and teachers throughout Pennsylvania in intervention approaches for children with physical impairments. She was in private practice from 1985 to 2002, involved in several modes of clinical practice and consultation. Between 1986 and 1991, Dolores served as Therapy Coordinator at Sebastian Riding Associates, a nonprofit center for therapeutic horseback riding. Through her efforts, many therapists were trained in making horseback riding safe and therapeutically sound for children and adults with disabilities, and she was able to conduct and publish the first scientific research study on the effects of riding on postural control. Between 1993 and 1996, Dolores served as a research associate on a team at the Shriners Hospital in Philadelphia investigating the efficacy of percutaneous intramuscular electrical stimulation as an intervention option for children with cerebral palsy, again publishing and presenting the findings. Presently, Dolores is a research mentor with the Thomas Jefferson University Occupational Therapy Program Project, Therapy in Natural Environments, as well as a peer mentor with the American Physical Therapy Association.

A respected and engaging lecturer, Dolores has been an invited speaker presenting continuing education workshops regionally, nationally, and internationally, totaling more than twenty-five presentations. Her presentation topics cover a wide range, including clinical practice in neurorehabilitation, electrotherapy, and pediatrics, with a focus on the application of motor control theory on evaluation and intervention. She most recently is presenting on topics pertaining to enhancement of student success and the importance of scholarly writing as an integral component of professional development. She routinely presents poster presentations at state, regional, and national conferences.

Dolores joined the faculty of Alvernia College in Reading, Pennsylvania in 1992, where she has served as department chair of the OT, PTA, and AT programs, program director of the PTA program, and interim

xiv About the Author

program director of the OT program. She taught in the Physical Therapist Assistant program between 1992 and 2001, and served as adjunct instructor at Arcadia University in Pediatric Physical Therapy between 1991 and 2000. At Alvernia, she is currently an associate professor in the areas of Movement Science, Kinesiology, Neuroscience, and Electrotherapy for the Occupational Therapy and Athletic Training pro- grams, and has been instrumental in the development of the programs. In addition, Dolores is Dean of Academic Advancement. Faculty Development and Student Success initiatives at the college are organized under her leadership. Known for her talent and energy in the classroom, Alvernia College awarded her the Annual St. Bernardine Award for Teaching Excellence in 1995.

About the Artist

Timothy Brough is a self-taught illustrator residing in Upper Darby, Pennsylvania with his wife, Andrea. With more than twenty years experience as a graphic artist, he is currently employed as Art Director with a nationally renowned decorator in the screen printing and embroidery industry. In addition to commercial graphics, Tim enjoys painting and drawing. His work is featured prominently in the annual Philadelphia St. Patrick's Day parade. Brother to the author, and this being his first venture as an illustrator for a medical textbook, Tim ascribes his success to his sister's compelling spirit, enthusiasm, and keen communication skills, making it possible for him to be able to create these unique images.

About the Photographer

Reginald Wickham is an internationally acclaimed photographer from Mount Laurel, New Jersey. A member of the prestigious Photographic Society of America, Reggie was awarded their John Doscher Award in 1999, which is given annually to only one photographer in the world. He is ranked fourth in North America for pictorial photography.

His work has been published in major photographic journals, magazines, catalogs, and brochures, including the Annual Report for the Staten Island Hospital in Staten Island, New York.

Numerous articles written about him praise his extraordinary talent, encompassing an artist's perspective with a highly developed skill.

Contents

Part 1

The Science Behind the Art of Patient Intervention

The Role of Occupational and Physical Therapy in Neurorehabilitation

Dolores B. Bertoti, MS, PT and
Penelope A. Moyers, EdD, OTR, FAOTA

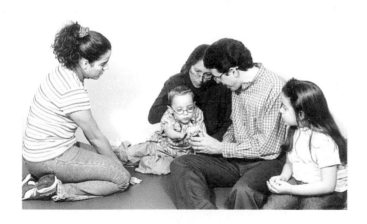

Cornerstone Concepts

- Relationship between basic science and theoretical intervention approaches in physical and occupational therapy

- The complementary roles of occupational and physical therapy in neurological rehabilitation

- Application of disablement model and focus on enablement

- The APTA and AOTA guides to practice and practice framework

- Clinical decision making and clinical reasoning

The common denominator between occupational and physical therapy is to focus on the value of a true therapeutic use of oneself in selfless giving. Working effectively with a client means that the client is always at the center of every team member's thoughts; requiring that each team member preserve autonomy, celebrate common backgrounds and unique insights, and remember that each perspective is contributory but not more important than another.

Introduction

Caring for patients is the single most important concern of rehabilitation professionals. Patient care and human service are probably the incentives that draw most aspiring clinicians to either occupational or physical therapy as a chosen profession. Regardless of the unique setting in which one works, caring for people is the very glue that binds all of us together and enthuses us as we approach every workday. Clinicians, managers, educators, researchers, and writers all literally do what they do *for the person entrusted to their care*. The patient gives meaning to who we are and what we do as health care professionals. As the fields of physical and occupational therapy develop, change, and mature, the patient or client remains at the center and provides the motivation for continued professional development.

In both occupational and physical therapy, several different terms may be used to identify the recipient of these professional services. In physical therapy, the traditional term *patient* continues to be most commonly used, especially when referring to individuals within the medical setting. With the broadening of services to include wellness, screening, education, and preventive care, use of the term *client* is gaining in popularity in both professions. In the field of occupational therapy, the word *client* is more often used than the word *patient* to indicate that many occupational therapists and occupational therapy assistants do not work in medical model settings (Moyers, 1999). The word *client* may indicate that therapists and their assistants provide population-based services in which the client may be a group of people, an organization, or a community. Even when the client is a group of people, occupational therapists and occupational therapy assistants still provide intervention based on the understanding of the occupational performance needs of a single individual.

In this book, the words *patient* and *client* are used interchangeably for both disciplines. Both professions commonly employ the words *intervention* and *intervention planning* to denote the collaborative role of the client in the treatment process. In the past, the word *treatment* was thought to imply something done *to* people rather than *with* people. However, even though the word *treatment* is used in this book at times to indicate the rehabilitation model, the authors stress the importance of the patient/client being involved in the decision making throughout the process of therapy, a philosophical orientation commonly referred to as patient-centered care.

Occupational and physical therapists and their assistants, depending on their caseload, may participate in the effective rehabilitation of patients who are neurologically impaired. The scope and limitations of practice are well defined and easily found in entry-level texts in both disciplines. It is *not* the intent of this text to blur the lines between the professions of occupational and physical therapy, although there are legitimate areas of overlap between the two professions. Rather, the intent is to reinforce the unique value of the contribution of each discipline to the overall management of the patient/client, given that the areas of overlap also contribute to our ability to understand each other and work together. This text is written for students and clinicians of both professions, with a focus on patient application.

The language and communication style throughout this text is friendly and direct. The author and contributors recognize the demanding task of the student to delve into a topic that is complex by nature. The author also recognizes, however, that it is the task and the responsibility of experienced therapists who are now also authors and teachers to make this material not only palatable but also exciting and interesting. It is a pleasure to make that attempt.

Neuroscience and Neurorehabilitation

Definitions and Scope

The orchestration of human movement is nothing short of miraculous. Whether the example is a baby reaching with accuracy for a parent's face, a young hockey player shooting a forceful goal, a ballet dancer expressing emotion artistically through graceful movement, a college student racing across campus to make class, or a professor struggling to carry armloads of books and papers, the human body is a constant marvel. The nervous system sends, refines, and changes expressions of movement as appropriate for the demand of the task. These movement commands are then filtered through the musculoskeletal system. Absolute intrigue with the mystery and marvel of human movement can ignite and excite the student of rehabilitation. It is true that rehabilitation is not limited to understanding only movement and that the nervous system is involved in the execution of multiple functions, such as cognitive processing, emotion, perception, sensory processing, vision, and psychological functioning, which occupational therapists and occupational therapy assistants also deal with. However, this text primarily focuses on movement.

By definition, **neuroscience** is the "quest to understand the nervous system," having evolved as an interdisciplinary science from several basic sciences, including medicine, biology, mathematics, physics, chemistry, and psychology (Lundy-Ekman, 2002). **Neurorehabilitation** is the application of neuroscience to the rehabilitation of patients with brain injury. A brief reflection on the history of the acquisition of neuroscience knowledge is helpful to set the tone for this text. It also helps the new professional to set foot on the current stage of neurorehabilitation as an applied science. A historical review is helpful to illustrate the ongoing nature of scientific inquiry. Today's rehabilitation professionals are at this point in history as a result of the efforts and discoveries of all their predecessors within the profession. *Our moment in history is now.* New discovery and advances will surely continue, built on the contributions of today's scientists and clinicians—you!

Historical Review

The ancient Egyptians recognized the brain as a space-occupying structure implicated in lesions associated with altered behavior. Recovered writings from the physicians of ancient Egypt, dating back almost 5000 years, indicate that they were well aware of the signs and symptoms of brain damage (Bear, Connor, & Paradiso, 2001). They did not, however, develop any theories about the specific relationship between the brain and behavior. In fact, they believed that the heart, not the brain, was the habitation of the soul. As evidence of this belief, although the rest of the body was preserved carefully and mummified for the afterlife, the brain of the deceased ancient Egyptian was simply scooped out through the nostrils and discarded because the heart, not the brain, was considered the seat of consciousness and memory.

In ancient Greece, some debate continued as to whether the heart or the brain was the center of the human intellect. Hippocrates (460–379 B.C.), the father of Western medicine, was the first to state that the brain was the seat of intelligence. Arguing against him with a still significant following, however, was the famous Greek philosopher Aristotle (384–322 B.C.), who clung to the belief that the heart was the center of the intellect. Aristotle proposed that the brain functioned as a radiator for the cooling of blood that was overheated by the emotional, seething heart (Bear et al., 2001).

These early observations and the limitations experienced by these observers as a result of lack of sophisticated methods of analysis illustrate an important lesson that is still relevant today for the student of neuroscience. These ancient scientists and students of neuroscience were all limited by the fact that their observations were not systematic and were not linked to a strategy for analysis and understanding. Of course, technology was not available to permit rigorous observation and sophisticated analysis, but the problem-solving strategies themselves were also shortsighted. The early observations, important as they were, were only that—observations. Early on, there was little

attempt to conduct systematic observations and little ability to analyze the observations. The focus was simply on recording the observations themselves.

The important lesson gleaned from the history of neuroscience for today's student and clinician is that, without a *theoretical* reference within which to organize and analyze observations, progress in the understanding of brain function is limited. **Theory** in its simplest form is defined as a statement of relationships among important concepts. The scope of theory may range from single statements meant to explain a specific phenomenon to a set of interrelated statements designed to address a broad range of phenomena (Domholdt, 2000). Normally, observation conducted without the organizational context of theory to guide interpretation (deduction) fails to further understanding. However, if observation follows a rigorous and systematic process to remove the influence of existing theory, it can be a major strategy for developing new and emerging theoretical concepts and relationships (induction). Equally important, theory that emerges from systematic observation must be tested to determine its validity and applicability (deduction). An untested theory is just as limiting as unsystematic observation that lacks rigor (Cohen, 1999). A fluid interaction between deduction and induction, in which one scientific process informs the other, is needed. Today's students of neuroscience should be warned against either wrongfully accepting observation alone without systematic and rigorous theory development or accepting theory as sacrosanct without further testing. Both types of acceptance may create difficulty in providing excellent patient/client care.

Several centuries after the ancient Egyptians and Greeks, Galen (A.D. 130–200), one of the greatest scientists in history, performed thousands of careful animal dissections in his attempt to learn about the brain. Galen was not only a famous Roman scientist but also a physician to the gladiators, and he undoubtedly witnessed the effects of brain and spinal cord injuries. He is credited with beginning to link systematic observation and theory development with methods to test his theories. Through his dissections, he noted the differences between the tissues in the cerebrum and cerebellum and was the first to try to ascribe separate functions to these areas. He was really the first to form a bridge between observation of structure and analysis of function. Galen also promoted the prevailing theory that the body functioned according to a balance of four vital fluids, or humors, a notion that prevailed for 1500 years (Bear et al., 2001).

During the Renaissance, Leonardo da Vinci (1452–1519) and René Descartes (1596–1650) developed methodologies for studying brain structures. Descartes introduced the concept that the brain could be dissected and demonstrated an early example of a flexor withdrawal reflex (to be discussed in subsequent text). After Descartes, Willis (for whom the circle of Willis, to be discussed in Chapter 2, is named) observed that some brain functions could be localized to specific areas of the brain. Still, however, the widespread belief was that the spirit was associated with the brain, but the structure itself was little understood. It was during this time that the "mind" was considered a separate anatomical entity housed outside the brain.

By the end of the 18th century, the nervous system had been completely dissected, and its gross anatomy was described in detail. It was known that injury to the brain could disrupt sensations, movement, and thought and even cause death. It was also known that the brain communicated via nerves with different identifiable parts and that there was a difference between white and gray matter.

During the 19th century, understanding increased to viewing the nerves as "wires," capable of conducting electricity, and knowledge expanded to include the brain's capacity to generate electricity. By this time, Benjamin Franklin had moved science forward by recognizing the phenomenon of electricity. In the 19th century, researchers demonstrated that nerves control motion and that sections of the spinal cord can control a reflex. Continued work by Broca, Jackson, and others extended the observations on localization of function. Advances in the study of evolution shed light on how adaptations are reflected in the structure and function of the brain of every species. Until late in the 19th century, investigators thought that the brain was made of a reticular network, an indivisible brain substance. By the end of the century, it was well accepted that many functions were localized to different parts of the brain (Bear et al., 2001).

In 1839, a German zoologist named Theodor Schwann proposed what became known as the cell theory, identifying the basic unit of the nervous system, the neuron. The cell theory of the brain, depicting the brain as made up of several different kinds of cells with individual characteristics, was widely accepted and expanded on only after technology, specifically the light microscope, allowed neuroanatomists such as Purkinje and Schwann to see and describe these cells. Simultaneously, investigators such as Sherrington, demonstrating the relationship between sensation and movement, were making important contributions (Bear et al., 2001). Many interventions in rehabilitation today continue to be based on findings from some of these early studies. Some of the names of the aforementioned scientists are still associated with structures or functions within the human nervous system. The reader will again hear of the names of some of these scientists, including Schwann, Broca, Sherrington, Willis, and Jackson, in subsequent text when neurological structures or functions named after these early scientists are described.

Relationship Between Neuroscience and Therapeutic Application

This text will present the essentials of the science of neuroanatomy and neurophysiology framed within a neurorehabilitation application approach. It actually presents a practical and therefore unique perspective to well-established and emergent rehabilitation practice. There is really no totally new information, but rather unusual and fresh combinations of material presented elsewhere. What *is* new and original is the lens through which the same material is viewed, the lens of an educator and a problem-solving, experienced clinician.

In many educational programs, the basic sciences are taught in courses separate from the clinical applied sciences. Although this is academically understandable, it can create a counterproductive gap in the mind of the student. This practice of academic but artificial separation of basic and clinical science unfortunately reinforces a separation in the mind of the student that may even remain so for the future practitioner. It is *vital* to establish an interrelationship between the two sciences from the beginning and to retain this relationship throughout study. For aspiring rehabilitation professionals, the basic sciences are somewhat dry and often difficult to learn. Clinical application to patient care establishes the meaningfulness of this information and therefore facilitates learning. This text will attempt to intertwine the two and to present them concurrently.

Therapeutic approaches always depend on the state of the basic science knowledge base and on the state of the applied science knowledge base. Any theoretical approach aimed at the rehabilitation of patients with neurological impairments is based on assumptions regarding how the central nervous system (CNS) controls movement in response to information from the internal environment of the body and from the environment external to the body. From these assumptions, a theoretical practice model is developed, guiding a particular theoretical approach, which is then verified through applied research. When current approaches are perceived as inadequate, both practically and theoretically, and when applied research fails to support the theory from which these approaches arise, optimal conditions for therapeutic innovation exist. It is important to remember that clinical frustration often forces new levels of insight and stimulates ideas for both applied and basic research. New ideas are born of theoretical advances, basic science research in neuroscience, and experimentation with practical application in the clinic (Carr & Shepherd, 2000). This intertwining of basic and applied science again illustrates the inseparable nature of both kinds of information to clinical practice. They are so interdependent that to present basic science and clinical application separately would be frustrating and meaningless.

The most exciting feature about the rehabilitation field is that today's educators are all teaching from a text that is unfinished. The last chapters cannot be written because of the dynamic, evolving nature of the field. As knowledge in the basic sciences increases, there will be a natural evolution of therapeutic approaches as practitioners develop their science of applying this new neuroscience knowledge to patient/client care. Concurrently, experienced practitioners will demand innovative answers and new ideas from the basic scientists to further develop the innovation that occurs in the science of application. This text, like others, will need ongoing revision as knowledge emerges and as clinicians and applied researchers strive for effectiveness in patient application.

The purpose of this text is to provide an integrated approach to basic neuroscience and applied neurorehabilitation, presented with practical applications illustrating the functional implications of neurological damage. Students and novice therapists and assistants can expect this text to give them useful answers to the most commonly voiced set of questions posed by new professionals, who may say something like: "Do not tell me only what is going on with the patient, but more importantly, what can I *do* to improve that patient's function, *where* do I start, and *how* do I know the patient's function really improved as the result of my treatment?"

This text will attempt to present the essentials of the science of neuroscience and movement and to cross the bridge directly to practical application by offering solutions to commonly encountered clinical dilemmas.

Neurorehabilitation: A Joint Effort

The professions of physical and occupational therapy really developed in parallel, prompted by medical and societal needs at the turn of the 20th century. In fact, a single pathological condition, the worldwide poliomyelitis epidemic, was the primary genesis of the physical therapy profession in the late 1800s and early 1900s. The first person to be formally recognized as a physical therapist was Mary McMillan, who, having studied corrective exercise science, worked primarily with children with poliomyelitis and other developmental disorders (Scott, 2002). Occupational therapy was developed in the early 1900s as an outgrowth of two social forces, Moral Treatment and the Arts and Crafts movement, occurring in reaction to specific health problems (Reed, 1993). Moral Treatment reformed the way in which persons with mental illness were treated, and the Arts and Crafts movement was a reaction to the poor health and living conditions created in large cities as the result of industrialization. Both movements placed an emphasis on using activities to keep the mind "occupied" and on developing these occupations as a daily habit as a way to promote health.

During World War I, these early occupational therapists joined a group of caring and dedicated volunteers who eventually became either physical therapists or occupational therapists or in some cases remained interested in both emerging disciplines. All these therapists were referred to by the common name "reconstruction aide." Some of these, as volunteers, received training that focused on working with soldiers with musculoskeletal disorders. However, the reconstruction aides with previous experience in mental health–related occupational therapy also worked with the soldiers who experienced "shell shock," now referred to as posttraumatic stress disorder. The occupational therapists, because of their experience in running "curative workshops" before the war, tended to focus their efforts on helping soldiers with residual musculoskeletal disabilities or those with mental illness find ways to take care of themselves independently and remain "productive" members of society.

Thus, we can see how the fields of occupational and physical therapy both evolved with an interest in human movement. We can also see how each developed specific interests as well. Occupational therapists maintained a strong focus on the roots of the profession in the area of mental health and the use of daily occupations to restore health, and physical therapists became experts in facilitating movement in individuals with movement disorders. Margaret Rood, for example, a well-known name in neurorehabilitation, was trained and registered as both an occupational therapist (OT) and a physical therapist (PT), first serving patients during World War I (Low, 1995).

Tremendous demands for therapy services continued to occur as a direct result of the polio epidemic from the 1920s through World War II, continuing until the discovery of polio vaccine in 1955. With medical advances also ensuring that children and adults with neurological impairment, such as spinal cord injury or stroke, could survive their actual injury and acute phases of rehabilitation, therapists became increasingly involved in the rehabilitation of these children and adults. From the 1940s through the 1960s, an interest in treating children with neurological problems and working with children who experienced learning disorders led to the development of several still well-accepted neurophysiological and developmental approaches to intervention, such as neurodevelopmental treatment (NDT) and sensory integration (SI). Most recently, an appreciation of motor control and motor learning has become a driving force behind intervention.

Currently, OTs are clarifying their professional focus as a result of the emerging discipline of occupational science, which emphasizes understanding the person as an occupational being who actively engages in meaningful and purposeful activity. Physical therapists, identifying themselves as movement scientists, are ensuring that helping patients to meet functional goals by minimizing or preventing functional limitations is a cornerstone to intervention. Both professions use the newest findings in motor control and motor learning to frame the clinical management of individuals with movement disorders. Most physical therapists and occupational therapists currently subscribe to an eclectic approach to intervention, one of deliberately selecting complementary aspects from several different intervention approaches to best meet the individual needs of the patient/client. The main emphasis in both physical and occupational therapy is on a functional, individualized approach to assessment and intervention.

Problem-Solving Approach to Patient/Client Intervention: Disablement Model

Current practice in physical and occupational therapy views the needs of the patient through the lens of a model of disablement so that the therapy process can address the interrelated variables that impact the quality of life and well-being of the patient and the patient's family (Table 1–1). The concept of **disablement** refers to the impact of pathological conditions on the functioning of body systems, on basic human performance, and on a person's ability to function in necessary, usual, expected, and personally desired roles in society (Jette, 1994; Verbrugge, 1994). The disablement model is used to delineate the consequences of disease and injury rather than focus on only the disease itself.

Rehabilitation professionals have accepted a disablement paradigm modified by principles of health as important for enabling patients to remain active within their communities regardless of disease, disability, or risk for these problems (Moyers, 1999). All these

models focus on the process of disablement—in other words, on the impact of conditions on function. Some models address the process of remaining healthy despite disability more than others. Be advised, though, that the word **function** has many meanings among health care professionals, and that function refers broadly to functioning of the body, as well as functioning in activities within specific environments necessary for participation in society (Moyers, 1999; WHO, 2001). Therefore physical therapists and occupational therapists may have slightly different ideas about what the term *function* entails, a difference reflecting their respective roles in the therapy process.

In the context of the disablement model, therapists provide services to persons at risk for, as well as to patients/clients with, impairments, functional limitations, and disabilities resulting from disease, injury, or factors in the environment. This framework partially rejects the medical model of disease that emphasizes diagnosis as the main focus of patient care. Although rehabilitation professionals must understand a variety of diagnoses, these professionals play only a minor role, as outlined in their scopes of practice, in addressing the actual symptoms of disease. More importantly, the role of the rehabilitation professional is to promote health through the maintenance of function, to address the functional consequence of disease, and to prevent these consequences from initially occurring. Therapeutic intervention is directed at enablement, or optimizing the best function for the patient/client.

Three major disablement models have emerged over the past three decades, all with similar terminology and all advocating for improved quality of life and life satisfaction for persons with disabling conditions. These models delineate the interrelationships among disease, impairments, functional limitations, disabilities, and handicaps or societal limitations. They stress the importance of the effect of these factors, or some facsimile of these factors, on the person's ability to interact with the environment to participate in society.

TABLE 1–1			
Disablement Model: Practical Application			
Pathology/ Pathophysiology	Impairment	Functional Limitation	Disability
Disease, condition, or disorder, usually consistent with the medical diagnosis	Typical consequences of disease or pathological processes; loss or abnormality of physiological, psychological, or anatomical structure or function	Restriction of the ability to perform at the level of the whole person—a physical action, activity, or task, in an efficient or typically expected manner	Inability to perform actions, tasks, or activities usually expected in social roles that are customary for the individual within a social-cultural context and physical environment
Cerebrovascular accident	Balance deficit	Frequent falls	Inability to keep up with peers

Saad Nagi proposed the first model in 1965 (Nagi, 1965). The World Health Organization (WHO) developed an alternative model in 1980, publishing the *International Classification of Impairments, Disabilities, and Handicaps* (ICIDH; WHO, 1980). WHO has revised this classification and released a version in 2001 as the *International Classification of Functioning, Disability, and Health* (ICF), which adds a significant focus on health and functioning. The third model was published by the National Center for Medical Rehabilitation and Research (NCMRR) in 1992, derived from both the Nagi and the 1980 WHO classifications (National Institutes of Health, 1992). This model rejected the negative connotation of the word *handicap* used in the 1980 WHO model, replacing it with the term *societal limitations.*

There are differences between the models, but all possess significant similarities. This text uses terminology based on the broadest application of the disablement model and terms developed by Nagi: pathology or pathophysiology, impairment, functional limitation, and disability. Both the American Occupational Therapy Association (AOTA) and the American Physical Therapy Association (APTA) have cited this model, with both organizations stressing the importance of function and prevention or minimization of functional limitations.

Currently, AOTA has primarily adopted the ICF model of the WHO (2001) and has adapted it to fit the functional emphasis of occupational therapy, which involves addressing the occupational performance needs of patients through the therapeutic use of meaningful occupations and purposeful activities (AOTA, 2002; Moyers, 1999). To help occupational therapists and occupational therapy assistants translate between the language adopted by this text and the language of the ICF model (WHO), there will be explanations of the similarity between model terminology.

The main differences in the two languages is that the new ICF language (WHO, 2001) extends the scope of the old 1980 WHO classification system in a way that allows positive experiences to be described in addition to the problems associated with disablement. The ICF classification has "moved away from being a 'consequences of disease' classification (1980 version) to become a 'components of health' classification" (WHO, 2001, p. 4). The ICF classification has two parts, each with two components. The first part involves functioning and disability and includes the body structure/body function component and the activity and participation component. The second part involves contextual factors and includes the environmental factors component and the personal factors component. Components can be expressed in positive terms to describe the relationship to health, such as structural and functional integrity, activities participation, and environmental facilitators. If disablement in the two functioning components occurs, the word *impairment* denotes a problem located in the body structure/body function component. Either the expression **activity limitation** or **participation restriction** applies at the next component level, depending on whether the activity performance of the person is generally limited or occurs in only specific environments, thus restricting the ability of the person to participate freely in society. Environmental factors can hinder activity participation.

Pathology/pathophysiology, synonymous with disease, condition, or disorder, is usually consistent with the medical diagnosis and is primarily identified at the cellular level. Pathology can be the result of many different etiologies, such as infection, trauma, or degenerative processes. Any single disorder may disrupt normal anatomical structures or physiological processes. Because the WHO also authors the *International Statistical Classification of Diseases and Related Health Problems, 10th Revision* (1994), its ICF model (2001) does not have a specific level of disablement that includes only pathology and pathophysiology. However, these documents are used together because it is understood that disease and its pathology contribute to impairments in body structure and function. Using the disablement model does not negate the importance of the medical diagnosis, but it takes it out of a position of central importance. It is certainly true that changes at the cellular, tissue, and organ levels associated with disease and injury may predict the range and severity of the impairments at the system level (APTA, 2001). For example, a diagnosis of multiple sclerosis certainly alerts the therapist to common factors associated with the disease and provides vital information in implementing preventive and therapeutic management strategies. However, the diagnosis alone tells the therapist very little about the impairments and functional limitations that need to be the focus of physical and occupational therapy intervention.

Impairments are the typical consequences of disease or pathological processes, further defined as the loss or abnormality of physiological, psychological, or anatomical structure or function. Impairments occur at the tissue, organ, and system levels, and signs and symptoms indicate them. Examples of impairments include abnormal muscle strength, range of motion, memory, and vestibular functions. Impairments can be classified as either primary or secondary. Primary impairments are expected, typical consequences of a pathological process; secondary impairments are not always typical and may be preventable. An example of a primary impairment for a patient with a peripheral neuropathy in the lower extremity is ankle muscle weakness; a secondary impairment may be a plantarflexion contracture that develops over time secondary to the weakness.

In the ICF model (WHO, 2001), this level of disablement is referred to as impairments in body structure/body function. Body structures and body functions include structures and functions in many domains, but the ones of most concern to occupational and physical therapists and their assistants are mental functions; sensory functions and pain; structures and function of the eye and ear; structures and functions of the cardiovascular, respiratory, and immunological systems; neuromusculoskeletal and movement-related structures and functions; and structures and functions of the skin. Thus, areas of overlap between the two professions often occur because the two professions may share some of the same strategies to treat impairments for which both possess similar expertise. However, each may have a stronger role in working with some of the structures and functions than the other profession. For example, physical therapists may have more expertise in musculoskeletal assessment and occupational therapists may have more expertise in addressing visual problems that lead to functional limitations.

Functional limitation is defined as restriction of the ability to perform—at the level of the whole person—a physical action, activity, or task in an efficient, typically expected, or competent manner. The corresponding ICF terminology (WHO, 2001) is activity limitation. The concept of activity limitation in occupational therapy is preferred over the concept of functional limitation because of the confusion in how the word *function* can be used. As indicated previously, *function* is an umbrella term and can refer to the body, as well as to the way a person performs in activities. Activity limitation is clearly differentiated from body structure/body function impairments because performance in activities is dependent not only on the person's body structure/body function but also on the way in which the task is designed and the way in which the environment supports or acts as a barrier to performance (AOTA, 2002).

Thus, it is important to remember that functional limitations are individually experienced, are measured at the personal level, and are not to be confused with signs and symptoms of disease. A functional limitation may include inability to remove a coat from a hanger, inability to roll over in bed, or difficulties with dressing, all of which are examples of **basic activities of daily living (BADL).** A functional limitation may also involve **instrumental activities of daily living (IADL),** such as shopping or using public transportation to go to work (AOTA, 2002). Occupational therapists and occupational therapy assistants are concerned with multiple areas of occupation or activities that may be limited. These areas of occupation, in addition to ADL and IADL, include the areas of education, work, play, leisure, and social participation (AOTA, 2002). Overlap between physical and occupational therapy most commonly occurs when facilitating movement or promoting postural stability during the performance of activities. Occupational therapists also address the cognitive, perceptual, and psychological aspects, as well as the task-specific skills and patterns of activity engagement needed for successful performance. The occupational therapy profession classifies ADLs as an area of occupation. Occupational and physical therapy are concerned with some of the same ADLs, whereas some are of more concern to one profession than to the other. For instance, occupational therapy might be more likely to address the use of communication devices and physical therapy might be more likely to address functional mobility.

Disability is defined as the inability to engage in age-specific and gender-specific roles in a particular social context and physical environment (APTA, 2001). Disability is a restricted ability to perform tasks and activities associated with self-care, home management, work, community, and leisure (APTA, 2001). The ICF model (WHO, 2001) refers to disability as participation restrictions and is combined with the activity component of functioning. Participation focuses on the way in which the contextual factors, either environmental or personal (age, gender, education, marital status, and so forth) enable or restrict performance in activity. Both occupational therapists and physical therapists are interested in the interaction of a person's function with the physical environment and social and personal contexts. Occupational therapists and occupational therapy assistants are also interested in how a broader set of contexts impacts performance and are additionally concerned with the influence of cultural, virtual, temporal, and spiritual contexts (AOTA, 2002).

Consequently, both the disablement models and the functioning model or ICF (WHO, 2001) have always included the concepts of preventing progression toward disability and promoting maximum functioning. However, it must be emphasized that these levels of functioning and their corresponding levels of problems in functioning are not linear in that pathology *does not* automatically produce an impairment, an impairment *does not* necessarily result in a functional limitation (activity limitation), and a functional limitation *may not* lead to a disability (participation restriction). Similarly, focusing in therapy on one problem level for patients with problems in all four levels of disablement, such as primarily emphasizing the impairment level, may not automatically lead to an improvement in function or prevention of a disability (Moyers, 1999).

Clinical Connection:

The following are two examples of the differences between pathology or pathophysiology, impairment, functional limitation, and disability as applied in physical therapy and then as applied in occupational therapy. An example from geriatric rehabilitation is a patient who has had a stroke. Physical and occupational therapists would understand the pathology as the cerebrovascular accident that led to the stroke. In physical therapy, an impairment may be limited ankle strength and voluntary motion, the functional limitation may be the toe drag during gait resulting from this lack of voluntary movement, and the disability may be an inability to ambulate on uneven terrain. In occupational therapy, the impairment may be perceptual processing problems leading to inability to accurately judge relationships between objects and among the objects and the self. The functional limitation created is misjudging the distance needed to accurately reach for a glass of water. A disability is created when the environment and the task fail to provide extra cues to help the person compensate for the difficulty in accurately judging distance. Without this compensation, the arm movement is inefficient and ineffective and activity performance is less than successful.

An example from pediatric rehabilitation is a child with cerebral palsy. The pathology is the etiology of the cerebral palsy. In physical therapy, an example of an impairment may be weakness with spasticity; a functional limitation is the inability to isolate shoulder flexion to reach overhead; and the disability may be the child's inability to raise his or her hand in a classroom to answer a teacher's question. In a slightly different fashion, the occupational therapist in working with this same child might consider the impairment as the weakness with spasticity and the inability to isolate shoulder flexion to reach overhead, the functional limitation as the inability to raise the hand to answer the teacher's question, and the disability as the failure of the classroom environment to provide alternative methods for the student to indicate his or her desire to participate.

The first example in the clinical connection shows that the clinical problems of concern to each profession may be diverse, which results in therapists from each profession possessing a unique set of skills and expertise. The second example illustrates the slight difference in interpreting these levels of disablement. These differences do not mean that one profession is more correct in its interpretation than the other. On the contrary, the differences are reflective of separate roles on the rehabilitation team. Instead of the professions being considered duplicative, these differences support the need for a close working relationship between the two professions to thoroughly solve the problems of functioning in a way that might not be achieved by a single discipline. However, because there is overlap in some skills and expertise, as well as differences in interpretation, occupational and physical therapists must communicate with each other so that the patient's clinical problems

are solved in a way that avoids unnecessary duplication and so that appreciation of each profession is maximized. The working relationship between occupational and physical therapists should not suffer from arguments over turf and from misunderstandings created by assumptions of having the same perspective. Perspectives between the two professions are similar but not the same. Celebrating the differences and deliberately assigning clinical problems to the therapist with the best expertise underscores the value of the contribution of each profession to the rehabilitation goals of the patient. Ultimately, the patient clearly benefits from this collegial relationship among professionals.

In general, the focus of rehabilitation professionals is on maximizing an effective interaction among the person, the activity, and the environment, thereby facilitating an "enabling" rather than a "disabling" process. Occupational and physical therapy professionals are locked arm in arm in helping their patients strive for the overarching goal of improved function. The professions of both physical and occupational therapy have adopted the disablement model and its concepts as a cornerstone to clinical reasoning (defined subsequently in this chapter). Both the *Guide to Physical Therapist Practice* (APTA, 1997, 2001) and the *Guide to Occupational Therapy Practice* (Moyers, 1999) were products of the widespread acceptance of the disablement model in rehabilitation. Both professions are in agreement with placing the emphasis of intervention on function. How these two professions define the meaning of function may differ, but again, these differences support the need for both professions to be involved together in providing a more holistic type of outcome for each patient/client.

The Guide to Physical Therapist Practice

The *Guide to Physical Therapist Practice,* a natural extension of the disablement model, is a consensus document developed in 1997 and most recently revised in 2001 by APTA (APTA, 2001). This guide standardizes terminology and delineates practice guidelines to assist therapists in physical therapy diagnosis and in the establishment of management strategies for commonly encountered diagnostic groups. The terminology selected for the *Guide* is based on the disablement terms developed initially by Nagi and incorporates the broadest possible interpretation of those terms (APTA, 2001). APTA developed the *Guide to Physical Therapist Practice* "as a resource not only for physical therapist clinicians, but also for educators, students, health care policy makers, managed care providers, third-party payers, and other professionals" (APTA, 2001, pp. 24–25). The *Guide* is therefore intended to be shared with collaborative disciplines in an effort to standardize terminology and delineate common preferred practice patterns. It is *not* intended to provide intervention protocols, but rather to give general clinical guidelines.

APTA defines "physical therapy as a dynamic profession with an established theoretical and scientific base and widespread clinical applications in the restoration, maintenance, and promotion of optimal physical function. The role of physical therapists is to diagnose and manage movement dysfunction and enhance physical and functional abilities, to restore, maintain, and promote not only optimal physical function but optimal wellness, fitness, and quality of life as it relates to movement and health, and to prevent the onset, symptoms, and progression of impairments, functional limitations, and disabilities that may result from diseases, disorders, conditions, or injuries" (APTA, 2001, p. 21). Physical therapist assistants are uniquely recognized as the collaborative paraprofessionals who assist in the provision of physical therapy interventions (APTA, 2001).

The *Guide* categorizes professional clinical practice into five specific parameters: examination, evaluation, diagnosis, prognosis, and intervention. Preferred practice patterns provide comprehensive, evidence-based management strategies for prevention and clinical care in the areas of musculoskeletal, neuromuscular, cardiopulmonary, and integumentary conditions (APTA, 2001; Scott, 2002). The *Guide* consists of two parts: Part One contains an overview of physical therapy and defines that profession's approach to patient management, and Part Two describes practice patterns grouped within the previously named four categories of conditions. There are several appendixes pertinent to key issues, including standards of practice and the code of ethics, standards of conduct for the physical therapist assistant, and guidelines for documentation. The *Guide* addresses the role of physical therapy not only in primary comprehensive care but also in the areas of prevention, patient and community education, and wellness. This text will adhere to the terminology used by this guide, subscribe to the disablement model as a cornerstone concept, and familiarize readers with appropriate practice patterns and procedural interventions, as presented in the *Guide to Physical Therapist Practice*. The practice patterns that are most relevant to the clinical management of individuals with neurological disorders are the neuromuscular and musculoskeletal patterns, predominately the neuromuscular pattern. The procedural interventions contained within the *Guide* that are most commonly utilized in neurorehabilitation are therapeutic exercise and functional training, to be expanded on in Chapters 6 through 10 of this text.

Occupational Therapy Practice Framework and The Guide to Occupational Therapy Practice

The occupational therapy profession, with its *Guide to Occupational Therapy Practice* (Moyers, 1999) and its recent adoption of the *Occupational Therapy Practice Framework* (AOTA, 2002), also a consensus document, has placed the patient's functional performance at the cornerstone of assessment and intervention. Functional performance in these documents is referred to as occupational performance or the engagement of the individual in meaningful occupations and purposeful activities. Occupations are the activities of "everyday life, named, organized, and given value and meaning by individuals and a culture. Occupation is everything people do to occupy themselves, including looking after themselves,...enjoying life,...and contributing to the social and economic fabric of their communities" (Law, Polatajko, Baptiste, & Townsend, 1997, p. 32). However, occupations and activities are distinguished from each other in the following way:

Occupations are generally viewed as activities having unique meaning and purpose in a person's life. Occupations are central to the person's identity and competence, and they influence how the person spends time and makes decisions. The term *activity* describes a general class of human actions that are goal directed. A person may participate in activities to achieve a goal, but these activities may not assume a place of central importance or meaning for the person (AOTA, 2002, p. 7).

The *Occupational Therapy Practice Framework* includes some of the language of the ICF model (WHO, 2001) and is the result of the work of the AOTA Commission on Practice to replace the profession's terminology standard, titled *Uniform Terminology for Occupational Therapy* (AOTA, 1994). The *Practice Framework* updates the *Guide to Occupational Therapy Practice* (Moyers, 1999) because the guide was not only based on *Uniform Terminology* but also had highlighted some confusion among commonly held occupational therapy concepts that previously had not been clearly defined.

This *Framework* outlines the enabling process and a structure for focusing occupational therapy's domain of concern on occupational performance (AOTA, 2002). The process of changing a person's performance in occupation begins with evaluation, which includes obtaining an occupational profile of a patient to understand the person's history of engagement in meaningful occupations and purposeful activities and to understand the person's current abilities in and problems with performance. Based on this profile, in-depth evaluation analyzes current performance and potential for desired occupational performance and highlights problems resulting from a combination of variables involving patient/client factors (body structure/body function), activity demands (e.g., task objects used, space and social demands, required actions and their timing and sequencing, and demands on patient factors), performance patterns (habits, routines, and roles), performance skills (motor, process, or communication/interaction), or the context (physical, personal, spiritual, social, temporal, cultural, and virtual).

According to the *Framework*, intervention follows evaluation and includes intervention planning (collaboratively establishing goals, selecting evidence-based methods, developing the discharge plan, and making referrals), intervention implementation, and intervention review to determine progress or the need for discharge from therapy services. It should be noted that intervention methods involve the use of therapeutic occupations/activities, which are specially selected and carefully analyzed and designed either to accommodate impairments or to remediate, resolve, or prevent impairments, functional limitations, or disability. In addition to therapeutic activities and occupations, intervention methods include strategies to prepare the patient for engagement in occupations, such as splinting, exercise, sensory input, and so forth. Therapeutic occupations and activities, however, are the "hallmark" of occupational therapy intervention and are thus both a means to therapy and the end result of therapy (AOTA, 2002). The occupational therapy process culminates in outcomes measured as improvement in occupational engagement to support participation in one's roles.

The *Occupational Therapy Practice Framework* (AOTA, 2002) provides definitions and descriptions of terms and constructs used by the profession. This textbook adheres primarily to the terminology published in the *Occupational Therapy Practice Framework* (AOTA, 2002). Exceptions to this have been explained previously and include using Nagi's disablement terms (1965) instead of the ICF language (WHO, 2001) and using the word *patient* in addition to *client* and the word *treatment* at times instead of *intervention*. This text familiarizes readers with appropriate interventions and techniques as presented in the *Guide to Occupational Therapy Practice* (Moyers, 1999). The intervention approaches presented in Chapters 6 through 10 of this text were derived from available practice models and frames of reference as appropriate for the treatment of the patient with a neurological impairment. There is a glossary at the end of both the *Guide to Physical Therapist Practice* (APTA, 2001) and the *Occupational Therapy Practice Framework*

(AOTA, 2002). The terminology used in this text is consistent with both guides.

Clinical Reasoning and Problem Solving

All professionals who treat patients must use some level of clinical reasoning to guide intervention application and patient/client interaction. Therapists and assistants need to develop keen reasoning and problem-solving skills. Every conversation, every observation, and, most certainly, every intervention requires some level of problem solving and clinical reasoning.

Clinical reasoning is the process of generating hypotheses, seeking answers, and making collaborative decisions with the patient on possible solutions for a clinical dilemma. All professionals involved with a patient use this clinical reasoning process. Therapists are engaged in the full process of clinical reasoning, beginning with the receipt of a referral, medical record review, evaluation, assessment, intervention plan development including the establishment of goals, intervention with concurrent reassessment, and, finally, decision making regarding termination of services and discharge planning. An in-depth discussion of this entire process of clinical reasoning is beyond the scope of this text, and most certainly, it is a core element of the professional education of therapists. Assistant personnel also participate in clinical reasoning and contribute those insights when performing measurements and carrying out an intervention with a patient. Clinical reasoning is a highly specialized cognitive process that includes some level of problem solving.

Therapists and assistants, from the moment when they learn they will be treating a patient until the moment when the patient leaves the clinical environment, continually implement problem solving (Umphred, 2001). During intervention, reassessment is ongoing. The treating therapist or assistant must understand the neurophysiological and motor control processes being utilized in *treatment/intervention* and must understand the rationale for the strategy being employed so that changes can be made when indicated. This **problem-solving** posture requires clinical flexibility, so that strategies can be constantly modified to meet the dynamic needs of the patient. Gifted therapists and assistants are often said to have intuition. Intuitive behavior is based on experience, a thorough knowledge of the problem area, sensitivity to the total environment, and the ability to integrate all three and respond optimally. Some of the skills required to develop effective problem solving include interactive reasoning, pattern recognition, and procedural reasoning.

Occupational therapists and occupational therapy assistants, because of their focus on engagement in occupations to support participation, may also use another type of reasoning, **narrative reasoning** (Schell, 1998). Narrative reasoning involves learning the patient's story, from which the occupational therapist can discern the role that occupational performance has played in the person's life. The emphasis in therapy is to help the patient rewrite the story so that he or she can project the self into the future; that is, imagine how he or she might still engage in meaningful occupations and purposeful activities regardless of the conditions created by impairments, functional limitations, and disability. Narrative reasoning by the occupational therapist can bring about the patient's understanding of what might be possible and lead to hope and motivation for the patient to continue on in spite of what may initially seem to be insurmountable difficulties.

Interactive reasoning takes place during any face-to-face encounter between the treating professional and the patient and the patient's family or caregivers. Information is gleaned by simply talking with the patient and caregivers, starting right at the time of greeting. This type of reasoning gives clinicians a way to gain insight into the patient as a person. There are several different categories of interaction that can be used, including body orientation, activity, eye contact, eye movement, nonverbal behavior, and direct verbal cues including voice elements. Therapists and assistants can use these strategies to convey numerous messages, such as support, encouragement, challenge, and reassurance (Fleming, 1993). These same cues given by the patient and the caregiver can then guide the therapist or assistant in determining the most effective way of motivating the patient throughout the therapy process. Effective use of interactive reasoning requires that the patient, and often the caregiver as well, be actively involved in the treatment.

Professionals can encourage participation by discussing goals and strategies together with the patient and caregiver, enlisting cooperation, and linking meaningfulness of therapy throughout the *treatment/intervention* interaction to the potential outcome. Occupational therapists and occupational therapy assistants also refer to interactive reasoning as **therapeutic use of self** (AOTA, 2002).

Pattern recognition is a problem-solving strategy typically employed in the initial problem identification phase. It is based on the ability to observe and interpret cues. Cues are aspects of the situation that one observes and interprets as potentially significant to understanding the person or the situation. Pattern recognition is this ability to observe a phenomenon, identify significant characteristics (cues), determine whether there is a relation among the cues, and make a comparison or

decision. Pattern recognition requires that a comparison can be made to an expectation or a familiar pattern. This is a vitally important skill for all practitioners to learn to make practice more efficient. Proficiency in pattern recognition usually accompanies experience. For example, an experienced therapist recognizes the probable impact of a visual deficit, expected to be seen in the new patient referred for functional mobility training after an amputation secondary to diabetes mellitus complications. The therapist not only recognizes but anticipates common practice patterns.

Procedural reasoning is the type of knowledge used when a practitioner applies learned professional or academic knowledge to a clinical problem, often involving knowledge of the human body, medical diagnoses, therapy practice models or theoretical frameworks, and therapy techniques, and knowledge from the biological, physical, social, and psychological sciences. The concepts presented previously from the disablement model and concepts from professional association documents illustrate some of the professional knowledge that guides procedural reasoning about the essential core of a clinical problem germane to each discipline (Fleming, 1993; Umphred, 2001).

Therapists and assistants enter even the first clinical experience with some hypotheses about what procedure or intervention might be most effective for a clinical problem. Procedural reasoning usually begins with problem identification, but equally important is the ability to then reevaluate the hypothesis in light of new or more complete information. Assistants and therapists alike need to be able to generate myriad "little" hypotheses during intervention about the array of details and factors needed to make fine-tuned adjustments or unique adaptations to an individual therapy session.

Practice experience is the best way to gain mastery in problem solving so that clinical reasoning can be a reliable tool used every day in the clinic. Problem solving is also a life skill, and intuitive reasoning is certainly a skill worth developing. Students and clinicians are encouraged to be open to learning as a *process*, so that the very attempt at learning (including successes and misses) is permitted to help gain insight into reasoning and intuition.

Clinical Connection:

The following clinical vignette demonstrates the different types of problem-solving strategies used by therapists in clinical practice.

A 52-year-old woman, Betsy, is visited at home by the therapist and the assistant. The specific referral is for teaching Betsy to perform activities in the kitchen in a safe and energy-conserving manner. Betsy has had a diagnosis of multiple sclerosis (MS) for the past 7 years. Because the specific findings of assessment and functional limitations are not relevant to this particular clinical connection, that information is not detailed here.

As the therapist and assistant travel to the home, they discuss the referral information sent by the referring agency, reviewing academic knowledge about the effect that MS has on all the body's systems. The clinicians develop a broad plan for a possible intervention approach (procedural reasoning). On arrival at the home, they are greeted by an obese woman in a manual wheelchair who demonstrates an obvious upper extremity tremor and slurred (dysarthric) speech. (Pattern recognition: These cues alert the clinicians to coordination difficulties and mobility limitations compounded by obesity.) Betsy appears to be delighted to have visitors, engaging readily in social conversation but denying that she requires any professional assistance because her "son's wife comes over daily to fix all of my meals." (Interactive reasoning: Clinicians gain insight into Betsy's perceived opinion of their visit, and her socialization attempts may be a ploy to delay attention to the task at hand—the purpose of the therapy visit; she seems to prefer to focus on the professionals as social visitors.) The therapist and assistant immediately engage Betsy in conversation about the role of (occupational or physical) therapy and listen carefully to Betsy as she is led into a conversation about her goals, hobbies, interests, and favorite purposeful activities (narrative reasoning). As the dialogue continues and assessment, intervention planning, and intervention begin, the clinicians continue to use all the problem-solving strategies as they interact with Betsy. An intervention plan is discussed (narrative reasoning), Betsy's response to the plan is carefully and respectfully assessed (interactive reasoning), and plans for intervention approaches are presented and tried (pattern recognition and procedural reasoning).

This vignette demonstrates the ongoing nature of clinical reasoning as professionals practice in a problem-solving state of mind, continually tuned in to the needs and cues offered by the patient.

In this text, the development of clinical reasoning skills is emphasized. Active learning experiences, presented in the companion workbook, offer the reader an opportunity to engage actively in the process of learning. Beginning in Part 2 (Chapters 5 through 10), case studies offer opportunities to practice problem solving. Discussion assists in the development of such skills as interactive reasoning, pattern recognition, and procedural reasoning.

Summary

This chapter serves as a foundation for the text, describing the history of neuroscience, as well as how basic science knowledge and therapeutic advances are codependent. Effective approaches to neurorehabilitation for patients/clients throughout the life span are a common goal of both occupational and physical therapists and their assistants, a common ground framed within the concept of the disablement model. Occupational and physical therapy practitioners possess unique but complementary skills and approaches to patient care. This text is offered for adoption by both disciplines, to be expanded on by discipline-specific study, which is beyond the scope of this text, but aptly left to the professors within the unique programs. The patient benefits best from the skills of both disciplines. It is not only possible but also vital for rehabilitation professionals to embrace some common terminology so that patient care is maximized. This text subscribes to the principles and guiding concepts presented in both the *Guide for Physical Therapist Practice* (APTA, 2001) and the *Guide for Occupational Therapy Practice* (Moyers, 1999). The chapter ends by summarizing clinical reasoning and problem solving, encouraging the reader to be open to the process of learning so that the "tuned-in" practitioner can then be most effective with patients.

References

American Occupational Therapy Association (1994). Uniform terminology for occupational therapy. *American Journal of Occupational Therapy, 48*, 1047–1054.

American Occupational Therapy Association (2002). *Occupational therapy practice framework: Domain and process.* Bethesda, MD: American Occupational Therapy Association.

American Physical Therapy Association (1997). Guide to physical therapist practice. *Physical Therapy, 77*, 1163–1165.

American Physical Therapy Association (2001). Guide to physical therapist practice (2nd ed.). *Physical Therapy, 81*(1).

Bear, M. F., Connors, B. W., & Paradiso, M. A. (2001). *Neuroscience: Exploring the brain* (2nd ed.). Baltimore: Lippincott Williams & Wilkins.

Carr, J., & Shepherd, R. (2000). *Movement science: Foundations for physical therapy in rehabilitation* (2nd ed.). Gaithersburg, MD: Aspen Publishers.

Cohen, H. (1999). *Neuroscience for Rehabilitation* (2nd ed.). Philadelphia: Lippincott Williams & Wilkins.

Domholdt, E. (2000). *Physical therapy research principles and applications* (2nd ed.). Philadelphia: W. B. Saunders.

Fleming, M. H. (1993). Aspects of clinical reasoning in occupational therapy. In H. L. Hopkins & H. D. Smith (Eds.), *Willard and Spackman's occupational therapy* (8th ed., pp. 867–881). Philadelphia: J. B. Lippincott.

Jette, A. M. (1994). Physical disablement concepts for physical therapy research and practice. *Physical Therapy, 74,* 380–386.

Law, M., Polatajko, H., Baptiste, W., & Townsend, E. (1997). Core concepts of occupational therapy. In E. Townsend (Ed.), *Enabling occupation and occupational therapy perspective* (pp. 29–56). Ottawa, ON: Canadian Association of Occupational Therapists.

Low, J. F. (1995). Historical and social foundation for practice. In C. A. Trombley (Ed.), *Occupational therapy for physical dysfunction* (4th ed., pp. 3–14). Baltimore: Williams & Wilkins.

Lundy-Ekman, L. (2002). *Neuroscience: Fundamentals for rehabilitation* (2nd ed.). Philadelphia: W. B. Saunders.

Moyers, P. (1999). Guide to occupational therapy practice. *American Journal of Occupational Therapy, 53,* 247–322.

Nagi, S. (1965). Some conceptual issues in disability and rehabilitation. In *Sociology and rehabilitation* (pp. 100–113). Washington, DC: American Sociological Association.

National Institutes of Health (1992). *Draft V: Report and plan for medical rehabilitation research.* Bethesda, MD: National Institutes of Health National Center for Rehabilitation and Research.

Reed, K. L. (1993). The beginnings of occupational therapy. In H. L. Hopkins & H. D. Smith (Eds.), *Willard & Spackman's occupational therapy* (8th ed., pp. 26–43). Philadelphia: J. B. Lippincott.

Schell, B. B. (1998). Clinical reasoning: The basis of practice. In M. E. Neistadt & E. B. Crepeau (Eds.), *Willard & Spackman's occupational therapy* (9th ed., pp. 90–100). Philadelphia: J. B. Lippincott.

Scott, R. (2002). The physical therapy profession. In Scott, R. (Ed.), *Foundations of physical therapy.* New York: McGraw-Hill.

Umphred, D. A. (2001). *Neurological rehabilitation* (4th ed.). St. Louis, MO: Mosby.

Verbrugge, L. (1994). The disablement process. *Social Science Medicine, 38,* 1–14.

World Health Organization (1980). *International classification of impairments, disabilities, and handicaps.* Geneva, Switzerland: World Health Organization.

World Health Organization (1994). *International statistical classification of diseases and related health problems, 10th Revision* (Vols 1–3). Geneva: Switzerland: World Health Organization.

World Health Organization (2001). *International classification of functioning, disability, and health.* Geneva, Switzerland: World Health Organization.

2

The Essentials of Neuroanatomy and Neurophysiology: A Neurorehabilitation Application Approach

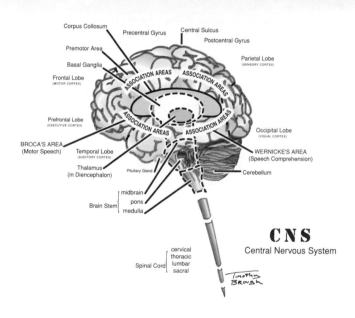

Corpus Collosum
Precentral Gyrus
Central Sulcus
Postcentral Gyrus
Premotor Area
Parietal Lobe
(SENSORY CORTEX)
Basal Ganglia
Frontal Lobe
(MOTOR CORTEX)
ASSOCIATION AREAS
ASSOCIATION AREAS
Prefrontal Lobe
(EXECUTIVE CORTEX)
ASSOCIATION AREAS
ASSOCIATION AREAS
Occipital Lobe
(VISUAL CORTEX)
BROCA'S AREA
(Motor Speech)
Temporal Lobe
(AUDITORY CORTEX)
WERNICKE'S AREA
(Speech Comprehension)
Thalamus
(in Diencephalon)
Pituitary Gland
Cerebellum
midbrain
pons
medulla
Brain Stem
CNS
Central Nervous System
cervical
thoracic
lumbar
sacral
Spinal Cord
Timothy Brough

The human brain is nothing short of a miracle.

Cornerstone Concepts

▪ The basic anatomical organization and key elements of the nervous system

▪ The basic physiological processes involved in nervous system signaling

▪ An overview of nervous system development and clinical implications

▪ The basics of motor and sensory functions vital to human movement

▪ An introduction to common signs and symptoms of neurological damage and various types of lesions

▪ A review of theories of recovery of function and a comparison of developmental and adult neuroplasticity

Introduction to the Nervous System

The Language of the Nervous System

As with the study of any professional discipline, specific language accompanies that area of study. If one were learning about computers, one would need to first get a grasp on terms such as *drives, bites,* and *memory,* specifically as used by computer scientists or technicians. The field of neurorehabilitation is therefore not unique in its need to have its own language. Upon first reading, the student of any of the areas of neurology may be totally overwhelmed by the mere number of syllables in the words. The student of neurorehabilitation can become comfortable with the language through an understanding of the geography or topography of the nervous system, a sense of direction, and of course, a sense of adventure. This sense of perspective lends itself to developing a user-friendly approach to not only learning the neuroscience but, more importantly, to knowing how to apply this knowledge to intervention with patients with neurological disorders.

The language of neuroscience is like a geography roadmap. The name given to the structure often tells the reader the location and often the function of the structure itself. The order of the term often indicates the order of the message transmission. For example, **corticospinal tract** indicates that the origin of the nervous signal is in the cortex and the destination is in the spinal cord. Further thought therefore also tells the student that if these are the origins and destinations of this signal, then the signaling message must be leaving the cortex as opposed to entering it; furthermore, it tells the student that the information being transmitted is an outgoing, or motor, action, or an efferent one. Conversely, *spinocerebellar* indicates that the origin of the signal is in the spinal cord and the destination is in the cerebellum. The student can then further deduce that the signaling message must be entering a higher level of the central nervous system as opposed to leaving it; furthermore, it can be deduced that the information being transmitted is an input, sensory, or afferent one. As you can see, the language of neuroscience is very descriptive, often providing hints about the location and the function of the named structure or process.

Other terms are derived from Latin or Greek, requiring that the student break the term into portions. Try to approach the word as a puzzle that usually has very recognizable pieces, such as a commonly used prefix, root, or suffix. The meaning and therefore the function of the term **neuromodulators** can be derived as follows. The prefix *neuro–* means that it has something to do

with a neuron, the root *mod* means that it has something to do with change (i.e., to modify), and a quick glance in any dictionary tells the reader that the suffix *–or* means a condition or quality. The reader has now determined that the term *neuromodulators* describes a substance that can change or alter the properties or qualities of a neuron. Indeed, neuromodulators do make neurons more or less responsive to incoming stimuli.

Last, a basic sense of direction will assist the student in understanding this fascinating language. Table 2–1 defines common directional terms used in neuroscience. **Dorsal horn,** for example, indicates that the structure or area is in the back or posterior region of something; whereas **ventral horn** indicates that the structure or area is in the front or anterior region.

General Plan of the Nervous System

When undertaking any subject of complexity, it is often helpful to first step back and take a wide-angle view of the entire picture. This approach is often helpful in gaining perspective on how the small details contribute to the overall function of something as complex as the human nervous system. The general layout of the human nervous system is organized in a practical, common sense manner.

Remember the difference between anatomy and physiology. Anatomy is the study of how the parts of the whole fit together. It describes the basic structure of a part of the body, answering the questions *what* and

TABLE 2–1	
Directional Terms Used in Neuroanatomy	
Ventral, anterior	Toward the front side
Dorsal, posterior	Toward the back
Rostral	Toward the head
Caudal	Toward the tail or coccyx, in the lowermost position
Superior	Toward the top, a part that is situated above another part
Inferior	On the lower side, a part that is situated below another part
Proximal	Near the point of origin
Distal	Farthest from the point of origin
Medial	Toward the middle
Lateral	Toward the side, away from midline
Ipsilateral	On the same side
Contralateral	On the opposite side
Bilateral	Involving two body sides

Source: Information compiled from multiple sources. See text and references for details.

where. Physiology offers answers to the questions *how* and *why,* by explaining the function of how body parts work and how parts of the whole function within an overall system. A **systems approach** to studying neuroanatomy and neurophysiology is an attempt to fuse these two study approaches by telling the story of structure and function simultaneously.

This chapter reviews the basics of neuroanatomy and neurophysiology, so that the student can become comfortable with the puzzle pieces and how they fit together. For the therapist student, this chapter serves as a review and summary. For the assistant student, this chapter contains sufficient depth to serve as an overview of the essential concepts of neuroanatomy and neurophysiology. The text then adheres to a systems approach, as described in the Chapter 3, because function and structure cannot be separated. A quick glance in a dictionary reveals that a system is simply an assemblage or combination of parts forming a whole, a group of body parts that form a functioning unit. A systems approach allows the practitioner to view the nervous system as subservient to functional purpose, where structures may contribute to more than one function and thereby be a part of more than one system. For the sake of simplicity and definition, this chapter covers only the basic neurophysiology and neuroanatomy.

The nervous system can be subdivided in two ways, based on either anatomical or physiological differences. Keeping these language concepts in mind, we now begin our journey into a study of the essentials of neuroanatomy and neurophysiology. The broadest perspective is first gained by examining the organizational divisions of the nervous system.

Anatomical Divisions

▪ Central Nervous System

The central nervous system (CNS), composed of the brain and spinal cord, is wrapped in protective coverings (meninges) encased in bone (cranium or vertebrae) and contains several fluid-filled spaces.

▪ Peripheral Nervous System

The cranial and spinal nerves, outside the CNS, form the peripheral nervous system (PNS).

Physiological Divisions

▪ Somatic Nervous System

The somatic nervous system is composed of all the receptors and nerves that innervate the muscles and skin.

▪ Autonomic Nervous System

The autonomic nervous system (ANS) can be described functionally as the visceral nervous system. Anatomically it contains portions of both the CNS and PNS. The ANS, divided into sympathetic and parasympathetic divisions, controls the activities of glands, smooth muscles, cardiac muscle, internal organs, and blood vessels. Functionally, this division of the nervous system is responsible for the regulation of homeostasis, as well as for responding to situations of stress, real or perceived. This important information about the state of the body is then shared with the brain (Waxman, 2000).

Building Blocks

The building blocks of the nervous system, neural tissue, consist of excitable neurons and nonexcitable support cells. Excitable cells can change in response to changes in their environment, whereas nonexcitable cells do not change.

▪ Excitable Cells or Neurons

A **neuron** (Fig. 2–1) is an excitable cell that receives and sends signals to other excitable cells. A neuron is composed of a cell body, or soma, dendrites, and an axon. The soma contains the cell nucleus.

Dendrites are cell processes that carry impulses toward the cell body. A neuron may have several dendrites. Dendrites can extend short or long distances and can branch repeatedly, communicating with either other dendrites or axons. As one learns, grows, and explores the world, the dendrites grow profusely (Leonard, 1998). Just as plants and trees branch and grow, the term used to describe this proliferative growth, thickening, and branching has been **dendritic arborization** (meaning leafy, intertwined vines). A correlation exists between the complexity of dendritic systems in the human brain and the type of work in which the individual participated during his or her lifetime (Scheibel, Conrad, Perdue, Tomiyasu, & Wechsler, 1990).

Clinical Connection:

Individuals involved in occupations that demand hand dexterity have been shown on autopsy to have increased dendritic branching within the primary motor areas of the brain; those who depended on talking and communication skills had increased thickening and branching in the brain areas devoted to speech. Conversely, the number and complexity of dendrite

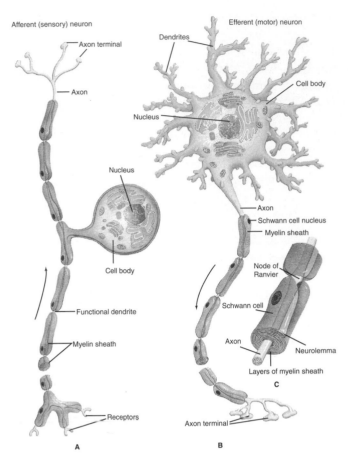

Figure 2–1. Neuron structure. (A) A typical sensory neuron. (B) A typical motor neuron. The arrows indicate the direction of impulse transmission. (C) Details of the myelin sheath and neurolemma formed by Schwann cells and the nodes of Ranvier. (From Scanlon, V. C., & Sanders, T. [2003]. *Essentials of anatomy and physiology* [4th ed., p. 157]. Philadelphia: F. A. Davis. Reprinted with permission from F. A. Davis Company, Philadelphia, PA.)

formation can be very limited in the brains of children with mental retardation (Bertoti, 1999). Alcohol ingestion during pregnancy can also have a devastating effect on the developing fetus, adversely affecting dendritic growth and neural maturation, resulting in *fetal alcohol syndrome*, a developmental disorder characterized by cognitive and motor deficits.

The axon is a single process that may extend for long distances, typically making contact with another neuron. Axons range in length from very short (only a few micrometers to another interneuron) to more than a meter in length (e.g., a lumbar motor neuron extending all the way from the low back to the muscles of the foot). Some axons are myelinated, which means covered in a fatty insulating substance that helps the axon conduct the message faster. Although only one axon leaves a soma, it may branch several times, so that a single axon can make contact with many neurons along the route to a specific target, such as a motor neuron pool in the spinal cord.

Neurons are often further classified by their function, so that a motor neuron innervates muscle, a sensory neuron carries sensory information, and an interneuron is literally just that, a neuron along the route to the intended target. There are slight anatomical differences in the structure of sensory and motor neurons, as depicted in Figure 2–1. Simply put, a neuron whose function is to respond to or convey a sensory signal is called an **afferent** neuron (remember that the prefix *a–* always denotes going toward—in this case, the CNS); an **efferent** neuron will respond to and convey a motor or action signal (remember that the prefix *e–* means to take something away from—in this case, the CNS again). Of the more than 100 billion neurons in the human nervous system, only about 5 million are sensory neurons, and only several hundred thousand are motor neurons (Leonard, 1998). The remaining 99 percent of neurons are interneurons, a fact indicative of the vast intercommunication and organizational tasks of the nervous system.

Inside the CNS, nerve cells serving a common function are often grouped together into something called **nuclei** (singular: **nucleus**). These nuclei may originate, relay, modify, or multiply information within the nervous system. Outside the CNS, nerve cells with common function, form, and connections are often grouped into **ganglia** (singular: **ganglion**). The general population is probably familiar with the distinction in the CNS between gray matter and white matter. The gray matter is made up of soma and groups of neurons (nuclei) and gives a gray appearance. White matter is the color of myelin therefore axons. Nerves travel in bundled **tracts,** therefore white matter, within the CNS. Comfort with the language of the nervous system helps with an understanding of the naming and therefore the origin, destination, and function of the tracts. For example, the corticospinal tract originates in the cortex, goes to the spinal cord, and therefore must carry descending, motor, or efferent information.

▪ Nonexcitable Cells or Neuroglia

Although there are billions of neurons in the human nervous system, neurons are outnumbered at least 10:1 by nonexcitable support cells called **neuroglia** (Waxman, 2000). The root word *glia,* meaning "glue," aptly describes the overall supportive function of these cell types. There are different types of neuroglia, each with specific support functions, such as formation of myelin, guidance of developing neurons, maintenance of extracellular ion levels, and reuptake of chemical transmitters following neuronal activity.

Astrocytes are found mostly in the gray matter of the CNS. They are directly in contact with blood vessels and involved in the exchange of substances in the bloodstream. They serve an important role in the maintenance of an effective blood-brain barrier, aiding in control from infection and maintaining optimal levels of various chemicals in the blood. **Oligodendrocytes,** found predominately in the white matter of the CNS, have long processes composed almost exclusively of myelin. They produce the myelin for the CNS and act as a support network. **Schwann cells** are found in the PNS and have a similar function there as the oligodendrocytes do in the CNS (Stokes, 1998). **Microglia** are phagocytic cells (a cleanup crew) that form part of the CNS's defense against infection and injury.

The Essential Neurophysiology

Signaling and Communication Between Structures

Neurons send and receive electrochemical signals, which is why they are said to be an *excitable* type of tissue.

▪ Resting Potential

Remember to apply a basic knowledge of the English language to the mastery of scientific terms when a term is first encountered. For example, the term *potential* simply means "capable of being or becoming; possible," just as every aspiring clinician has the *potential* to learn this material and become a great therapist or assistant! When applied to a cell membrane, *potential* simply means that there is an opportunity to become different or to change.

The fluid within the cell (intracellular) and outside the cell (extracellular) contains ions. Ions are charged particles that are electrically active. Extracellular fluid has a high concentration of sodium ions (Na^+) and chloride ions (Cl^-), whereas intracellular fluid contains predominantly potassium ions (K^+) and large positively charged proteins. The membranes of all cells are structured so that a difference in electrical potential (or readiness to change) exists between the inside (negative) and the outside (positive) (Fig. 2–2).

Under resting conditions, the permeability (ability to be crossed) of the cell membrane to K^+ and Cl^- is much greater than that to Na^+. The concentration gradients that exist across the cell membrane mean that if the ion is permeable (can pass easily through the cell membrane), there will always be a passive diffusion of ions from an area of greater concentration to an area of less concentration. Under resting conditions, Na^+ ions will continue to move into the cell; they are driven to do so because of a concentration difference, as well as the attraction of the negative intracellular potential. This

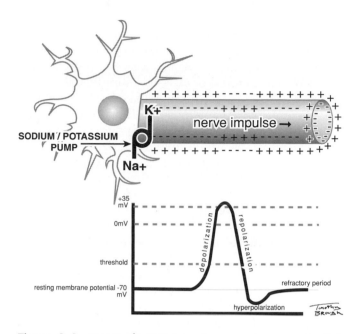

Figure 2–2. Figure depicting resting membrane potential, NA/K pump, and generation of an action potential.

diffusion of charged particles generates an electromotive force opposing it. This **electromotive force,** created by the differences in potential, gives rise to an electric current (Waxman, 2000).

Keeping this system in check, however, is the active expulsion of Na^+ through a metabolically fueled pump situated within the cell membrane. This Na^+/K^+ pump, which is one of many pumps in the human body, ensures that the exchange of Na^+ and K^+ is regulated in such a way that a **resting membrane potential** is always maintained at -70 to -90 mV for nerves (up to -90 mV inside a muscle fiber). It is important to remember that this state of rest is not a state of inactivity but rather a period when the cell is not signaling. The cell is expending energy to stay in this alert state of rest, maintaining the resting potential difference across the cell membrane. This active resting state is responsible for maintaining a state of responsiveness to change. The functional implication of the resting potential is that it creates an environment of readiness to respond to any change in the cell's environment. This is why only nerves and muscles are characterized as possessing the property of cell membrane excitability. These excitable membranes keep the cells in a constant state of irritability.

▪ Action Potential

An **action potential,** as the name implies, is an action event occurring when the cell membrane undergoes a change in its state of rest. It is a temporary reversal (lasting only about 1 millisecond) of the resting membrane potential that is then sufficient enough to be propagated (transmitted; hence the word *action*) as an electrochemical signal along the length of the axon. When the excitable cell membrane of a nerve or muscle cell is exposed to a chemical or electrical stimulus, the membrane will change in response. A decrease in membrane potential, making it more positive, is called **depolarization,** whereas an increase in resting potential, making it more negative, is called **hyperpolarization.** Hyperpolarization makes a neuron less likely to reach an action potential threshold and is therefore referred to as **inhibitory.** Any input that depolarizes a neuron, making it more likely to reach action potential threshold, is called excitatory or **facilitatory.**

How can the resting membrane read and respond to stimuli it is exposed to? There are several different kinds of ion channels that can be activated and in turn disturb the resting potential. These channels can best be envisioned as multisubunit proteins that span the cell membrane and are selectively permeable either to ions, a neurotransmitter (called ligand gated channels), or a change in voltage (called voltage gated channels). The channel possesses a voltage sensor, which, in response to changes in potential across the membrane, either opens (activates) or closes (inactivates) the channel (Waxman, 2000). Such channels open or close in response to a specific type of stimulus and thereby effect changes in neuronal activity by changing the distribution of ions between the inside and outside of the cell (Gilman & Newman, 1996).

Threshold (see Fig. 2–2) is a critical voltage level that must be reached before rapid depolarization can occur. If an axon is depolarized to a critical threshold, voltage sensitive channels for Na^+ in the membrane will open, causing a movement of Na^+ inward. Depolarization is followed by a period of **repolarization,** when the Na^+ gates close and gates allowing movement of K^+ open, resulting in a movement of K^+ outward. The membrane voltage then becomes more negative, actually passing the resting membrane potential to a more negative level, called hyperpolarization, finally followed by a swift return of the membrane potential to rest. This complete process of depolarization, to a maximum voltage of +30 mV, followed by a hyperpolarization and then a re-established rest, constitutes the action potential. Immediately following the action potential is a very short refractory period, a time during which the membrane is unable to respond to any new stimulus.

This action potential then generates an electric current that depolarizes the adjacent membrane further along the cell membrane and generates a new action potential. In this manner, the action potential then becomes a transmitted, or propagated, signal. The action potential is followed by a period of **refractoriness,** which means that the membrane is resistant to

stimulation (Taber's, 2001). Immediately after the action potential, the membrane is in an **absolute refractory period,** a very brief period during which the membrane cannot respond to any stimulus, regardless of how strong. This is followed by a **relative refractory period,** when excitability is depressed but a response can be triggered by either repeated or intensified stimuli. The presence of these refractory periods helps to ensure that action potentials always travel along the axon in one direction. Another crucial aspect of an action potential is that once depolarization reaches a critical threshold, an action potential occurs—thus, the infamous all-or-none quality ascribed to such an event.

Conduction speed of impulses along axons is directly related to the structural characteristics of that axon, specifically whether the axon is insulated or not and the size or diameter of that axon. Myelinated axons conduct action potentials more quickly than unmyelinated axons or muscle fibers. The myelin acts as an electrical insulator. Current can only be dissipated at the breaks in the myelin, anatomical locations called **nodes of Ranvier** (see Fig. 2–1). The current actually is able to conduct quickly, jumping efficiently from node to node, a process known as saltatory conduction. The greater the diameter of the axon, the faster an action potential signal will be transmitted. An analogy can be made if one envisions how a given amount of water will pass through a larger diameter garden hose faster than through a smaller hose. The threshold for stimulation is also related to axon size, with the largest axons having the lowest threshold, allowing them to be more readily stimulated (Stokes, 1998).

Table 2–2 lists the great variety of nerve fibers found within the human nervous system, of varying diameters, some myelinated and others unmyelinated, with varying conduction velocities. This rich anatomical diversity within the nervous system allows for signaling to be constantly modified so that complex information can be transmitted and utilized at many levels of the nervous system. Survival and arrival of the signal at the termination point within the nervous system are also dependent on the concurrent speed of supporting or competing messages reaching their neural destination.

■ Synapses

Communication between neurons occurs at a **synapse** (Fig. 2–3), a specialized zone where neurons communicate with each other. The number of synaptic connections in the human brain has been estimated at 100,000,000,000,000 (a hundred billion) (Carper, 2000). Synapses can occur between two axons (axoaxonic), between the cell body and axon (axosomatic), or between dendrites and axons (axodendritic). Synapses

TABLE 2-2
Nerve Fiber Types and Functions

Fiber Type	Fiber Diameter (μm)	Conduction Velocity (m/sec)	Peripheral Organ	Function
A alpha (α) (motor)	12–20	70–120	Skeletal muscle	Motor, skeletal muscle efferent
A alpha Ia (sensory)	12–20	70–120	Muscle spindle afferent	Proprioception
A alpha Ib (sensory)	12–20	70–120	Golgi tendon organs afferent	Proprioception
A beta II (sensory)	5–12	30–70	Muscle spindle and touch/pressure receptors	Touch, pressure, vibration
A gamma (γ) (motor)	3–6	15–30	Intrafusal muscle fibers of muscle spindle	Motor, muscle spindle efferent
A delta (δ) (sensory)	2–5	12–30	Skin	Pain and temperature afferent
B fibers	1–3	3–15	Autonomic sympathetic	Autonomic efferent

Source: Information compiled from multiple sources. See text and references for details.

can be further classified as either electrical or chemical, depending on whether a chemical or electrical communication process is used. The human nervous system contains mostly chemical synapses, which is the type to be discussed here.

Chemical synapses consist of presynaptic and postsynaptic neurons completely separated by a **synaptic cleft** (space), about 200 Å wide. The presynaptic terminal usually has synaptic vesicles containing a chemical transmitter called a **neurotransmitter.** The postsynaptic membrane active zone contains specialized receptors, which are complex proteins capable of mediating the effect of these neurotransmitters. When an action potential moves down the axon and enters the axon terminal on the presynaptic side of the synapse, Ca^{++} voltage-dependent channels open, which then allow neurotransmitter release. The released neurotransmitter diffuses across the synaptic cleft. The transmitter diffuses across the cleft and binds to postsynaptic receptors. This transmission can only occur in a single direction, from presynaptic cell to postsynaptic cell. Many single neurons, however, will be receiving thousands of connections from other neurons.

Some of these chemical connections are excitatory, others inhibitory, depending on the type of neurotransmitter. An example of an excitatory neurotransmitter is glutamate, a substance found in the cerebral cortex and cerebellum. Acetylcholine is another example of an excitatory neurotransmitter, vitally important at the synapse between nerve and muscle. Examples of inhibitory chemicals in the CNS include gamma-aminobutyric acid (GABA), glycine, and dopamine (the key neurotransmitter lacking in patients with Parkinson's disease). Serotonin is another key neurochemical, actually a vasoconstrictor, playing a key role in sleep-wake cycles, mood regulation, and appetite regulation (Gilman & Newman, 1996).

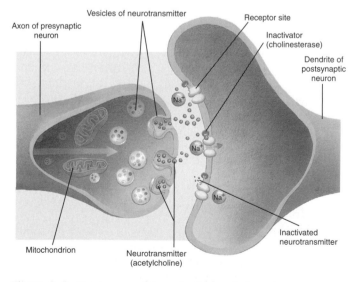

Figure 2–3. Synapse and impulse transmission at a synapse. The arrow indicates the direction of the electrical impulse. The entry of NA$^+$ ions stimulates an electrical charge in the postsynaptic neuron. (From Scanlon, V. C., & Sanders, T. [2003]. *Essentials of anatomy and physiology* [4th ed., p. 159]. Philadelphia: F. A. Davis. Reprinted with permission from F. A. Davis Company, Philadelphia, PA.)

Clinical Connection:

The following are illustrations of conditions where synaptic function is impaired. *Presynaptically*, botulinum toxin is currently used quite successfully in rehabilitation to purposely block neurotransmitter release in patients with a heightened state of muscle contraction, known as spasticity. As you would expect, botulinum toxin, which causes some forms of food poisoning, contributes to weakness and paralysis. Used judiciously as a clinical intervention, botulinum toxin injections (Botox) can therapeutically decrease undesired muscle activity so that voluntary strengthening or stretching programs can be effective. Currently Botox injections are gaining in popularity as a cosmetic intervention to decrease the facial signs of aging by relaxing the muscles, thereby decreasing wrinkles.

A disease that affects the *postsynaptic* area of the synapse is myasthenia gravis. This disease disrupts the transmission of neural impulses across the neuromuscular junction, causing impaired functioning of skeletal muscle. There are a decreased number of receptor sites for the neurotransmitter acetylcholine on the muscle membrane. Patients with myasthenia gravis present with weakness, fatigue, impaired chewing and swallowing, **diplopia** (double vision), drooping eyelids, and impaired breathing. These signs worsen with prolonged activity and fatigue.

In another example, cocaine addiction appears to interfere with the uptake of neurotransmitter within the *synaptic cleft*. In the presence of cocaine, the neurotransmitter dopamine is not cleared, resulting in an elevation in dopamine level in the synaptic cleft, producing the addictive high sought by drug addicts. ▪

As mentioned previously, many neurons will receive countless connections from other neurons, some excitatory and others inhibitory. These connections may cause a depolarization (excitation) or hyperpolarization (inhibition). One action potential makes only a small depolarization. Stimulation of a single presynaptic excitatory neuron evokes in the postsynaptic neuron an **excitatory postsynaptic potential (EPSP),** a small, local, and nontransmitted or nonpropagated depolarization. When increasing numbers of presynaptic neurons make connections and transmit simultaneously, the EPSPs can progressively increase in amplitude until they bring the neuronal membrane to threshold, resulting in the generation of an action potential. Stimulation of a single presynaptic inhibitory neuron contacting a single postsynaptic neuron evokes an **inhibitory postsynaptic potential (IPSP),** a small, local, and nontransmitted or nonpropagated hyperpolarization (Gilman &Newman, 1996). Multiple IPSPs result in inhibition.

At any given time, the dendrites and neuron can receive EPSPs and IPSPs simultaneously from the axons of thousands of other neurons. Therefore, the response of the target neuron is determined by the net effect of all the incoming potentials, or stimuli. These postsynaptic potentials are local events that diminish over time as they travel. The actual survival, intensity, or integration of these potentials depends on timing and the arrival sites on the target neuron. Remember that when a target neuron is depolarized, this change in membrane potential is transient, and with time the membrane returns again to rest.

If the target neuron receives additional EPSPs at the same location quickly enough, the potentials can add to each other, a phenomenon called **temporal summation.** The target neurons are also capable of integrating multiple postsynaptic potentials that arrive simultaneously but at different locations, a phenomenon called **spatial summation** (Cohen, 1999). This electrical integration of incoming information allows neurons to process huge amounts of information. It also permits the nervous system to discriminate at multiple levels regarding whether a signal is meaningful enough to continue for further transmission or whether it will simply be allowed to dissipate.

▪ Receptor Potentials and Stimulus Transduction

Receptors that are not associated with the special senses (such as vision and hearing) are called somatic receptors (because they detect information about the body, or soma). They give the nervous system information about the body, including temperature, touch, and pain.

These receptors will be described later in this chapter, but it is fitting to describe here how these receptors detect and transmit their information within the nervous system. Most receptors respond preferentially to a specific stimulus much like a key fitting into a specific lock. The end organs of the receptors convert the stimulus into electrical energy so it can be transmitted, after first converting the energy into a local **receptor potential.** The term *transduction* simply means "conversion or change" of one form of energy to another. In this case, therefore, stimulus transduction means that the mechanical energy of touch or pressure or the thermal energy of temperature is converted into an electrical energy so that it can be sent throughout the nervous system. This transduction involves the production of another type of local, unpropagated potential, called a **generator potential,** in the terminal part of the sensory nerve axon (Stokes, 1998). This local depolarization is graded and additive if summation occurs. Current from the generator potential flows along the axon, and if sufficient numbers of stimuli occur or if the stimulus persists, an action potential may then be generated and the impulse is then transmitted.

The Essential Neuroanatomy

Development of the Nervous System

An appreciation of the human nervous system and ultimately the effects of damage to either the developing baby or the aging adult first requires just a cursory familiarity with evolutionary science and embryology. This section is simply intended to offer a basic sense of perspective and highlight key points as they relate to neurorehabilitation.

As the human CNS evolved, it increased in size and complexity by adding on to more primitive brain structures. The modern human brain, weighing typically 3.5 pounds in the adult male, still retains the structural organizational patterns that are reflections of its evolutionary past (Katz, Mills, & Cassidy, 1997). Classical anatomists consider the whole human brain to consist of five major subdivisions, each with a main behavioral regulation task, based on their evolutionary and embryologic origins. A more functional approach, however, divides the brain into three main components:

- Brainstem: serves vegetative functions such as breathing, blood pressure, and heart rate. It includes the basal ganglia, which serves many volitional behaviors directed toward individual preservation and propagation of the species, such as feeding and sexual aggression. These areas are grouped by evolutionists into the reptilian brain.
- Limbic system: serving primitive but distinctly mammalian behaviors such as caring for offspring and hoarding. These areas are grouped by evolutionists into the paleomammalian brain.
- Cerebral cortex: outermost area of the cerebrum, serving the uniquely human behaviors of cognition and speech. Evolutionists designated this area as the neocortex (Katz et al., 1997).

This functional framework is helpful to keep in mind when studying the implications of brain damage on activity and behavior.

The human nervous system starts forming when the human embryo is approximately 21 to 22 days of age and measures less than 4 mm in length (Cohen, 1999). The development of the human nervous system begins with the formation of the neural groove appearing along the midline of the embryo, derived from the ectoderm. This neural groove is flanked by neural folds, which then close to form a neural tube (Fig. 2–4)

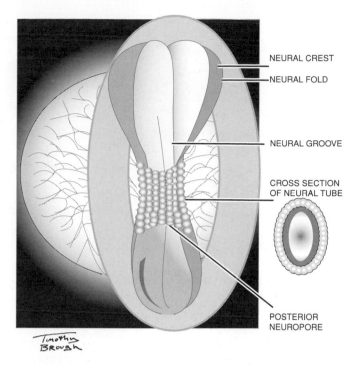

NEURAL CREST

NEURAL FOLD

NEURAL GROOVE

CROSS SECTION OF NEURAL TUBE

POSTERIOR NEUROPORE

Figure 2–4. Dorsal view of the CNS in a human embryo at the end of the third week showing key aspects of the neural tube: the beginning formation of the human brain.

(Gilman & Newman, 1996). The superior end of this tube develops into the brain, with the remainder differentiating into the spinal cord. The tube closes first at the level destined to become the cervical region of the spinal cord. From there, closure proceeds caudally (inferiorly). The ends of the neural tube, called the anterior and posterior neuropores, remain open through the fourth week of embryonic life to allow for circulation of amniotic fluid around the developing nervous system (Gilman & Newman, 1996; Cohen, 1999).

Clinical Connection:

Failure of the posterior neuropore to close results in spina bifida, a developmental anomaly, causing complete or partial paralysis. Because of the direction and timing of closure of the neural tube, the most common site of spina bifida is in the lumbar area, resulting in paralysis of lower extremity muscles. Less commonly, failure of the anterior neuropore leads to anencephaly, where a large portion of the brain does not develop, rendering the fetus unable to survive. Think about how early these serious defects arise, in only the first month of pregnancy, sometimes before a woman may even know that she is pregnant! ▪

Lateral to the neural tube is an area of tissue known as the neural crest. The tissue in this area eventually

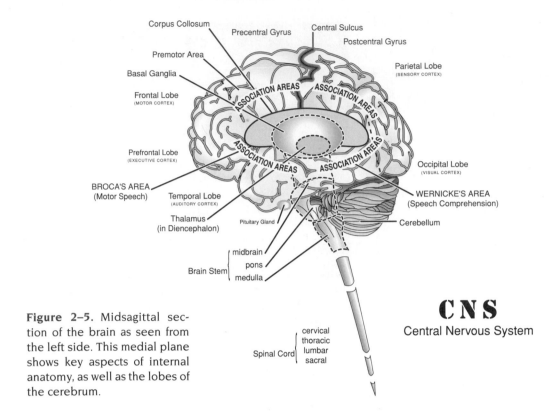

Figure 2–5. Midsagittal section of the brain as seen from the left side. This medial plane shows key aspects of internal anatomy, as well as the lobes of the cerebrum.

differentiates into neurons and neuroglial cells and into most of the autonomic and sensory ganglia. Development of the brain begins with differentiation of the superior (or rostral) end of the neural tube into first an area of three, then a five-area stage where the brain consists of the embryonic telencephalon, diencephalon, mesencephalon, metencephalon, and myelencephalon. The first three of these areas eventually differentiate into the cerebral hemispheres, the diencephalon (thalamus and hypothalamus), and the midbrain. The metencephalon becomes the cerebellum and the pons. The myelencephalon becomes the medulla (Gilman & Newman, 1996). This basic arrangement of the brain is established by the time the embryo is 6 weeks of age! After 6 weeks, the major changes are increases in the size and differentiation of the cerebral hemispheres and cerebellum (Fig. 2–5).

Clinical Connection:

Think of the implications of early brain development for children with developmental disabilities. Many of the most severe forms of cerebral palsy and mental retardation, secondary to abnormal brain development, occur probably within the first trimester of pregnancy. Children with Down syndrome, the most common form of mental retardation, have underdeveloped brains and less dendritic formation than normally developed children. Children with disorders affecting early formation of the brain may have difficulty with many nervous system functions; hence a general developmental delay will result, impacting all areas of development. ▪

Central Nervous System

The CNS includes the brain and spinal cord.

▪ Brain

The brain consists of the cerebrum, the cerebellum, and the brainstem.

▪ Cerebrum

The cerebrum (Fig. 2–5) is divided into two cerebral hemispheres (right and left), further divided into four main lobes, frontal, parietal, temporal, and occipital, each having unique functions. The surface of the cerebrum, called the cerebral cortex, is comprised of depressions, called **sulci** (singular: **sulcus**), and ridges, called **gyri** (singular: **gyrus**). These convolutions are a fascinating anatomical feature in that they serve to increase the surface area of the cerebrum without increasing the actual size. The outer surface of the cerebrum, the cortex, is comprised of gray matter, whereas the inner area is composed of white matter. This means that information is conveyed by the white matter (axons) and integrated and processed within the gray matter (soma and nuclei).

Frontal Lobe

The frontal lobe is responsible for voluntary control of complex motor activities and cognitive functions such as judgment, attention, mood, abstract thinking, and aggression. The frontal lobe, often referred to as the **motor cortex,** is further subdivided into the primary motor cortex, the premotor cortex, and the supplementary motor area. All three of these areas have their own somatotopic maps of the body, so that if different areas are stimulated, different muscles and body parts move. This is represented by the motor homunculus, depicted in Figure 2–6. Areas requiring more detailed control, such as the mouth and hand, are most highly represented (Shumway-Cook & Woollacott, 2001).

The primary motor cortex is responsible for contralateral (opposite side of the body) voluntary control of the upper extremity and facial movements. The supplemental motor cortex controls the initiation of movement, orientation of the head and eyes, and bilateral (involving both body sides) movements (Morecraft & Van Hoesen, 1996; Martin & Kessler, 2000). The supplemental area also controls the sequencing of movement and plays a role in the preprogramming of movement sequences that are familiar and part of an individual's memory repertoire (Lundy-Ekman, 2002). The premotor cortex controls the muscles of the trunk and muscles used in anticipatory postural adjustments, such as required in establishing the correct "postural set" in preparation for standing up from a chair (see Fig. 2–5).

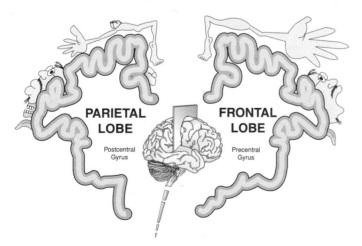

Figure 2–6. Sensory and motor homunculus.

PARIETAL LOBE

Postcentral Gyrus

FRONTAL LOBE

Precentral Gyrus

Clinical Connection:

Lesions of the primary motor cortex (as seen following a stroke) usually give rise to contralateral weakness or paresis, typically seen as a period of initial **flaccidity**, where muscle tone is absent. Postural reactions and stretch reflexes are reduced in the acute phase, but slow recovery and eventually overactivity, such that stretch reflexes become hyperactive, are the typical clinical picture. This clinical presentation has classically been defined as **upper motor neuron** dysfunction, the upper motor neurons being those that arise from the cortex and the **lower motor neurons** those that arise from the spinal cord and brainstem. After the acute phase, recovery is typically gradual but incomplete. Proximal movements usually show the greatest recovery, whereas fine distal movements remain weak and fractionated (jerky or decomposed movement characterized by lack of smooth and isolated muscle action).

Lesions of the supplemental motor cortex result in complex motor dysfunction, including severe **akinesia** (lack of movement), loss of facial expression, and difficulty with tasks requiring the cooperative use of both hands. Patients also have difficulty performing self-initiated tasks but are able to benefit from therapeutic approaches that teach them to use additional sensory cues to start a movement.

Lesions of the premotor cortex result in nonspecific motor disturbances or **apraxia**, where the patient's movements are slow and clumsy with mild proximal weakness and loss of coordination around the proximal joints. Rhythmic movements such as typing or tapping are disrupted, and **perseveration** (stammering or repeating) may occur. Unlike patients with lesions of the supplemental motor cortex, these patients are able to perform self-initiated tasks, but have difficulty with sensory-triggered tasks. Previously acquired sequential tasks deteriorate, even though individual components of the sequenced task can be performed (Cohen, 1999).

The main motor region responsible for speech is also located in the frontal lobe. In the right hemisphere, this area is responsible for nonverbal communication such as tone of voice and the use of gestures, whereas in the left hemisphere, this area, specifically called Broca's area, plans the movements of the mouth needed to produce speech.

The prefrontal cortex, an area in the anterior-most aspect of the frontal lobe, serves a set of executive functions integral for the planning, prioritizing, and sequencing of actions into a goal-directed stream of behavior (Waxman, 2000). When prefrontal areas are impaired, as in traumatic brain injury or accompanying senile dementia, patients can become either apathetic (exhibiting the inability to plan or initiate a goal-directed activity) or uninhibited and distractible, with loss of judgment and the inability to adhere to social graces.

Parietal Lobe

The parietal lobe is the primary **sensory cortex.** Incoming sensory information is processed and given meaning, the difference between reception and perception. Perception is the process of actually attaching meaning to sensory information. Different areas of the body are assigned locations within different regions of the parietal lobe, represented by the familiar sensory homunculus (see Fig. 2–6). The parietal lobe is also involved in short-term memory (Martin & Kessler, 2000).

The somatosensory cortex, located in the parietal lobe, is the major processing center for all **somatosensory** (feelings from or awareness of the body) modalities, marking the beginning of conscious awareness. It is in this area that we see cross-modality processing occur, meaning that information from many different types of receptors is now integrated to give aggregate information about a specific body part. The somatosensory cortex is also able to assign distinctiveness and meaningfulness to incoming sensory information by a process known as contrast sensitivity. Contrast sensitivity means that somatosensory neurons have a peripheral area described as an excitatory or inhibitory surround. An inhibitory surround, for example, inhibits lateral input so that specific input is then accentuated in comparison. Sensory capabilities such as **two-point discrimination** (the ability to detect that the skin is being touched by two points or objects at once) are made possible through this mechanism (Shumway-Cook & Woollacott, 2001).

Clinical Connection:

Individuals with damage or disease affecting the parietal lobe often demonstrate difficulties in the areas of sensory awareness, perception, and interpretation. There will be evidence of disturbed interpretation of peripheral sensations such as proprioception, localization, and the discrimination of stimuli. Because effective reach and grasp is made possible as a result of the integration of information within the somatosensory cortex, adults with parietal lobe damage have abnormal patterns of reaching and grasping and difficulties shifting movements in response to somatosensory information. Difficulties in differentiating between right and left, up and down, around, under, or beside and applying these directional concepts to an individual or an object's orientation in space will have obvious implications to movement planning and movement success. ▪

The somatosensory cortex also has descending connections to the thalamus, dorsal columns, and spinal cord, thereby having the ability to change (or modulate) the incoming information ascending through these structures (Shumway-Cook & Woollacott, 2001).

Temporal Lobe

The temporal lobe is the primary auditory cortex. It is responsible for auditory discrimination and speech comprehension. Auditory impulses travel from the inner ear, along the eighth cranial nerve, to the temporal lobe. Wernicke's area, a specialized region of this lobe, is responsible for hearing and comprehension of spoken language. The speech areas in the brain are concerned with not only the mechanics of speech production but also with the thinking that precedes speech. This area also interprets sounds and assigns meaning to those sounds. Wernicke's **aphasia**, characterized by fluent, nonsensical speech, is specifically associated with lesions of the left temporal lobe (Christiansen, Lopez, & Phillips, 2001; Umphred, 2001). The temporal lobe also processes visual perceptual information, music, and long-term memory.

Clinical Connection:

Research suggests that in humans, lesions in the temporal lobe may interfere with the laying down of new memory (Milner, 1966). In the past, patients with temporal lobe areas removed as a surgical treatment for epilepsy were observed to no longer be able to acquire long-term memories, although they did retain old memories. Their short-term memory was also normal, but if they were distracted from an item being held in short-term memory, they forgot it completely. Skill learning, however, was unaffected in these patients. They would be able to learn a complex task but be unable to remember the steps, tasks, or environmental setting that surrounded learning the new skill (Shumway-Cook & Woollacott, 2001).   ▪

Occipital Lobe

The occipital lobe is the primary visual cortex. It is responsible for the processing and interpretation of visual information, including judging distances and seeing in three dimensions. Visual impulses travel via the optic nerve, crossing to the contralateral side of the brain. The left hemisphere receives visual information

TABLE 2–3	
Possible Outcome of Brain Damage to the Four Lobes of the Brain	
Frontal lobe	Motor paralysis, inability to sequence multitask movements, loss of spontaneity in interacting with others, loss of flexibility in thinking, persistence of a single thought (perseveration), inability to focus on a task, mood changes **(emotional lability)**, changes in personality, difficulty with problem solving, inability to express language (Broca's area aphasia)
Parietal lobe	Inability to name an object **(anomia)**, difficulty with writing **(agraphia)**, problems with reading **(alexia)**, difficulty in distinguishing right from left, difficulty with doing math **(dyscalculia)**, lack of awareness of certain body parts and surrounding space, inability to focus visual attention, difficulties with eye and hand coordination
Temporal lobe	Difficulty recognizing faces, disturbance of selective attention to what is seen and heard, short-term memory loss, interference with long-term memory, inability to categorize objects, increased aggressive behavior, difficulty in understanding spoken language (Wernicke's area aphasia)
Occipital lobe	Deficits in vision (visual field cuts), difficulty locating objects in environment, difficulty recognizing colors, visual hallucinations and illusions, difficulty in recognizing words and drawn objects, difficulties with reading and writing

Source: Information compiled from multiple sources. See text and references for detail.

about the right half of the visual world and vice versa. There is an orderly mapping of the visual world onto the visual cortex. The physiology of the cells within this lobe allows for sensitivity to visual detail, permitting recognition and interpretation of visual information. An in-depth presentation of the importance of the visual system as it relates to the control of movement is presented in the next chapter and in Chapters 8 and 9 on postural and balance and upper extremity control, respectively.

Clinical Connection:

Patients with damage to their occipital cortex, even though the eyes are undamaged, are sometimes described as "cortically blind," a condition in which they can *receive* but not *perceive* visual information. Unless the occipital lobe of the brain can interpret and assign meaning to visual information, the reception of the stimulus by the camera-like eye is meaningless. Lesions of the occipital lobe can also result in disorders of eye movement, visual **agnosia** (inability to comprehend visual stimuli), or other visual processing disorders.

Table 2–3 describes common possible outcomes due to damage to any of the four lobes of the brain.

Association Cortexes

Within each of the four lobes are association areas that literally do just as their name implies. They associate, provide additional information from, and link together different regions of the cortex. These areas integrate and interpret information from all the lobes, allowing an individual to perceive and attach meaning to specific sensory experiences. It is in the association cortexes that a transition occurs between perception and action. Synaptic connections within the association areas allow someone to associate a specific kind of touch with its meaning. For example, the association cortex allows an individual to identify a certain touch with tenderness versus danger and to subsequently begin to retrieve the most appropriate action. The association areas also are involved in personality, intelligence, memory, spatial relationships, mood, and emotional affect (Lundy-Ekman, 2002).

Hemispheric Specialization

The cerebrum is divided into a right and a left hemisphere, with some gross anatomical differences permitting neuroanatomists to generalize that certain functions are predominantly associated with the right hemisphere, whereas other functions are usually associated with the left hemisphere. Generally speaking, the right hemisphere is associated functionally with perceptual abilities and the left hemisphere is associated with language functions. Table 2–4 lists the primary functions of the two hemispheres and common behaviors associated with damage to either hemisphere.

Connections Between the Hemispheres

Even though the cerebrum can be anatomically subdivided into two hemispheres, it is obviously of vital importance that the two hemispheres communicate with each other. Association fibers connect the various portions of a cerebral hemisphere and permit the cortex to function as an integrated whole (Waxman, 2000).

TABLE 2–4		
Behaviors Attributed to the Left and Right Hemispheres		
Behavior	Left Hemisphere	Right Hemisphere
Cognitive style	Processing information in a sequential, linear manner Observing and analyzing details	Processing information in a simultaneous or holistic manner Grasping overall organization or pattern
Perception/cognition	Processing and producing language	Processing nonverbal stimuli (environmental sounds, speech intonation, complex shapes, and designs)
Academic skills	Reading: sound-symbol relationships, word recognition, reading comprehension Performing mathematical calculations	Mathematical reasoning and judgment Alignment of numerals in calculations
Motor	Sequencing movements Performing movements and gestures to command	Sustaining a movement or posture
Emotions	Expressing positive emotions	Expressing negative emotions Perceiving emotion

Source: Adapted from O'Sullivan, S. B. (2001). Stroke. In S. B. O'Sullivan & T. J. Schmitz (Eds.). *Physical rehabilitation: Assessment and treatment* (4th ed.). Philadelphia: F. A. Davis, with permission.

Although there are several opportunities for hemispheric communication, the largest anatomical connection is through the corpus callosum. The corpus callosum is a large group of axons (therefore this is white matter) that connect the two hemispheres, allowing communication between the two. Yes, it literally is not only possible but also important that the right hand know what the left hand is doing! Furthermore, it *is* possible to walk and chew gum at the same time!

▪ Deeper Brain Structures

Internal Capsule

All axons leaving the motor areas of the frontal lobe travel through the internal capsule, a structure located deep within the cerebral hemispheres. The internal capsule is thus made up of axons traveling to and from the cerebral cortex, the brainstem, and the spinal cord. Geographically, the capsule is made up of an anterior and a posterior limb, each containing axons from specific nerve tracts. For example, the corticospinal tract, carrying information commanding contralateral limb movement and conscious sensation about the body, travels in the posterior limb. Damage to this area, then, will cause deficits in those functions.

Diencephalon

The diencephalon, situated very deep within the cerebrum, is composed of the thalamus and hypothalamus. Cranial nerve II, the optic nerve, is also located in the diencephalon. This is the area where all the major sensory and motor tracts synapse.

The thalamus actually consists of a large collection of nuclei and synapses. It acts as a central relay station for all sensory information coming in from other parts of the body to the cerebrum. The thalamus then relays information to the appropriate association cortex. Motor information received from areas such as the cerebellum and basal ganglia are also relayed through the thalamus to the correct motor region of the cortex. The function of the thalamus is likened to that of an efficient office administrator, filtering information and dispatching it to the appropriate area. Lesions in this area can be catastrophic, resulting in both sensory and motor deficits. Projections from the thalamus to the frontal lobes and limbic system are concerned with interpretation of pain, allowing an individual to perceive pain as hurting. Projections from the thalamus and sensory cortical areas to the temporal lobes are responsible for pain memory, and projections to the hypothalamus trigger an autonomic response to pain (Christiansen et al., 2001; Wessel, Vieregge, Kessler, & Kompf, 1994).

The hypothalamus is a group of nuclei that lie at the base of the brain. The term *hypothalamus* denotes that this structure must lie underneath the thalamus. The hypothalamus regulates homeostasis (equilibrium) and several autonomic functions, such as the regulation of hunger, sleep-wake cycles, body temperature, and blood pressure. These body functions are regulated through the production and secretion of hormones through the autonomic nervous system.

Basal Ganglia

What does *basal ganglia* mean? It literally names this region as a group of structures located at the base of the cerebrum ("basal" and "ganglia"). The group is made up of the caudate, putamen, globus pallidus, substantia nigra, and subthalamic nuclei. The basal ganglia is responsible for the regulation of posture and muscle tone. It plays a very important role in the control of both automatic and voluntary movement, exerting effects on the motor planning areas of the motor cortex.

Clinical Connection:

The most common clinical condition that results from pathology in the basal ganglia is Parkinson's disease, where patients exhibit a **resting tremor**, difficulty initiating movement **(akinesia)**, slowness of movement **(bradykinesia)**, muscular rigidity, and a stooped posture. This progressive disease, with a mean onset age of 58 years, is caused by a gradual loss of dopamine-producing neurons in the basal ganglia. ▪

▪ Cerebellum

The cerebellum is located posterior to the brainstem, beneath the occipital lobe, filling the posterior fossa of the cranium. Like the cerebrum, the cerebellum is further divided into two hemispheres. The cerebellum regulates balance and coordination. It is responsible for regulating and adjusting the accuracy, intensity, and timing of movement as required by the specific movement task. It sequences the order of muscle firing when a group of muscles work together to perform a complex task such as stepping or reaching (Martin & Kessler, 2000). The cerebellar pathways control balance, coordination, and movement accuracy on the same or ipsilateral body side, as opposed to the contralateral control feature associated with the cerebral cortex. The cerebellum is often called the great comparator, because it constantly monitors and compares the movement requested with the actual output, making adjustments as necessary. The cerebellum has the ability to receive sensory feedback from receptors about the movements as the movement is occurring, a property called **reafference.**

Clinical Connection:

Cerebellar lesions cause distinctive motor symptoms. Cerebellar symptomology often includes deficits in balance and coordination, including ataxia (wide-based movements), intention tremor (tremor accompanying purposeful movement), and **dysmetria** (inability to gauge distance in reaching or stepping). Cerebellar damage can cause any number of errors in the kinematic parameters of movement control, including difficulties with timing, accuracy, coordination, and regulation of intensity. ▪

▪ Brainstem

The brainstem is located at the base of the brain above the spinal cord and is composed of three parts: the midbrain, the pons, and the medulla. All the descending motor pathways except the corticospinal tract originate in the brainstem. In addition to being a major relay area, however, each area is responsible for different functions.

The midbrain is the most superior and is largely a relay area for tracts passing among the cerebrum, cerebellum, and the spinal cord. It also houses reflex centers for visual, auditory, and tactile responses (Martin & Kessler, 2000). Cranial nerves III and IV are located in the midbrain.

The middle area, the pons, contains axons that travel between the cerebellum and the rest of the CNS. Along with the medulla, it regulates respiratory rate. The pons contains reflex centers associated with the orientation of the head in relation to visual and auditory stimuli. The nuclei of cranial nerves V through VIII are also located here.

The area of the brainstem right above the spinal cord is called the medulla oblongata. Anatomically, the medulla is actually an extension of the spinal cord, containing the tracts running through the spinal cord. The medulla also contains motor and sensory nuclei for the neck and mouth, control centers for respiration and heart rate, and reflex centers for vomiting, sneezing, and swallowing (Martin & Kessler, 2000). Cranial nerves IX through XII are located in the medulla.

Extending vertically throughout the brainstem is the reticular activating system, a system vital for regulating an individual's state of arousal and sleep-wake cycles. So if your eyelids are feeling heavy and you are drifting off right about now, blame it on your reticular activating system!

Clinical Connection:

Damage to the brainstem can result in paralysis to the opposite body side; cranial nerve symptoms, such as paralysis of the tongue; and disruption of life-sustaining functions, including the control of heart rate and respiration. Because the brainstem regulates these vital functions of heart rate, blood pressure, and respiration, damage to this area can result in various levels of stupor or coma, as seen in severe head injuries or encephalitis. ▪

▪ *Spinal Cord*

The spinal cord is a direct continuation of the brainstem, specifically the medulla. It is housed within the vertebral column and extends caudally (to the bottom) to approximately the site of the second lumbar vertebrae. After this L2 level, the spinal cord tapers to form the conus medullaris. Below that level, the spinal cord becomes a bundled mass of lumbar and sacral spinal nerves, called the cauda equina (Fig. 2–7).

The spinal cord has two major functions: communication of sensory information and communication and coordination of motor information and movement patterns. The spinal cord provides a means of communication between the brain and the peripheral nerves. The circuitry of the spinal cord is involved in the initial reception and processing of somatosensory information (from the muscles, joints, and skin), contributing to the

control of posture and movement (Shumway-Cook & Woollacott, 2001). Sensory and motor tracts travel to and from the brain within the spinal cord. At the level of spinal cord processing, one can expect to see a fairly simple relationship between sensory input and motor output. Some subconscious reflexes, such as the stretch reflex and the withdrawal reflex, both to be discussed later, are integrated within the spinal cord (Martin & Kessler, 2000). At this level, the most stereotypical responses to sensory stimuli are organized, including basic flexion and extension patterns of the muscles involved in leg movements, such as kicking and locomotion (Kandel, 1991).

The internal anatomy of the spinal cord is best viewed as a cross-section, as depicted in Figure 2–8. Like the brain, the spinal cord is composed of gray and white matter. The gray area is in the central area of the crosssection (and therefore composed of motor neuron cell bodies and synapses), whereas the surrounding white areas are composed of axons arriving to and leaving the CNS. The cell bodies of the sensory neurons lie within the dorsal root ganglia outside the spinal cord.

The central gray area is quite distinguishable with its characteristic butterfly or H shape. The limbs of the H are called horns. The posterior or dorsal horns, in the back of the H, contain the synapses of incoming sensory (afferent) information. The anterior or ventral horns, in the front of the H, contain the cell bodies of lower motor neurons, which, as their name implies, transmit motor impulses directly to muscles. There is also a lateral horn

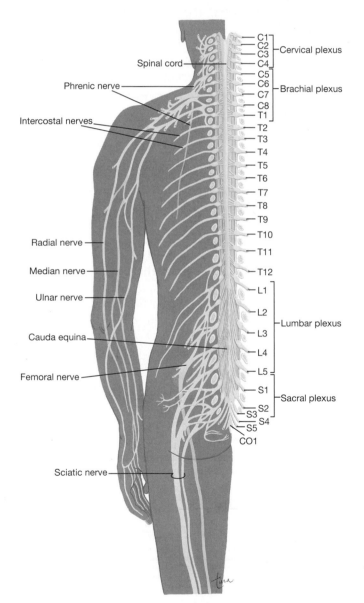

Figure 2–7. The spinal cord, spinal nerves, plexuses, and cauda equina. (From Scanlon, V. C., & Sanders, T. [2003]. *Essentials of anatomy and physiology* [4th ed., p. 163]. Philadelphia: F. A. Davis. Reprinted with permission from F. A. Davis Company, Philadelphia, PA.)

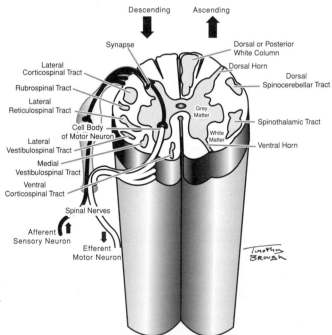

Figure 2–8. A typical cross-section of the spinal cord showing the dorsal and ventral horn, afferent and efferent neurons, and the location of the main tracts primarily involved in the control of movement as discussed in this text.

present at the T1 to L2 levels, containing cell bodies of preganglionic sympathetic neurons for the processing of autonomic information.

The peripheral white area is composed of sensory (ascending or afferent) and motor (descending or efferent) fiber tracts. A tract is a group of nerve fibers that are similar in origin, destination, and function. They carry impulses to and from various areas within the nervous system (Martin & Kessler, 2000). Sometimes these tracts travel on one side of the cord (ipsilateral), and sometimes they cross (contralateral). This anatomical fact is important to remember when seeing the result of injury; sometimes an injury to the right side of the spinal cord or brain will produce loss of motor or sensory function on the left side of the body.

▪ Afferent Tracts

There are two main sensory or ascending tracts, carrying sensory (afferent) information to the CNS. These pathways synapse at various levels within the CNS, ensuring the ability to modulate (change) incoming information at every level of the CNS. Although each tract is anatomically separate, there is some redundancy (overlap) of function between the two, another example of the CNS ensuring that more than one structure bears the responsibility for a function. One of these pathways crosses in the medulla to the other side of the brain and the other crosses immediately after entering the spinal cord, with subsequent clinical consequences as described in the text.

The **posterior (or dorsal) white columns** carry information about position sense (**proprioception**), vibration, two-point discrimination, and deep touch. The fibers of this tract enter the spinal cord in the dorsal horn, ascend the spinal cord, and then cross to the other side of the brain at the level of the brainstem, specifically in the medulla. These sensations from the left side of the body, for example, are received and processed on the right side of the brain. The **anterior spinothalamic tract** carries information about pain and temperature. The fibers of this tract enter the dorsal horn, synapse, and cross to the other side of the spinal cord within three segments. Its name tells you that the information first is relayed to the thalamus. Sensory information from all ascending tracts is then processed by the cerebral cortex for discrimination, association, and integration to occur.

Clinical Connection:

The pathways of the tracts in the human nervous system give rise to the constellation of clinical symptoms presented by the patient. Depending on the location of the lesion and whether or not the nerve tract crosses or not, the symptoms may be on the same side (ipsilateral) or opposite from (contralateral) the location of the lesion. For example, damage to one side of the spinal cord (as in a stab or puncture wound) will result in loss of kinesthetic and proprioceptive sensation on the same side of the body (posterior or dorsal white column) and loss of pain and temperature sensation on the opposite side of the body (spinothalamic tract). This unique syndrome due to a spinal cord hemisection is known as the Brown-Séquard syndrome. There are a few other syndromes easily recognized in neurorehabilitation for which the reader is referred to other sources (Schmitz & O'Sullivan, 2001; Trombly, 2001). For the purposes of this chapter, the reader is cautioned to remember that the clinical presentation of the patient will certainly reflect neuroanatomical structure and the results of anatomical damage, but rarely are lesions and injuries "classic textbook examples." Rather, injuries and lesions are often asymmetrical and somewhat diffuse, affecting perhaps different tracts or even portions of tracts unevenly. As always, a thorough physical and occupational therapy evaluation, in concert with medical tests and diagnoses, will uncover the unique presentation of any individual patient. ▪

▪ Efferent Tracts

The main motor or descending tract is the corticospinal tract (also called the pyramidal tract). This tract originates in the frontal lobe, specifically in the primary and premotor cortices, crosses to the opposite side in the brainstem, and continues through many interconnections and synapses to its final destination, onto a nerve in the anterior or ventral horn of the spinal cord, fittingly called the anterior horn cell.

The **anterior horn cell** is a large neuron, located in the gray matter of the spinal cord, that sends axons out through the anterior or ventral spinal root, eventually giving rise to peripheral nerves that innervate muscle fibers. **Alpha motor neurons** (so named for their large size) are a specific type of cell, found in the anterior (or ventral) horn, that innervates skeletal muscle. Because axons can branch sometimes extensively, several muscle fibers can be innervated by one neuron. A **motor unit** is defined as the alpha motor neuron and all the muscle fibers it innervates. A smaller motor neuron, called the gamma motor neuron, is also located within the ventral or anterior horn of the spinal cord. **Gamma motor neurons** innervate small muscle fibers within a specialized receptor called the muscle spindle. Muscle spindles are specialized receptors located within the muscle, to be discussed later in this chapter.

Other descending motor pathways that affect muscle control and posture are the rubrospinal, reticulospinal, tectospinal, and vestibulospinal tracts (Martin

& Kessler, 2000). The rubrospinal tract originates in the red nucleus of the midbrain (hence the prefix *rubro–*) and ends on the lower motor neurons going to the upper extremities. This tract functions to facilitate (activate) muscles of the flexors and inhibit (suppress) muscles of the extensors. The reticulospinal tract originates in the reticular formation, which runs vertically throughout the brainstem. Part of it facilitates limb extensors, and another portion of it facilitates flexors and inhibits extensors. The tectospinal tract provides for orientation of the head toward a sound or moving object, to be discussed with the visual system in Chapter 3. The vestibulospinal tract has a lateral and medial component, with a close anatomical relationship to the mechanisms of the inner ear. The lateral vestibulospinal tract assists in postural adjustments by facilitating proximal extensor muscles, whereas the medial vestibulospinal regulates muscle tone in the neck and upper back and helps to keep the head balanced on the trunk as the body moves. Normal adult control of posture and movement is made possible by interplay and convergence of all these varying inputs.

Peripheral Nervous System

The PNS is made up of the nerves leading to and from the different regions of the CNS. These include the spinal nerves exiting the spinal cord, the receptors detecting sensory stimuli, and the cranial nerves. The PNS can also be subdivided into two major components, the somatic (about the body) nervous system and the autonomic nervous system. The somatic nervous system is concerned with reaction to outside stimuli, innervates skeletal muscle, and is under voluntary control. The ANS is an involuntary system that innervates the viscera, glands, smooth muscle, and the heart. The ANS will be discussed later. This section covers the somatic nervous system.

Within the somatic nervous system, there are 12 pairs of cranial nerves, 31 pairs of spinal nerves, and several different kinds of peripheral receptors.

▪ Cranial Nerves

The cranial nerves are located in the brainstem and brain, numbered according to the site of attachment, from anterior to posterior. Some cranial nerves are purely sensory, some are motor, and some are mixed. The primary functions of cranial nerves include smell, eye movement, vision, and sensation perceived by the face and tongue, with the exception of the vagus nerve, which has an autonomic function. The sternocleidomastoid and upper trapezius muscles are also partially innervated by the accessory nerve, which is a cranial

nerve. This is a good example of the redundancy of the nervous system, which allows for preservation of function in the incidence of some injuries. Table 2–5 lists the cranial nerves and their locations and functions.

▪ Spinal Nerves

The spinal nerves, exiting from the spinal cord, are shown in Figures 2–7 and 2–8. Spinal nerves, made up of both sensory and motor components, exit through the intervertebral foramen. Once through the foramen, the nerve divides into anterior and posterior rami (branch), this division representing the anatomical beginning of the PNS (Martin & Kessler, 2000). The ventral or anterior rami innervate the anterior and lateral trunk, the intercostals, and the muscles and skin of the extremities. The dorsal or posterior rami innervate the paraspinal muscles and the overlying skin. The 12 pairs of thoracic nerves maintain their segmental relationship. The anterior rami of the cervical, lumbar, and sacral spinal nerves join together to form local nerve networks, identified as the cervical plexus, brachial plexus, and lumbosacral plexus.

A **plexus** is a network of nerves, bundled and subdivided so that the branching allows for a rich representation of spinal nerve origin in the peripheral nerve terminal. This is another way that the anatomy of the nervous system allows for redundancy and therefore preservation of some semblance of innervation in the face of some injuries. The cervical plexus is composed of the spinal nerves of C1 through C5. The anterior rami of C5 through T1 form the brachial plexus, giving rise to the axillary, musculocutaneous, radial, median, and ulnar nerves, which innervate the upper extremity. The lumbosacral plexus is formed from the rami of L1 through S3, innervating the musculature of the lower extremities.

The spinal nerves are named according to their respective vertebrae: 8 cervical pairs, 12 thoracic pairs, 5 lumbar pairs, 5 sacral pairs, and 1 very small coccygeal pair. The first seven cervical nerves exit above the corresponding vertebrae; the eighth cervical nerve and all the thoracic and sacral nerves exit below the corresponding vertebrae. Each of these spinal nerves has two roots, which are neurons either entering or leaving the spinal cord.

▪ Peripheral Nerves

Peripheral nerves contain both afferent (sensory) and efferent (motor) nerve fibers. Motor fibers originate in the anterior or ventral horn and have large cell bodies, several dendrites, and usually one long axon. This axon eventually becomes part of a peripheral nerve, innervating a motor end plate of a muscle. A sensory neuron, on the other hand, has a dendrite that originates as a

TABLE 2-5

Cranial Nerves, Functions, and Locations

Number	Name	Type	Function	Anatomical Location
I	Olfactory	Sensory	Smell	Inferior frontal lobe
II	Optic	Sensory	Vision	Diencephalon
III	Oculomotor	Motor	Innervates extraocular muscles to move eye up, down, and medially and raise eyelid; constricts pupil	Midbrain
IV	Trochlear	Motor	Innervates extraocular muscles to move eye up and down	Midbrain
V	Trigeminal	Mixed	Chewing, sensation from face, cornea, and temporomandibular joint	Pons
VI	Abducens	Motor	Abducts the eye	Between pons and medulla
VII	Facial	Mixed	Facial expression, closes eye, tears, salivation, and taste	Between pons and medulla
VIII	Vestibulocochlear	Sensory	Sensation of head movements and head position in relation to gravity; hearing	Between pons and medulla
IX	Glossopharyngeal	Mixed	Taste, swallowing, and salivation	Medulla
X	Vagus	Mixed	Regulates viscera, speech, swallowing, and taste	Medulla
XI	Accessory	Motor	Shoulder elevation by innervation of trapezius muscle; turns head by innervation of sternocleidomastoid muscle	Spinal cord and medulla
XII	Hypoglossal	Motor	Innervation of tongue	Medulla

Sources: Adapted from Cohen, H. (1999). *Neuroscience for rehabilitation* (2nd ed.). Philadelphia: Lippincott Williams & Wilkins; Lundy-Ekman, L. (2002). *Neuroscience: Fundamentals for rehabilitation* (2nd ed.). Philadelphia: W. B. Saunders; and Martin, S., & Kessler, M. (2000). *Neurologic intervention for physical therapist assistants.* Philadelphia: W. B. Saunders.

receptor in the skin, muscle, or tendon. This dendrite then travels all the way to its cell body (soma), located in the dorsal horn of the spinal cord. The cell body then sends an impulse along an axon, which may either terminate at the spinal cord level or synapse with higher-order neurons as the stimulus enters the white matter in the ascending tracts to different levels of the CNS.

Clinical Connection:

Because most peripheral nerves are mixed, injuries to a peripheral nerve produce both sensory and motor deficits. A common consequence of advanced diabetes mellitus is peripheral nerve neuropathy. Numbness, tingling, and weakness accompany diabetic neuropathy, most commonly seen in the distal extremities. Carpal tunnel syndrome is a common clinical example of weakness and sensory symptoms caused by compression of the median nerve as it passes under the flexor retinaculum (ligament on palmar aspect of wrist) within the carpal tunnel. ▪

▪ Receptors

Information about the external world and the internal body environment is communicated to the CNS through afferent impulses. The impulses first arise from the stimulation of various sensory receptors, these receptors acting as energy transducers, converting the energy of the stimuli into electrical activity for transmission and communication. Most receptors respond preferentially to one form of stimulus, such as mechanical, chemical, or thermal. In order for the stimulus, such as pressure or temperature, to be converted into an electrical impulse, the stimulus is first converted by the receptor into a generator potential. This generator potential is a local, unpropagated event, which, if sufficient in number, timing, or intensity, will then cause depolarization of the afferent axon for transmission into the CNS.

This afferent information can be transmitted to many levels of the CNS, including the spinal cord, brainstem, cerebellum, and cerebrum. The information transmitted along the afferent axon can be coded in two ways: the frequency of nerve impulses and the number of channels opened. Such an arrangement allows afferent axons to signal a wide range of stimulus intensities (Stokes, 1998). Sensory information is received and able to be modulated (turned up or turned down) at all these levels, giving rise to both conscious and subconscious sensation.

Clinical Connection:

Perhaps you are reading this while sitting in a wicker chair, wearing a sweatshirt and pair of pants. You are not conscious of the wicker pattern of the chair beneath you, nor are you paying any attention to the clothing tag on the inside of your shirt or even the hole in the knee of your pants. You could divert your attention to these sensations, but your nervous system maintains them at a subconscious level so that you can pay attention to the more relevant task at hand, learning about the nervous system by reading this text! ▪

Sensory receptors are distributed over the body surface, within the musculoskeletal system, within the special senses, and deep within the viscera. These different types can be subcategorized functionally into three groups: **exteroceptors,** which give the CNS information about the external world, such as touch; **interoceptors,** which give the CNS information about the viscera and the inside of the body; and proprioceptors, which give the CNS information about the state and position of the musculoskeletal system. Although all receptors are the same in their functional ability to respond to stimulation and to change that stimulus into an electrical signal, they vary tremendously in their complexity. The simplest receptors are free nerve endings and the most complex comprise complicated sense organs.

▪ Special Senses and Receptors

The receptors for taste, smell, vision, hearing, and the vestibular system are highly specialized. The impulses from these receptors are transmitted through the cranial nerves. (Refer to a basic anatomy text for review of taste and smell.) The visual and vestibular systems are detailed in Chapter 3, which describes the major systems that contribute to human movement control.

▪ Cutaneous Receptors

The skin has several different types of receptors that respond to touch, pressure, or stretch of the skin during movement or interaction. Skin receptors, sometimes called cutaneous receptors, are a type of exteroceptor. The particular area or region of the skin in which it is possible to excite that receptor and then activate the

afferent nerve fiber is called the **receptive field** (Cohen, 1999). Receptive field size and the density of receptors within a given area of skin determine the degree of discrimination. For example, the fingertips are able to discriminate two points only 1 mm apart, whereas skin on the abdomen cannot discriminate points closer than 5 to 10 mm (Stokes, 1998). The receptive fields have corresponding representation in the somatosensory cortex, as represented by the sensory homunculus (see Fig. 2–6), where large representation in the sensory cortex corresponds to those neurons with the smallest, most discriminative receptive fields (as in the fingertips and tongue).

Clinical Connection:

I'm sure you've experienced an injury, perhaps an ankle sprain or a hand injury, that was accompanied by swelling. Do you remember how clumsy you felt while trying to grasp something with a swollen hand or trying to step accurately with a swollen ankle? This experience occurs because swelling, a primary sign of inflammation, also distorts the receptive fields in the swollen area, so that the fine discrimination ability is sacrificed. Think, then, of the patient with congestive heart failure or diabetes, where the ankles are chronically swollen, or the patient with shoulder-hand syndrome, where the hand is grossly edematous (swollen). These patients have difficulty executing simple tasks and may require assistance or visual feedback. ▪

Examples of cutaneous (skin) receptors include Ruffini endings, Meissner's corpuscles, Pacinian corpuscles, and tactile discs, graphically depicted in Figure 2–9 (Schmitz, 2001). Some receptors, such as the Paciniform corpuscles, adapt rapidly to a stimulus and therefore only signal when there is a change in stimulus, such an initial touch. Others, such as Meissner's corpuscles and Merkel's discs, adapt slowly and continue to fire as long as the stimulus persists (Stokes, 1998). In hairy skin, a multitude of receptors exist with terminals attached to hair follicles, allowing them to respond to the movement of hairs. These are typically rapidly adapting and exquisitely sensitive (Stokes, 1998). Most of the afferent axons from these cutaneous receptors are myelinated. The skin also has free nerve endings that are innervated by slower-conducting unmyelinated axons. These are the receptors that respond to changes in temperature and to noxious stimuli that cause pain.

▪ Proprioceptors

The main **proprioceptors** are the muscle spindle, the Golgi tendon organs (GTO), and joint receptors (Fig. 2–10). All these receptors contribute to overall proprio-

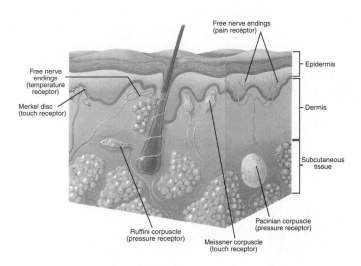

Figure 2–9. Cutaneous sensory receptors in a section of the skin. (From Scanlon, V. C., & Sanders, T. [2003]. *Essentials of anatomy and physiology* [4th ed., p. 189]. Philadelphia: F. A. Davis. Reprinted with permission from F. A. Davis Company, Philadelphia, PA.)

ceptive function, knowledge about one's own body and its position, static and dynamic.

Muscle Spindle

The **muscle spindle** (so named for its shape) is a unique receptor, located between the fibers of skeletal muscle (also called extrafusal muscle fibers because they lie outside the spindle), which has both sensory and motor

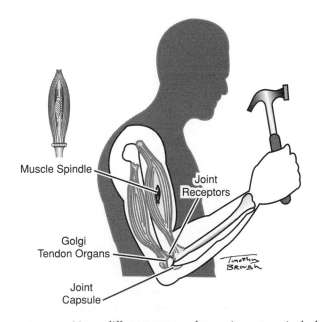

Figure 2–10. Many different types of proprioceptors, including muscle spindles, tendon organs, and joint receptors, all contribute to proprioceptive function

properties. Within this spindle, at either ends of a broadened fuse-shaped center, are muscle fibers called intrafusal muscle fibers. Intrafusal muscle fibers are much smaller than extrafusal (skeletal) muscle fibers. There are two types, nuclear bag and nuclear chain fibers, terms descriptive of their specific anatomical configuration. It is easiest to explain the anatomy and the function of the muscle spindle simultaneously.

As depicted in Figure 2–11, the receptor function of the muscle spindle is provided for by the location of the spindle in parallel alignment with the extrafusal or skeletal muscle fibers (EFMF). In humans, there are varying amounts of spindles located within different muscles. For example, the extraocular, hand, and neck muscles have a very high spindle density because of the importance of those muscles being constantly alerted to even small changes. As the EFMF changes length, such as during muscle contraction or stretch, the spindle detects this length change and depolarizes an afferent sensory nerve wrapped around it, called a Ia sensory nerve (again, a size classification depicting a large myelinated sensory nerve; pronounced "one a"). This Ia nerve also has a critical velocity threshold, meaning that it will also only detect a length change if this change exceeds a certain rate, or velocity. If this sensory nerve depolarizes, noting a muscle stretch of a sufficient velocity, it will send this impulse into the dorsal horn (where all sensory information enters the spinal cord), where it can connect with other neurons. It makes a direct connection (monosynaptic) to an efferent nerve, an alpha motor neuron (the anterior horn cell), which then transmits a signal back to the same EFMF, signaling the skeletal muscle to contract. The incoming sensory afferent nerve also makes an additional connection, this time through an interneuron (disynaptic) to another efferent alpha motor neuron, which then transmits a signal to the antagonist muscle, signaling that muscle to relax.

The monosynaptic component of this example is also known as the **stretch reflex**, a simple reflex arc mediated at the spinal cord level, without cerebral influence (Fig. 2–12). We have all experienced having the integrity of this reflex connection tested when a doctor taps a reflex hammer on a muscle tendon, typically the patellar tendon, producing a knee jerk.

Equally important are the functional ramifications of the fact that when an agonist muscle is signaled to contract, its antagonist is signaled to relax. This **reciprocal innervation** allows for some of the fluidity seen in human movement, for example, allowing for relaxation of the hamstrings to permit passive elongation while the quadriceps are being actively recruited to give a forceful kick. This anatomical fact also provides the basis for the rationale behind active stretching, where a patient is asked to actively contract a muscle to shut off its antagonist, allowing both active and passive stretching to be effective.

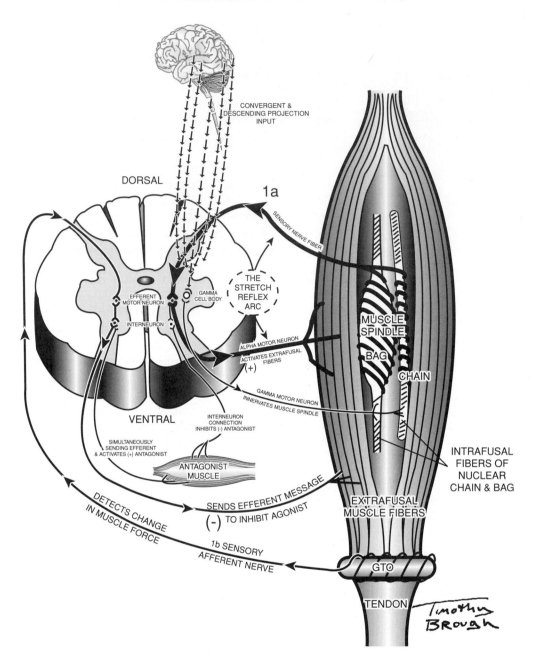

Figure 2–11. A cross-section of the spinal cord shows Ia afferent fiber originating in a muscle spindle, entering a dorsal root, and making synaptic connection with an alpha motoneuron. The axon of the alpha motoneuron emerges through the ventral root, terminating in the extrafusal muscles fibers. This figure also depicts reciprocal inhibition. Ib afferent fiber is seen originating at the Golgi tendon organ, and the connections involved in autogenic inhibition are depicted. The axon of the gamma motoneuron, receiving various inputs, including from the descending corticospinal tract, terminates in the intrafusal fibers within the muscle spindle. (Adapted from original drawing by Rich Milan, BS, CP, PTA, with permission.)

Clinical Connection:

Active and passive stretching techniques utilize the neuroanatomical connections described earlier. For example, if a patient presents with tight hamstring muscles, an active contraction of the quadriceps muscles will induce relaxation of the hamstrings, allowing them to be effectively stretched. In this clinical example, the limb would be taken to the position of gentle stretch; the patient is asked to actively contract the agonist (the quadriceps), facilitating the stretch by inhibiting the muscle undergoing the stretch (the hamstring as the antagonist in this example).

The motor function of the muscle spindle is conceptualized by further study of Figure 2–11. The muscle fibers at either ends of the spindle, called intrafusal muscle fibers (IFMF), are innervated by gamma efferent nerves, whose cell bodies are located in the ventral or anterior horn of the spinal cord. These gamma cells, however, receive synaptic connections and influences from throughout the human nervous system, such as the cortex, cerebellum, and brainstem. This constant volley of regulatory input onto the IFMF of the muscle spindle through the collective input onto the gamma nerves sets up a constant resting state of readiness, so that skeletal muscle is literally on a steady state of alert or arousal for the task demands to be placed on it. This

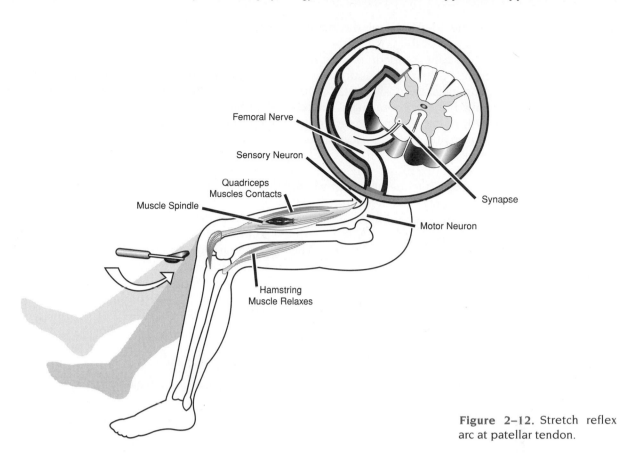

Femoral Nerve

Sensory Neuron

Quadriceps
Muscles Contacts

Muscle Spindle

Synapse

Motor Neuron

Hamstring
Muscle Relaxes

Figure 2–12. Stretch reflex arc at patellar tendon.

constant state of readiness is called **muscle tone,** further clarified as normal muscle tone where the inputs onto this system are absent of pathology. Tone is determined by the level of excitability of the entire pool of motor neurons controlling a muscle, the intrinsic stiffness of the muscle itself, and the level of sensitivity of many different reflexes. The contribution of the muscle spindle is only one piece of the puzzle contributing to the phenomenon called muscle tone. The spindles, however, do play a vital role by providing ongoing feedback to the nervous system about the changing conditions of muscle length.

Golgi Tendon Organs

Golgi tendon organs (GTO) are located at the musculotendinous junction of skeletal muscle, arranged perpendicular to the pull of the muscle (see Fig. 2–11). This anatomical location allows for the GTO to constantly monitor tension and detect fatigue, as a muscle contracts and pulls on its tendon. The afferent nerve from the GTO is called a Ib (remember the size classification in Table 2–2; this nerve is therefore smaller than the larger Ia, which is the muscle spindle afferent) and enters the spinal cord dorsal horn. It then synapses with several interneurons (disynaptic or

polysynaptic), dispatching several efferent messages, including one to the agonist muscle to be inhibited and another to that muscle's antagonist to be facilitated. This connection allows the GTO, through the Ib afferents, to mediate nonreciprocal inhibition, also called **autogenic inhibition.** This autogenic inhibition refers to an inhibitory input to an agonist muscle (the prime mover) and an excitatory message to the antagonist (opposing) muscle.

Clinical Connection:

Autogenic inhibition can be effectively applied to therapeutic stretching techniques, especially in situations where the patient is extremely anxious about movement due to pain. In this technique, called hold-relax, the limb is held by the therapist or assistant at the end of the agonist range (e.g., the hamstrings) and the patient is asked to perform an isometric "holding" contraction. After the ensuing relaxation of the agonist, the therapist or assistant can then move the limb further into the newly achieved range. ■

The Ib interneurons, however, can be either facilitory or inhibitory. Therefore, GTO activation results in myriad responses in addition to autogenic inhibition. It was once thought that the inhibition of the agonist muscle was the main function of the GTO. Although it certainly was the first described function, it is now known that it is only one of many functions, all basically concerned with detecting tension. A single GTO has many muscle fibers from different motor units associated with it, typically 10 to 15. Within a given motor unit (an alpha motor neuron and all the muscle fibers it innervates), only one muscle fiber acts on the GTO. A single GTO therefore receives one muscle fiber from 10 to 15 different motor units. GTOs therefore appear to monitor whole muscle tension rather than individual fiber tension. The CNS probably relies on the aggregate information provided by a group of GTOs from each muscle to extract information about muscle force. The GTO therefore gives important feedback to the CNS.

Joint Receptors

Joint receptors are also located within the structure of the joint, the joint capsule, and its ligaments (see Fig. 2–10). There are a number of different types, including Ruffini-type endings or spray endings, Paciniform endings, ligament receptors, and free nerve endings, all distributed throughout various portions of the joint capsule. These receptors signal joint position, detect the end of a joint range, and give very accurate information to the CNS about even the most minute fractionation (small increments) of joint range of motion.

Autonomic Nervous System

The ANS can be described functionally as the visceral nervous system, actually anatomically containing portions of both the CNS and PNS. The ANS controls the activities of glands, smooth muscles, internal organs, and blood vessels. This important information about the state of the body is then shared with the brain (Waxman, 2000).

The ANS regulates circulation, respiration, digestion, metabolism, secretion, body temperature, and reproduction (Martin & Kessler, 2000).

Anatomically, the ANS consists of control centers located in the brainstem and hypothalamus, some cranial nerves, and motor nerves within the spinal nerves that then innervate the smooth muscles of glands, the viscera, and the heart. The CNS exerts influence over the ANS. Specifically, the hypothalamus regulates digestion and the medulla houses important respiration and cardiac centers. The ANS is divided into the sympathetic and the parasympathetic system. Both systems innervate internal organs, use a two-neuron relay pathway connecting impulses through a single ganglion, and function automatically (Martin & Kessler, 2000).

The **sympathetic nervous system** is composed of fibers that arise from the thoracic and lumbar portions of the spinal cord. The axons of the preganglionic neurons then terminate in the sympathetic chain ganglia or the prevertebral ganglia in the abdomen. This system is commonly known as being responsible for fight-or-flight responses, because it assists in responding to stressful situations. These sympathetic responses help us to cope with stressful situations by maintaining an optimal blood supply to skeletal muscle; increasing the secretion of the neurotransmitters epinephrine and norepinephrine, which raise heart rate and blood pressure; and diverting blood flow from the gastrointestinal tract (Martin & Kessler, 2000). These are certainly important responses if the stress is real and short lived. Imagine, however, the negative consequences of long-term stress, especially perceived stress, on optimal health. Current increases in heart disease and mental illness may be due to a society immersed in a stress-filled lifestyle.

Clinical Connection:

When a person sustains a spinal cord injury above the level of T6, a common accompanying impairment may be periods of **autonomic dysreflexia**. Autonomic dysreflexia, as the term implies, is a situation in which the autonomic nervous system is no longer under effective CNS control because of the spinal cord injury; a state of disarray, or dysreflexia, can result from otherwise minimal disturbances perceived by the body. Autonomic dysreflexia can be caused by overdistension of the bladder, a urinary tract infection, a pinched catheter tube, or even monthly menstrual cramps. The body perceives, incorrectly, an emergency situation and signals a massive sympathetic response. The signs are a pounding headache, increased blood pressure, and a feeling of anxiousness. Swift recognition of this medical emergency is crucial because it can be life threatening. Removal of the irritant will reverse the symptoms. When encountered clinically, clinicians are advised to immediately seek assistance and sit the patient up in an effort to bring the elevated blood pressure down. ▪

The **parasympathetic nervous system** maintains homeostasis and balanced body functions. This division receives information from the brainstem, several cranial nerves, and from lower sacral segments of the spinal cord. The vagus nerve (cranial nerve X) is an important parasympathetic nerve, innervating the myocardium and smooth muscles of the digestive tract and lungs. Acetylcholine, a vasodilator, is the main neurotransmitter of the parasympathetic system. When an individual is calm, parasympathetic activity decreases heart rate and maintains normal gastrointestinal activity (Martin & Kessler, 2000).

Support Systems: Meninges, Ventricular System, Circulation

▪ Meninges, Ventricular System, and Cerebrospinal Fluid

Inside its armor of bone, the nervous system is encased and protected by membranes called **meninges** (Cohen, 1999). These meninges, the pia mater, arachnoid mater, and dura mater, offer protection from infection and contusion. The nervous system is cushioned by **cerebrospinal fluid (CSF),** formed within cavities in the brain called ventricles. CSF is formed primarily by specialized tissue located within the ventricles, called the choroid plexus. The CSF circulates around the brain and spinal cord within the subarachnoid space of the meninges, offering support, transportation of nutrients, and removal of metabolic wastes. Unimpaired flow of CSF is vital to maintaining normal support of the CNS. Any pathological increase in CSF volume or obstruction of flow can cause enlarged ventricles and compression of brain tissue.

Clinical Connection:

Obstruction in the flow of CSF produces enlargement of the ventricles, resulting in a condition known as **hydrocephalus**. Hydrocephalus can be treated very successfully through the surgical placement of a shunt, typically a ventriculoperitoneal shunt. A shunt is plastic tubing that redirects the overflow fluid from the ventricles into the peritoneal area for reabsorption and excretion. As the shunt tubing exits the lateral ventricle, it can be palpated distally along the neck, under the clavicle, and down the chest wall, just underneath the superficial fascia. Hydrocephalus, left undetected and untreated, or a blocked shunt can cause pressure on brain structures, secondary brain damage, and even death.

In children, hydrocephalus often accompanies neural tube defects such as spina bifida. In this case, a shunt is placed very early, sometimes even in utero, thus preventing any chance of secondary brain damage. In young children, before the cranial sutures close (at approximately age 2), signs of a newly developing hydrocephalus or a blocked shunt may include swelling of the forehead or fontanel, irritability, nausea, change in eye position, or sleepiness. In the older child or adult, once the cranium is fused, the signs may be more subtle but the results more catastrophic because there is literally nowhere for the swelling or increased pressure to go. In adults, hydrocephalus usually is the result of a traumatic brain injury or the presence of a space-occupying lesion, such as a brain tumor. Once again, placement of a shunt will prevent secondary brain damage and help to preserve function. ▪

▪ Circulation

Just as anywhere else in the body, the cells of the nervous system rely on an adequate blood supply for delivery of nutrients, such as glucose and oxygen. All arteries to the brain arise first from the aortic arch, with a first major division into the carotid arteries in the neck. The carotid arteries offer the main blood supply for the cerebellum. The carotid arteries then bifurcate (divide) behind the jaw to form the internal and external carotids. The internal carotids then enter the cranium and supply the cerebral hemispheres, including the frontal lobe, parietal lobe, and parts of the temporal lobe; the optic nerve; and the retinas of the eyes. At the base of the brain, the internal carotid bifurcates into the right and left anterior and middle cerebral arteries. The middle cerebral artery, supplying the deepest portions of the frontal and parietal lobes and the lateral aspect of the brain, is the largest and the most often occluded. The anterior cerebral artery supplies the superior portions of the frontal and parietal lobe.

In the posterior region, two vertebral arteries branch off the subclavian artery and arise to supply the brainstem and cerebellum. Upon entrance into the cranium through the foramen magnum, the vertebral arteries first unite to form the basilar artery, which supplies the brainstem and part of the occipital and temporal lobes. This artery also bifurcates into a pair of posterior cerebral arteries, supplying the main portions of the occipital and temporal lobes.

The carotid arteries, through the anterior cerebral artery, and the vertebral arteries, through the posterior cerebral arteries, are interconnected at the base of the brain, forming the **circle of Willis** (Fig. 2–13) (Martin & Kessler, 2000). This circular arrangement is another method whereby the CNS preserves function in the face of injury or pathology. In the face of an occlusion (block) in one area, blood supply can be rerouted so that the metabolic and nutritional needs of that tissue can be met, at least partially, by an alternate blood supply. Arising from the circle of Willis are several large vessels, which provide blood supply to surface areas and deep structures of the brain. One of the largest of these vessels is the middle cerebral artery, a major branch of the internal carotid, which supplies blood to the surface and deep layers of both cerebral hemispheres (Cohen, 1999). In a stroke (**cerebrovascular accident [CVA]**), this is the most common site of occlusion. Table 2–6 describes resultant deficits associated with stroke involving the main cerebral arteries.

Clinical Connection:

A stroke, from the Greek term *streich*, meaning "to strike," is the well-known expression associated with a CVA. In its early Greek use, people used the term *streich* to describe the casualty that befell such an individual, thinking that it was a "stroke of God" (McKeough, 1999). A CVA is caused by either a hemorrhage or occlusion in any of the cerebral blood vessels (Cohen, 1999). The symptoms presented by a patient following a CVA are a direct result of the blood vessel involved and hence the areas of the brain that are damaged. The most commonly encountered patient with a CVA has a lesion from occlusion or hemorrhage of the middle cerebral artery, manifested by motor disturbances on the side opposite the brain damage; impaired language and spatial perception; and impaired cognition. ▪

Clinical Thinking: Relationship Between Clinical Signs and Lesions

What and Where Is the Lesion: Clinical Implications

For rehabilitation professionals, the main concern in studying the nervous system is to understand the effects of nervous system damage to effectively plan and execute a rehabilitation program. A **lesion** is an area of damage or dysfunction. Signs and symptoms following a lesion depend on both the location and the severity of the lesion. Lesions can be physiological, reflecting physiological dysfunction in the absence of demonstrable anatomical abnormalities, such as meta-

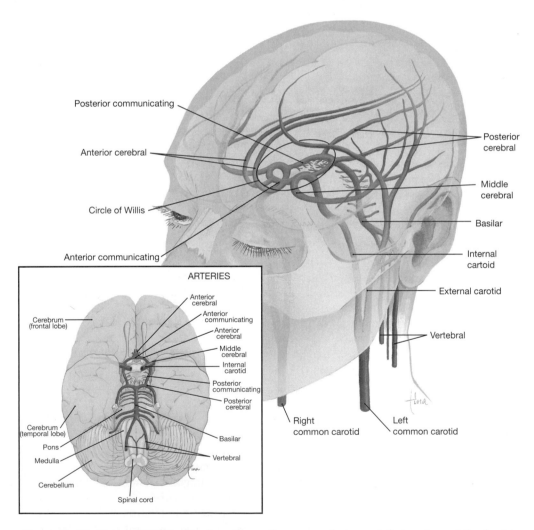

Figure 2–13. Circle of Willis. The box shows these vessels in an inferior view of the brain. (From Scanlon, V. C., & Sanders, T. [2003]. *Essentials of anatomy and physiology* [4th ed., p. 289]. Philadelphia: F. A. Davis. Reprinted with permission from F. A. Davis Company, Philadelphia, PA.)

TABLE 2-6

Cerebral Circulation and Resultant Deficits Associated with Stoke

Anterior cerebral artery	Contralateral weakness and sensory loss primarily in lower extremity, aphasia, memory and behavioral deficits, incontinence
Middle cerebral artery	Contralateral weakness and sensory loss in the face and upper extremity with less involvement in the lower extremity, **homonymous hemianopsia** (loss of contralateral half of each visual field; the nasal half of one eye and the temporal half of the other, corresponding to the hemiplegic side of each eye)
Posterior cerebral artery	Contralateral sensory loss, thalamic pain syndrome, homonymous hemianopsia, visual **agnosia** (inability to recognize common objects), cortical blindness
Vertebrobasilar artery	Cranial nerve involvement, difficulty swallowing (dysphagia), **dysarthria** (speech difficulties associated with coordination of respiration, phonation, and articulation), ataxia, coordination deficits, dizziness, headaches

Sources: Adapted from Fredericks, C., & Saladin, L. (1996). *Pathophysiology of the motor systems.* Philadelphia: F. A. Davis; Martin, S., & Kessler, M. (2000). *Neurologic intervention for physical therapist assistants.* Philadelphia: W. B. Saunders; and O'Sullivan, S. B., & Schmitz, T. J. (Eds.), *Physical rehabilitation: Assessment and treatment* (4th ed.). Philadelphia: F. A. Davis, with permission from Elsevier, 2000.

bolic diseases or even commonly occurring transient ischemic attacks (TIAs or "mini-strokes"), which produce deficits without structural neuronal damage. Anatomically, lesions can be categorized as follows (Daube, Sandok, Reagan, & Westmoreland, 1986; Lundy-Ekman, 2002):

- **Focal lesion:** limited to a single location
- **Multifocal lesion:** limited to several nonsymmetrical locations
- **Diffuse lesion:** affecting bilaterally symmetrical structures but not crossing midline as a single lesion

A tumor in the cerebellum is an example of a focal lesion, whereas such a tumor that has metastasized to several locations in the CNS, would be considered multifocal. Down syndrome and Alzheimer's disease, affecting several cognitive, memory, and motor areas, are examples of diffuse damage. Regardless of the cause of nervous system damage, the signs and symptoms depend on the site and the type of the lesion (Lundy-Ekman, 2002).

Focal lesions cause signs and symptoms on the basis of a single geographically contiguous lesion. The most common example is a stroke, where blood supply is occluded and a specific area of the brain loses its blood supply, a situation termed ischemia. In this situation, it is entirely possible to be able to ascribe most of the patient's symptoms to a loss of function in that specific area of the brain. *Multifocal* pathology results in damage to the nervous system at numerous, separate locations. The best example is multiple sclerosis (MS), where lesions develop over time in different areas. The signs and symptoms presented by this patient will be multiple, with the presentation of new signs an indication of spread or progression of the disease process. *Diffuse* dysfunction of the nervous system can be produced by a number of toxins or metabolic disturbances, often

alerting the examiner to look for a systemic disorder giving rise to such a multitude of signs, sometimes indicative of global dysfunction (Waxman, 2000).

The extent and location of the lesion; whether or not the lesion is localized or diffuse, symmetrical or asymmetrical; and the rapidity with which the lesion is produced all affect the degree of deficit and recovery (Cohen, 1999). The significance of size is not a simple matter. It is not correct to say that the smaller the lesion, the smaller the deficit. Size of the lesion is relative to the area of the brain involved. More importantly, size relates to whether an entire area or only a portion of that area is damaged. Size also relates to how strictly localized the functions or subfunctions of the areas are (Cohen, 1999).

Signs and Symptoms of Neurological Impairments Affecting Movement

To effectively treat patients with movement problems, therapists and assistants must have an operational understanding of the pathophysiology of neurological disorders and accompanying impairments. Remember the disablement model presented in Chapter 1 with the classifications of pathology, impairments, functional limitations, and disability.

Brain pathology produces a unique pattern of signs and symptoms associated with the nature and area of the neurological damage. CNS lesions can result in a variety of primary impairments affecting motor, sensory, perceptual, and cognitive systems. In addition to primary impairments, secondary impairments also contribute to the movement problems demonstrated by patients. Secondary impairments do not result from the

CNS pathology directly but rather develop as a result of the consequences of the pathology or primary impairment. For example, a child with cerebral palsy (CP) may have a lesion in the descending motor pathways, causing a primary impairment of muscular weakness and abnormal muscle tone. The child presenting for therapy may have secondary impairments of a hip flexion contracture and a dislocating hip because of the abnormal muscle pull caused by these primary impairments. It is important to realize that function can be limited by the abnormal muscle tone and weakness, as well as by the unstable hip and flexion contracture.

According to Shumway-Cook & Woollacott (2001), the following section describes in general terms the major motor system impairments that commonly accompany neurological damage. These motor system impairments are presented briefly in this chapter to assist the reader in establishing an immediate connection between pathology in the neuromotor systems and subsequent movement impairments. These common impairments and their functional consequences will be expanded on in the last four chapters of this text, with detailed clinical management suggestions.

■ Primary Neuromuscular Impairments

■ Muscle Weakness

Weakness is defined as an inability to generate normal levels of muscular force. Depending on the extent of the lesion, weakness in the patient with a cerebral cortex lesion can vary in severity from total loss of muscle activity, called paralysis or plegia, to a mild or partial loss of muscle activity, called paresis (Shumway-Cook & Woollacott, 2001). Paresis and plegia are described by their distribution: **hemiparesis** or **hemiplegia** affects one body side; **paraplegia** or **diplegia** affects primarily the lower extremities; and **tetraplegia** or **quadriplegia** affects all four extremities and the trunk. Paresis results from damage to the descending motor pathways, which interferes with the central (from the brain) excitatory drive to the motor units (Ghez, 1991). The end result is an inability to recruit and modulate the motor neurons, leading to a loss of movement.

■ Muscle Tone Abnormalities

Normal muscle tone is defined as a state of readiness of skeletal muscle so that the muscular system is in a state of arousal, prepared for the task demands to be placed on it. It is determined by the level of excitability of the entire pool of motor neurons controlling a muscle, the intrinsic stiffness of the muscle itself, the absence of neuropathology, and the level of sensitivity of many different reflexes. A hallmark of CNS pathology is the presence of abnormal tone. Muscle tone can be viewed as a continuum, according to the following diagram (Shumway-Cook & Woollacott, 2001):

FLACCIDITY↔HYPOTONIA↔NORMAL↔
SPASTICITY↔RIGIDITY

Flaccidity and hypotonia are states of muscle hypotonicity, and spasticity and rigidity are states of hypertonicity.

Flaccidity

Flaccidity is characterized as the complete loss of muscle tone. Flaccidity is often seen in the acute stage, immediately following a CNS injury, but it can also be secondary to a lower motor neuron lesion. In patients with flaccidity, deep tendon reflexes (DTRs) are absent. In the CNS, flaccidity is often but not always a transient stage. Clinically, it is vital that therapists and assistants offer additional support, either manually or with a physical aid such as an orthotic device or splint, to flaccid extremities to prevent injury.

Hypotonia

Hypotonia is defined as a reduction in muscle stiffness, often seen in spinocerebellar lesions and in developmental disorders such as a type of CP or Down syndrome. Hypotonia is characterized by low muscle tone, weak neck and trunk control, poor muscular cocontraction, and limited stability.

Spasticity

Spasticity is a state of hypertonicity of the muscle. It is defined as a motor disorder characterized by a velocity-dependent increase in the stretch reflex with exaggerated tendon jerks, resulting from hyperexcitability (Lance, 1980). Spasticity is typically seen as part of the upper motor neuron syndrome. The predominant hypothesis regarding the neural mechanism underlying spasticity is that it is due to changes in the descending activity, which results in abnormalities within the stretch reflex. Disorders in the stretch reflex mechanism result in increased resistance to passive movement, especially when moving the limb quickly. A common clinical sign is clonus, spasmodic alternations of muscle contractions between antagonistic muscle groups, caused by hyperactive stretch reflexes. DTRs are hyperactive.

Because the stretch reflex is velocity dependent, spasticity limits a patient's ability to move quickly. Current research is also showing that inadequate recruitment of agonist motor neurons, rather than increased activity in antagonist motor neurons, is the primary basis for the spasticity accompanying CNS lesions. It is important to remember that spasticity is simply one of several symptoms of neurological damage and should therefore be treated as it interferes with function. Typically, voluntary active muscle control is severely weakened in the patient with spasticity. Functional intervention approaches should be focused on improving active muscle control in addition to reduction of spasticity when it is severe enough to limit movement.

Rigidity

Rigidity is another form of hypertonicity, characterized by a heightened resistance to passive movement, but independent of the velocity of that stretch or movement. Rigidity tends to be predominant in the flexor muscles of the trunk and limbs and results in severe functional limitations. There are two types of rigidity: **lead pipe** and **cogwheel.** A constant resistance to movement throughout the range characterizes lead pipe rigidity, whereas cogwheel rigidity is characterized by alternate episodes of resistance and relaxation. Rigidity is often associated with lesions of the basal ganglia, commonly seen in Parkinson's disease.

■ Coordination Problems

Coordinated movement involves multiple joints and muscles that are activated at the appropriate time and with the correct amount of force so that smooth, efficient, and accurate movement occurs (Shumway-Cook & Woollacott, 2001). The essence of coordinated movement therefore is the synergistic organization of multiple muscles, not just the capacity to fire an isolated muscle contraction. Incoordination can result from pathology in a variety of neural structures, including the motor cortex, basal ganglia, and cerebellum. Uncoordinated movement may be displayed through the manifestation of abnormal synergies, inappropriate coactivation patterns, and timing problems.

Abnormal Synergies

In rehabilitation literature, the word *synergy* has often been used in describing abnormal or disordered motor control (Bobath, 1978; Brunnstrom, 1970). A synergy is a group of muscles that often act together as if in a bound unit. Abnormal synergies are stereotypical patterns of movement that don't change or adapt to environmental or task demands. Abnormal synergies reflect an inability to move a single joint without simultaneously generating movement in other joints. Movement out of the fixed pattern is often difficult if not impossible.

There is a flexion and extension synergy of both the upper and the lower extremity (see Chapter 6 and Fig. 6-7) In the patient with hemiplegia secondary to a CVA,

the flexor synergy in the upper extremity and the extensor synergy in the lower extremity often dominate the patient's movement. In the upper extremity, the flexion synergy is characterized by scapular retraction and elevation, shoulder abduction and external rotation, elbow flexion, and wrist and finger flexion. The scapular and elbow components are usually the first to emerge after the CVA and stay the strongest. In the lower extremity, the extensor synergy is characterized by pelvic retraction; hip extension, adduction, and internal rotation; knee extension; and ankle plantar flexion and inversion. The pelvic retraction and ankle plantar flexion components can be quite strong.

Coactivation

Inappropriate coactivation of muscles is an example of a sequencing problem. Coactivation means that the agonist and antagonist muscles both fire, preventing functional movement. Coactivation is commonly seen in CNS disorders in both children and adults.

Timing Problems

Uncoordinated movement can also be manifested as an inability to appropriately time the action of muscles and thus the movement itself. There can be many facets to timing errors, including problems initiating the movement, slowed movement execution, and problems terminating a movement. All these timing errors have been observed in patients with neurological damage.

■ Involuntary Movements

Involuntary movements are a common sign of neurological damage and can take many forms.

Dystonia

Dystonia is defined as a syndrome dominated by sustained muscle contractions, often causing abnormal postures, twisting or writhing movements, and repetitive abnormal postures. The abnormal postures associated with dystonia are diverse and can range from athetoid (slow involuntary writhing or twisting, usually involving the upper extremities more than the lower extremities) to quick **choreiform movements** (involuntary, jerky, rapid, and irregular). Dystonic movements usually result from basal ganglia disturbances.

Associated Movements

We have all experienced mild demonstrations of associated movements, when under stress or engaged in a novel or difficult activity. **Associated movements** are characterized by involuntary movement of one body part during the voluntary movement of another body part. In some situations, an unimpaired individual may demonstrate an associated movement, such as flexing the toes within the ski boots while moving down an unusually challenging slope. Associated movements are often seen in the presence of abnormal muscle tone, especially spasticity. They are probably seen as the result of lost supraspinal inhibitory mechanisms that normally suppress the coupling of movements between limbs (Lasarus, 1992). Associated movements are easily observable in patients with CNS damage and are often evident during times of effort, stress, or fatigue.

An example of an associated reaction is a response known as **Raimiste's phenomenon,** where resistance applied to hip abduction or adduction on one side of the body causes a similar response in the contralateral lower extremity. In the companion workbook, there is an active learning experience presented that will illustrate this phenomenon. Another associated reaction seen in individuals with hemiplegia is **Souques' phenomenon,** whereby elevation of the hemiplegic upper extremity (UE) with the elbow extended above the horizontal may elicit an extension and abduction response of the fingers. **Homolateral limb synkinesis** is a term used to describe the dependency that often is observed between hemiplegic limbs: Flexion of the UE elicits flexion of the lower extremity (LE) on the hemiplegic side. These are all examples of abnormal associated reactions, which, when severe enough, can significantly impair function.

Tremor

Tremor is defined as a rhythmical, involuntary, oscillatory movement of a body part (Deuschl, Bain, & Brin, 1998). Tremor results from damage to the CNS. Resting tremor is a tremor occurring in a body part that is not being voluntarily activated and is supported against gravity. Resting tremor is a symptom of Parkinson's disease, secondary to basal ganglia dysfunction. Intention tremor is tremor evidenced on purposeful movement of the body part, typically seen during reaching with the upper extremity or stepping with the lower extremity. Intention tremors often accompany cerebellar lesions.

Neuroplasticity and Recovery of Function

A number of factors influence the effects of brain damage, the clinical presentation and implications, and the hope for recovery. The nature of the damage itself, the age of the person, and the experiences of the person

before and after the injury are all known to influence the patient presentation, as well as the outcome.

Contemporary thinking favoring a systems model of movement control views the nervous system as a somewhat flexible system, with numerous reciprocal connections and redundant representations. In this model, the effect of brain damage is less catastrophic and the system has greater potential for recovery of function.

Effect of Age

The age of the individual at the time of brain damage is a very complex matter. Injury in some brain areas show similar deficits whether it occurs in the infant or adult; damage to other areas show little effect in infancy, but problems develop later in life (Held, 1987). Why? It has been hypothesized that if an area is mature, injury will cause similar damage in infants and adults. However, if another area that is functionally related is not yet mature, it may assume the function of the injured area. In addition, if an immature area is damaged and no other area assumes its function, no problems may be seen in infancy but will be seen in later years, when deficits become apparent. The brain definitely reacts differently to injury at different stages of development (Stein, Brailowsky, & Will, 1995; Shumway-Cook & Woollacott, 2001).

Recovery of Function

There are several theoretical mechanisms proposed to contribute to recovery of function in the human nervous system. One popular concept is that unassigned regions of the brain can learn, or take over, the function lost through damage to another area. Another mechanism is based on the concept of redundancy; that is, functions are represented throughout the nervous system, so that when one area is damaged, several others still retain the capacity to control the function (Cohen, 1999). These theories of recovery are summarized as follows (Leonard, 1998):

- Vicarious function theory: contends that undamaged CNS regions have latent capabilities that can respond to or control actions originally handled by the damaged areas.
- Equipotentiality (again, that "potential" thing): asserts that various parts of the nervous system can mediate the same motor function.
- Functional reorganization theory: suggests that a neural system can alter its function depending on the need and secondary to damage to related areas.
- Theory of substitution: proposes that a motor behav-

ior can be performed by a different mechanism than that which originally controlled the behavior. In other words, the end can be achieved through different means.

When damage to the CNS occurs in regions that are mature and are primarily composed of cell bodies, those cells will die. Those neurons cannot be replaced because the remaining intact cells in the area will have withdrawn from normal physiological function and can no longer divide. Many types of insults to the CNS, however, occur in regions where the axons are injured rather than the cell bodies. Some of these axonal recovery mechanisms are based on anatomical rearrangements and physiological readjustments. Anatomically, regenerative or collateral neuronal sprouts can arise in an area of injury, occurring within 5 days of the injury. **Collateral sprouting** arises from nearby undamaged neurons. Although these collateral (meaning "additional or auxiliary") sprouts don't replace the original circuitry, they don't occur randomly either. These new inputs occur only from systems most closely associated with the injured area. **Regenerative sprouts** grow from the distal end of the cut axon, near the injury site, sometimes traveling over great distances in attempting to reconnect to their target (Cohen, 1999; Leonard, 1998; Martin & Kessler, 2000).

Neuroplasticity

Neuroplasticity is a term used to describe the ability of the nervous system to change in response to experience, changing conditions (including injury), and repeated stimuli (Waxman, 2000). Plasticity is clearly evident in the developing nervous system. From conception through the second year of life, the human nervous system is in a tremendous wave of development and change. The processes guiding these changes are many, involving such things as cell migration and differentiation, axonal growth, dendritic formation and branching, neurotransmitter synthesis, and synaptogenesis (*genesis* means "beginning"; therefore, this word simply means the beginning formation of synapses).

In early childhood, the CNS actually overgrows. Regressive processes such as cell death and projection retraction are an equally important part of child development (Leonard, 1998). Some of these developmental processes, including neural organization, are dependent on activity. Activity conducive to neuronal growth, development, and maturation begins in utero and continues with postnatal sensory and motor experiences. Herein lies the rationale for early intervention to promote optimal child development and minimize secondary functional impairments that may accompany a developmental disability. Environmental

enrichment and varied, stimulating experiences definitely have a positive impact on brain development and maturation.

There are differences between developmental and adult neuroplasticity. The dramatic changes that occur in the developing brain don't occur again in later life. The growth of adult axons is very restricted. Dendrite formation occurs throughout life, but not to the extent that it occurs during development. In fact, once a critical period of development has passed, changes become limited. The plasticity that is associated with early development is heavily reliant on structural changes, such as cell growth, migration, and the formation of axons, dendrites, and synapses. The plastic changes available to adults are generally considered due not to actual structural change but rather to changes in synaptic strength and efficiency (Leonard, 1998).

In both developmental and adult learning and neuroplasticity, repetitive stimulation and activity within a neural pathway are of vital importance. A synapse that is used is preferred over one receiving less activity (Coleman, Nabekura, & Lichtman, 1997). A synapse that is used over and over again will undergo **long-term potentiation (LTP)** and thus strengthen its synaptic connection. Whereas in the child, enhanced synaptic activity contributes to the very survival of that connection, in the adult an established synapse is likely to survive regardless of its level of activity. It is the strength of the synapse that actually increases with activity during adulthood. LTP has been found to exist in the cerebellum, motor cortex, and other CNS regions (Iriki, Pavlides, Keller, & Asanuma, 1989; Leonard, 1998). Training, experience, and, yes, neurorehabilitation, can have a positive impact on recovery of function in the both the developing and adult nervous system.

Clinical Connection:

All these theories and facts are supportive of the value of early intervention as a sound approach for therapists. Whether it is with a young child or an acutely injured adult, the earlier rehabilitation professionals become involved in training or retraining, the greater the possibility of maximizing the patient's functional outcome.

Summary

This chapter described the essentials of neuroanatomy and neurophysiology, presented by first defining the language of the nervous system, then describing and defining the basic building block processes and structures. The evolutionary and embryological development of the human brain was presented to give the reader an appreciation of the overall plan of the nervous system. The systems approach to how the nervous system controls movement was defined and introduced, to be elaborated on in the next chapter. An organizational framework was offered to help the reader make the connection between location, size, and type of brain damage to how patients may present in the clinic. The ability of the developing, immature, and mature nervous system to recover from damage was presented.

It is hoped that this chapter helps aspiring therapists and assistants to relax about embarking on such a complicated study by immediately attempting to make the neuroanatomy and neurophysiology organized and meaningful, ready to be applied to patient care.

References

Bertoti, D. B. (1999). Mental retardation: Focus on Down syndrome. In J. S. Tecklin (Ed.), *Pediatric physical therapy* (3rd ed., pp. 283–313). Philadelphia: Lippincott Williams & Wilkins.

Bobath, B. (1978). *Adult hemiplegia: Evaluation and treatment.* London, UK: Wm. Heinemann Medical Books.

Brunnstrom, S. (1970). *Movement therapy in hemiplegia: A neurophysiological approach.* New York: Harper & Row.

Carper, J. (2000). *Your miracle brain.* New York: HarperCollins.

Christiansen, C. J., Lopez, R. O., & Phillips, K. M. (2001). Brain tumors. In D. A. Umphred (Ed.), *Neurological rehabilitation* (4th ed). St. Louis, MO: Mosby.

Cohen, H. (1999). *Neuroscience for rehabilitation* (2nd ed.). Philadelphia: Lippincott Williams & Wilkins.

Coleman, H., Nabekura, J., & Lichtman, J. W. (1997). Alterations in synaptic strength preceding axon withdrawal. *Science, 275,* 356–361.

Daube, J. R., Sandok, B. A., Reagan, T. J., & Westmoreland, B. F. (1986). *Medical neurosciences: An approach to anatomy, pathology, and physiology by systems and levels* (2nd ed.). Boston: Little, Brown.

Deuschl, G., Bain, P., & Brin, M. (1998). Consensus statement of the Movement Disorder Society on tremor. *Movement Disorders, 13,* 2–23.

Fredericks, C., & Saladin, L. (1996). *Pathophysiology of the motor systems.* Philadelphia: F. A. Davis.

Ghez, C. (1991). Voluntary movement. In E. Kandel, J. H. Schwartz, & T. M. Jessell (Eds.), *Principles of neuroscience* (3rd ed., pp. 609–625). New York: Elsevier.

Gilman, S., & Newman, S. W. (1996). *Manter and Gatz's essentials of clinical neuroanatomy and neurophysiology* (9th ed.). Philadelphia: F. A. Davis.

Held, J. M. (1987). Recovery of function after brain damage: theoretical implications for therapeutic intervention. In J. H. Carr, R. B. Shepherd, & J. Gordon (Eds.), *Movement sciences: Foundations or physical therapy in rehabilitation* (pp. 155–177). Gaithersburg, MD: Aspen Publishers.

Iriki, A., Pavlides, C., Keller, A., & Asanuma, H. (1989). Long-term potentiation in the motor cortex. *Science, 245,* 1385–1388.

Kandel, E. (1991). Brain and behavior. In E. Kandel & J. H. Schwartz (Eds.), *Principles of neuroscience* (3rd ed., pp. 5–17). New York: Elsevier.

Katz, D. I., Mills, V. M., & Cassidy, J. W. (1997). The neurologic rehabilitation model in clinical practice. In V. M. Mills, J. W. Cassidy, & D. I. Katz (Eds.), *Neurologic rehabilitation: A guide to diagnosis, prognosis, and treatment planning* (6th ed., pp. 1–27). Malden, MA: Blackwell Science.

Lance, J. W. (1980). Symposium synopsis. In R. G. Feldman, R. R. Young, & W. P. Koella (Eds.), *Spasticity: Disordered motor control.* Chicago: Year Book.

Lasarus, J. C. (1992). Associated movement in hemiplegia: The effects of force exerted, limb usage, and inhibitory training. *Archives of Physical and Medical Rehabilitation, 73,* 1044–1052.

Leonard, C. T. (1998). *The neuroscience of human movement.* St. Louis, MO: Mosby.

Lundy-Ekman, L. (2002). *Neuroscience: Fundamentals for rehabilitation* (2nd ed.). Philadelphia: W. B. Saunders.

Martin, S., & Kessler, M. (2000). *Neurologic intervention for physical therapist assistants.* Philadelphia: W. B. Saunders.

McKeough, D. M. (1999). Neuroscience review of stroke: typical patterns. In C. B. Royeen (Ed.), *Neuroscience and occupation: Links to practice.* Bethesda, MD: American Occupational Therapy Association.

Milner, B. (1966). Amnesia following operation on the temporal lobes. In C. W. M. Whitty & O. L. Zangwill (Eds.), *Amnesia* (pp. 109–133). London, UK: Butterworth.

Morecraft, R. J., & Van Hoesen, G. W. (1996). Cortical motor systems. In C. M. Fredericks & L. K. Saladin (Eds.), *Pathophysiology of the motor systems: Principles and clinical presentations* (pp. 158–180). Philadelphia: F. A. Davis.

O'Sullivan, S. B., & Schmitz, T. J. (Eds.). *Physical rehabilitation: Assessment and treatment* (4th ed.). Philadelphia: F. A. Davis.

Scheibel, A. B., Conrad, T., Perdue, S., Tomiyasu, U., & Wechsler, A. (1990). A quantitative study of dendrite complexity in selected areas of the human cerebral cortex. *Brain Cognition, 12,* 85–101.

Schmitz, T. J. (2001). Sensory assessment. In S. B. O'Sullivan & T. J. Schmitz (Eds.), *Physical rehabilitation: Assessment and treatment* (4th ed., pp. 133–175). Philadelphia: F. A. Davis.

Shumway-Cook, A., & Woollacott, M. (2001). *Motor control: Theory and practical applications* (2nd ed.). Philadelphia: Lippincott Williams & Wilkins.

Stein, D. G., Brailowsky, S, & Will B. (1995). *Brain repair.* New York: Oxford Press.

Stokes, M. (1998). *Neurological physiotherapy.* London, UK: Mosby International Limited.

Taber's cyclopedic medical dictionary (19th ed). (2001). Philadelphia: F. A. Davis.

Trombly, C. A. & Radomski, M. V. (Eds.). (2001). *Occupational therapy in physical disfunction* (5th ed.). Philadelphia: Lippincott Williams & Wilkins.

Umphred, D. A. (2001). *Neurological rehabilitation* (4th ed.). St. Louis, MO: Mosby.

Waxman, S. (2000). *Correlative neuroanatomy* (24th ed.). New York: McGraw-Hill.

Wessel, K., Vieregge, P., Kessler, C., & Kompf, D. (1994). Thalamic stroke: Correlation of clinical symptoms, somatosensory evoked potentials, and CT findings. *Acta Neurologica Scandinavica, 90,* 167–173.

3

A Life Span Approach to the Systems That Produce Human Movement

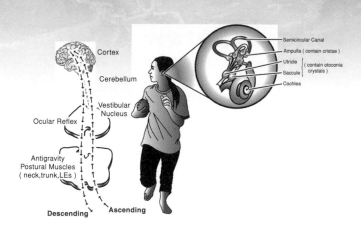

It does not yet appear what ye shall be—New Testament

Life offers us each the opportunity to develop and change constantly as each individual continually and uniquely unfolds.

Cornerstone Concepts

- The relationship among theoretical assumptions, practice models, and intervention concepts

- A description of the evolution of the dynamic systems approach to understanding human movement

- Application of a systems approach to movement science and neurorehabilitation

- A functional anatomical overview of the nervous system, somatosensory system, visual system, vestibular system, and motor system

- The life span view of development

- Developmental changes of the nervous system, somatosensory system, visual system, vestibular system, and motor system

Introduction

In Chapters 1 and 2, some basic information was presented to orient the student or clinician to the applied field of neurorehabilitation. This chapter is a cornerstone chapter in that it moves forward from the basic neuroanatomy and neurophysiology and presents the information within a functional framework. This chapter presents human movement as a system made up of several subsystems that develop, mature, and age over the life of the individual. Movement is a product of the contributions of many systems, working together within their own maturational level, to produce movement tailored for that particular individual, at that particular time, within that unique environment, to perform a specific task.

This chapter not only presents a functional, dynamic systems approach to the study of human movement production but will frame it within an ever-evolving process of life span development. Picture the following: an infant drinking from a baby bottle, a child drinking from a cup, a teen drinking from a sports bottle, a 30 year old downing a cold can of soda, an executive drinking coffee from a travel mug, and a grandmother sipping tea from a porcelain cup. Picture further that the infant is being cradled by a caring mother, the child is sitting stabilized in a high chair, the teen is balanced precariously on the edge of the team bench, the 30 year old is standing at the helm of a fast-moving fishing boat, the executive is seated comfortably in an office chair, and the grandmother is lying in bed propped by pillows. Continue imagining just a moment further: The infant is full term and healthy, the child has cerebral palsy and is sitting in an adapted highchair, the teen has juvenile rheumatoid arthritis, the 30 year old is in excellent physical health, the executive is visually impaired, and the grandmother has just suffered a stroke requiring her to drink the tea with her unimpaired but nondominant hand.

There is no disputing the fact that all these individuals are engaged in the task of drinking. However, we all know that the described task of drinking is very different in each circumstance. Each individual presents within a specific environmental context at a specific time of the life span, with unique opportunities and limitations. The environment that each individual is in, the parameters of the task (baby bottle versus cup, sports bottle, soda can, travel mug, or porcelain cup), make the task unique to that individual. Furthermore, some of these individuals present with limitations or constraints imposed by a pathological condition. The point of this visual travelogue is to illustrate the importance of viewing movement—as in this example, the holding of a container of liquid and drinking it—within its specific context, which includes the task itself, the environment, and the developmental stage of the individual. The drinking of the liquid is tailored for the unique situation and made possible by the contributions of the individual's nervous system, motor system, and sensory system to the execution of the task. The task of drinking is not simply just that; rather it is unique to the who, the how, and the when of task execution.

The movement system is made up of contributing systems that are capable of incredible changes and adaptation. An understanding of the mechanisms that change across the life span offers a framework within which therapists and assistants can then view the patient, his or her pathophysiology, possible subsequent impairments, and available movement solutions. More importantly, this perspective helps the clinician to appreciate the patient's functional capabilities and limitations and the potential effects of rehabilitation and recovery. This perspective will increase effectiveness as a clinician, allowing therapists and assistants to treat patients at whatever life stage the patient presents, across a variety of environments.

This author acknowledges the immenseness of the human nervous system and the multiple processes that are vital to normal function. The sensory, cognitive, and perceptual input that is associated with movement cannot be separated from the movement it produces. Some of these systems, such as the systems supportive of perception, consciousness, and cognition, are not covered in this chapter, not because of less importance, but because that information is contained in other texts and is not within the scope or purpose of this text. This chapter focuses on the functional significance and the life span developmental changes of the major subsystems crucial to the production of human movement.

Motor Control: A Historical Review

Therapeutic intervention in neurorehabilitation is often directed at changing the capacity to move or assisting with determining strategies for improving the quality of postures and movement essential for function. **Motor control** is a field of study directed at the study of movement as the result of a complex set of neurological, physical, and behavioral processes. Motor control is the ability of the individual to maintain and change posture and movement based on an interaction among the individual, the task, and the environment. Physical and occupational therapists are "applied motor control physiologists" (Brooks, 1986).

Current theories on motor control evolved first from a reflex model, to a hierarchical or neuromaturational model, and most recently to a systems or a dynamic action model. It is valuable to reflect briefly on this evolution because the development of practice models in occupational therapy and physical therapy reflects this history. It is very important to remember that models and consequent practice approaches will continue to evolve in a constant attempt to improve patient care. A **model** is nothing more than a schematic representation of theory; in this case, how the nervous system regulates movement behavior.

The reader is reminded that all models offer both insights and limitations. By their very nature, models, as well as theories, are constantly changing as they undergo scrutiny, clinical application, and reassessment. Clinical practices are constantly changing, in part to reflect new knowledge and newer views on the physiological basis of movement control. Therapists and assistants should never be afraid of something that is changing. It is better to constantly change and reach for new solutions than to rigidly adhere to an outdated model or one that only can be applied in certain circumstances. Chapter 5 (Motor Learning Through the Life Span) and Chapter 6 (Neurorehabilitation Intervention Approaches) will expand on practice models and intervention concepts within both physical therapy and occupational therapy. One of the greatest characteristics of the therapy professions is the dynamic nature of the knowledge base, as practitioners engage in problem solving in an effort to best serve patients/clients.

The traditional model of motor control originated from the reflex model, which viewed reflex chaining as a basis for action, based on Sherrington's work in the early 1900s (Sherrington, 1906). This model suggested that movement was the result of a summation of sensory input to the central nervous system (CNS) and that the CNS controlled the execution of movement based on the sensory feedback it received (Tse & Spaulding, 1998). This **closed-loop theory of motor control** proposed that errors in motor performance were compared with an internal reference of correctness (stored within the brain), which in turn could influence subsequent movement (Adams, 1971). Many of the early neurophysiological intervention approaches in physical therapy and occupational therapy had their roots in this model, with clinical strategies focusing on methods to reduce spasticity and reflex influence to enhance normal movement capacity. Some valuable intervention concepts still in use today, based on the knowledge gained from this model, will be presented in current form in Chapter 6. This theory had its limitations, however, in explaining how movement could occur without sensory feedback and how anticipatory movements were elicited (Schmidt, 1988). The hierarchical model and the neuromaturational models suggested then that movements were controlled in a top-down fashion, originating from the CNS, differing from the reflex model, which had said that movement was controlled peripherally.

Clinical Connection:

When therapists were first exploring ways to evaluate and treat children and adults with neurological damage, this view of the nervous system as being arranged in a "top-down" hierarchy was the commonly accepted theory. Berta Bobath (1965) and Signe Brunnstrom (1970) were therapists who became famous for their contributions to intervention with children with cerebral palsy or adults who had suffered a cerebrovascular accident (CVA). Bobath, for example, stated that "the

release of motor responses integrated at lower levels from restraining influences of higher level, especially that of the cortex, leads to abnormal…[motor] activity" (Bobath, 1965). Although contemporary views based on more current research have abandoned this strict hierarchical view, these early theorists offered clinicians useful intervention strategies that can be adapted even today. Some of these tools and strategies will be discussed in Chapter 6. ▪

The concept of motor programs then emerged, conceptualizing that hierarchically organized motor programs store rules for generating movements so that tasks could be accomplished with a variety of musculoskeletal effectors. These theories viewed the human nervous system as an **open-loop feedforward motor control system,** proposing that movements are selected, planned, and initiated based on a central reference, called a **schema,** that was established by past experience (Schmidt, 1975). Although this theory could explain how movements could occur without sensory feedback and how anticipatory motions could occur, it still had limitations, such as describing how novel movements could occur. These theories, however, had a significant impact on patient intervention by directing therapists to be focused on retraining movements important to a functional task, rather than on reeducating specific muscles in isolation.

Clinical Connection:

Clinically, schema would include such things as the initial conditions of a movement (e.g., body position, height or weight of an assistive device), the parameters of the movement components themselves (e.g., trunk, head, and all extremity ranges required), the environmental outcome, and the consequences of the movement (e.g., what it felt like, presence of feelings of accuracy or inaccuracy). Therapists and assistants incorporate these ideas into intervention by ensuring that patients practice a variety of movements so that the patient can develop expanded schema or rules able to be applied to a variety of task modifications or across a broader range of environmental conditions. ▪

Today, contemporary motor control knowledge reflects a shift from either a reflex or hierarchical model to a systems model of motor control, which recognizes the dynamic nature of movement and the adaptable contributions of many subsystems to the orchestration of human movement. Physical and occupational therapists have adopted the term *systems* from the engineering field to describe the relationship of various brain, spinal, and peripheral structures that work together, with the ongoing use of feedback, to produce an outcome. These systems are not arranged in a **hierarchy,** where one is more important than the other. Rather, they are a functioning **heterarchy,** where the contributing systems work parallel to each other.

A Systems Approach to the Nature of Movement

Definition

A quick glance in a dictionary tells you that a system is an assemblage or combination of parts forming a whole—a group of body parts that form a functioning unit. A systems approach allows the practitioner to view the nervous system as subservient to functional purpose, where structures may contribute to more than one function and thereby be a part of more than one system.

Nicolai Bernstein developed the first systems model in 1932, but the information wasn't widely read until it was translated into English in 1967. This model focuses on the interaction of the many systems that contribute to movement. This author's depiction of the systems model is seen in Figure 3–1, illustrating all the subsystems within an individual working in concert to complete a given task, given the constraints and affordances of the environment within which the movement is occurring. It is important to note that included in this complex of interactive systems are systems related to

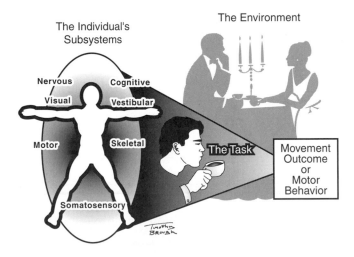

Figure 3–1. The systems model can currently be visualized as all the subsystems (somatosensory, visual, vestibular, and motor) within an individual, dynamically working in concert to complete a given task, given the constraints (limitations) or affordances (allowances or opportunities) of the environment within which the movement needs to occur.

the environment and to the task itself, both crucially important to movement execution. According to Horak (1991), a major assumption of the systems model is that the nervous system is organized to control the end points of behavior, the accomplishments of task goals, within a given environment.

Normal movements are coordinated not because of muscle activation patterns prescribed by sensory and motor pathways but because the strategies of motion emerge from the interaction of the systems. Multiple subsystems interact to produce a given motor behavior, within a context appropriate for the environment and the task. These different performer systems compose a set of structural functional units that are fairly flexible, interacting with the individual, the task, and the environment. Functions are shared among the systems. The interactions among these subsystems within the individual, the requirements of the task, and the unique aspects of the environment all affect the movement outcome. The human nervous system is viewed as tremendously flexible, capable of adapting to changes within the individual, the task, and the environment in an effort to produce the most effective movement possible. Motor behaviors are conceived of as functional **synergies** (groups of muscles working together) rather than specific muscles or individual muscle groups.

Movement is made possible by the contributions of many systems. Bernstein suggested that the control of integrated movement was probably distributed throughout many interacting systems working cooperatively to achieve movement (Bernstein, 1967). Not only is movement not the product of any one system, no system acts in isolation from the others to produce movement (Cech & Martin, 1995). Movement emerges through the interaction and self-organization of many subsystems, and a movement behavior is greater than the sum of its individual parts (Thelen, Kelso, & Fogel, 1987). Absence of movement may result from a problem in the nervous, motor, skeletal, or sensory system or from a difficulty encountered within the environment. The patient's movement that a clinician observes is the end result of all the possibilities and **constraints** (limitations or restrictions) offered by all the contributing systems. Most importantly, this functional systems approach to the study of human movement lends itself well to understanding not only commonly encountered patient problems but also clinical solutions to common patient problems.

Clinical Connection:

This viewpoint clarifies for clinicians the importance of examining the patient/client in a holistic manner, where the status of every subsystem within the individual patient may affect the movement outcome. The attempted task, performed within the specific environment with its unique variables, also is defined by specific characteristics. The movement that the clinician observes as demonstrated by the patient represents the sum of the interaction of all these contributing systems, both within and surrounding the patient as he or she engages in a movement activity. Clinical examples illustrating this systems approach will be expanded on in subsequent chapters. ■

It is important to realize that these contributing systems change over time and are therefore best viewed as dynamic in nature. The systems model was expanded on in the 1980s when researchers and clinicians began to look at the moving person within the newer perspective of changing over and within time (Thelen et al., 1987). According to Cohen (1989), "control systems theory relates movement of any part of the body to the *entire system,* which continually adapts to the changing conditions." A **dynamic action system** is any system that demonstrates change over time (Heriza, 1991).

This dynamic action system model, inspired by the work of Bernstein and expanded by Thelen and colleagues, views movement not as the unfolding of predetermined or prescribed patterns in the CNS, but as emerging from the dynamic cooperation of many subsystems in a task-specific context (Thelen et al., 1987). The many systems then self-organize to produce movement and do not depend on prior instructions embodied in one hierarchically important subsystem, such as the CNS (Heriza, 1991). Motor behavior emerges from the dynamic cooperation of all subsystems within the context of a specific task—CNS, biomechanical, psychological, and social-emotional components. Each component is perceived as necessary but insufficient, by itself, to explain movement (Larin, 2000). The movement outcome emerges in a self-organizing fashion as a function of the many subsystems in a task-specific context.

Movement can then be expressed from among a variety of movement combinations, represented by the possible **degrees of freedom.** Degrees of freedom represent the variety of potential movement combinations in the human body. For example, the shoulder can move within three planes and therefore has three degrees of freedom, the elbow and the forearm each have one, and the wrist has two degrees of freedom. These compose seven degrees of freedom for the upper extremity, excluding the fingers and thumb. If one were to add all the degrees of freedom available and all the different directions of muscle pull across those joints, the total number of possible movement combinations is

extremely numerous (Janeschild, 1996). Every joint contributes a certain number of degrees of freedom to a movement, so that the movement emerges as the sum of all the possible combinations that can occur. These functional movement synergies are self-assembled according to the interaction among the individual, the task, and the environment.

Observed movement, then, will be the outcome of the interplay of all system components in time, including developmental time. Thus, at every stage of development, movement is assembled with whatever subsystems are maturationally available with respect to the particular environment and task-specific context (Heriza, 1991). The systems develop and change dynamically, changes perhaps required as a response to growth, maturation, aging, disease, or the requirements of the environment or the task. This theory also offers an assumption that new movements emerge because of readiness within the system, an idea that will be explored in Chapter 6 of this text, expanding on intervention concepts.

An appreciation of the dynamic nature of constantly developing subsystems will offer the clinician a unique perspective on how to view the patient with a movement problem. Effective practitioners can treat a patient/client presenting at any age, within a variety of environments, if the clinician can step back and take a wide-angle view of the contributing systems, their functional contributions to movement production, and how these systems change over the life span.

The Movement System

Consistent with the tone and definitions established in this text, it is reasonable to speak of movement as a physiological system. Remembering that physiology describes how body parts function and that a system describes how the parts of a whole function in combination, it becomes easy to then take the next logical step and view movement as a physiological system. Sahrmann in the American Physical Therapy Association (APTA) Mary McMillan Lecture voiced the value of this perspective in 1998: "Clinicians who focus on the **movement system** must consider the effects of all the components involved in system function rather than just considering the specific part of the anatomical system affected by a lesion" (Sahrmann, 1998). Sahrmann has further proposed the widespread adoption of a definition of the movement system as the functional interaction of structures that contribute to the act of moving (Stedman, 2001).

The movement system, like any other system, is made up of an assemblage of parts. The following major systems are considered to be vital components of the movement system controlling human movement: the nervous system; the motor system, including the musculoskeletal system; and the sensory systems, including the somatosensory system, visual system, and vestibular system. These systems are primarily within the scope of physical and occupational therapists. These main subsystems, which contribute to the control of movement, will be explored in this chapter, including viewing them as they change over the course of the life span. The important roles of cognition and perception as contributing to motor control will be discussed in Chapter 5 on motor learning and throughout the intervention application chapters in Part 2 of this text.

Life Span Perspective

The systems that contribute to human movement develop and change over the life span of the individual. **Development** is a lifelong process beginning at conception and ceasing only at death (Gallahue & Ozmun, 2002). This concept of life span development encompasses all developmental changes—those generally associated with childhood and adolescence, as well as the changes that take place with aging. Because functional demands are different at different ages, the movement forms that emerge throughout development also change. The life span itself can be thought of as a long chain of interactions between the organism and the environment (Hasselkus, 1974; Welford, 1958). Each such interaction *modifies* the organism so that when it confronts later situations it is different from what it was before.

Changes occur on many levels. Age-related change in motor behavior is a lifelong phenomenon (VanSant, 1990). The changes that occur can be viewed as responsive to basically four processes: growth, maturation, adaptation, and learning. Structural and functional changes are a normal part of this developmental process. Changes in body systems can be progressive, reorganizational, or regressive (Cech & Martin, 1995). A life span perspective encompasses all the changes that naturally occur as part of the lifelong developmental process—those that are progressive, those that are regressive, and those that result in reorganization.

The form of expressed movement will reflect the morphological (structure and form) characteristics of the individual, as well as the specific developmental stage within which the individual is functioning. Across the life span, the physical capacity of the individual changes and helps to define functional capacity (Cech & Martin, 1995). Development occurs not only as a result of physical changes within the body but also because of environmental influences. Development and functional tasks are interwoven. Development cannot be viewed linearly. Rather, development implies change over time, which can be viewed both negatively and positively, throughout the course of an individual's life.

For the purpose of study, it is helpful to have some method for dividing and defining the different phases of the life span. The life span is most often divided into age-related segments. Although there are variations in the age levels presented by different experts, this text will adhere to universally applicable terminology describing the following four main developmental stages: infancy and childhood; adolescence; adulthood; and older adulthood. These broad categories are considered adequate for the scope of this text. Infancy and childhood includes birth through approximately age 10, or the onset of puberty. Adolescence begins at puberty and lasts until maturity; approximately spanning ages 10 through 21. In this text, adulthood encompasses both young and middle adulthood, including approximately age 20 through 60, with young adulthood spanning 20 to 40 and middle adulthood 40 through 60. The period of older adulthood includes the older adult, as well as the old-old, or late adulthood, spanning from 60 through 80-plus years. Typical age periods are just that—typical, and no more. Each individual person has a unique timetable for the acquisition and development of movement abilities (Gallahue & Ozmun, 2002). Age periods merely represent the *approximate* time ranges during which certain behaviors can be typically observed.

Rather than a strict adherence to age ranges, a broader, more functional perspective will be presented in this text (Fig. 3–2). This text will present the developmental changes of the subsystems of movement by organizing the broad divisions of life corresponding to the age periods and functional changes in the following way:

- **Maturation** occurs during infancy and childhood continuing through adolescence. *Maturation* refers to the qualitative changes that enable one to progress to a higher level of functioning, characterized by a fairly fixed order of progression, which may vary in pace and sequence between individuals (Gallahue & Ozmun, 2002).
- **Maturity** is associated with adulthood, including both young and middle adulthood. Maturity implies a period of relative stability, with most changes driven by individual responses to environmental or task demands.
- **Aging** is the predominant developmental occurrence during the older adult years. *Aging* refers to the changes in physical, sensory, and psychosocial performance that occur to some degree in all elderly persons with the passage of time. Although aging can occur at different rates, the structural and func-

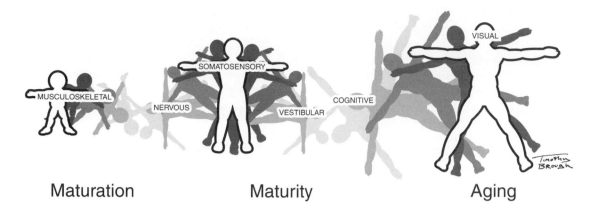

Maturation   **Maturity**   **Aging**

Developmental Time

Figure 3–2. Development is a lifelong process whereby each subsystem changes, cumulating in a unique developmental timeline for the individual. Generally, the lifelong developmental phases can be described as *maturation* (including infancy and childhood and adolescence), *maturity* (including early and middle adulthood), and *aging* (the older adult).

tional consequences are surprisingly consistent across the different physiological systems, with profound behavioral consequences (Bonder & Wagner, 2001).

Development is a continuous process, best defined by Keogh and Sugden (1985) as "adaptive change towards competence." This definition aptly implies that development is a lifelong process, with adults equally engaged in the process, as are children and adolescents. In this chapter, however, the term **early development** will also be more discretely applied to describe the beginning prenatal growth and organization of each system.

For rehabilitation professionals, it is important to recognize the parallel value of the patient's/client's age at the time of neurological damage, as well as the state of wellness of the individual. At one time, it was thought that early brain injury was less catastrophic than the same injury occurring in adulthood. We now know that the effect of damage is closely related to the functional maturity of the damaged area. For example, if the area was mature at the time of damage, regardless of the age of the patient, the consequences are the same. If, on the other hand, the damaged area was not mature when damaged, no initial deficit may be apparent and several subsequent possibilities may occur. Another region could assume the functional responsibilities of the damaged area, or the deficits can become apparent when the damaged area would normally have matured (Cohen, 1999).

What follows is a review of the functional significance and the developmental changes of each of the main subsystems of the movement system: nervous system, somatosensory system, visual system, vestibular system, and musculoskeletal system. As the life span changes of each system are discussed, think about the clinical implications of these changes at each life stage. The role of the cognitive system and its vital contribution to movement production will be discussed in Chapter 5.

The Nervous System: Life Span Changes

Clinical Relevance

The human nervous system is incredibly adaptable and flexible. The way that the nervous system manages and processes all the information being conveyed by multiple sources is through a process described as parallel processing. **Parallel processing** refers to similar information being conveyed by multiple sources. The fact that different pathways convey similar information does not necessarily mean that they will result in the same outcomes. Perhaps the pathways convey the same information to different regions of the CNS. Perhaps the different pathways synapse on different neurons within the same or different areas. Parallel processing increases the information-carrying capabilities of the human nervous system. It also results in some degree of redundancy within the CNS, an important feature if one area becomes dysfunctional because of injury or disease (Leonard, 1998).

The consequences of damage to the immature developing brain are different from those manifested in the mature adult. Certain motor behaviors (such as grasping and locomotion) may appear to be unaffected in infancy, but deficits in these areas may be displayed during subsequent development. This phenomenon is termed "growing into the deficit" (Goldman & Galkin, 1978). During early development, one type of behavior may be subserved by several different neural structures. During this immature period, the actual motor skill, such as grasping or locomotion, would not have yet occurred. The deficit then appears to become present only later because that is when the evidence of that behavior becomes observable.

Recovery or even maintenance of a function appears to depend on the stage of development of the damaged pathway and also on the stage of development of the undamaged pathways. It is well accepted that **critical periods** exist whereby damage to various parts of the CNS will have different behavioral effects depending on whether the damage occurs before or after this critical period (Leonard, 1994). Critical periods are times when axons are competing for synaptic sites and pathways are organizing. The concept of critical periods has important clinical implications. For example, if input from one area or sensory receptor is dysfunctional during the critical period for that region or structure, the axons are at a disadvantage as they compete for synaptic space. Permanent neural change will result. Various CNS structures have different critical periods of different durations (Haines, 1997).

The following describes some of the developmental changes of the human nervous system, summarized in Table 3–1. It is important for therapists and assistants to appreciate the developmental changes of the nervous system, because it will help the clinician to view the patient/client as he or she presents in his or her own developmental time line. Remember, however, that these are simply guideposts, subject to individual variation.

Early Development of the Nervous System

From conception through the second year of life, the human nervous system is undergoing a tremendous wave of development and change. The main processes guiding these early changes are cell migration and differentiation, axonal growth, dendritic formation, neurotransmitter synthesis, and the formation of synapses. These dramatic changes that occur in the developing brain don't occur again in later life. In early development, the CNS actually overgrows. Regressive processes such as cell death and the retraction of some projections, which follow subsequent to this initial overgrowth, are an equally important part of early development (Leonard, 1998).

Clinical Connection:

Some of these initial developmental processes, including neural organization, are dependent on activity. Physiological activity leads to neuronal growth, development, and maturation, beginning in utero and continuing as fostered by postnatal sensory and motor experiences. Brain development is actually shaped by experiences. Brain development and the observable behavioral changes seen in the developing infant are mutually influential, not just concurrent in timing. ▪

TABLE 3–1			
Nervous System Changes Through the Life Span: Functional Implications			
Developmental Phase	**Major Changes**	**Functional Implications**	**Rehabilitation Implications**
Early development	CNS overgrowth with subsequent regressive processes Axon, dendritic formation and growth Cell proliferation and migration Synapse formation Regional differentiation Myelination of sensory and motor nerve fibers, cranial nerves, beginning myelination of tracts	Beginning sensory-motor matching allows for first fetal movements, predominantly reflex in nature. Sensory and motor tracts myelinate first; myelination in a caudal to cephalic order. Areas of CNS to be used first, such as brainstem and cranial nerves, allowing for sucking and swallowing, are myelinated first.	Abnormalities in cell migration can result in seizure disorders. Poor prenatal nutrition results in decreased myelination, decreased number of synapses, and limited dendritic branching. Neural connections and maturation highly dependent on use of pathway.

TABLE 3–1

Nervous System Changes Through the Life Span: Functional Implications

Developmental Phase	Major Changes	Functional Implications	Rehabilitation Implications
Maturation (infancy and childhood)	By end of first postnatal month, evidence of myelination in cerebral hemispheres Corticospinal tract myelinated by end of year 1, sensory tracts by age 2; frontal and parietal lobes by birth, occipital lobes soon after, temporal and frontal lobes during first year Neuronal growth and maturation Increasing complexity of neuronal processes	Function is highly dependent on postnatal sensory and motor experiences. Myelination and CNS development closely match Piaget's cognitive stages. Myelination and development of parietal, occipital, and temporal lobes related to development of visuosensorimotor functions; that of frontal lobes is related to motor and emotional development. Critical period for growth is birth to 2; areas of brain growth coincide with developmental maturation.	Neural maturation highly dependent on use of pathway. "Growing into deficit" may appear to be the case, where deficits are displayed during subsequent development when the behavior or lack of functional ability becomes observable.
Maturation (adolescence)	Continued brain growth until age 12–15; critical growth periods at 6–8, 10–12, and age 18 Increased complexity of fiber systems and increased conduction velocity Continued myelination but at a slower rate	Motor control becomes more automatic. Motor skills attain maximum precision by age 18–21.	Competence and individual ability highly dependent on innate abilities, motivation, and practice.
Maturity (adulthood)	Continued myelination of association areas Continued synaptic remodeling and growth Declining nerve conduction velocities after age 30 Beginning decline in brain weight and volume	IQ peaks at age 20–30. Learning continues to be able to be maximized because of ongoing development of association areas. Reaction time peaks between 20–60 years. First areas to show neuronal loss and shrinkage are sensory and motor cortexes and hippocampus.	Built-in redundancy offers great implications for recovery. Plasticity in adulthood is highly dependent on use, which increases synaptic strength and efficiency. Short-term memory beginning to decline.
Aging (older adult)	Continued growth of dendrites into old age Decreased number of neurons, shrinkage of neurons, especially in higher-order association areas Decrease in temporal and frontal lobe volume Decrease in size of brainstem and cerebellum Myelin loss with consequent slowed conduction velocity and slowed neuronal processing	Higher-level cognitive functioning declines and memory deficits increase. Reaction time decreased, reflex responses slowed, acuity of senses decreased, and motor performance diminished. Basic intellectual ability maintained until at least age 75.	Learning continues to be possible well into old age. Due to maintained plasticity, functional decline not evident until critical threshold of cell loss/shrinkage is crossed. Acquisition of new information and conversion of new information from working memory to long-term memory is significantly declined. Balance problems. "Use it or lose it!"

Source: Information compiled from multiple sources. See text and references for details.

The human nervous system starts forming when the human embryo is approximately 21 to 22 days of age and measures less than 4 mm in length. The cardiovascular system and the nervous system are the first systems to function in an embryo (Afifi & Bergman, 1998). The formation of the neural tube, the establishment of the ventricular system, division of the nervous system into main regions, and differentiation into neurons and neuroglial cells are the hallmarks of prenatal development (see Chapter 2). The neural tube is formed by 4 weeks of age, and the basic arrangement of the brain is established by the time the embryo is 6 weeks of age (see Fig. 2–4). Motor nerve fibers begin to appear in the spinal cord at the end of the fourth week, forming the spinal nerves. Shortly thereafter, the dorsal nerve roots, consisting of sensory fibers, appear. Synapse formation occurs by week 7 (Cech & Martin, 1995).

After 6 weeks, the major changes are increases in size and differentiation of the cerebral hemispheres and cerebellum. The regional brain enlargements are complete by the third prenatal month. Months 3 through 5 are characterized by cell proliferation (increase) and migration of neurons to destination points. By birth, the human newborn has the full complement of neurons, all which have migrated to their final destination point. The following example illustrates how migration of neurons occurs in the developing nervous system. By approximately 8 weeks' gestation, cortical cells have migrated toward their target. Thalamic projections, having already arrived, have anxiously awaited the arrival of cortical neurons. Thalamic sensory inputs attach themselves to these migrated cortical neurons and travel outward with them to the cortex. This allows for the beginning of sensory-motor matching. Interestingly, it is at about 8 weeks of gestational age that the first fetal movements are demonstrated (Prechtl, 1985).

Clinical Connection:

Seizure disorders are a common problem for children with developmental disabilities. When cell migration goes awry, cells fail to reach their normal destination. In the cerebral cortex, this results in an abnormal number of cells and displacement of the gray matter, a condition known as **heterotopia.** This displaced gray matter commonly goes into the deeper white matter. Heterotopia is often associated with developmental seizure disorders. ▪

From 5 months' **gestational age** (before birth), the nervous system is constantly organizing itself, manifested by growth of axons and dendrites and synapse formation. As differentiation proceeds, neurons become more widely separated due to an increase in size and complexity of dendrites and axons and the enlargement of synaptic surfaces. These organizational changes continue to occur through early adulthood (Adams, Victor, & Ropper, 1997).

These earliest synaptic connections allow for the appearance of **spinal reflexes,** the pairing of sensory inputs and motor responses. Many of these spinal reflexes are permanent, "hard-wiring" the developing human quite early, equipping the fetus with survival capabilities such as the ability to suck and gag. Reflex movements in response to touch have been chronicled as early as 8 weeks of gestation. Touching the lips at 11 weeks gestation elicits swallowing movements. By 14 weeks gestational age, the **reflexogenic zones** (stimulus area that elicits a reflex response) spread so that touching the face of the embryo results in a complex sequence of movements consisting of head rotation, grimacing, stretching of the body, and extension of the extremities. Reflexes connections are established in utero in a **cephalocaudal** (head to toe) direction (Cech & Martin, 1995).

From 8 weeks' gestation through age 3 years, myelination is the main nervous system task (Lundy-Ekman, 2002). The acquisition of myelin sheaths by the spinal nerves and roots by the 10th week of life is also associated with the beginning of the first reflex motor activities, such as sucking and fetal kicking. Myelination occurs first in those areas of the nervous system that will be used first, initially laid down in the areas of the brainstem and cranial nerves involved in reflexive sucking and swallowing.

Clinical Connection:

Many of a baby's first movements are reflexive in nature. Reflexes, as first movements, serve many purposes, such as providing for basic survival reactions and allowing for use of the immature pathways, which then mature and develop further with use. Chapter 4 will present an in-depth study of the functional purposes and clinical significance of understanding automatic movement responses, including reflexes. ▪

Myelin formation in the CNS begins at the sixth month of gestation, continuing into adulthood. Myelin formation appears to be initiated by a combination of cellular chemical mechanisms and neural impulses. Different fiber systems myelinate at different developmental periods. Generally, motor and sensory tracts myelinate before association fibers, those fibers that develop and myelinate secondary to experience and processing from among a rich variety of sensory and motor experiences. Myelination proceeds on a caudal to cephalic order (Cech & Martin, 1995).

Maturation of the Nervous System

▪ Infancy and Childhood

At birth, the human infant brain is far from a finished product, weighing one quarter the weight of the adult brain. The human newborn brain weight is approximately 10 percent of its body weight. This difference in weight is accounted for by the laying down of myelin, which occurs mainly in the first 2 years of life; increase in neuron size; increase in the number of glial elements; and the increasing complexity of neuronal processes (Afifi & Bergman, 1998).

The brainstem and spinal cord are the most advanced portions of the brain in terms of myelination at birth, hence the reflexive capabilities of the newborn's movement. Within the cerebrum, the posterior frontal and parietal lobes are myelinated around the time of birth, the occipital lobes soon after, and the frontal and temporal lobes during the first year. These findings are important because they closely correlate with the importance of visual stimulation in the youngest infant and with beginning language development, which occurs toward the later half of year 1.

The corticospinal tract, which conducts efferent messages to skeletal muscle, is myelinated by age 1, and the sensory tracts are complete by age 2, facts indicative of the importance of the tasks of movement and sensory exploration engaged in during the first years of life. As the child continues to develop an increased repertoire of sensory, motor, and cognitive skills, the CNS continues to develop nerve processes, synaptic connections, and myelinated pathways.

Clinical Connection:

Nervous system maturation changes are another example of how early experiences and movement both reflect and support the developmental changes that occur. Early experience and neurological development are not a cause and effect relationship; rather, they are *mutually influential*. Early experiences influence neural development and organization and neural development and organization influence early experiences. Herein lies the rationale for early intervention to promote optimal child development and minimize secondary functional limitations that may accompany a developmental disability. ▪

Brain growth during childhood is thought to coincide with the stages of cognitive development described by Piaget and with the development of language (Piaget, 1952; Thelen & Fogel, 1989). Structural change and functional development and maturation are inter-

woven, as highlighted in Table 3–1. The parietal, occipital, and temporal lobes are developing dramatically during early infancy, coincident with the development of visual spatial skills and visuosensorimotor integrative functions. Between 8 and 12 months of age, the frontal cortex is undergoing rapid development, coincident with the demonstration of higher cortical functions, emotional development, and motor skills. The cerebellum undergoes a growth spurt from 30 weeks' gestation through the end of the first prenatal year, reflective of major developmental advances in balance and coordination (Afifi & Bergman, 1998).

Although the brain continues to develop until approximately age 10, the critical period for postnatal brain growth is considered to be from birth until age 2 (McKeough, 1995). The first 2 months after birth are considered a period of tremendous CNS organization (Cech & Martin, 1995). The primary motor cortex develops ahead of the primary sensory cortex. The cerebellum, which has remained relatively small throughout prenatal development, experiences its main growth spurt from 30 weeks' gestation through the first year of life.

Clinical Connection:

Poor prenatal nutrition results in a decrease in the number of synapses formed and in the amount of dendritic branching and myelination (Herschkowitz, 1989). Pregnancy education, good prenatal care, and maternal health are paramount to the developing fetus. Malnutrition during the first 2 years of life limits the number of synapses forming, decreases dendritic branching and myelination, and decreases glial cell formation, having a significant impact on future neurological functioning. Because there are no fats that originate from within the brain, the developing and immature nervous system requires lipids in the form of fatty acids. Prenatally, these must be supplied nutritionally from the mother and transported through the blood-brain barrier for adequate nervous cell formation. Postnatally, fat is an important nutritional element of an infant's diet. ▪

Naturally occurring cell overgrowth, followed by neuronal death and axon retraction, is a major feature of human brain development (Leonard, 1994). These processes appear to be selective, mainly used for the matching of neural populations with the appropriate target. This allows for functionally redundant neurons and projections to be eliminated. There is approximately a 50-percent loss of neurons during early brain development in most of the structures studied. The establishment and continued survival of neural connection is highly dependent on use of the pathway.

This dependence on sensory (afferent) input is of significant clinical significance for therapists and assistants.

Clinical Connection:

Early brain development is very dependent on the input received by the brain. For example, a child with damage to the motor areas of the brain will be restricted in his or her movement experiences. This lack of activity results in less afferent input and may cause further deficits in the development of brain structures. Intense physical and occupational therapy may lessen these effects by utilizing afferent and efferent pathways so that brain development is optimized. ▪

▪ Adolescence

The brain continues to grow, although at a much slower rate, until 12 to 15 years, when the average adult weight is attained. Myelination also continues, although at a slower rate, during this period. The tripling of brain weight, which has occurred by adolescence, is due to myelination, increases in glia, and increases in complexity of processes. Emergence of the skills associated with throwing, catching, and balancing are observed as the nervous system continues to mature and increase the speed of conduction of nerve impulses through ongoing myelination. Motor control becomes more automatic, complex, and sophisticated (Cech & Martin, 1995).

The brain undergoes additional critical periods during growth spurts at 6 to 8 years, 10 to 12 years, and around age 18. Fiber systems continue to increase in complexity as late as middle adult life. Motor skills attain their maximal precision in performance, peaking at maturity, age 18 to 21 (Adams et al., 1997). Individual levels of motor skill proficiency, with subsequent nervous system change, are highly variable, dependent on practice, instruction, motivation, and of course, innate ability. The years from 18 through 30 are peak years for speed and agility.

The Mature Nervous System

▪ Adulthood

Myelination continues into adulthood in those areas responsible for integrating information necessary for purposeful action, the association areas of the brain. This fact is a reminder to all therapy professionals about the value of purposeful activity and its impact on brain development! Intellectual ability, as reflected by IQ

measures, actually peaks between the ages of 20 and 30 (Katzman & Terry, 1983). The nervous system's built-in redundancy serves us well throughout adulthood, such that, even if neurons are lost in one area, other connections can be gained. Most areas of the brainstem, the area responsible for vital functions, and the basal ganglia, responsible for implementing motor programs, are stable throughout adulthood and show minimal changes throughout middle adulthood.

The nervous system on the whole, however, begins to decline in middle adulthood. Brain weight and volume decline linearly with age (Cech & Martin, 1995; Duara, London, & Rapoport, 1985). Structurally, the brain experiences a continual loss of neurons that are not replaced (Gallahue & Ozmun, 2002). Beginning at age 20, brain weight decreases, the cortex thins, and the number of glia cells increase (Earnest, Heaton, & Wilkinson, 1986; Whitbourne, 1985). The speed with which sensory nerves conduct impulses begins to decline at age 30 (Buchtal, Rosenfalck, & Behse, 1984; Cech & Martin, 1995).

Losses in brain weight and volume are not uniform; rather, there are differences in the losses experienced within certain regions compared with others (Cech & Martin, 1995). The primary motor and sensory areas of the cortex are susceptible to neuron loss beginning as early as age 20. The hippocampus, associated with memory, has been reported to show a 30-percent decrease in neurons after 30 years of age (Ball, 1977). The acquisition of new information and the conversion of that information from working memory into long-term memory significantly decline with age (Koroshetz & Moskowitz, 1996; LeVere, 1980). On average, the decline in short-term memory is gradual and slow through age 60, after which time it becomes more rapid. Long-term, memory, on the other hand, seems to be largely unaffected as one gets older (DiGiovanna, 1994). Reaction time reaches its optimum at age 25 and is maintained until age 60, when it slows secondary to decline in central processing and decreased conduction velocities.

The growth of adult axons is very restricted. Dendrite formation occurs throughout life, but not to the extent that it occurs during early development. In fact, once a critical period of development has passed, changes become limited. The plasticity that is associated with early development was heavily reliant on structural changes, such as cell growth, migration, and the formation of axons, dendrites, and synapses. The plastic changes available to adults are generally considered due not to actual structural change but rather to changes in synaptic strength and efficiency (Leonard, 1998). Synaptic remodeling and growth occur late into adulthood. New research has discovered some evidence that the adult nervous system has the ability to grow new neurons, and dendritic sprouting has been observed up until old age (Papalia, Olds, & Feldman, 2001).

Clinical Connection:

There certainly appears to be some truth to the well-known adage "Use it or lose it!" (Cech & Martin, 1995). Continued use of pathways causes synaptic facilitation due to increased synaptic strength and efficiency. Therapists and assistants can have a significant impact on the wellness of patients of all ages, especially adults, by maximizing purposeful activity, directly affecting neural processing. It is also helpful to share with patients/clients the rationale for purposeful and continued activity. If a patient can understand the profound affect that activity has on neuronal processing, compliance with activity is certain to increase. ▪

The Aging Nervous System

▪ Older Adult

The most obvious characteristic of the aging nervous system is the great variability seen (Mortimer, Pirozzolo, & Maletta, 1982). Therapists and assistants always need to remember the individuality of the patient and the uniqueness of each person's own developmental process. Generally, however, people experience some decline in functionality associated with aging of the nervous system. Death of brain cells and slowing of conduction speed along nerves accompany normal aging. There are decreases in reflex response times, reaction times, and acuity of the senses. With aging, reflexes require more stimulation to be activated and it takes longer for a response to be elicited. As an illustration of slowed responses, most adults over 70 do not demonstrate a knee jerk; by 90, all deep tendon reflexes are gone (Papalia et al., 2001).

CNS changes related to aging are not the same for every part of the brain. Changes in the brain vary considerably between individuals. Aging affects the temporal and frontal lobes more than the parietal lobes (Brody & Vijayashanker, 1977). The volumes of the frontal and temporal lobes decrease significantly with age (Coffey, Wilkinson, & Parashos, 1992; Sullivan, Marsh, Mathalon, Lim, & Pfefferbaum, 1995). This decrease in size is currently thought to be due to neuronal shrinkage more than actual loss of neurons. Shrinkage seems to begin earliest and advance most rapidly in the frontal cortex, an area vital for memory and higher-level cognitive functioning (Papalia et al., 2001).

The acquisition of new information and the conversion of that new information from working memory to long-term memory significantly decline with age (LeVere, 1980; Koroshetz et al., 1996). There is an age-related reduction in size of the brainstem and cerebellum, perhaps with functional significance pertaining to balance problems so often seen in the elderly (Hasselkus, 1974). Studies have shown that higher-order association areas lose more neurons than the primary motor or visual cortex during aging (Kemper, 1984). Many current studies conclude that the total number of neurons in the cortex does not significantly change during the aging process and that the dominant age-related change in brain volume is really due to neuronal shrinkage (Cech & Martin, 1995). This loss of neuron size may be a possible explanation for forgetfulness in older adulthood (Morgan, 1989).

On a biochemical level, the loss of enzymes involved in neurotransmitter synthesis has been documented along with a moderate loss of receptor sites for certain neurotransmitters in both the CNS and the peripheral nervous system (PNS). A decline in motor system performance has been linked to a decrease in dopamine uptake sites due to age-related loss of axons in basal ganglia pathways (DeKeyser, Ebinger, & Vauquelin, 1990). Research has also demonstrated an age-related decrease in the number of receptors and the desensitization of the remaining receptors, both factors influencing synaptic transmission (Antonini & Leenders, 1993; Cohen, 1999). The most significant changes are seen after 65 to 70 years of age. Myelin loss is thought to be a part of normal aging process, with obvious implications for stimulus transmission and nervous system processing. Nerve conduction velocities decrease after age 60 with obvious consequences for sensory and motor performance (Mortimer et al., 1982). Because conscious sensation and voluntary movement use many CNS synapses and interneurons, age-related changes have a great impact on these functions (DiGiovanna, 1994). Aging is also associated with degeneration of dendrites in cortical cells (Cohen, 1999; Jacobs & Scheibel, 1993).

Clinical Connection:

All these normal changes in the nervous system of the older adult contribute to the functional limitations so often seen: deficits in memory, decline in higher-level cognitive processing, decreased reaction time, balance difficulties, and delayed information processing. Clinicians are reminded that although these changes are real, older adults can continue to learn new skills well into old age. Practice and increased meaningful, purposeful activity slow these aging processes. ▪

Despite all these changes, few overall changes in the structure of the brain and nervous system exceed 25 percent of the total area, except in disease states, and only during the last few months of life (Cotman & Hotlets, 1985). In fact, it is not until around age 80 that the brain has lost 15 percent of its weight (Waxman, 2000). There are also areas of the brain that demonstrate an absence of significant age-related neuron cell loss. The basal ganglia and brainstem nuclei show little or no neuron loss as a result of aging (Konigsmark & Murphy, 1970). Dendrites continue to grow into old age (Herschkowitz, 1989). The number of synapses in various brain areas may increase or decrease depending on the use of that area. Therapists and assistants are reminded: "Use it or lose it!" In the absence of impairment, intellectual ability, as reflected by measurements of IQ, is maintained until at least 75 years of age (Cech & Martin, 1995; Katzman & Terry, 1983).

The main functional implications associated with age-related nervous system changes are changes in reaction time, defined as nervous system efficiency during movement, and cognitive decline, which enables interaction with the environment (Cech & Martin, 1995). With normal aging, cerebral blood supply is decreased by approximately 20 percent (McKeough, 1995). The walls of cerebral blood vessels also thicken (Afifi & Bergman, 1998). The decrease in cerebral blood flow and subsequent oxygen utilization by brain tissues is not only responsible for some slowing of neural processing but also puts the older adult at risk for CVA.

Because of maintained plasticity, decline in function may not become evident until very old age. It has been proposed that loss of function may not occur until a critical number of cells are lost for a threshold to be crossed. For example, it has been demonstrated that critical nuclei in the motor system may lose as many as half their neurons without obvious clinical impairment, suggesting that a great deal of redundancy exists. This plasticity protects the individual against adverse consequences of neuronal functional loss with aging (Mortimer et al., 1982). The human brain certainly is incredible, offering tremendous opportunity for preservation of optimal function well into the golden years.

Somatosensory System: Life Span Changes

Contribution to Movement Control

The function of the sensory system is to provide the CNS with the information necessary to regulate behavior. This information can be broadly divided into two main categories: information from our external world (exteroception) and from our internal world (interoception and proprioception). **Somatosensation** literally means sensory information about the body (soma), therefore including the cutaneous sensations of touch and the proprioceptive sensations from ligaments, muscles, joints, and tendons. A discussion of somatosensation, then, involves sensory information from the skin and from the musculoskeletal system. Put simply, somatic sensation enables our body to feel, ache, chill, and know what its parts are doing.

The **somatosensory system** is unique in two very important ways:

1. The receptors for the somatosensory system are distributed throughout the body.
2. It can respond to many different types of stimuli.

The somatosensory system is really a catchall name for the four senses of touch, pain, temperature, and body position, excluding the sensations of hearing, seeing, tasting, smelling, and the vestibular sense of equilibrium (Bear, Connors, & Paradiso, 2001). This chapter focuses on the functional somatosensory integration from touch and body position because these somatosensations are such an integral part of the movement system. Refer to other sources for a discussion on pain and temperature.

Current neuroscience research suggests that sensory information plays many roles in the control of movement (Shumway-Cook & Woollacott, 2001). Sensory stimuli serve as a primary stimulus for reflexive movement organized at the spinal cord level. Reflexes such as the flexor withdrawal and crossed extension reflex are wired at the level of the spinal cord (see Chapter 4). Additionally, sensory information has a role in modulating (changing or refining) the output of movement, whether the movement command is generated from the spinal cord or from a higher center. The reason that sensation can **modulate** all these different types of movement commands is because sensory receptors converge (come together) on the motor neurons, considered the final common pathway to the musculoskeletal system (Shumway-Cook & Woollacott, 2001).

The somatosensory system, from the lowest to the highest level of CNS hierarchy, includes all those structures involved in the reception of signals from the periphery to the integration and interpretation of those signals relative to all the simultaneous incoming information (Fig. 3–3). At every level of this system, there is a great deal of not only hierarchical organization but parallel distributed processing, so that signaling can be modified at any time. The somatosensory system, like other movement subsystems, is arranged as a heterarchy rather than a hierarchy.

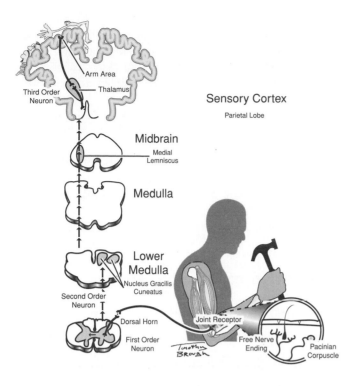

Figure 3–3. Key elements of the somatosensory system, emphasizing the following functional anatomical components of the somatosensory system as a major subsystem of the human movement system: peripheral cutaneous receptors and proprioceptors, dorsal column afferent pathway, spinal cord including dorsal horn, brainstem (medulla and midbrain), thalamus, and somatosensory cortex within the parietal lobe.

Clinical Connection:

The following example illustrates the value and complexity of the somatosensory system as not simply a hierarchical arrangement of neurons and pathways with one set of response capabilities. If you were walking across the floor in your bare feet and you stepped on a sharp piece of glass, we can all surmise that you would immediately withdraw your foot into a flexor withdrawal posture, cry out in pain, and perhaps hop to the nearest chair to inspect your injury. This automatic set of responses would happen quickly and without a great deal of conscious thought. In fact, you might even utter a profanity, and it is only afterward that you'd wish you hadn't said such a thing out loud. The key point is that the movement, verbal, and emotional responses all occur quickly and in a fairly predictable way, but not necessarily as consciously planned. If, on the other hand, you were walking across the same floor barefoot and this time you happened to notice that the baby at the table was about to fall out of her highchair and you then stepped on a piece of glass, we all know that the response to the glass would be different. You would undoubtedly suppress the urge to withdraw your foot and continue to move toward the baby, even though the glass was still embedded within your foot. Your brain would override (modulate) the reflexive response to the pain in your foot, because it is more important to run to the baby and prevent her from falling. Amazingly enough, our brain is able to discern this for us, make the appropriate response decision, and effect the best response for that situation, also without conscious thought! This is only one example of how the somatosensory system can modify its response as appropriate for the situation and the task at hand. ▪

Sensory integration is the combining or pulling together of information from two or more sensory systems for use, possible because of mature cross-modality processing. **Cross-modality processing** means the assimilation of information from more than one sensory modality into a composite sensory picture. Ayres defines sensory integration as the neurological process whereby the spatial and temporal aspects of inputs from different sensory modalities are integrated, associated, and unified. The brain processes sensory information and then is able to select, enhance, inhibit, compare, and associate the information for use in a flexible, constantly changing pattern (Ayres, 1989; Bundy, Lane, & Murray, 2002; Fisher & Murray, 1991). The development of sensory integration occurs simultaneously with the development of the individual senses. During normal development, integration is partially functional at birth, improves as the child grows, and then may begin to decline as one enters adulthood. As a result, individuals of different ages may require a different configuration of cutaneous, proprioceptive, vestibular, and visual information for different tasks (Poole, 1991).

Functionally, somatosensation contributes to the production of smooth, purposeful movement. In addition to visual and vestibular inputs, the somatosensory inputs provide crucial information to the CNS for effective postural control and movement execution. The role of sensation in movement changes over the life span. First, sensation is paired with movement in the form of reflexes. Sensation is used as feedback to refine movement and as a stimulus for postural responses. Eventually, sensation is fed forward in anticipation of a movement and is used less for feedback during familiar actions. With age, sensation is still used to reinforce or refine new movements, but the speed of processing sensory information declines.

Functional Anatomy Overview

In general, the somatic sensory systems consist of a three-neuron projection system. **First-order neurons** extend from the sensory receptor and enter the CNS, with the cell body located in the dorsal route ganglion. The **second-order neurons** then transport the information to the thalamus, usually crossing in the brainstem or spinal cord where its cell body lies. The **third-order neuron** arises from a cell body in the thalamus and projects to the sensory cortex (Lundy-Ekman, 2002).

As discussed in Chapter 2, somatic sensory information is carried along either of two main pathways: the dorsal column/medial lemniscal system or the anterolateral system. The basic anatomy of these peripheral receptors, processes, and tracts has been presented previously in that chapter of this text. Centrally, the somatosensory cortex, located in the parietal lobe, is the major processing center for all somatosensory (feelings from or awareness of the body) modalities, marking the beginning of conscious awareness. It is in this area that we see cross-modality processing, so that information from many different types of receptors is now integrated to give aggregate information about a specific body part. The somatosensory cortex is also able to assign distinctiveness and meaningfulness to incoming sensory information. Different areas of the body are assigned locations within different regions of the parietal lobe, represented by the familiar sensory homunculus (Figs. 2–6 and 3–3). The somatosensory cortex has descending connecions to the thalamus, dorsal columns, and spinal cord, thereby having the ability to change (or modulate) the incoming information ascending through these structures (Shumway-Cook & Woollacott, 2001).

The following describes some of the developmental changes of the somatosensory system, summarized in Table 3–2.

Early Development of the Somatosensory System

Defined as "to be in contact with," touch is our first language (Weber, 1984, p. 3). It is the first system to function in utero, allowing for communication and attachment (Fisher, Murray, & Bundy, 1991). It is the "oldest and most primitive expressive channel," a primary system for "making contact with the outside world" (Cech & Martin, 1995; Collier, 1985). In utero, the sensory systems develop in the following order: touch, motion detection, smell, hearing, vision, taste, and proprioception (Cech & Martin, 1995). The fetus develops the ability to respond to touch around the mouth as early as 7 weeks' gestation (Hooker, 1952). By 17 weeks, cutaneous sensation spreads to the entire body, with the exception of the top and back of the head; these areas are preserved because they are subject to so much stressful touch during delivery.

Proprioceptive receptors are well developed by mid-fetal life (Lowery, 1986). Tapping, stretching, and even the pressure of a change in amniotic fluid elicit a response from the fetus (Cech & Martin, 1995). Muscle spindles are formed by 12 weeks, Pacinian corpuscles can be found in the distal portions of the limbs by 20 weeks, and the Golgi tendon organs are also formed by this time (Wyke, 1975).

Maturation of the Somatosensory System

▪ Infancy and Childhood

The senses of touch and proprioception are ready to function at birth, evidenced by the complete myelination of the involved neural pathways. For the first several months of life, the somatosensory system is the most mature system. Physiological changes occur after birth in all sensory systems, as evidenced by increases in nerve conduction velocity, myelination, redistribution of axon branching, and increased synaptic efficiency. Structural and functional changes result as the infant and child interact with the world (Cech & Martin, 1995).

Although the defensive movements to light touch fade by birth, the newborn can reflexively turn his or her head to clear the airways of the nose and mouth in order to breathe. The first responses to touch are random arm and leg movements. Information from touch is first used by the infant to locate food. Early tactile input plays a crucial role not only in survival behaviors but in parent-infant attachment, sociability, and cognitive development (Gottfried, 1984). The use of touch to recognize shape differences develops gradually; a 1-month-old baby is already able to distinguish between different pacifier shapes (Meltzoff & Borton, 1979).

The receptive fields for different sensations develop over the first months. In the newborn, touch to any part of the leg elicits a flexor withdrawal response. Gradually the receptive field becomes limited to the sole of the foot. Specific touch localization is demonstrated by 12 to 16 months of age (Lowrey, 1986). Children can usually identify familiar objects by touch at 5 years of age. Two-point discrimination is possible by age 7 (Cech & Martin, 1995). Knowledge of

TABLE 3–2

Somatosensory System Changes Through the Life Span: Functional Implications

Developmental Phase	Major Changes	Functional Implications	Rehabilitation Implications
Early development	First sensory system to develop in utero. Proprioceptors well developed by mid-fetal life. Somatosensory pathways completely myelinated by birth.	Ability to respond to touch first seen around mouth by 7 weeks' gestation.	Infant is born prepared to receive and transmit somatosensory information, highlighting the importance of early touch and attachment.
Maturation (infancy and childhood)	Most mature system for first few months of life. Conduction velocities increase, myelination continues rapidly, synapses increase in efficiency. Proprioceptive pathways highly developed in early childhood.	Early tactile input crucial for survival behaviors, sociability, and emotional attachment in early infancy. Interaction with world produces physiological changes in neuronal structure and efficiency. Receptor fields narrow as touch becomes increasingly discriminative. Somatosensory information integrates with vestibular and visual information, contributing to beginning sensory-motor mastery.	Early intervention stimulation activities need to emphasize both motor and sensory experiences; sensory experience does not "drive" motor ability; rather, sensory and motor development are intertwined. Integration of somatosensory information with other sensory modalities develops the ability to plan motor action and move about in space, called praxis; difficulty with this ability can result in developmental **dyspraxia.**
Maturation (adolescence)	Myelination continues. Maturation and integration of somatosensory processing continue.	Maturing sensory abilities contribute to refinement of skill and emerging body image. Somatosensory system keenest in late adolescence.	Integration of somatosensory information will contribute to development of an intact body image. Lack of experience and exposure to novel opportunities will limit skill refinement.
Maturity (adulthood)	Small, almost imperceptible changes not noticeable until after age 40. Skin changes, such as dryness and decreased elasticity, affect precision of cutaneous receptors.	Reaction time is decreased.	Knowledge based on experience will make up for any minimal sensory and motor decline, minimizing any functional impact. Clinicians can maximize rehabilitation at this life stage by choosing tasks from patient's past experience and knowledge repertoire.
Aging (older adult)	Number of receptors decreased, structural distortion of receptors, proprioceptor atrophy, and weakening of impulse conduction occur. Skin changes such as wrinkling, increased toughness, and changes in hair distribution affect accuracy of reception.	Tactile sensitivity decreases, especially fine touch, pressure, and vibration sense, predominately in fingertips, palms, and lower extremities. Decrease in feedback to CNS secondary to proprioception loss, contributing to movement inaccuracies, instability, incoordination, gait disturbances, and falls.	High incidence of peripheral neuropathy. Need to compensate with additional sensory or external cues. Need to make purposeful, more deliberate movement.

Source: Information compiled from multiple sources. See text and references for details.

where the body is in space and the sequence of movements that must be planned to perform a motor task are based on the interaction of tactile, vestibular, and proprioceptive information. This ability to plan a motor action, termed **praxis**, develops during childhood.

Proprioception, vital for the execution of purposeful movements such as imitation, reaching, and locomotion, is used very early after birth. Newborn infants imitate mouth opening and tongue protrusion, evidence of the interactive development of visual and proprioceptive information. Research has shown that reaching in 5-month-old babies depends more on the infant's motor and somatosensory ability than on visual control (Sugden, 1986). Ability to achieve and maintain upright postures depends on the infant's ability to interpret and respond to information about **body sway,** derived from vestibular, visual, and proprioceptive input. The baby uses all the senses while learning to combat the force of gravity and to either maintain alignment or move the body through space.

Clinical Connection:

Movement and sensation are intimately intertwined during development. Experience with one does not cause an effect in the other; rather, they develop in parallel and are mutually influential. Sensory experiences do not "drive" motor development. Early intervention stimulation activities need to emphasize both sensory and motor experiences. Current early intervention efforts attempt to work with the child and caregiver in natural environments, allowing the child to explore, with assistance or adaptation as needed, familiar, natural environments rich with sensory and motor opportunities. ▪

Proprioceptive acuity and memory for movements improves vastly in children between the ages of 5 and 12, allowing for beginning mastery in such skills as hopping, dancing, and gymnastic routines (Bairstow & Laszlow, 1981).

▪ Adolescence

Tactile and proprioceptive information are crucially important for refining the changing adolescent's body scheme and affective view of the body. No new events are specific to adolescence beyond the continued maturation and integration of somatosensation processing. Maturing sensory abilities during adolescence guide motor abilities and the refinement of skill. The sensory system is considered to be its keenest during late adolescence into early adulthood.

The Mature Somatosensory System

▪ Adulthood

Despite the continued development of intersensory associations, sensory function begins a slow decline in adulthood. These changes are not always related to a decline in function, nor are they universal in significance or rate. From young through middle adulthood, these sensory changes are small, gradual, and almost imperceptible, until one day the 45-year-old man mentions that his reaction time seems slower or the 60-year-old woman realizes she's not as quick on her feet as she used to be (Papalia et al., 2001). In many activities, knowledge based on experience may more than make up for these sensory and motor changes.

Clinical Connection:

An important consideration in therapy is to retrain adults using familiar tasks and past experiences. Knowledge based on experience will minimize the functional effects of age-related declines in sensory and motor function. This previous knowledge will also have a positive effect on rehabilitation success. The chapter on motor learning through the life span (Chapter 5) will discuss further the value of past experience and familiarity on motor learning with adults. ▪

Simple reaction time peaks in the mid-20s but then slows by 20 percent during middle adulthood, between 20 and 60 years of age (Hodgins, 1963; Papalia et al., 2001). The skin becomes dry and less elastic, affecting the precision of the cutaneous receptors located there. Awareness of vibration begins to decline at age 50, but only in the lower extremities (Potvin, Syndulko, & Tourtellotte, 1980; Steiness, 1957).

The Aging Somatosensory System

▪ Older Adult

Age changes that affect the sensory systems are important because by providing monitoring and communication, this system is vital in the successful execution or modification of movement. Aging causes a gradual decline in sensory functioning as a result of a decrease in the numbers of several types of sensory neurons, a decline in functioning of the remaining sensory neurons, and actual structural and physiological changes within the CNS (DiGiovanna, 1994).

Tactile sensitivity decreases with age, as demonstrated by a measurably changed threshold to touch stimuli (Bruce, 1980). Meissner's corpuscles and Pacinian corpuscles decrease in number and become structurally distorted, resulting in a decline in fine touch, pressure, and vibration sense. By age 80, only 8 corpuscles/mm^2 of skin surface are found, compared with 24 at 20 years of age. In addition to actual receptor loss, there is a decline of up to 30 percent of the sensory fibers innervating the peripheral receptors, eventually causing **peripheral neuropathy** (Shumway-Cook & Woollacott, 2001). Further reduction in cutaneous sensation seems to result from a weakening of the action potentials that conduct impulses to the CNS. The skin, as a sense organ itself, undergoes changes in structure in thickness, wrinkling, and toughening, differences in subcutaneous layers, and changes in the hair pattern and distribution on the skin's surface. Reduced touch sensitivity is especially prevalent in the fingertips and palms and in the lower extremities (Hooyman & Kiyak, 1991; Verillo, 1980).

Proprioceptive sense declines with age. The proprioceptive receptors—the muscle spindle, joint receptors, and Golgi tendon organs—atrophy with age. One functional consequence of muscle spindle degeneration is a decrease in the feedback that the CNS normally receives regarding a movement. Additionally, arthritic changes might affect how precisely joint receptors detect joint position. These changes can obviously adversely affect the efficiency of the proprioceptive system (Hasselkus, 1974).

The redundancy of sensory information normally available is decreased by age-related changes in older adults. This causes more situations in which older adults have reduced input and are then forced to compensate when decreased or even conflicting inputs occurs in one of the sensory systems. Age-related declines also simply limit the amount of sensory information received and therefore available for association or integration.

Clinical Connection:

Therapists and assistants may need to use additional cues for the older adult who is experiencing some of these age-related changes in the somatosensory system. Use of additional visual or touch cues, or even the use of biofeedback to augment visual or auditory feedback, are possible options for clinicians to consider. The provision of adaptive equipment or assistive devices can help to provide additional support in the absence of reliable somatosensory feedback.

Decreases in the ability to detect, locate, and identify objects touching or pressing on the skin results in decreases in the ability to respond to these sensations. Functionally, the decline in proprioception in the lower extremities could contribute to falls in the elderly. Because of the proprioceptive changes, older people demonstrate a decreased ability to orient their body in space and to detect externally induced changes in body or limb position. These changes therefore contribute to the observed behavioral adaptation on the part of elderly persons to move slower, take more time, and make deliberate, careful movements. Older persons need more external cues to make up for these functional losses. ■

Proprioceptive and exteroceptive sensory decline, in combination with age-related changes in the visual, hearing, and vestibular system, may impose a variety of functional limitations for the older adult. These functional consequences may include postural instability, exaggerated body sway, balance problems, gait disturbances, diminished fine motor coordination, the tendency to drop things held in the hands, and difficulty recognizing body or limb positions in space (Maguire, 1996; Schmitz, 2001). Reaction time is sharply decreased in the older adult (Gallahue & Ozmun, 2002; Hodgins, 1963).

Visual System: Life Span Changes

Contribution to Movement Control

The visual system is the dominant sensory modality in humans. It is truly remarkable because it allows us to focus on a tiny mosquito as close as the tip of our nose or as immense and far away as the distant stars of the galaxy (Leonard, 1998). The visual system serves movement in many ways. Vision allows an individual to identify objects in space and to determine their movement. Vision also gives someone information about where the body is in space, the relation of one body part to another, and the motion of one's own body. Vision therefore not only gives someone information about the external world but also plays a vital role in the control of posture, locomotion, balance, and hand function.

Functional Anatomy Overview

The visual system is divided into a peripheral portion and the central visual pathway (Fig. 3–4). The peripheral structures include the eye, its photoreceptors, and several different cells that either respond to stimuli or relay visual information once transduced into communicable electrical impulses. (Remember that nerve cells all have to transduce and signal information.) The eye itself consists of the lens, cornea, pupil, retina, and six extraocular muscles. For a visual image to be formed, the eyes must be positioned so that the photoreceptors, located in the retina, can sense the electromagnetic waves of light reflected from the visual target. The six extraocular muscles direct the eyes to specific targets in the visual field so that images fall on corresponding parts of both retinas. Eye movements are accomplished by the contractions of these muscles, innervated by cranial nerves III, IV, and VI. There are basically four types of eye movements:

- Fast saccadic: fast **conjugate** (paired) eye movements used during voluntary searching motions to track a moving object
- Slow pursuit or tracking: slow conjugate eye movements used while following a moving object
- **Vestibuloocular reflex** (VOR) eye movement: uses vestibular signals to move the eyes in an equal and opposite direction if the viewer's head or body moves, serving to maintain the fixation of the eyes on a visual target while the head is moving
- Vergence: used while maintaining fixation on a moving target when it moves from the far visual field to the near visual field (Gilman & Newman, 1996).

Clinical Connection:

It is important to recognize the importance of head position as it relates to the ability for the eyes to fixate, focus, or track an object. The head can be considered to be the base of support for the eyes. For therapists and assistants, this illustrates the importance of accurate positioning for patients to provide them with the best opportunity for optimal visual functioning. Patients with poor head control need adapted seating to stabilize their head position so that the patient has the best opportunity to use their visual system. ■

The **visual field** is the extent of space seen by one eye (see Fig. 3–4). (See the active learning experience in the companion workbook.) The image seen by an eye is inverted when projected onto the retina, so that the left visual field is imaged on the right side of the retina and the right visual field is imaged on the left side of the retina (Bear et al., 2001).

The central visual pathway includes the optic nerve, optic chiasm, optic tract, and lateral geniculate body of the diencephalon; superior colliculus within the midbrain; optic radiations; and visual cortex of the cerebrum. Like other sensory systems, the pathway of the visual system **decussates** (crosses) so that information from the left visual field is projected to the right visual

cortex. The optic nerves from each eye combine to form the optic chiasm, which lies at the base of the brain, near the pituitary gland. At the **optic chiasm**, axons originating from the nasal portions (adjacent to the nose) of both retinas cross, whereas those from the temporal portions (adjacent to the temple) do not. Because the fibers from the nasal portion of the left retina cross to the right side at the optic chiasm, all the information from this left half of the visual field is directed to the right side of the brain. The left visual **hemifield** (half of one eye's visual field) is therefore "viewed" by the right hemisphere and the right visual hemifield is "viewed" by the left hemisphere (see Fig. 3–4) (Bear et al., 2001; Lundy-Ekman, 2002).

Clinical Connection:

It is important to mention here some of the commonly encountered manifestations of lesions in the optic nerve versus the optic tract. Lesions of the optic nerve are associated with **monocular vision** (one eye) blindness. Because of the visual field projections and the decussation as discussed earlier, lesions of the optic

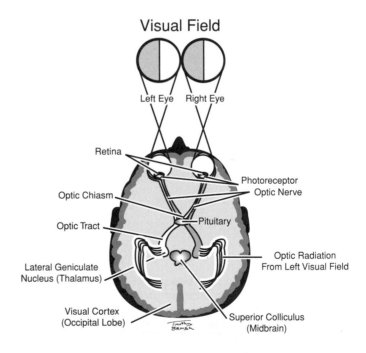

Figure 3–4. Key elements of the visual system, emphasizing the following functional anatomical components of the visual system as a major subsystem of the human movement system: eye including retina, optic nerve, optic tract, optic chiasm, lateral geniculate body of the diencephalon (thalamus), and primary visual cortex in the occipital lobe. The temporal and nasal regions of the visual fields are also depicted, showing the paths of the afferent axons from these retinal regions to the brain.

tract are associated with a contralateral homonymous hemianopsia, often seen after a stroke (Fig. 3–5). Remember how to break down words, as described in Chapter 2. This long word has its origins in Greek: *homos*, meaning "the same"; *onoma*, meaning "name"; *hemi*, meaning half; *a*, meaning "without"; and *opia*, meaning "eye." Lesions at the level of the optic tract or higher cause degeneration of optic nerve fibers from the temporal half of the ipsilateral (same side) retina and the nasal half of the contralateral (opposite side) retina. The patient loses half the visual field from each eye. For example, a patient with a right CVA, resulting in a left hemiplegia, will lose the left visual hemifield from each eye—in this case, the left temporal half from the left eye and the right nasal half from the right eye. Simply put, a loss of the left half of the visual field accompanies left hemiplegia, and loss of the right visual field accompanies right hemiplegia (Unsworth & Warburg, 2001) (Fig. 3–5).

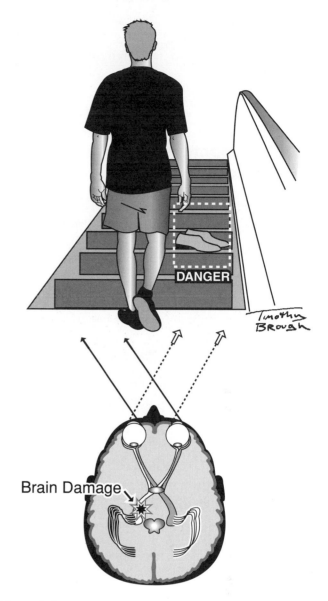

Figure 3–5. The functional significance of homonymous hemianopsia—in this case, accompanying a left hemiplegia.

The signals from the periphery travel in the optic tract, then project through visual pathways to the primary visual cortex in the occipital lobe. Visual information reaching the visual cortex stimulates neurons that discriminate the shape, size, or texture of objects. Information conveyed to the adjacent cortical areas, the visual association cortex, is analyzed for color and motion. From the visual association cortex, information flows to other areas of the cortex where the information is used to visually identify objects, adjust movements, or initiate a response to the visual stimulus (Lundy-Ekman, 2002). Central visual processing pathways also include cells in the temporal and parietal lobes, where somatosensory and visual information is integrated, giving rise to spatial and perceptual information.

The cells within the visual pathways contribute to a hierarchy within the visual system, with each level of the hierarchy increasing the visual abstraction (Hubel, 1988). Visual perceptual abilities develop with experience in time and space, giving meaning to the visual world as a visual input is integrated with other sensory experiences (deBenabib & Nelson, 1991). From the time light hits the cornea and a visual image is projected onto the retina and the brain receives the image, a whole host of processing and subsequent perceptual problems can occur. Further analysis of this complex system is beyond the scope of this book; refer to other sources for further information.

It is not only visual information that arrives in the parietal and temporal cortical areas. Information from several sources converges in those areas. Areas that respond to visual motion, eye movement, and head movement are all located in close proximity to one another (Leonard, 1998). The sensory information is then projected so that the sensory information is associated with other neural information and then transformed into an appropriate motor sequence if indicated. Current research supports the model that the visual system consists of parallel pathways through which visual information is processed, assimilated, and then contributes to motor control. Dynamic visual perception considers not just the seeing eye and its associated neural structures and functions, but rather a visual system that coordinates the anatomical location of the eyes in the head, the head on the shoulders, and an articulated muscle-joint system. The role of vision in both calibrating and maintaining posture and balance provides support for the dynamic systems theory, where the coordination of human movement is created through the organism's ability to self-organize as a function of the task and the environment (Wade & Jones, 1997).

The following describes some of the developmental changes of the visual system, summarized in Table 3–3.

Early Development of the Visual System

Embryonically the visual apparatus is derived from a portion of the diencephalon that migrates to the periphery. The most peripheral structure develops into the eyeball, which maintains its innervation during migration. Once in place, the visual system extends to the occipital poles, forming the horizontal axis of the brain (McKeough, 1995). The eye itself is formed by the fourth week. Myelination begins at the optic chiasm at around 13 weeks. Neurons in the occipital cortex are organized into their adult layers during the second half of gestation, so that they are ready to receive input by birth (Boothe, 1988). The fetus demonstrates reflex eye blinking by six months' gestation (Cech & Martin, 1995).

Maturation of the Visual System

■ Infancy and Childhood

Central visual pathways develop postnatally even though the neurons that constitute these pathways are formed prenatally. This is an excellent example of how use of the neuronal structures actually drives the development and maturation of those structures. Utilization and stimulation of neuronal structures must occur before synaptic pathways are functional. Thalamic connections begin to myelinate and continue to until 5 months of age (Cech & Martin, 1995).

Sustained ocular fixation on an object is observed at birth and even preterm. It has been observed that the neonate will consistently gaze at some stimuli more than others. Newborns definitely have pattern preference and can maintain attention if the stimulus is novel enough or, better yet, resembles a human face. Because the lenses are fixed in focus for the first month, infants can best fixate on a face or an object at about 7 to 9 inches away from the eyes (Bronson, 1994; VanderZanden, 2000). Infants see initially in black and white; 2-month-old babies can see two colors, and full color vision is developed by 4 months. Preference for a colored object seems apparent by the end of the third month (Cech & Martin, 1995).

Clinical Connection:

Parents should be educated about how best to visually stimulate their newborn baby, especially the premature infant. Nursery items should be bright, of sharp contrast, and placed at a distance of 7 to 9 inches from the baby's face. It is also important not to overwhelm the baby with an excess of stimulation; rather, parents should be advised to select a few items and to then change these items from time to time. Babies especially enjoy looking at the complex human face, an important fact to share with new parents because face gazing encourages emotional bonding and attachment.

By 2 months, infants can tract vertically and horizontally, as well as in a circular path. Perception of form, judged by the length of time spent looking at different visual representations, is evident at 2 or 3 months of age (Adams et al., 1997; Fantz, 1961). **Binocular vision** (the ability to tell the distances of objects and experience the world three-dimensionally) has a maturation burst between 3 and 5 months of age. Binocular vision allows for depth perception, which then is fortunately in place by the time a baby starts to creep on all fours (Yonas, Granrud, & Pettersen, 1985). Adult levels of visual acuity (20/20) are achieved by 1 year of age (Nelson, Rubin, & Wagner, 1984).

Head control contributes to the ability of the infant to visually fix on objects. By 3 months, most infants have discovered their hands and spend considerable time watching their own movement. In the first 3 months of life, it is easy to observe the postures that are used by the infant to visually explore the world. The infant uses the whole body to stabilize and permit maintenance of visual contact with an object or person. The baby's postural adjustments maintain a position in space that supports visual exploration of the environment. In other words, postural control subserves visual interest (deBenabib & Nelson, 1991). Much of early development involves looking at objects, judging their position, reaching for them, and manipulating them.

The role of visual feedback in the development of postural control has been studied. The requirement for visual feedback is greatest the first 3 months after an infant has acquired the ability to sit or stand, and this need declines afterward. This has been demonstrated for both typically developing infants and infants with Down syndrome (Butterworth & Cicchetti, 1978; Stokes, 1998). In the development of postural control, children between the ages of 4 and 6 years were found to be highly dependent on visual feedback and less dependent on somatosensory input (Poole, 1991; Woollacott, Shumway-Cook & Nashner, 1986). Preschoolers are also highly dependent on visual feedback for the develop-

TABLE 3-3

Visual System Changes Through the Life Span: Functional Implications

Developmental Phase	Major Changes	Functional Implications	Rehabilitation Implications
Early development	Eye formed by fourth week gestation. Neurons in occipital cortex are arranged in columns by birth, ready to receive visual input.	Fetus demonstrates reflexive eye blinking by 6 weeks' gestation.	
Maturation (infancy and childhood)	Central visual pathways, including thalamic connections, develop early. Adult levels of visual acuity (20/20) attained by end of first year. Binocular vision (for depth) matures between 3 and 5 months.	Newborns prefer patterns and can focus on objects 7–9 inches from face, such as a parent's face. Infants see initially in black and white; full color vision present by 4 months. Young infants can fixate, converge, and track by 2 months. Head and antigravity postural control promotes visual development. Postural control subserves visual interest. Depth perception in place by the time infant learns to creep. Development of postural control is highly dependent on vision through age 6.	Neonatal stimulation and parent education programs should include guiding parents in how to best visually stimulate the newborn, including how to arrange an appropriately stimulating nursery environment. Movement and visual development are subservient to each other Early intervention programming should reinforce the connection between vision and motor development in infants and young children.
Maturation (adolescence)	Maturation and processing increase. Adult levels of depth perception attained by age 12. Eyesight sharpest at age 20.	Sensory abilities and motor skill continue to contribute to advanced capabilities, allowing for success with sports and leisure activities.	This is an age of tremendous opportunity for motor learning and reeducation.
Maturity (adulthood)	Visual acuity continues to improve during 20s and 30s. At age 45 there is a tendency for presbyopia, caused by age-related inability of lens to change its curvature. Lens elasticity and transparency decrease. Incidence of cataract formation increases over age 30.	Sharp decline in ability to quickly adapt to change from light to dark environment after age 40.	Difficulty with reading small print and adapting quickly to lighting between environments are issues for clinicians to be aware of with patient instruction.
Aging (older adult)	Eye structure changes so that less light is transmitted to the retina and pupil size decreases. Both macular degeneration and cataracts are common. Visual acuity decreases between the ages of 60 and 80; at 80% of normal at age 85.	Because less light is transmitted, visual threshold is increased, requiring more light to see. Ability to adapt when moving from a dark to a light environment decreases and incidence of glare is high. Depth perception, contrast sensitivity, and peripheral vision decline.	Significant implications for safety, mobility, and functional independence. Older adults may require additional sensory or external cues, especially when in unfamiliar environments. Clinicians should be aware that approximately 10% of elderly persons have undetected eye disease or visual impairment.

Source: Information compiled from multiple sources. See text and references for details.

ment of postural control. Group play, which encourages not only social skills but also opportunity for imitation and modeling, is to be encouraged for this age group. Children ages 7 to 10 show similar responses to adults, an integrated reliance on somatosensory, visual, and vestibular input (Poole, 1991).

Clinical Connection:

Babies are highly dependent on visual feedback during these first months of life. Parents and therapists should be encouraged to use imitation and mirrors to help tap into this preference for vision as a learning tool. It is also vital to remember that infants require additional visual feedback, especially during the beginning practice of a new postural skill, another helpful hint for therapists and parents. ▪

Perception of size becomes increasingly accurate during the preschool years. By 2 years of age, adultlike binocular vision, crucial for accurate depth perception, is present. Many aspects of visual perception develop during childhood. The development of mature spatial skills is made possible through the ongoing maturation of visual perception. By age 5, children demonstrate visual closure, the ability to discern a shape when seeing only part of it. Figure ground perception (Fig. 3–6), the ability to separate the figure from the background, improves with age, fully developing by age 8 (Williams, 1983).

▪ Adolescence

The visual system continues to mature and become increasingly sophisticated during adolescence. Sensory abilities in adolescence continue to guide motor abilities. Adolescents can smoothly track small moving objects, allowing for success in activities such as baseball, pinball, and computer games. Perceptual judgments regarding the size of various objects at different distances become mature by age 11 (Collins, 1976). Adult levels of depth perception are developed by 12 years of age (Cech & Martin, 1995). Eyesight is the sharpest at age 20 (Zastrow, 1997).

The Mature Visual System

▪ Adulthood

Visual acuity continues to increase during the 20s and 30s, remains stable during the 40s and 50s, and then declines (Pitts, 1982). A decline in visual acuity is not significant until age 45, when there is the tendency

toward **presbyopia** (farsightedness). Presbyopia is a normal age-related change that occurs because the lens of the eye loses some of its elasticity, so that the lens is unable to adjust its curvature to focus on objects on the very near points of vision. After the age of 40, there is a sharp decline in the ability to quickly adapt from light to dark environments. **Cataracts,** an age-related decrease in the transparency of the lens, begin to form in everyone over the age of 30 (Kollarits, 1986).

The Aging Visual System

▪ Older Adult

The incidence of visual deficits in adults over 65 is 101 per 1000 persons (Poole, 1991). Therapists and assistants should be alert to the fact that approximately 10 percent of elderly persons have undetected eye disease or visual impairment (Bernstein-Lewis, 1996; Maguire, 1996).

By age 85, there is an 80-percent loss in visual acuity from that present at 40 years of age (Weale, 1975). Because of changes within the structure of the eye itself, less light is transmitted to the retina; therefore, visual threshold increases with age, requiring more light to see

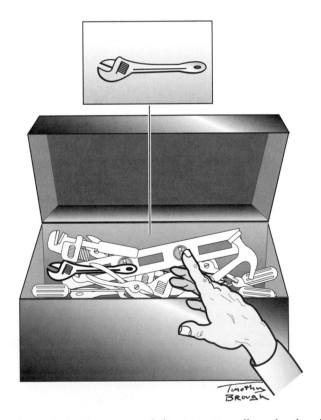

Figure 3–6. Figure ground discrimination allows for the ability to visually discriminate and choose a specific object from among a complex background.

an object (Shumway-Cook & Woollacott, 2001). Pupil size decreases with age, allowing less light into the eye. Glare introduces extraneous light into the eye and may be particularly troublesome for elderly persons (Cech & Martin, 1995). There is a decline in the ability to adapt from dark to light environments. When entering a dark house or a room that is not well illuminated, a teenager needs only 6 or 7 minutes to adapt, whereas the older adult needs almost three quarters of an hour (Williams, 1990).

The period of most rapid decrease in acuity is between the ages of 60 and 80 years. Sixty percent of all people over 65 have some degree of cataract formation. A major source of visual impairment in older adults is from **macular degeneration,** affecting 28 percent of adults over the age of 75. Macular degeneration is a pigmentary change of the central (macular) portion of the retina, produced by small hemorrhages, which then causes the individual to have blurred vision or to experience a "blind spot" (Chalifoux, 1991).

Older adults demonstrate narrower peripheral vision. The field of vision may be as wide as 270 degrees in the adolescent or young adult, but then may become as narrow as 120 degrees in the older adult (Hooyman & Kiyak, 1991). Depth perception and contrast sensitivity decreases sharply between the ages of 60 to 75 years. Losses in depth perception and contrast sensitivity have significant implication for safe mobility, especially climbing stairs. Clinicians may observe the tendency for older adults to require additional support, such as a handrail.

Older adults are slower than younger adults, with a significant decline in central processing. These deficits in the visual system, both in the central and the peripheral system, have significant functional implications, especially in the area of postural control, balance, safety, and independence. Studies show that older adults seem to be actively engaged in adaptation, and that they do not generally use visual input to stabilize posture. Instead, studies have demonstrated that they rely more on somatosensory input (Poole, 1991; Woollacott, Shumway-Cook, & Nashner, 1986; Woollacott, 1993). Vision is more often relied on when proprioceptive input is diminished or absent.

Clinical Connection:

Older persons may require additional sensory, verbal, or physical cues to execute tasks and maintain successful independence. These age-related changes need not handicap the older adult if therapists and assistants are able to help them adapt their activities and environment to fit their current level of functioning and needs.

Vestibular System: Life Span Changes

Contribution to Movement Control

The function of the vestibular system is to signal changes in head position or motion, referenced by the pull of gravity. Vestibular input is integrated with visual and proprioceptive information to provide the CNS with information to maintain equilibrium and develop an ever-accurate sense of spatial awareness, this system again demonstrating a wonderful example of parallel processing (Fig. 3–7). The vestibular system provides information concerning gravity, rotation, and acceleration. This information is crucial for the development of a subjective sensation of motion and regulating the orientation of the body in space. Even though the vestibular system does project to the cerebral cortex, it is primarily a subcortical system, with powerful influence on the spinal cord, affecting muscle tone and reflex activity (Burt, 1993; McKeough, 1995). The vestibular system is both a sensory and a motor system. As a sensory system, it provides information about position and movement of the body; as a motor system, it controls head position and coordinated postural movements (Fig. 3–8).

The vestibular system is sensitive to two types of information: the position of the head in space and sudden changes (including acceleration and decelera-

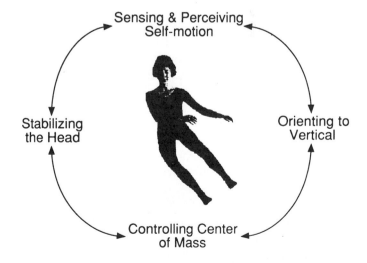

Figure 3–7. Four important roles of the vestibular system in postural control interact with other sensory and motor systems to accomplish tasks such as maintaining equilibrium and body alignment on an unstable surface. (From Herdman, S. J. [2000]. *Vestibular rehabilitation* [2nd ed., p. 26]. Philadelphia: F. A. Davis.)

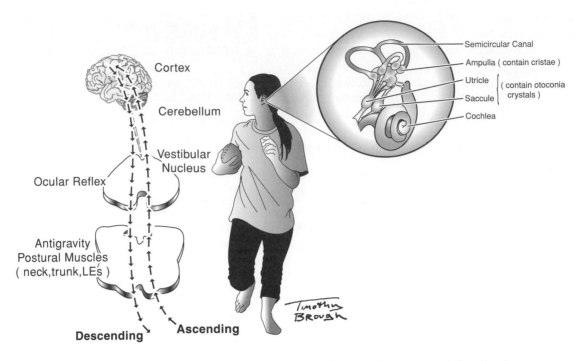

Figure 3–8. Key elements of the vestibular system, emphasizing the major peripheral and central components and the sensory and motor functions of this system, a crucial subsystem contributing to the human movement system.

tion) in the direction of head movement. The vestibular system is part of the labyrinth of the inner ear, separate but closely associated with the cochlea, which is concerned with hearing. Vestibular inputs, integrated subconsciously, are important for the coordination of several motor responses, helping to stabilize the eye and maintain postural stability during standing and walking (see Fig. 3–7).

Functional Anatomy Overview

The vestibular system originates from sensory receptors located in each ear, projects directly into the brainstem, divides, and extends as far superiorly as the cerebral cortex and as far caudally as the spinal cord. Anatomically this system can be divided into a peripheral and a central component (see Fig. 3–8).

The peripheral vestibular system, located within the inner ear, consists of membranous and bony labyrinths, the motion sensors of the vestibular system, the hair cells, and the eighth cranial nerve. The bony labyrinth consists of three semicircular canals, the cochlea, and a central chamber called the vestibule. The membranous labyrinth is suspended within the bony labyrinth by fluid and connective tissue. It contains five sensory organs: the membranous portions of the semicircular canals and the two otolith organs, the utricle and saccule (Herdman, 2000). One end of each semicircular canal is widened to form an ampulla.

The semicircular canals serve as angular accelerom-eters (Shumway-Cook & Woollacott, 2001). When the head starts to rotate, fluid within these canals disturbs tiny hair cells and motion is detected. The three pairs of semicircular canals are oriented in three planes, so that pairs work together, giving rise to composite signals representing the movement. The utricle and saccule provide information about body and head position with reference to gravity and linear acceleration of the head in a straight line. Within the utricle and saccule, otoconia crystals are suspended above the hair cells. The vertical downward force of gravity on these crystals stimulates the hair cells, which then provide information about the pull of gravity on the head. These peripheral receptors all send impulses through the eighth cranial nerve, which then enters the vestibular nuclei in the brainstem, the beginning of the central component of this system (Hain, Ramaswamy, & Hillman, 2000).

The central portion of the vestibular system is structured so that there are two main targets from the primary afferents: the vestibular nuclear complex within the brainstem and the cerebellum; both areas are involved in processing vestibular information with somatosensory and visual input. The vestibular nuclear complex is the primary processor of vestibular input and implements direct, fast connections between incoming afferent information and motor output efferent neurons. It is here that vestibular sensory input is processed concurrently with the processing of other sensory information, including proprioceptive, tactile, visual, and auditory information. This complex contains the relays for the VOR, so vital for allowing the eyes to remain fixed on an object while moving. Connections then proceed through ascending and descending tracts to the oculomotor complex. This area is also involved in vestibulospinal reflexes and in coordinating head and eye movements that occur together. (Some of these reflexes and automatic movements are discussed in Chapter 4.) The cerebellum is the adaptive processor, monitoring vestibular performance and readjusting central vestibular processing if necessary (Herdman, 2000).

The motor output from the vestibular system includes the motor neurons to the extraocular eye muscles, as part of the VOR, and the motor neurons within the spinal cord, which drive skeletal muscle. There are three efferent tracts that connect the vestibular nucleus to the spinal cord: the lateral vestibulospinal, medial vestibulospinal, and reticulospinal tracts. Generally, they all generate antigravity postural activity, primarily to the cervical muscles and muscles of the trunk and lower extremities. These antigravity responses are triggered in response to head position changes that occur with respect to gravity (Herdman, 2000). In Chapters 4 and 8, some of these automatic responses, including righting and equilibrium responses, will be described.

The implications of vestibular disorders to movement control are obvious, to be elaborated on in Chapter 8. Because this system helps to maintain the upright position, pathology impairs this ability and causes disequilibrium. Because vestibular signals are used to detect gravity, loss of this input can lead to disorientation (Cohen, 1994). Abnormalities within the vestibular system result in sensations such as dizziness, unsteadiness, problems with focusing the eyes, **nystagmus,** and balance impairments. Functional limitations, including difficulty with driving a car, dressing, or walking, can be significant. Disorders of the vestibular system can be due to pathology in either the peripheral or central component of the system. Both can present with vertigo, dizziness, loss of balance, and gait unsteadiness, but central vestibular disorders are more likely than peripheral to cause imbalance (Furman & Whitney, 2000). Central disorders are also often associated with additional neurological symptoms. The most common peripheral vestibular disorder is benign paroxysmal vertigo (see Chapter 8).

Clinical Connection:

Vestibular disorders are characteristically accompanied by blurred vision, poor balance, spatial disorders such as past-pointing or veering off course when attempting to walk a straight line, and autonomic symptoms such as nausea, increased heart rate, and respiratory difficulties. The most common peripheral vestibular disorder,

benign positional **vertigo**, causes patients to experience a false sense of motion. Vertigo is caused by unequal signals from the two vestibular nerves projecting to the vestibular nuclei. The vestibular nuclei then misinterpret the difference between the signals as indicating movement, when there really is no movement. These patients may demonstrate impaired postural control, impairments or loss of the VOR, nystagmus, and disorientation. ▪

Vestibular nystagmus is the rapid alternating movement of the eyes in response to continued rotation of the body. Nystagmus is characterized by alternating slow movement of the eyes in the direction opposite to head movement and then the rapid resetting of the eyes in the direction of the head movement. This is a normal consequence of head movement, one you may observe on a friend while that friend is on a spinning amusement ride at a fair or amusement park. **Postrotatory nystagmus,** a reversal in this movement when the spinning stops, has been used as a clinical assessment tool to evaluate the intactness of the vestibular system.

Clinical Connection:

In some children and adults with severe brain damage, a condition known as resting nystagmus can be observed, where there is a constant horizontal flickering of the eyes, suggestive of neurological impairment at the brainstem level. ▪

Following are some of the developmental changes of the vestibular system, summarized in Table 3–4. This section is noticeably shorter that the previous sections on the other subsystems related to movement control. Few studies have been performed on changes in the human vestibular system, presumably due to the difficulty in isolating or selectively stimulating vestibular receptors as opposed to those that are visual or somatosensory in origin. The vestibular system is also the most widely dispersed subsystem in the body.

Early Development of the Vestibular System

The vestibular apparatus begins as a thickening of the ectoderm within the primitive ear early in the fourth week of gestation. The semicircular canals, utricle, and saccule are completely formed by 10 weeks (Humphrey, 1965). The fetus moves constantly in utero, and the vestibular apparatus provides information about that movement. The fetus shows a generalized body response to changes in body position, including the ability to right the head. Movement in utero has been linked to later movement competence (Milani-Comparetti, 1981).

TABLE 3-4
Vestibular System Changes Through the Life Span: Functional Implications

Developmental Phase	Major Changes	Functional Implications	Rehabilitation Implications
Early development	Peripheral receptors formed by 10 weeks' gestation. Vestibular system operational in utero, providing information about fetal movement.	Fetus able to show generalized body responses to changes in position, such as head righting. Uterine movement has been linked to later movement competence.	It is reasonable to be concerned about lack of or paucity of fetal movement as an indicator of movement dysfunction.
Maturation (infancy and childhood)	Completely myelinated at birth, prepared to transmit information regarding movement and gravity. Continuing maturation and sensory integration of this system ongoing throughout childhood.	Development of equilibrium reactions and the ability to right the body develop as vestibular system mature and becomes integrated with other movement subsystems. Early movement activities are related to development of competence over gravity and postural stability.	Preterm infants have delayed vestibular responses to movement. Infants with vestibular problems demonstrate delays in attainment of motor skills.
Maturation (adolescence)	Vestibular system continues to mature, with full maturity attained between ages 10–14.	Normal maturation and integration contribute to healthy body scheme and gravitational security. Vestibular system coordinates with visual and somatosensory system, contributing to refined static and dynamic balance. Balance performance peaks between ages 9–12.	Refinement of this system is related to experience and exposure.
Maturity (adulthood)	Beginning at age 40, number of sensory fibers and cells decrease.	No specific significant functional implications.	As with other systems, knowledge and past experience will make up for any minimal decline, maximizing rehabilitation potential.
Aging (older adult)	Age-related changes include reduction in number of receptor and motor fibers, loss of hair cells. Centrally, vestibular nuclei have decreased electrical excitability and deterioration in central processing.	Decline in vestibular abilities contributes to postural control deficits. Incidence of dizziness, vertigo, unsteadiness, and balance disorders increases. Increased threshold for vestibular activation could contribute to increased body sway.	Ability to function adequately in new or unfamiliar environments, or where other sensory cues are unpredictable, decreases. Falls in the elderly are caused by a constellation of factors, including decline in vestibular functioning.

Source: Information compiled from multiple sources. See text and references for details.

Maturation of the Vestibular System

■ Infancy and Childhood

The vestibular system is completely myelinated at birth. It has been demonstrated that preterm infants have delayed vestibular responses to movement, especially preterm infants who are also small for gestational age (Eviatar, Eviatar, & Naray, 1974). This delay is due to immaturity of the vestibular system, not pathology. The VOR is not present until a few weeks after birth. Righting reactions of the head, mediated by the labyrinths, are possible at birth. The ability to move against gravity continues with the development of trunk righting and progresses to the development of equilibrium reactions. The body appears to seek the most efficient posture to support reaching, manipulation, and locomotion (Cech & Martin, 1995). Infant and children with vestibular problems demonstrate delays in motor function (Kaga, Maeda, & Suzuki, 1988). Many of the infant's early activities are related to the task of attaining and maintaining postures against gravity.

Clinical Connection:

Movement, as a learning experience in it's own right, is a vital part of early childhood development. Children should be encouraged to explore and experience different varieties of movement experiences. In the case of children with motor delays, therapists and assistants can advise parents and caregivers by offering suggestions as to how to provide safe, effective movement experiences for children who cannot move independently.

During childhood, it is typical to observe children engaging in repetitive self-stimulation, such as rocking and spinning. This activity is thought to contribute to maturing of the vestibular system and disappears by middle childhood. Children have a stronger response to vestibular stimulation than adults. Studies on postural control demonstrate that there is a clear difference between the relative weighting of somatosensory input or visual input in cueing for postural control. Children are more reliant on vision than on somatosensory input when making automatic postural adjustments (Woollacott et al., 1982).

■ Adolescence

The vestibular system continues to mature during early adolescence, with full maturity achieved between 10 and 14 years of age. Normal maturation and integration of the vestibular system is thought to contribute to a healthy body scheme and gravitational security (Fisher et al., 1991). The vestibular apparatus coordinates with the visual and somatosensory systems in governing balance. Static and dynamic balance can be used as an indicator of vestibular system maturity and integration of the many subsystems contributing to the complex nature of balance. **Static balance** refers to the ability of the body to maintain equilibrium while in a stationary position. **Dynamic balance** refers to the ability to maintain equilibrium when moving from point to point. Abilities in the area of static balance performance surge between the ages of 9 and 12. Rapid gains are also made in the area of dynamic balance at around age 12 (Gallahue & Ozmun, 2002). Activities typically engaged in throughout adolescence, such as sports and dancing,

contribute to the continuing maturation and refinement of this system.

The Mature Vestibular System

■ Adulthood

There are minimal beginning signs of age-related changes in this system that become evident during adulthood. In the peripheral vestibular system in adults over 40, the number of sensory cells and nerve fibers reduces progressively (Rosenhall & Rubin, 1975). Neural changes in the vestibular nerve may begin as early as age 40 years (Cech & Martin, 1995).

The Aging Vestibular System

■ Older Adults

The vestibular system shows a decline in function with aging. Adults over 70 show a 40-percent reduction in hair cells and a 36-percent reduction in nerve fibers in the peripheral vestibular system (Rosenhall & Rubin, 1975). By age 75, the number of myelinated vestibular nerve fibers is decreased by almost 40 percent (Bergstrom, 1973). Adults over 60 have been found to show decreased sensitivity for nystagmus and longer effects after rotation has ceased (VanderLaan & Oosterveld, 1974). It is theorized that the vestibular nuclei demonstrate decreased electrical excitability and therefore increased thresholds for excitation with aging. Increased thresholds for vestibular activation could contribute to increased body sway in elderly persons (Woollacott et al., 1982). Disordered balance in the elderly is probably due to a manifestation of deterioration in central vestibular integrative functions, rather than deterioration in the peripheral apparatus (Marsh & Geel, 2000).

Because one of the functions of the vestibular system is to provide an absolute reference for the somatosensory and visual systems, it is especially important during times of visual and somatosensory conflict, when information coming in from the different sensory sources seems to give conflicting information (Black & Nashner, 1985). Studies on postural control demonstrate that there is a clear difference between the relative weighting of somatosensory input or visual input in cueing for postural control. In contrast to children, adults are more reliant on somatosensory than on visual input when making automatic postural adjustments (Woollacott et al., 1982). A decline in vestibular function with age causes this absolute reference system to be unreliable, as evidenced by the nervous system's experiencing difficulty dealing with the conflict. This may be the reason that older adults with vestibular disorders have problems with dizziness and unsteadiness when they are in environments with conflicting or unfamiliar visual and somatosensory inputs (Shumway-Cook & Woollacott, 2001). This may result in situations where individuals can function adequately in the more restricted home environment but have difficulty maneuvering in unfamiliar situations where unpredictable and unexpected challenges to postural stability may occur (McClenaghan et al., 1995). Dizziness and vertigo are common disturbances in the older adult. Falls in elderly persons appear to be caused by the combination of several factors, including a less reliable vestibular system.

Motor or Action Systems: Life Span Changes

Contribution to Movement Control

Dynamic systems theory views the brain's function on movement as a whole, proposing that the nervous system functions as a heterarchy rather than a hierarchy (Case-Smith, 1996). Even so, it is academically helpful to view the nervous system as controlling movement within three task levels: the strategy level, the tactics level, and the execution level. Remember, however, that the processing, feedback, and modulation capability between levels is constant and that any strict division of levels is academic. Strategies are organized at the higher levels, such as the association areas and the basal ganglia. The tactics are determined by the motor cortex with continual modulation from the cerebellum. The execution of the movement is fed through the brainstem and spinal cord to the muscles acting on the skeleton (Drubach, 2000). This section focuses on the functional contribution of these strategy and tactical areas to the overall control of movement and then the life span changes seen in the execution structures, the musculoskeletal system. The functional contributions from the areas of the brainstem and spinal cord will be explored further in Chapter 4, where reflexes and automatic movements are discussed.

The actual output of the brain to the external world is manifested as movement. The motor or action systems, like the other subsystems, demonstrate tremendous ability to adapt to the changing needs of the movement, individual, task, or environment. The action system includes the higher centers of the nervous system, such as the motor cortex, cerebellum, and basal ganglia, which perform processing essential to the coor-

dination of movement. The motor or action system also includes the actual effector organs of movement, the muscular system acting on a skeletal system so that movement occurs (Fig. 3–9). The actual anatomy of many of these structures has previously been discussed (see Chapter 2) or can be found in basic anatomy texts.

Functional Anatomy Overview

▪ The Higher Centers

The motor cortex, including the primary motor cortex, the supplementary motor area, and the premotor cortex, all in the frontal lobe, interact with sensory processing areas in the parietal lobe and with basal ganglia and cerebellar areas to identify where we want to move, to plan the movement, and finally to execute the movement (Ghez, 1991). All three of these areas have their own somatotopic maps of the body, so that if different regions are stimulated, different muscles and body parts move (Shumway-Cook & Woollacott, 2001). The motor map, or motor homunculus (Figs. 2–6 and 3–9), is similar to the sensory map in the way that the represen-

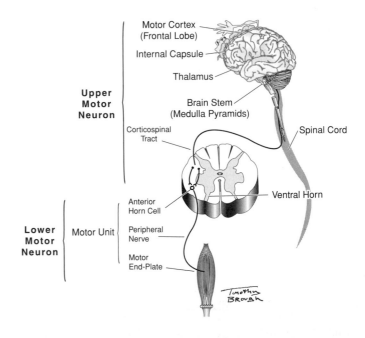

Figure 3–9. Key elements of the motor system, emphasizing the following functional anatomical components of the motor system as a major subsystem of the human movement system: primary motor cortex, which includes the premotor and supplementary motor areas of the frontal lobe, through the internal capsule and brainstem (medulla/pyramids) as the corticospinal efferent pathway innervating the muscular system acting on the skeletal system. Differentiation between upper and lower motor neuron is clarified.

tations are distorted so that areas requiring more detailed control (such as the mouth and hand) are most highly represented. Inputs to the motor areas come from the basal ganglia, cerebellum, and all the sensory areas.

Outputs from the motor cortex contribute mainly to the corticospinal tract, also called the pyramidal tract because its fibers concentrate to form pyramids at the level of the medulla. These axons then descend to enter the ventral horn, terminating on interneurons and motor neurons. The primary motor cortex and the corticospinal tract function to control the speed of movement and absolute force of that movement. There are, however, many parallel motor pathways for carrying out an action sequence, just as there are parallel pathways for sensory processing

Clinical Connection:

It is extremely important for therapists and assistants to remember that there are many parallel motor pathways available for carrying out a movement sequence. Simply by training a patient/client in one situation, one cannot automatically assume that the training will transfer to all other activities requiring the same set of muscles. In fact, one should assume otherwise. Training needs to be task specific. For example, if the goal is to reestablish the ability to flex the lower extremity (LE) adequately to step up onto a step, training should be done in standing and in contexts similar to actually stepping up onto a step. Training or practice of LE flexion in sitting or lying down will not necessarily carry over to an improved ability to flex the LE as required for stepping. Additional examples of task-specific training will be expanded on in Chapters 5 and 6. ■

The supplementary motor area is active when a sequence of remembered movements is planned, when movement is initiated, and when this area participates in the assembly of a central motor program or motor subroutine. Premotor neurons are more active when the action is visually guided, such as in reaching, and is therefore more important for the generation of a new movement not previously in the movement repertoire (Shumway-Cook & Woollacott, 2001).

The cerebellum has an important role in movement coordination, receiving information from almost every sensory system, consistent with its role as a regulator of motor output. Through its circuitry and neuronal connections, this great comparator compensates for errors by comparing intention with performance. Vital to its role as an error detector is the ability of the cerebellum to receive sensory feedback, called **reafference**, from the receptors about the movements as the move-

ment is occurring. The cerebellum collects a tremendous amount of both sensory and motor information and constantly readjusts and refines movement. It is responsible for judging and monitoring movement accuracy, timing, and intensity.

The basal ganglia, consisting of a set of nuclei at the base of the cerebral cortex, have major afferent, internal, and efferent connections, permitting widespread functions in sensory, motor, and association areas. Much of the output from the basal ganglia, as well as the brainstem, is filtered through what is called the extrapyramidal system, a set of subcortical circuits and pathways. It is now hypothesized that the basal ganglia play a role in selectively activating some movement while suppressing others. It is concerned with internally generated movements and automatic postural control. It appears that the basal ganglia is very involved in determining and specifying the nature of the movement pattern required for the task and the environment and altering aspects of movement to accommodate changed task demands or environmental changes (Connor & Abbs, 1990). The basal ganglia appear to have a prominent role in the initiation and coordination of simple and complex movement and the maintenance of muscle tone.

Clinical Connection:

Diseases of the basal ganglia, such as Parkinson's disease, typically produce some form of dystonia, disorders of muscle tone and postural control, in addition to involuntary movements (**dyskinesia**) and evidence of poverty and slowness of movement (**bradykinesia**). Patients with Parkinson's disease demonstrate symptoms such as a resting tremor (called "pill-rolling" because of its characteristic look), rigidity, and slowness in initiating movement (**akinesia**). The tremor and rigidity may be due to the loss of regulatory, inhibitory influences within the basal ganglia. ■

■ Musculoskeletal System

The basic anatomy of the muscular and skeletal systems is found in anatomy and physiology texts. The following describes some of the developmental changes of the musculoskeletal system, summarized in Tables 3–5 and 3–6. Of all the subsystems, the musculoskeletal system, because the other subsystems act on or through it, demonstrates tremendous ability to adapt to physical demands, or lack of physical demands, placed on it. Aspiring or practicing clinicians are reminded to study the following section with ongoing reflection about the clinical significance of not only the influence of normal

TABLE 3-5

Muscular System Changes Through the Life Span: Functional Implications

Developmental Phase	Major Changes	Functional Implications	Rehabilitation Implications
Early development	Motor units form and skeletal muscles mature by 8 weeks. Different fiber types developed by 30 weeks. Number and size of fiber increases during last half of gestation.	First fetal movements seen by 8 weeks.	Lack of fetal movement may be a worrisome indicator of future motor problems.
Maturation (infancy and childhood)	At birth, most fibers are fast twitch; slow twitch develops between ages 1–2; adult ratio reached by end of second year. Fourteenfold increase in fiber number between birth and age 16; rapid growth spurt at age 2.	Development of slow twitch fiber type corresponds with developing postural control as mastery over gravity continues to become evident.	Children with delayed attainment of motor skills and poor postural control may never attain the normal adult fiber type ratio. The value of early intervention and movement stimulation is tremendous.
Maturation (adolescence)	Greatest strength development occurs between ages 6–18. Number of fibers doubles between 10–16.	Increase in strength is directly related to increase in mass.	Boys have greater strength than girls at all ages.
Maturity (adulthood)	Fiber numbers continue to increase through age 50, after which decline begins.	Maximum strength begins to peak during 20s, maximal in men between 30–35, staying constant until 50; 20% loss by age 60.	Physically active adults maintain and increase strength. There is considerable variation in strength and endurance between individuals.
Aging (older adult)	Senile muscular atrophy occurs, due to decrease in fibers, decrease in muscle mass, and decline in number of functional motor units.	Strength and speed of muscle contraction decrease; 50% loss by age 70. Rate of decline in muscle strength less in upper extremities than in trunk and lower extremities, this distribution contributing to changes in postural alignment and perhaps causing functional instability. Trunk weakness may contribute to less effective equilibrium reactions.	Degree of atrophy highly variable, dependent on activity level and level of fitness. Strength losses can be minimized with exercise, including moderate weight training. Rehabilitation program success is highly dependent on premorbid fitness level.

Source: Information compiled from multiple sources. See text and references for details.

or abnormal movement on the musculoskeletal system, but also the value of wellness programs and preventive management in keeping these effector systems in top functioning condition.

Early Development of the Musculoskeletal System

The muscular system develops from the mesoderm. Muscle tissue develops from primitive cells called myoblasts, derived from mesenchymal cells. Before 30 weeks' gestation, most muscle fibers are undifferentiated. Some type I fibers (slow-twitch tonic type) can be distinguished as early as 21 weeks, and type II fibers (fast-twitch phasic type) are generally recognizable by 30 weeks. Studies have concluded that between 31 and 37 weeks' gestation, type II fibers constitute about 25 percent of fetal muscle tissue (Malina & Bouchard, 1991). The motor unit, which consists of an efferent motor neuron and all the muscle fibers it innervates, begins to develop by 8 weeks' gestation. This corresponds to the earliest fetal movements (Gajdosik & Gajdosik, 2000).

TABLE 3–6

Skeletal System Changes Through the Life Span: Functional Implications

Developmental Phase	Major Changes	Functional Implications	Rehabilitation Implications
Early development	Cartilage model of long bones formed by week 6; primary ossification centers emerge by week 12.	Malleable, cartilaginous skeleton models in response to forces acting on it.	Confines of uterus limit fetal movement; may result in modeling deformities, such as clubfoot, which respond well to early intervention.
Maturation (infancy and childhood)	Epiphysis is an active site of bone formation. Vertebral column responds to gravitational forces by developing secondary lordotic curves in cervical and lumbar areas.	Rotational, angular, and torsional changes to pelvis and LEs are in response to movement and muscular forces. Weight bearing promotes bone growth and density. Development of head control in prone leads to development of cervical lordosis; sitting and standing contribute to lumbar lordosis.	Fractures of epiphyseal plate may interfere with bone growth pattern and may result in deformity. Abnormal forces, either from limited movement or excessive force, such as in spasticity, may result in abnormal skeletal development and deformity.
Maturation (adolescence)	Sudden increase in height and weight producing "growth spurt," lasting two years, at 12–13 for girls, 13–15 for boys. Skeletal maturity attained when epiphyseal plate closes; complete closure may take up until age 25.	Girls demonstrate greater flexibility than boys. Boys tend to make rapid gains in strength throughout adolescence, whereas girls peak at puberty and regress by end of adolescence.	Bone grows before muscle often contributing to muscular tightness, limited range of motion giving credence to common complaint of "growing pains." Stress fractures and avulsion fractures are common. Scoliosis commonly appears during adolescence.
Maturity (adulthood)	Bone remodeling and increases in density continue. After age 40, bone resorption begins to exceed bone replacement. Intervertebral disc becomes more fibrous, less hydrated; vertebral bodies are less dense. Menopause creates a great impetus for bone loss in women.	Changes in density and modeling occur as response to weight bearing and muscular contraction. Due to changes in vertebral column, some degree of shortening in height may become evident.	High incidence of back pain secondary to disc changes. Physical activity, including weight training and weight bearing, will contribute to less bone resorption and decrease osteoporosis.
Aging (older adult)	Collagen is less elastic and slower to respond to stretch changes. Loss of bone mass continues.	Loss in flexibility may contribute to hypokinesis. Declines in both strength and flexibility can contribute to poor posture.	Range of motion can be maintained but stretching needs to be done more slowly. Incidence of osteoporosis and osteoarthritis is high. Age-related bone loss decreases with physical fitness, including moderate weight training.

Source: Information compiled from multiple sources. See text and references for details.

Nearly all the skeletal muscles are present and are reasonably mature by 8 weeks' gestation. During the last half of gestational growth, the number and size of muscle fibers increases rapidly so that most of the skeletal muscle has been developed by birth. Some of the developmental changes that occur in order to arrive at this reasonably mature state are as follows. The directions of the muscle fibers change; in fact, only a few muscles retain their original fiber orientation of parallel to the long axis of the body (rectus abdominis and erector spinae). A myotome may split so that two or more parts become portions of the final muscle, such as the trapezius with three parts, or the sternocleidomastoid with two. The original myotome may also split into two or more layers, such as the intercostal muscles and the abdominal obliques. Portions of the muscle also degenerate, leaving behind a sheath of connective tissue known as an aponeurosis. This process is a good example of the overgrowth, selective regeneration, and reorganizational change so characteristic of early development (Crelin, 1981). The greatest increase in the number of muscle fibers occurs before birth, as a result of an increase in both number of fibers and size of the individual fibers (Cech & Martin, 1995).

Bone and cartilage are also derived from the mesoderm. Development of bone begins between the third and eighth week. By the fifth week, mesenchymal models of the bones appear in the extremities, with upper extremity preceding lower extremity development. By the sixth week, mesenchymal cells have differentiated into chondroblasts, which form the cartilage model of all the long bones. Primary centers of ossification have emerged between the 7th and 12th week (Moore, 1988). The diaphyses are fairly well ossified by birth, but the epiphyses remain cartilaginous. The confining intrauterine environment in the later weeks of gestation limits the fetus's positioning options and applies forces to this developing, malleable skeletal system (Cech & Martin, 1995). The term *malleable* literally means able to be shaped by pressure, descriptive of how forces shape the bony skeleton (Taber's, 2001). Intrauterine molding may result in deformities such as clubfoot, tibial bowing, or congenital hip dislocation, all of which respond fairly favorably to early orthopedic or therapeutic intervention.

Maturation of the Musculoskeletal System

■ Infancy and Childhood

After birth, the growth of the muscle comes mainly from an increase in size of the individual fibers, although there is also an increase in number. There is

approximately a 14-fold increase in fiber number between 2 months and 16 years of age. In childhood, there is a rapid growth spurt at 2 years. The fiber size also shows a steady increase until adolescence, with a potential 10-fold increase. In girls, the increase in fiber size is more rapid than boys, peaking between 3 and 10 years of age. At birth, skeletal muscles tend to be predominantly fast twitch and have a high rate of contraction and brief relaxation time. Between 1 and 2 years of age, the characteristics of slow twitch (slow contraction speed and longer relaxation times) are acquired (Cech & Martin, 1995). Types I and II gradually increase in number throughout the first 2 years of life. By the second birthday, the relative fiber distribution ratio between fiber types is at the adult level (Cech & Martin, 1995). Generally speaking, the contractile properties of skeletal muscle mature early in infancy. These facts give credence to the importance of early development and movement. Muscular strength increases steadily during infancy and early childhood. Although only a few studies are available on strength in this young age range, it appears that the development of strength is greatest in childhood between the ages of 6 through 18 years.

Throughout infancy and early childhood, bone growth occurs rapidly, affected by such factors as genetic makeup, general health, and nutrition. The bones of the skull do not fuse until age 2, allowing for expansion and molding of the cranium, as well as brain growth. The epiphysis is an active site for new bone formation, playing an important role in early skeletal development. Fractures of the epiphyseal plate interfere with bone growth patterns, resulting in asymmetry and possible deformity (Cech & Martin, 1995). The pelvis and lower extremities undergo rotational, angular, and torsional changes in addition to length changes. Many of these changes are a direct response to early motor development and movement, creating modeling of this changeable skeleton. These changes include changes in the femoral angles of inclination and torsion, as well as tibial torsion changes. Weight bearing and movement are the significant driving forces behind these developmental changes. The level of compressive forces, as seen in normal weight bearing, directly affects the thickness and density of the bone shaft. Functional movement development also contributes to vital changes in the vertebral column, as the infant develops mastery over gravity. The cervical lordosis develops in response to the development of head control in the prone position, and the lumbar lordosis develops in response to the attainment of sitting and standing.

This dynamic quality of bone growth contributes to the spontaneous correction of skeletal abnormalities and the responsiveness to early intervention seen in young children. On the other hand, abnormal skeletal development also results from the effect of abnormal forces pulling on this malleable skeleton, as seen in developmental disorders such as cerebral palsy.

▪ Adolescence

There is a growth spurt and significant rate of increase in number of muscle fibers between 10 and 16 years of age, when the number of fibers doubles (Crelin, 1981). Increases in strength are directly related to increases in mass during growth. Strength increases significantly in early to middle adolescence, through age 16. Boys tend to demonstrate a strength spurt during the adolescent years, secondary to hormonal influences. Boys tend to make rapid gains in muscular strength and endurance throughout adolescence, whereas girls tend to peak at the onset of puberty and regress slightly by the end of adolescence (Gallahue & Ozmun, 2002; Stout, 2000). Boys have greater strength than do girls at all ages (Blimkie, 1989; Gajdosik & Gajdosik, 2000; Malina, 1986).

During adolescence, bone continues to grow and remodel in response to mechanical stress. The adolescent experiences sudden increases in height and weight, with growth of the trunk preceding that of the lower extremities (Cech & Martin, 1995). The adolescent growth spurt, lasting 2 years, occurs at around 12 to 13 years for girls, 2 years later for boys. Skeletal growth precedes muscular growth, leading to the common complaint of "growing pains" experienced as the longer bone tugs on the temporarily shortened muscles. Scoliosis is commonly seen during adolescence, with this risk decreasing after the onset of puberty. Girls tend to display greater joint flexibility throughout adolescence than their male counterparts. Girls steadily gain in percent body fat throughout adolescence. Skeletal maturity is attained when the epiphyseal plate closes. Closure begins in childhood but may continue as late as into the 25th year (Moore, 1988).

The Mature Musculoskeletal System

▪ Adulthood

Muscle fiber numbers continue to increase through age 50, after which a steady decline begins (Crelin, 1981). Studies confirm that maximal physical strength is highest in the 20s (Rikli & Busch, 1986). Strength continues to increase into the third decade of life, especially for males. Strength is maximal in men between the ages of 30 and 35, remaining relatively constant through age 50 (Larsson, Grimby, & Karlsson, 1982). Some studies show a 20-percent loss in strength by age 60

(Gallahue & Ozmun, 2002). Complex sensorimotor coordination begins to slow in the 30s, although considerable variation is found among individuals (Welford, 1977). Adults who are physically active reap many benefits. Physical activity builds muscle, strengthens heart and lungs, lowers blood pressure, and relieves anxiety and stress. Therapists and assistants should consider a patient's **premorbid** (before the development of the disease) physical fitness level as a valuable indicator about rehabilitation prognosis and possible outcome.

Throughout adulthood, bone remodeling and increases in bone density continue to occur secondary to weight bearing and muscle contraction (Whitbourne, 1985). After age 40, bone resorption begins to exceed bone replacement. Cancellous bone loss begins in the third decade and cortical loss in the fourth decade (Borner, Dillworth, & Sullivan, 1988). Skeletal changes experienced during adulthood may result in beginning shortening in height due to compression of the intervertebral discs secondary to the disks becoming more fibrous and less hydrated and to decreased density of the vertebrae themselves. Menopause creates a great impetus for bone loss for women. It is estimated that women lose 1 percent of bone mass per year before menopause and then 2 to 4 percent during the first 5 years after menopause (Raub & Smith, 1985). After this time, the rate returns to 1 percent per year. Men lose 0.5 percent of bone mass per year.

The Aging Musculoskeletal System

▪ Older Adult

As humans age, the strength or force-generating capacity of skeletal muscles is reduced (Williams, Higgins, & Lewek, 2002). The muscular wasting associated with the aging process is generally referred to as **senile muscular atrophy** (Schultz & Lipton, 1982). The degree of atrophy is certainly individual and dependent on the activity level and physical fitness of the person. Decrease in strength is a consequence of many changes, including decreases in fibers, muscle mass, and the number of functional motor units (Frontera et al., 2000). Motor units decline due to a decrease in the number of motor neurons; a muscle cell degenerates if it does not receive stimulation from a motor neuron. Researchers have found a significant reduction in motoneurons in subjects after age 60; by age 70, motor unit means were less than 40 percent of normal (McComas, Upton, and Sica, 1973). Speed and strength of muscle contraction decline with age. It is generally considered that about 50 percent of an individual's strength is lost by age 70

(Bohannon, 1996). As muscle fibers degenerate, fat cells replace it, so that by age 70, fat may make up perhaps one-third the weight of the gastrocnemius (Hasselkus, 1974). Losses in strength can be minimized in older adults with exercise programs and moderate weight training.

Researchers agree that the rate of decline in muscular strength with age appears to be less in the upper extremities than in the trunk and lower extremities (Grimby, Danneskiold-Samsoe, Hvid, & Saltin 1982). Weakness and increased muscle fatigability is most striking in the muscles of the back, abdominals, and quadriceps. Weakness is also generalized in the pelvic girdle and neck musculature. This pattern of proximal weakness results in a weakening of the trunk muscles that would normally provide the stability on which movement takes place. Decreases in these postural muscles may contribute to diminished effectiveness of the individual's balance and equilibrium reactions (Hasselkus, 1974; Stelmach, Zelaznik, & Lowe, 1990).

There appears to be an age-related loss of both fiber types; however, type II fast-twitch fibers may be lost at a rate greater than type I slow-twitch fibers (Timiras, 1994). This loss of fast-twitch fibers, resulting in slower rates and magnitudes of contraction, places important constraints on what kinds of movements can be accomplished within the bounds of postural stability (Mortimer et al., 1982). Muscle response latencies are slower and temporal organization of muscle synergies is disrupted in older individuals, seen during both postural perturbations and initiation of voluntary movement (Woollacott, Shumway-Cook, & Nashner, 1986; Marsh and Geel, 2000). Movement time becomes important when the response consists of movement of the whole body or of an entire limb.

Changes in flexibility as one ages can be the result of collagen changes, **hypokinesis** (decreased activity), the effect of arthritis, or a combination of all these factors. Collagen in older people is less mobile and slower to respond to stretch, although it does stretch (Bernstein-Lewis, 1996). Declines in strength and flexibility lead to poor posture. The most common age-related changes in posture are forward head position, rounded shoulders, increased thoracic kyphosis, decreased lumbar lordosis, increased knee flexion angle, and more posterior hip position (Wagner & Kauffman, 2001; Bonder & Wagner, 2001).

With aging, the skeletal system becomes increasingly more compromised. Loss of bone mass continues and can be related to a wide incidence of osteoporosis in the older adult. **Osteoporosis** is characterized by a reduction of bone mineral density severe enough to increase vulnerability to fractures. This age-related bone loss may be related to the activity level of the individual. Current studies show that moderate exercise, especially weight bearing that delivers a mechanical load to the bone, decreases the rate of bone loss. Osteoarthritis affects 70 percent of people by the age of 70 (Gradisar & Porterfield, 1989).

Summary

Movement production and postural control are made possible through a complex interplay among many subsystems that each develop, mature, and age during an individual's lifetime. The multidimensionality of human movement required during different tasks within varying environments involves a complex set of processes that require successful integration of many subsystems. A person must rely on input from several different systems to effectively move. Somatosensory information is gathered from receptors in the skin, muscles, and joints about the position and motion of the body. Visual information gives feedback about the changing environment; the vestibuloocular reflex is one of many mechanisms that helps to keep the visual image focused during head and body motion. The vestibular system detects position and motion of the head in space, subconsciously helping the body to discriminate whole body movement from movement of the surrounding environment (Sherlock, 1996). The motor system enacts the movement, but only as constantly refined and modulated by feedback received from the individual and the environment. All systems that play a vital role in the production of human movement, including the nervous system itself, develop, mature, and age over the course of the life span.

An appreciation of the systems as dynamic, developmentally changing subsystems, offers the therapist and assistant a broad perspective from which to appreciate the movement problems encountered by patients/clients of any age. Effective assessment and intervention with any patient at any age require that the clinician view each individual patient as presenting with a dynamic set of subsystems, each of which may present at differing points within a unique developmental timeline. It is important to remember that an individual will approach a movement task within a specific environment, calling forth the contributions from several subsystems (the nervous, somatosensory, visual, vestibular, motor, and musculoskeletal systems), which may be at varying stages of maturation and aging or may be compromised by pathology.

References

Adams, J. A. (1971). A closed-loop theory of motor learning. *Journal of Motor Behavior, 3,* 111–150.

Adams, R. D., Victor, M., & Ropper, A. H. (1997). *Principles of neurology* (6th ed.). New York: McGraw-Hill.

Afifi, A. K., & Bergman, R. A. (1998). *Functional neuroanatomy: Text and atlas.* New York: McGraw-Hill.

Antonini, A., & Leenders, K. L. (1993). Dopamine D2 receptors in normal human brain: Effect of age as measured by positron emission tomography (PET) and (11C)-raclopride. *Annals of the New York Academy of Sciences, 695,* 81–85.

Ayres, A. J. (1989). *Sensory integration and praxis tests.* Los Angeles: Western Psychological Services.

Bairstow, P. J., & Laszlow, J. I. (1981). Kinaesthetic sensitivity to passive movement and its relationship to motor development and motor control. *Developmental Medicine and Child Neurology, 23,*606–616.

Ball, M. J. (1977). Neuronal loss, neurofibrillary tangles and granulovacuolar degeneration in the hippocampus with aging and dementia. *Acta Neuropatholigica, 37,* 111–118.

Bear, M. F., Connors, B. W., & Paradiso, M. A. (2001). *Neuroscience: Exploring the brain* (2nd ed.). Baltimore: Lippincott Williams & Wilkins.

Bergstrom, B. (1973). Morphology of the vestibular nerve: The number of myelinated vestibular nerve fibers in man at various ages. *Acta Oto-laryngologica Supplement, 406,* 173–179.

Bernstein, N. (1967). The coordination and regulation of movement. London: Pergaman.

Bernstein-Lewis, C. (1996a). *Aging and the health care challenge* (3rd ed.). Philadelphia: F. A. Davis.

Bernstein-Lewis, C. (1996b). Musculoskeletal changes with age: Clinical implications. In C. Bernstein-Lewis (Ed.), *Aging and the health care challenge* (3rd ed., pp. 147–176). Philadelphia: F. A. Davis.

Black, F. O., & Nashner, L. M. (1985). Postural control in four classes of vestibular abnormalities. In M. Igarshi & F. O. Black (Eds.), *Vestibular and visual control of posture and locomotor equilibrium* (pp. 271–281). Basel: Karger.

Blimkie, C. J. R. (1989). Age and sex associated variation in strength during childhood: Anthropometric, morphologic, neurologic, biomechanical, endocrinologic, genetic, and physical activity correlates. In C. V. Gisolfi & D. R. Lamb (Eds.), *Perspectives in exercise science and sports medicine: Vol. 2. Youth, exercise, and sport* (pp. 183–197). Indianapolis, IN: Benchmark Press.

Bobath, B. (1965). *Abnormal postural reflex activity caused by brain lesions.* London: William Heinemann Medical Books.

Bohannon, R. W. (1996). Clinical implications of neurologic changes during the aging process. In C. Bernstein-Lewis (Ed.), *Aging and the health care challenge* (3rd ed., pp. 177–195). Philadelphia: F. A. Davis.

Bonder, B. R., & Wagner, M. B. (Eds.). (2001). *Functional performance in older adults* (2nd ed.). Philadelphia: F. A. Davis.

Boothe, R. G. (1988). Visual development: Central neural aspects. In E. Meisami & P. S. Tirimas (Eds.), *Handbook of human growth and developmental biology* (Vol. 1, Part B, pp. 179–191). Boca Raton, FL: CRC Press.

Borner, J. A., Dillworth, B. B., & Sullivan, K. M. (1988). Exercise and osteoporosis: A critique of the literature. *Physiotherapy Canada, 40,* 146–155.

Brody, H., & Vijayashanker, N. (1977). Anatomical changes in the nervous system. In C. E. Finch & L. Hayflick (Eds.), *Handbook of biology and aging* (pp. 241–256). New York: Van Nostrand Reinhold.

Bronson, G. W. (1994). Infants' transitions toward adult-like scanning. *Child Development, 65,* 1243–1261.

Brooks, V. B. (1986). *The neural basis of motor control.* New York: Oxford University.

Bruce, M. F. (1980). The relation of tactile thresholds to histology in the fingers of the elderly. *Journal of Neurology, Neurosurgery, and Psychiatry, 43,* 730.

Brunnstrom, S. (1970). Movement therapy in hemiplegia: A neurophysiological approach. New York: Harper & Row.

Buchtal, F., Rosenfalck, A., & Behse, F. (1984). Sensory potentials of normal and diseased nerves. In P. J. Dyck, P. K. Thomas, & E. H. Lambert (Eds.), *Peripheral neuropathy* (Vol. 1, 2nd ed., pp. 981–1015). Philadelphia: W. B. Saunders.

Bundy, A. C., Lane, S. G., & Murray, E. A. (2002). *Sensory integration: Theory and practice* (2nd ed.). Philadelphia: F. A. Davis.

Burt, A. M. (1993). *Textbook of neuroanatomy.* Philadelphia: W. B. Saunders.

Butterworth, G., & Cicchetti, D. (1978). Visual calibration of posture in normal and motor retarded Down's syndrome infants. *Perception, 7,* 513–525.

Case-Smith, J. (1996). Analysis of current motor development theory and recently published infant motor assessments. *Infants & Young Children, 9,* 29–41.

Cech, D., & Martin, S. (1995). *Functional movement development across the life span.* Philadelphia: W.B. Saunders.

Chalifoux, L. M. (1991). Macular degeneration: an overview. *Journal of Visual Impairment & Blindness, 85,* 249.

Coffey, C. E., Wilkinson, W. E., & Parashos, I. A. (1992). Quantitative cerebral anatomy of the aging human brain: a cross-sectional study using magnetic resonance imaging. *Neurology, 42,*527–536.

Cohen, H. (1989). Occupational therapy and motor control. *American Journal of Occupational Therapy, 43,* 5, 289–290.

Cohen, H. (1994). Vestibular rehabilitation improves daily life function. *American Journal of Occupational Therapy, 48,* 919–925.

Cohen, H. (1999). *Neuroscience for rehabilitation* (2nd ed.). Philadelphia: Lippincott Williams & Wilkins.

Collier, G. (1985). *Emotional expression.* Hillsdale, NJ: Lawrence Erlbaum Associates.

Collins, J. K. (1976). Distance perception as a function of age. *Australian Journal of Psychology, 28,* 109–113.

Connor, N. P., & Abbs, J. H. (1990). Sensorimotor contributions of the basal ganglia: Recent advances. *Physical Therapy, 70,* 12, 864–872.

Cotman, C. W., & Holets, V. R. (1985). Structural changes at synapses with age: Plasticity and regeneration. In C.E. Finch & E. L. Schneider (Eds.), *Handbook of the biology of aging* (pp. 617–644). New York: Van Nostrand Reinhold.

Crelin, E. S. (1981). Development of the musculoskeletal system. *Clinical Symposia, 33,* 2–36.

deBenabib, R. M., & Nelson, C. A. (1991). Efficiency in visual skills and postural control: A dynamic interaction. *Occupational Therapy Practice, 3,* 57–68.

DeKeyser, J., Ebinger, G., & Vauquelin, G. (1990). Age-related changes in the human nigrostriatal dopaminergic system. *Annals of Neurology, 27,* 157–161.

DiGiovanna, A. G. (1994). *Human aging: Biological perspectives.* New York: McGraw-Hill.

Drubach, D. (2000). *The brain explained.* Upper Saddle River, NJ: Prentice-Hall.

Duara, R., London, E. D., & Rapoport, S. I. (1985). Changes in structure and energy metabolism of the aging brain. In C. E. Finch & E. L. Schneider (Eds.), *Handbook of the biology of aging* (pp. 595–616). New York: Van Nostrand Reinhold.

Earnest, M. P., Heaton, R. K., & Wilkinson, W. E. (1986). Cortical atrophy, ventricular enlargement and intellectual impairment in the aged. *Acta Physiologica Scandinavia, 126,* 107–114.

Eviatar, L., Eviatar, A., & Naray, I. (1974). Maturation of neurovestibular responses in infants. *Developmental Medicine and Child Neurology, 16,* 435–446.

Fantz, R. L. (1961). The origin of form perception. *Scientific American, 204,* 66.

Fisher, A.G., & Murray, E.A. (1991). Introduction to sensory integration theory. In A.G. Fisher, E. A. Murray, & A. C. Bundy (Eds.), *Sensory integration: Theory and practice.* Philadelphia: F. A. Davis.

Fisher, A. G., Murray, E. A., & Bundy, A. C. (1991). *Sensory integration: Theory and practice.* Philadelphia: F. A. Davis.

Frontera, W. R., Hughes, V. A., Fielding, R. A., Fiatarone M. A., Evans W. J., & Roubenoff R.(2000). Aging of skeletal muscle: A 12-year longitudinal study. *Journal of Applied Physiology, 88,* 1321–1326.

Furman, J. M., & Whitney, S. L. (2000). Central causes of dizziness. *Physical Therapy, 80,* 179–187.

Gajdosik, C. G., & Gajdosik, R. L. (2000). Musculoskeletal development and adaptation. In S. K. Campbell, D. W. Vander Linden, & R. J. Palisano, (Eds.), *Physical therapy for children* (2nd ed.). Philadelphia: W. B. Saunders.

Gallahue, D. L., & Ozmun, J. C. (2002). *Understanding motor development: Infants, children, adolescents, adults* (5th ed.). Boston: McGraw-Hill.

Ghez, C. (1991). Voluntary movement. In E. Kandel, J. H. Schwartz, & T. M. Jessell (Eds.), *Principles of neuroscience* (3rd ed., pp. 609–625). New York: Elsevier.

Gilman, S., & Newman, S. W. (1996). *Essentials of clinical neuroanatomy and neurophysiology.* (9th ed.). Philadelphia: F. A. Davis.

Goldman, P.S., & Galkin, T. W. (1978). Prenatal removal of frontal association cortex in the fetal rhesus monkey: Anatomical and functional consequences in postnatal life. *Brain Research, 152,* 451-485.

Gottfried, A. W. (1984). Touch as an organizer for learning and development. In C. C. Brown (Ed.), *The many facets of touch* (pp. 114–122). Skillman, NJ: Johnson & Johnson.

Gradisar, I. A., & Porterfield, J. A. (1989). Articular cartilage: Structure and function. *Topics in Geriatric Rehabilitation, 4,* 1–9.

Grimby, G, Danneskiold-Samsoe, B., Hvid, K., & Saltin, B. (1982). Morphology and enzymatic capacity in arm and leg muscles in 78-81 year old men and women. *Acta Physiologica Scandinavia, 115,* 125–134.

Hain, T. C., Ramaswamy, T. S., & Hillman, M. A. (2000). Anatomy and physiology of the normal vestibular system. In S. J. Herdman (Ed.), *Vestibular rehabilitation* (2nd ed.) Philadelphia: F. A. Davis.

Haines, D. E. (Ed.). (1997). *Fundamental neuroscience.* New York: Churchill Livingstone.

Hasselkus, B. R. (1974). Aging and the human nervous system. *Journal of Occupational Therapy, 28,* 16–21.

Herdman, S. J. (2000). *Vestibular rehabilitation* (2nd ed.). Philadelphia: F. A. Davis.

Heriza, C. (1991). Implications of a dynamical systems approach to understanding infant kicking behavior. *Physical Therapy, 71,* 222–234.

Heriza, C. (1991). Motor development: traditional and contemporary theories. In M. Lister (Ed.), *Contemporary management of motor control problems. Proceedings of the II-Step Conference.* (pp. 99–126). Alexandria, VA: Foundation for Physical Therapy.

Herschkowitz, N. (1989). Brain development and nutrition. In P. Evard & A. Minkowski (Eds.), *Developmental neurobiology* (Nestle Nutrition Workshop Series Vol. 12). New York: Raven Press.

Hodgins, J. (1963). Reaction time and speed of movement in males and females of various ages. *Research Quarterly, 34,* 335–343.

Hooker, D. (1952). *The prenatal origin of behavior.* Lawrence, KS: University of Kansas Press.

Hooyman, N. R., & Kiyak, H. A. (Eds.) (1991). *Social gerontology: A multidisciplinary perspective* (2nd ed.). Needham Heights, MA: Allyn & Bacon.

Horak, F. (1991). Assumptions underlying motor control for neurologic rehabilitation. In M. Lister (Ed.), *Contemporary management of motor control problems. Proceedings of the II-Step Conference* (pp. 11–27). Alexandria, VA: Foundation for Physical Therapy.

Hubel, D. H. (1988). *Eye, brain and vision.* New York: Scientific American.

Humphrey, T. (1965). The embryologic differentiation of the vestibular nuclei in man correlated with functional development. In *International symposium on vestibular and oculomotor problems.* Tokyo: 51.

Jacobs, B., & Scheibel, A. B. (1993). A quantitative dendritic analysis of Wernicke's area in humans: Lifespan changes. *Journal of Comparative Neurology, 327,* 83–96.

Janeschild, M. E. (1996). Integrating the dynamical systems theory with the neurodevelopmental approach. *Developmental Disabilities Special Interest Newsletter, 19,* 1–4.

Kaga, K., Maeda, H., & Suzuki, J. (1988). Development of righting reflexes, gross motor responses and balance in infants and labyrinth hypoactivity with or without mental retardation. *Advances in Oto-rhino-laryngology, 41,* 152–161.

Katzman, R., & Terry, R. D. (1983). Normal aging of the nervous system. In R. Katzman & R. D. Terry (Eds.), *The neurology of aging* (pp. 15–50). Philadelphia: F. A. Davis.

Kemper, T. (1984). Neuroanatomical and neuropathological changes in normal aging and dementia. In M. L. Albert (Ed.), *The neurology of aging.* Philadelphia: F. A. Davis.

Keogh, J., & Sugden, D. (1985). *Movement skill development.* New York: Macmillan.

Kollarits, C. R. (1986). The aging eye. In E. Calkins, P. J. Davis, & A. B. Ford (Eds.), *The practice of geriatrics.* (pp. 248–259). Philadelphia: W. B. Saunders.

Konigsmark, B. W., & Murphy, E. A. (1970). Neuronal population in the human brain. *Nature, 228,* 1335–1336.

Koroshetz, W. J., & Moskowitz, M. A. (1996). Emerging treatments for stroke in humans. *Trends in Pharmacological Sciences, 17,* 227–233.

Larin, H. M. (2000). Motor learning: Theories and strategies for the practitioner. In S. K. Campbell, D. W. Vander Linden, & R. J. Palisano, *Physical therapy for children* (2nd ed.). Philadelphia: W. B. Saunders.

Larsson, L., Grimby, G., & Karlsson, J. (1982). Muscle strength and speed of movement in relation to age and muscle morphology. *Journal of Applied Physiology, 46,* 451–456.

Leonard, C. T. (1994). Major behavior and neural changes following perinatal and adult-onset brain damage: Implications for therapeutic interventions. *Physical Therapy, 74,* 753–767.

Leonard, C. T. (1998). *The neuroscience of human movement.* St. Louis, MO: Mosby.

LeVere, T. E. (1980). Recovery of function after brain damage: A theory of the behavioral deficit. *Physiology and Psychology, 8,* 297–308.

Lowrey, G. H. (1986). *Growth and development of children* (8th ed.) Chicago: Year Book.

Lundy-Ekman, L. (2002). *Neuroscience: Fundamentals for rehabilitation.* Philadelphia: W. B. Saunders.

Maguire, G. H. (1996). The changing realm of the senses. In C. Bernstein-Lewis (Ed.), *Aging: The health care challenge* (3rd ed.). Philadelphia: F. A. Davis.

Malina, R. M. (1986). Growth of muscle and muscle mass. In F. Falkner & J. M. Tanner (Eds.), *Human growth: A comprehensive treatise: Vol. 2. Postnatal growth* (pp. 77–99). New York: Plenum Press.

Malina, R. M., & Bouchard, C. (1991). *Growth, maturation, and physical activity.* Champaign, IL: Human Kinetics.

Marsh, A. P., & Geel, S. E. (2000). The effect of age on the attentional demands of postural control. *Gait and Posture, July*, 105–113.

McClenaghan, B. A., Williams, H. G., Dickerson, J., Dowda, M., Thombs, L., & Eleazer, P. (1995). Spectral characteristics of aging postural control. *Gait and Posture, 4*, 112–121.

McComas, A. J., Upton, A. R., & Sica, R. E. (1973). Motoneurone disease and aging. *Lancet*, 1477–1480.

McKeough, D. (1995). *The coloring review of neuroscience* (2nd ed.). Boston: Little, Brown.

Meltzoff, A. N., & Borton, R. (1979). Intermodal matching by human neonates. *Nature, 282*, 403–404.

Milani-Comparetti, A. (1981). The neurophysiological and clinical implications of studies on fetal motor behavior. *Seminars in Perinatology, 5*, 183–189.

Moore, K. L. (1988). *The developing human: Clinically oriented embryology* (4th ed.) Philadelphia: W. B. Saunders.

Morgan, D. G. (1989). Consideration in the treatment of neurological disorders with trophic factors. *Neurobiology of Aging, 10*, 547–549.

Mortimer, J. A., Pirozzolo, F. J., & Maletta, G. J. (1982). Overview of the aging motor system. In F. J. Pirozzolo & G. J. Maletta (Eds.), *The aging motor system* (pp. 1–6). New York: Praeger Publishers.

Nelson, L. B., Rubin, S. E., Wagner, R. S. (1984). Developmental aspects in the assessment of visual function in young children. *Pediatrics, 73*, 375–381.

Papalia, D. E., Olds, S., & Feldman, R. (2001). *Human development* (8th ed.). New York: McGraw-Hill.

Pitts, D. G. (1982). Visual acuity as a function of age. *Journal of the American Optometric Association, 53*, 117–124.

Piaget, J. (1952). *The origins of intelligence*. New York: W. W. Norton.

Poole, J. L. (1991). Age related changes in sensory system dynamics related to balance. *Physical & Occupational Therapy in Geriatrics, 10*, 55–66.

Potvin, A. R., Syndulko, K., & Tourtellotte, W. W. (1980). Human neurologic function and the aging process. *Journal of the American Geriatric Society, 28*, 1–9.

Prechtl, H. F. R. (1985). Ultrasound studies of human fetal behaviour. *Early Human Development, 12*, 91–98.

Raub, D. M., & Smith, E. L. (1985). Exercise and aging: Effects on bone. *Topics in Geriatric Rehabilitation, 1*, 31–39.

Rikli, R., & Busch, S. (1986). Motor performance of women as a function of age and physical activity level. *Journal of Gerontology, 41*, 645–649.

Rosenhall, U., & Rubin, W. (1975). Degenerative changes in the human vestibular sensory epithelia. *Acta Oto-laryngologica, 79*, 67–80.

Sahrmann, S. (1998). The twenty-ninth Mary McMillan lecture: Moving precisely? Or taking the path of least resistance? *Physical Therapy, 78*(11), 1208–1218.

Schmidt, R. A. (1975). A schema theory of discrete motor skill learning. *Psychological Review 82*, 225–260.

Schmidt, R. A. (1988). *Motor control and learning* (2nd ed.). Champaign, IL: Human Kinetics.

Schmitz, T. J. (2001). Sensory assessment. In S. B. O'Sullivan & T. J. Schmitz (Eds.), *Physical rehabilitation: Assessment and treatment* (4th ed., pp. 133–175). Philadelphia: F. A. Davis.

Schultz, E., & Lipton, B. H. (1982). Skeletal muscle satellite cells: Changes in proliferation potential as a function of age. *Mechanisms of Aging and Development, 20*, 377–383.

Sherlock, J. (1996). Getting into balance. *Rehabilitation Management, Dec/Jan*, 33–36.

Sherrington, C.S. (1906). *The integrative action of the nervous system*. New Haven, CT: Yale University Press.

Shumway-Cook, A., & Woollacott, M. (2001). *Motor control: Theory and practical applications* (2nd ed.). Philadelphia: Lippincott Williams & Wilkins.

Stedman's concise medical dictionary for the health professions (4th ed.). (2001). Philadelphia: Lippincott Williams & Wilkins.

Steiness, I. (1957). Vibratory perception in normal subjects. *Acta Medica Scandinavica, 158*, 315–325.

Stelmach, G. E., Zelaznik, H. N., & Lowe, D. (1990). The influence of aging and attentional demands on recovery from postural instability. *Aging, 2*, 155–161.

Stokes, M. *Neurological physiotherapy*. (1998). London: Mosby International Limited.

Stout, J. L. (2000). Physical fitness during childhood and adolescence. In S. K. Campbell, D. W. Vander Linden, & R. J. Palisano (Eds.), *Physical therapy for children* (2nd ed.). Philadelphia: W. B. Saunders.

Sugden, D. A. (1986). The development of proprioceptive control. In H. T. A. Whiting & M. G. Wade (Eds.), *Themes in motor development* (pp. 21–39). Boston: Nijhoff.

Sullivan, E. V., March, L., Mathalon, D. H., Lim, K. O., & Pfefferbaum, A. (1995). Age-related decline in MRI volumes of temporal lobe gray matter but not hippocampus. *Neurobiology of Aging, 16*, 591–606.

Taber's cyclopedic medical dictionary (2001). Philadelphia: F. A. Davis.

Thelen, E., & Fogel, A. (1989). Toward an action based theory of infant development. In J. Lockman & N. Hazen (Eds.). *Action in social context* (pp. 23–63). New York: Plenum.

Thelen, E., Kelso, S., & Fogel, A. (1987). Self-organizing systems and infant motor development. *Development Review, 39–65*.

Timiras, P. (1994). Aging of the skeleton, joints and muscles. In P. S. Timiras (Ed.), *Physiological basis of aging and geriatrics* (2nd ed.). Ann Arbor, MI: CRS.

Tse, D. W., & Spaulding, S. J. (1998). Review of motor control and motor learning: implications for occupational therapy with individuals with Parkinson's disease. *Physical & Occupational Therapy in Geriatrics, 15*, 19–38.

Unsworth, C., & Warburg, C. L. (2001). Assessment and intervention strategies for cognitive and perceptual dysfunction. In S. B. O'Sullivan & T. J. Schmitz (Eds.), *Physical rehabilitation: Assessment and treatment* (4th ed., pp. 133–175). Philadelphia: F. A. Davis.

VanderLaan, F. L., & Oosterveld, W. J. (1974). Age and vestibular function. *Aerospace Medicine, 45*, 540–547.

VanderZanden, J. W. (2000). T. J. Crandell & C. H. Crandell (Eds.), *Human development* (7th ed.). Boston: McGraw-Hill.

VanSant, A. (1990). Life-span development in functional tasks. *Physical Therapy, 70*, 788–798.

Verillo, R. T. (1980). Age-related changes to the sensitivity of vibration. *Journal of Gerontology, 35*, 185–193.

Wade, M. G., & Jones, G. (1997). The role of vision and spatial orientation in the maintenance of posture. *Physical Therapy, 77*, 619–627.

Wagner, M. B., & Kauffman, T. L. (2001). The aging process: mobility. In B. R. Bonder & M. B. Wagner (Eds.), *Functional performance in older adults* (2nd ed.). Philadelphia: F. A. Davis.

Waxman, S. (2000). *Correlative Neuroanatomy* (24th ed.). New York: McGraw-Hill.

Weale, R. A. (1975). Senile changes in visual acuity. *Transactions of the Ophthalmology Society of the United Kingdom, 95*, 36–38.

Weber, R. (1984). Philosophers on touch. In C. C. Brown, *The many facets of touch* (p. 3). Skillman, NJ: Johnson & Johnson.

Welford, A. T. (1958). *Aging and human skill*. Oxford: Oxford University Press.

Welford, A. T. (1977). Motor performance. In J. E. Birren & K. W. Schaie (Eds.), *Handbook of the psychology of aging*. New York: Van Nostrand.

Whitbourne, S. K. (1985). *The aging body-physiological changes and psychological consequences*. New York: Springer-Verlag.

Williams, G. N., Higgins, M. J., & Lewek, M. D. (2002). Aging skeletal muscle physiologic changes and the effects of training. *Physical Therapy, 82*, 62–68.

Williams, H. G. (1983). *Perceptual and motor development.* Englewood Cliffs, NJ: Prentice Hall.

Williams, H. G. (1990). Aging and eye-hand coordination. In C. Bard, M. Fleury, & L. Hay (Eds.), *Development of eye-hand coordination.* (pp. 327–357).Columbia, SC: University of South Carolina Press.

Woollacott, M. J. (1993). Age-related changes in posture and movement. *Journal of Gerontology 48,* 56–60.

Woollacott, M., Shumway-Cook, A., & Nashner, L. (1982). Postural reflexes and aging. In F. J. Pirozzolo & G. J. Maletta (Eds.), *The aging motor system* (pp. 99–119). New York: Praeger Publishers.

Woollacott, M. H., Shumway-Cook, A., & Nashner, L. M. (1986). Aging and posture control: changes in sensory organization and muscular coordination. *International Journal of Aging and Human Development, 23,* 97–114.

Wyke, B. (1975). The neurological basis of movement: a developmental review. In K. S. Holt (Ed.), *Movement and child development* (pp. 19–33). Philadelphia: J. B. Lippincott.

Yonas, A., Granrud, C. E., & Pettersen, L. (1985). Infants: sensitivity to relative size information at distance. *Developmental Psychology, 21,* 161–167.

Zastrow, C., & Kirst-Ashman, K. K. (1997). *Understanding human behavior and the social environment* (4th ed.). Chicago: Nelson-Hall.

Life Span Motor Development

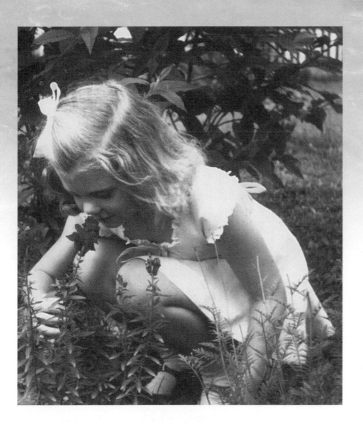

The gift of physical movement offers us the opportunity to either reach toward the stars or stoop to sniff a spring flower: Opportunities and blessings abound. This chapter is dedicated to my mentor and friend, Bonnie Marsden, PT. She taught me the value of keen observation and tireless inquiry, so that I would be challenged to always give my best, stay inquisitive, and therefore be delighted with my work. Thank you, Bonnie.

Cornerstone Concepts

▢ Motor development as a lifelong nonlinear process generally divided into the phases of early development, maturation (infancy, childhood, and adolescence), maturity (adulthood), and aging

▢ Overview of classic development theories: Piaget, Erikson, and neuromaturational; dynamic system perspective on motor development and therapeutic intervention

▢ Current usefulness of motor milestone charts and developmental milestones

▢ Functional movement components needed for upper and lower extremity control and postural control

▢ Development during infancy and childhood as a process model

▢ Major developmental changes in upper and lower extremity control and postural control encountered during maturation, maturity, and aging

Introduction

Physical and occupational therapists have historically studied human motor development as a keystone concept guiding assessment and intervention with patients/clients with neurological or developmental disabilities. Traditionally, the study of motor development focused on the development of the child and acquired motor components were then presented as milestones, hallmarks of "normal" or typical motor development. Developmental change was thought to correlate only with maturation of the central nervous system (CNS). This narrow view has now been expanded because it has been realized that the nervous system is not the only system that determines developmental change. As detailed in the previous chapter, changes in other systems, such as the musculoskeletal and sensory systems, also influence motor development. Each system interacts with each other, within the environment, in complex and fascinating ways to effect changes in motor behavior that continue throughout the life span. Movement expression, then, comes about as a result of all the convergent influences and changes acting on the individual at any point, as that individual moves to perform a task within a specific environmental context.

Development can be thought of as a change in form and function, where form and function are intertwined (Cech & Martin, 1995; Higgins, 1985). The form a movement takes is largely determined by the function for which it is intended. Simultaneously, the function, which emerges or becomes possible, is largely dependent on the available forms of movement and the developmental phase of the structures. Development is not simply growth. Developmental changes occur through the processes of growth, maturation, adaptation, and learning. **Growth** refers to an increase in size and weight—changes in the physical dimensions of the body (Cech & Martin, 1995). Growth is an important parameter of developmental change because some changes are linked to changes in body size; for example, a taller child can typically jump and throw farther than a small toddler. **Maturation** is an increase in complexity within body systems, allowing for more sophisticated functioning. Maturation includes such processes as the myelination of nerves, increasing complexity of internal organs, and emergence of secondary sexual characteristics. **Adaptation** occurs secondary to stimuli placed on the system, such as the modeling that occurs within bone secondary to muscle pull. Remember the life span changes of the muscular and skeletal systems as described in the previous chapter. **Learning** can certainly be considered as a type of adaptation, resulting in a relatively permanent change in behavior, usually as a result of practice. Growth, maturation, adaptation, and learning all contribute to an ongoing developmental change process that unfolds over the course of the life span of each one of us. All the systems that contribute to human movement production grow, mature, change, and adapt over the course of developmental time (Cech & Martin, 1995). The number of influences on a moving human being are tremendous, including all the influences within the individual, the environment, and pertaining to the task to be performed. Reflect on the information presented in the previous chapter and try to integrate that information along with the new information to be presented in this chapter.

Definition of Motor Development

Motor development is the process of change in motor behavior that is related to the age of the individual. A life span approach to the study of motor development assumes that age-related change in motor behavior is an ongoing, lifelong phenomenon, hallmarked by the consideration of all the processes and factors that contribute to these age-related changes. Contrary to traditional views of motor development, this contemporary view on motor development sees maturity not as a pinnacle reached, after which decline occurs, but rather as a passing point in time, to be valued no more or less than infancy, adolescence, or any other age periods (VanSant, 1990). Motor development is a dynamic, nonlinear process, occurring within a self-organizing system. Development proceeds in a continuous but spiral rather than linear fashion, with relative periods of stability and instability (Heriza, 1991). This current view is consistent with a dynamic systems approach.

Life Span Perspective on Motor Development

As described in the previous chapter, all the subsystems of the movement system develop, mature, and age over time. Motor development unfolds through an ongoing interaction between intrinsic and extrinsic factors. Intrinsic factors include variables within all the continually developing systems as described in Chapter 3 (somatosensory, visual, vestibular, musculoskeletal, and so forth), whereas extrinsic factors include such variables as culture, environment, and socioeconomic factors. A life span view on motor development encompasses any change in movement abilities that occurs across the span of life, from infancy through old age. VanSant (1990) aptly describes this viewpoint by describing the following. Consider the intrinsic factor of physical growth. We grow taller and heavier as we move from infancy through childhood and adolescence and into adulthood. During adolescence, body shape changes; in the middle adult years, body shape may change again. Later in the life span, during aging, height and weight typically decrease. Additional examples of intrinsic factors affecting motor development are the loss in flexibility experienced by adolescents during growth spurts and the increase in muscular endurance and power experienced by young men during their 20s. As detailed in Chapter 3, progressive, as well as regressive, changes are a natural part of any stage of the life span. All these changes contribute to certain movement capabilities and constraints, as seen in the individual's movement expression at a particular age stage.

Extrinsic factors also vary systematically with age. Extrinsic factors that affect age-related change in motor behavior are as dynamically related to age as are intrinsic factors. Early in life, children make transitions from drinking while cradled in their mothers' arms to drinking independently from a cup. Such transitions create the opportunity for the development of different motor behaviors. On the other hand, old age may bring along other age-related changes in lifestyle and activity patterns that affect motor behaviors. The influences of culture, opportunity afforded by socioeconomic condition, and the environment can all extrinsically (externally) affect motor behavior.

Clinical Connection:

An interesting current example of how extrinsic factors affect motor development is the following. Recently it has been recommended that parents avoid allowing infants to sleep in a prone position to decrease the incidence of sudden infant death syndrome. Because this practice is now so widely followed, children attain the motor skill of rolling prone to supine at a later age than previously, when prone positioning was commonplace for young babies. Interestingly, motor development charts may soon begin to reflect this change, with the expectation for rolling occurring at a later age than before.

A life span perspective on motor development offers the opportunity to examine a broad range of change processes. Baltes (1987) recognized four key characteristics that identify a theoretical approach as having a life span perspective:

- *Development is lifelong.* Each period of life is influenced by what has happened before and will affect what is to come. Each period has its own unique characteristics and value; none is more or less important than the other. Individual rates of change are variable. Motor skills can change in response to different physical, cognitive, or environmental requirements. Each of us has lifelong opportunities for learning.
- *Development depends on history and is contextual.* Each individual develops within a specific time and set of circumstances. Individuals do not only respond to their physical and social environments but also interact with and change them.
- *Development is multidimensional and multidirectional.* Throughout life, development is a constant interplay between growth and decline, regression and progression. As growth or progression occurs in one area, perhaps a decline or regression occurs in another.

Regressive changes are not always to be viewed as negative, nor are progressive changes to be always assumed to be positive. Individuals have a tremendous capacity to maximize gains and minimize losses through adaptation and learned compensation.
- *Development is plastic and flexible.* The ability to change, adapt, and learn is available at different levels throughout life (Papalia, Olds, & Feldman, 2001).

Motor development, similar to what has been demonstrated in cognitive and visual development, has **sensitive periods,** times when the individual is more sensitive to certain kinds of stimulation. Normal development in later periods may be hindered if a child fails to receive the proper stimulation during a sensitive period. For example, inadequate nutrition, inconsistent parenting, or inadequate environmental influences may have a negative impact on development if they occur early in life rather than at a later age. This concept of sensitive periods has important implications for therapeutic intervention. It suggests that appropriate intervention during a specific period tends to facilitate more positive forms of development at later stages than if the same intervention occurs at a later time. Although this concept of sensitive periods deserves important consideration, it is also crucial to remember that sensitive periods should not be too narrowly defined. A sensitive period is not a universal point in time. It is rather to be applied as a broad guideline, accounting for individual differences and for specific environmental circumstances. The human organism is also tremendously resilient, able to adapt and change in response to demands placed on it. As highlighted in Chapters 2 and 3, the human nervous system is incredibly adaptable and flexible, as illustrated by the parallel distributed processing that occurs at all levels within the CNS. This redundancy and resiliency are important features to remember when working with an individual with neurological impairments.

Clinical Relevance

The changes that occur over the life span of an individual are nothing short of remarkable. At birth, the infant needs full support for all life-sustaining needs to be met. By only the first birthday, an impressive amount of functional independence has developed. Throughout childhood, more and more independence and mastery over the environment emerge. This natural pattern of progression toward functional independence and mastery over the environment offers a useful guide for therapists and assistants when assessing and engaging patients/clients in interventions designed to promote independence. In physical and occupational therapy, an understanding of the natural process by which physical independence is acquired facilitates assessment and intervention with the patient with an impairment and functional challenge encountered at any age stage (VanSant & Goldberg, 1999). It is crucial that therapists and assistants have an understanding of how physical functioning changes over time, the relationship of physical function to other domains of function, and the components of physical function that contribute to the quality and efficiency of movement (Cech & Martin, 1995).

Review of Motor Development Theories

Development theories can be classified into three broad categories: cognitive, neuromaturational, and dynamic systems. A review of the main tenets and an overview of their history have clinical, as well as academic, value for clinicians and students. Although this text focuses mainly on the movement system, in order to be thorough and complete, it is crucial to include a review of cognitive theories, because cognition and personality certainly have a tremendous effect on all aspects of human movement behavior.

Cognitive Theories

There are two main cognitive theories on development that have broad implications for application by physical and occupational therapists. Although the cognitive system is not a focal point in this text, an appreciation of these theories is important for clinicians as they treat individuals at various times in the life span. As individuals struggle to define themselves and their role in society, the issues at different phases of the life span will have an affect on self-esteem, perceived independence, and mobility, especially when an individual encounters an impairment issue during any period of the life span. Because clinicians will work with individuals of many different ages, an active learning experience in the companion workbook offers the reader an opportunity to understand the relevance of appreciating the main concepts of cognitive theory and applying these concepts to interactions with patients/clients.

▪ Piaget

Through a study of his own children, Piaget developed a theory of intelligence whereby cognitive development is divided into four discreet stages (Piaget, 1952):

- *Sensorimotor stage: birth until age 2.* This stage is characterized predominantly by sensorimotor experience, allowing the infant to develop schemas (see Glossary) by associating sensory experiences with physical action. Repetition in action is a major factor at this stage, as is imitation and experimentation.
- *Preoperational stage or stage of representational thought: age 2 through 7.* The child now starts to represent the world by symbols, hallmarked by significant advances in language as symbolism for thought. Logical one-way thought processes develop during this stage.
- *Concrete operations: age 7 through 11.* During this stage, children develop the ability to classify objects according to their characteristics and to solve concrete problems. Thinking is mostly concrete, bound by stimulus and experience.
- *Formal operations: throughout adolescence.* This highest form of cognitive development allows for individuals to effectively deal with hypothetical, as well as concrete, situations. The ability to generate a hypothesis, demonstrate deductive reasoning, and engage in creative problem solving and decision making are all evidence of formal operations.

The impact of Piaget on physical and occupational therapy is significant. It is vital to include problem-solving activities within the intervention setting to assist in the cognitive and motivational aspects of facilitating motor development. Piaget reminds clinicians that movement does not occur spontaneously or without purpose (Rainville, 1999). Movement and purposeful activity are subservient to each other. Occupationally embedded activity and meaningfulness directly affect motor performance (see Chapter 5).

▪ Erikson

Erikson described the developmental stages that a person goes through to establish personality. He linked each of eight stages to chronological age, with each stage characterized by a conflict between two opposite traits. The eight stages are summarized in Table 4–1. Therapists and assistants working with individuals at different times of the life span should be sensitive to what primary developmental tasks are the main focuses at that age stage. For example, an appreciation of the importance of feeling purposeful and worthwhile throughout the adult years, when adults are actively solving the conflict between **generativity** (being worthwhile) and self-absorption, can sensitize therapists and families to the emotional, difficult issues being faced by an adult with a disability.

Neuromaturational Development Theories

Gesell first formulated the principle of developmental direction in 1954 as a means of explaining increasing coordination and motor control as a function of the maturing nervous system. Through observations, Gesell (1954) noted that an orderly, predictable sequence of physical development proceeds from the head to the feet (cephalocaudal) and from the center of the body to its periphery (proximodistal).

Gesell also is responsible for using the term **reciprocal interweaving** as descriptive of the spiraling process of development, made up of periods that alternate between states of equilibrium and disequilibrium. Periods of equilibrium are marked by fairly stable behavior, whereas periods of disequilibrium are marked by instability (Cech & Martin, 1995). He describes the process of coordinated and progressive intricate interweaving of opposing muscle groups into an increasingly mature relationship. Neuromaturational theory proposes that this reciprocal interweaving is a characteristic of motor development in children. The neuromotor maturation that occurs is evidenced through increased functional complexity, where motor and sensory mechanisms differentiate and integrate to interact with one another (Gallahue & Ozmun, 2002).

TABLE 4–1

Erikson's Eight Stages of Personality Development: Implications for Therapists and Assistants

Erikson's Psychosocial Stage	Age Stage	Developmental Task	Important Influences	Implications for Therapists and Assistants
Trust vs. mistrust	0–18 mo	Attachment; developing trust in self, parents, and world	Involved caregivers with loving interaction	Development of trust allows for interest in world and ability to explore it; very important for infant to feel secure and safe, including while practicing new movement skills.
Autonomy vs. shame and doubt	18 mo to 2–3 y	Developing feeling of control over behavior; realizing that intentions can be acted out; beginning independence and learning of self-control	Supportive parents and caregivers; therapist who is supportive, firm, but not threatening	As children become mobile, acting out becomes possible; imitation and modeling of others and supportive parents crucial at this time; caregivers, including therapists, should set reasonable limits.
Initiative vs. guilt	2–3 y to 6 y	Developing a sense of self and responsibility for one's own actions; initiates own activity; a time when active exploration can be either encouraged or made to produce guilt	Supportive parents, caregivers, and therapists	Children need to be able to make some decisions and exercise some choices regarding activity; activities need to have a purpose and direction; therapist should allow children some degree of choice in activity.
Industry vs. inferiority	6–11 y	Developing sense of self-worth through interaction with peers; works on projects for recognition; develops mastery and competence	Encouraging educational setting and supportive teachers, caregivers, and therapists	Children need to participate in therapy program choices, including goals; children should be allowed to record their own participation and progress and note achievements in competence; therapist can set up incentive programs to reward compliance; remember to accentuate the ability not the disability.

(Continued on following page)

TABLE 4–1

Erikson's Eight Stages of Personality Development: Implications for Therapists and Assistants (*Continued*)

Erikson's Psychosocial Stage	Age Stage	Developmental Task	Important Influences	Implications for Therapists and Assistants
Identity vs. identity diffusion or role confusion	11 y–late adolescence	Developing a strong sense of identity; selecting from among many potential selves	Supportive caregivers and teachers, role models, and peers	Self-esteem and body image are key issues; exploration of available vocational choices occurs.
Intimacy vs. isolation	Young adulthood	Developing close relationships with others; intimacy and partnership; working toward establishing a career	Supportive peers, colleagues, family (including spouse and children), society, community	Continuing concern regarding self-esteem and sexuality; some degree of vocational success is important.
Generativity vs. self-absorption or stagnation	Adulthood	Assuming responsible adult roles in community; being worthwhile; looking beyond oneself and embracing future generations	Supportive peers, colleagues, family (including spouse and children), society, community	Important time to include adult in exerting some guiding influence for the next generation, community, and social leadership roles.
Integrity vs. despair	Older adulthood	Coming to terms with meaning of life; facing mortality and potential despair; feeling satisfaction with one's life	Supportive family (spouse, children, other relatives), friends; religious and community support	Need for a sense of wholeness and vitality, wisdom, and respect from others, especially younger persons.

Source: Adapted from Porr, S. M., & Rainville, E. B. (1999). *Pediatric therapy: A systems approach* (p. 87). Philadelphia: F. A. Davis.

This theory has encountered criticism in recent years, because it is now appreciated that a strict developmental sequence or direction should not be viewed as hierarchically operational at all levels of development or for all individuals. We now know that this observed tendency toward developmental direction is not exclusively a function of nervous system maturation, as Gesell originally thought. It is due, at least in part, to the developmental changes of many systems and the demands of the task itself within a unique environment. For example, the task demands for upright walking are greater than those for creeping on all fours. It is mechanically and posturally easier to creep than to walk. The apparent cephalocaudal progression in development is not only due to maturation of the systems but also to the performance demands of the task itself.

Neuromaturational theory viewed development as occurring along a sequence of stages, with reflexes as the basic building block of movement. Gesell believed that neural maturation was the primary catalyst for developmental change and the development of postural control. New insights dispute this simplistic view, recognizing the complexity and adaptability of the human nervous system. If in fact the development of

postural control were simply a matter of neuromaturation, therapeutic intervention would most certainly have a limited effect on recovery. Neuromaturational theories, pioneered by Gesell's work, were an important steppingstone in the applied neuroscience knowledge base. These theories resulted in the development of important tests of motor milestones and have had a profound influence in the area of diagnosis of developmental delay. Therapists today are urged not to "throw the baby out with the bath water" by disregarding the valuable assessment and intervention insights and tools that emerged from these theorists. Functional outcomes, we now know, are dependent on a much more complex set of interdependent variables, bringing us to today's contemporary views.

Dynamic Systems Perspective on Motor Development

The previously presented theories all offer a stage or phase view of studying development. It is now understood that development is never static, with discrete stages of change and then relative stability. It is also now accepted that development does not occur on a hierarchical timeline but rather across systems, with a continually changing and adaptable individual functioning within an ever-changing environment. It is typical, however, that the use of academic stages or phases continues to offer a user-friendly concept for understanding development. Although contemporary views appear to criticize the use of artificial stages, the reader is advised not to totally disregard the value of that academic model, but rather to use it as a framework from which to step back and view the larger and more complex picture.

A dynamic systems approach provides a more holistic approach to the understanding of human motor development. This theory, as discussed in Chapter 3, suggests that control of movement is the result of many contributing subsystems working together dynamically. Coordination of movement, and therefore motor development, is affected by several factors, including arousal, neurological status, musculoskeletal factors, sensory status, and environmental factors. The model implies that no one factor has greater influence than the others, but that all systems interact in such a way that motor behavior emerges that is not specific to any one set of subsystems. This ability of the systems to self-organize is a dynamic characteristic of such a nonlinear system. In a self-organizing system, preferred patterns of behavior develop. Although functional skills can be achieved with a variety of possible combinations of factors, the patterns that reflect the most efficient subsystem interaction and that require the least amount of energy are utilized (Alexander, Boehme, & Cupps, 1993). It is usual, therefore, for the most frequently chosen movement patterns to have some degree of universality.

Clinical Connection:

"There are approximately 793 separate muscle groups in the human body, each made up of thousands of muscle fibers, that may be assembled in a nearly infinite number of combinations and sequences" (Thelen & Fogel, 1987, p. 28). Motor actions can be composed of an infinite number of combinations and sequences, within an infinite variety of settings, performed by a constantly changing individual. Yet within this variety, many movements retain a recognizable form: There are certain characteristics that make us recognize a kick, a smile, or a tennis swing. At the same time, the movement system is capable of generating novel movements, such as this author learning to play the flute in her 50s. Dynamic systems theory, forming the cornerstone theory of this text, emphasizes the ability of muscle synergies to self-organize within a dynamic, nonlinear relationship between all the contributing systems able to generate movement solutions of innumerable varieties and form. ▪

The complexity of the dynamic systems implies that there are many elements that can vary or change. These elements, the degrees of freedom, include neuromotor, as well as musculoskeletal and biomechanical, factors. The dynamic pattern theory offers a way of understanding how degrees of freedom can be constrained or expanded in a complex system. This theory suggests that the principles of pattern organization transcend specific structures. In other words, the specific subsystems provide a supporting framework for movement but do not dictate the pattern (Scholz, 1990). **Preferred patterns of movement** exist but are reorganized or altered when demands on the system change. For example, movement in all fours on the floor is a typical, preferred movement pattern utilized by infants and young toddlers, but one that is rarely seen at any other period of the life span. The transition from one preferred pattern of coordination to another is called a **phase shift.** During this phase shift, the system is in a relative state of instability until a new preferred pattern is established. Although pattern changes occur as part of daily functioning, such as changing from walking to running, they also occur during the development or reacquisition of motor skills (Alexander et al., 1993).

Dynamic systems theory emphasizes *process* rather than product. During motor development, the contributing subsystems become progressively integrated in an effort to gradually optimize skilled functioning. In this theoretical approach, both these internal components of the individual and the external context of the task and environment are equivalent in determining the outcome of behavior. This model views infant motor development as the infant solving the motor task within an environment, given the contributions of all subsystems as they self-organize and then demonstrate a preferred motor pattern. Because, however, the infant's cooperating subsystems do not develop at the same rate, certain components are seen as limiting or constraining to the performance of a specific behavior at any given developmental time. Each subsystem develops at its own rate but is constrained or supported by physical and environmental factors, such as opportunities to practice extension against the force of gravity while prone and standing upright (Campbell, 2000). The focus of control for function shifts over time, depending on the dominance of constraints of various subsystems. Spontaneous exploration of movement possibilities and flexible selection of the most appropriate movement synergy or preferred pattern for accomplishing goal-directed behavior are key concepts in viewing development from a dynamic systems perspective (Thelen & Corbetta, 1994). Transitional periods, when movement patterns appear to be unstable or more variable, are thought to be times when intervention might be particularly effective. Based on dynamic systems theory, developmental change is not seen as a series of discrete stages but as a series of states of stability, instability, and phase shifts (Thelen, 1995).

Viewed from a systems perspective, numerous elements can change as one grows and develops. Dynamic systems theory attempts to answer the "why" or process questions that result in the observable product of motor development. The key concepts and assumptions of this perspective are summarized in Figure 3–2. Remember to view the changing, ever-developing individual as a dynamic being, as this chapter now describes some of the common components of human movement production.

Key Concepts Related to Motor Development

Perspective

The following key concepts and terminology are presented to assist the clinician and student to visualize movement and motor development within a general working framework. As with all areas of study, it is imperative that some universality in language is adhered to for the purposes of discussion. Motor development has traditionally used observational analysis of a child's movement acquisition as a guidepost in understanding motor development. The following summarizes the main concepts related to motor development, useful for discussing key aspects of motor behavior. These are not rigid laws of development but are offered rather as a method for organizing thoughts and communicating with each other in a universal language.

Terminology Related to Direction

Development tends to proceed in characteristic directions: cephalocaudal, proximal to distal, gross to fine, and undifferentiated to specific.

▪ Cephalocaudal

The term **cephalocaudal** is used to describe the developmental direction of head to foot. This term is most appropriately used to describe the typical direction of development of postural responses in the infant (Woollacott & Shumway-Cook, 1990). Cephalocaudal development is related to the observation that head control precedes trunk control and control of the lower extremities. It does not mean that control of the head is *perfected or mastered* before any development of the trunk or lower extremities occurs. Skillful use of the head precedes skillful use of the trunk or lower extrem-

ities, even though the infant is working on different tasks with varying levels of mastery simultaneously.

Clinical Connection:

When I was a young therapist in the 1970s, the most widely used theoretical concept in neurorehabilitation advocated following the sequence of motor development as observed in the development of typical babies, then called "normal development." It was typical to try to meet therapeutic milestone goals in a fairly rigid order, striving first for head control when working with a patient. Many colleagues and I spent countless therapy hours trying to establish head control in the prone position by working with the individual of any age in prone, over ramps, with bolsters, in laps, or with a large therapy ball. We know now that the attainment of head control is important not only in prone but in every other body position and that the mastery of head control in the prone position does not necessarily carry over to control of the head in other positions, such as sitting or standing. We also now recognize that the development of *functional* control of the head is not a strictly hierarchical achievement. It is important to view the individual within his or her unique presentation within the life span, complete with the possibilities and constraints unique to that person. It is more valuable to establish head control in the most functional positions for that unique person. A 6-year-old child starting school who uses a power chair as primary mobility needs to have head control when sitting, perhaps aided by adaptive seating in the chair. Work on head control in the prone position is probably meaningless for that child at that age. ■

▪ Proximal to Distal

Developmental change is observed as proceeding in a proximal to distal direction, in reference to the midline of the body. Because the body is a linked structure, the midline must provide a stable base for head, eye, and extremity movement. The trunk is the stable base for the head above, as well as the lower extremities below and the arms projecting outward to the world. Control of the trunk is a requirement for control of the shoulder or pelvic girdles; shoulder girdle control is required for controlled use of the upper extremity; and control of the pelvis is necessary for controlled use of the lower extremities. Although some degree of proximal control appears to be a prerequisite for the refinement of distal control, this is not a cause-and-effect relationship. Although proximal stability and control *does not cause* the development of distal skill, there is a functional relationship between proximal and distal functions (Case-Smith, Fisher, & Bauer, 1989).

Clinical Connection:

Imagine how difficult it would be for me to use the computer if my trunk wasn't stabilized ensuring that my head could maintain my visual focus and my arms could be stabilized in order for my fingers to accurately strike the keys. The next time you are working on the computer, sit on a high stool so that you lower extremities are not stabilized on the ground and experience the lack of stability. ▪

▪ Gross to Fine

This developmental concept uses the term **gross movement** to describe large, undefined, or mass movements and **fine movement** to describe more refined, precise movements. In general, large mass movements occur before discrete ones. The infant will swipe at an object using the entire upper extremity before isolating first the hand for gross reach and then finally demonstrating more precise reaching with refined discriminative use of the fingers in isolation from the rest of the upper extremity.

Clinical Connection:

The infant will first swipe at objects using the entire upper extremity. Reaching then becomes more refined, characterized by stabilization of the shoulder girdle and a movement pattern requiring more elbow, forearm, and hand control. Finally, reach becomes very refined, allowing the infant to pick up the tiniest of items. These changes in upper extremity control will be expanded on in Chapter 9. ▪

▪ Undifferentiated to Specific

The concept of undifferentiated to specific movement describes how the infant first moves the entire body in response to a stimulus before a more specific response emerges. For example, the young infant will roll in a mass, loglike fashion, where the entire body moves as a unit, before more specific motions emerge. In excitement at seeing a mobile suspended above, the young infant will randomly move both upper extremities and the entire body seems to be involved in this initial attempt to swipe at the novel toy. Eventually, the arms will move separately from each other and arm movement will occur without associated motions of the trunk or head. This breaking up of the mass pattern is called **dissociation,** the ability to separate movement in one body part from associated movement in another. Mature movements are characterized by dissociation, with typical motor development providing many exam-

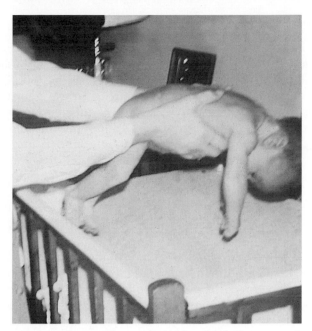

Figure 4–1. The posture assumed by the full-term newborn baby is one of physiological flexion, characterized by a completely flexed posture with no extension against the newly confronted force of gravity.

ples. When an infant learns to turn the head in all directions without trunk movement, the head can be said to be dissociated from the trunk. When the infant can reach with the upper extremity while in the prone position, the upper extremity is said to be dissociated from the trunk. In mature walking, the shoulders are dissociated from the trunk, the trunk is dissociated from both the pelvic and the shoulder girdles, and the lower extremities are dissociated from each other.

Kinesiological Concepts

▪ Physiological Flexion to Antigravity Extension to Antigravity Flexion

Full-term babies are born in **physiological flexion,** a term used to describe the predominantly flexed posture of a full-term newborn infant (Fig. 4–1). This flexed posture is precipitated by the position assumed secondary to the confines of the womb as the baby grew in size during the last prenatal weeks. The newborn baby naturally assumes a position of flexion, so much so that there is a normal neonatal hip flexion contracture of 30 degrees and knee flexion contracture of 20 degrees and the ankle is fixed in dorsiflexion (Bertoti & Stanger, 1994). If you were to try to straighten or uncoil any of the extremities of a newborn baby, they would immediately recoil to their original flexed position. Newborn infants also demonstrate a primary kyphotic curve of the spine.

Clinical Connection:

Prematurely born infants do not demonstrate a physiologically flexed posture, because they are born before the womb becomes too constraining. In the neonatal nursery, this is further complicated by the need to have the infant monitored, often requiring mechanical equipment that has to be closely monitored by nursing staff. The infant often must be in a supine position so that all the medical care can be closely administered. Neonatal nursery care staff attempt to balance these paramount medical needs with positioning and cradling of the infant.

The first developmental task of the newborn infant is to deal with the first encounters with gravity, having been in a gravity-free world while in utero. The effective development of antigravity control has profound effects on the successful development of postural control (Sellers, 1988). Movement against gravity begins during the first month of life and continues to be a main developmental task during the first year. **Antigravity extension** is the voluntary, active movement, first of the neck and then of the trunk, against the force of gravity. Antigravity extension is first evidenced in prone with head lifting and then extension of the trunk. Nature sets the stage for antigravity extension to occur because the physiologically flexed posture puts the extensors in a lengthened range, at a range optimal for developing active tension and voluntary force. The extensors are best prepared to develop voluntary force and controlled functioning rather than the positionally shortened flexors. Some of the infantile reflexes (to be discussed later in this chapter), such as primitive stepping, as well as the baby's body weight, also contribute to extension control success.

Practice and time spent in extended postures against gravity naturally lengthen the shortened flexors. The neonatal hip and knee flexion contracture naturally dissipate, and the foot assumes a neutral position. **Antigravity flexion** develops as the baby combats the force of gravity first in the supine and side-lying positions, evidenced by head lifting, foot play in supine, beginning bridging, and successful voluntary movement out of the supine position. A balanced control develops between the flexors and extensors, as evidenced by the ability to co-contract both muscle groups when holding a position (such as reaching forward from prone on the floor) or as seen in a dynamically balanced use of the trunk flexors and extensors, allowing the infant to play while in a side-lying position.

▪ Mobility and Stability

All human movement is characterized by a fascinating relationship between the need for stability and mobility.

This relationship between **stability** (holding a posture) and **mobility** (moving) is called **postural control** (Cech & Martin, 1995). Margaret Rood first presented this developmental concept of mobility preceding stability, followed by controlled mobility, and finally the emergence of skill (Stockmeyer, 1966). Mobility is present before stability, as evidenced by newborn infants' lack of ability to stabilize their own head, as well as random movements of the arms and legs. Infants are very mobile, able to assume postures but only holding them briefly. Stability occurs with the development of synergistic muscle control, evidenced by cocontraction and isometric control. Success is gained in the holding of postures such as prone on elbows.

Proximal stability is the ability to stabilize in antigravity positions with simultaneous functional mobility. This term is used to describe the required cocontraction around shoulder and pelvic girdles required for successful, coordinated use of the upper or lower extremities, respectively. Proximal stability requires a balance of flexor and extensor voluntary control, the ability to move in all three planes, and the ability to shift weight and demonstrate balance.

Controlled mobility utilizes the functional contributions of both mobility and stability, allowing for such motor activities as reaching accurately while prone, stabilized with one extremity with a stable head and trunk posture. Controlled mobility is often seen in successful open-chain activities, whereby proximal stability allows for successful movement of the upper or lower extremity through space. Skill emerges through a constant interplay between mobility, stability, and controlled mobility, evidenced by successful open-chain movements, where the proximal segments are stabilized, permitting freedom of movement of the distal segment, such as in manipulation. Application of these concepts to intervention will be explored in Chapters 6 through 10 of this text.

▪ Asymmetry to Symmetry to Controlled Asymmetry

According to *Taber's* (2001), **symmetry** is defined as a position or posture characterized by correspondence in relative position of parts on opposite sides of the body, whereas **asymmetry** is characterized by a lack of such correspondence. A newborn baby's posture is rather asymmetrical, with the head to the side apparently seeming to gaze at one outstretched arm. This asymmetry is replaced by relative symmetry at around 4 months of age. Symmetry is evident at this time by infants' ability to play with their own hands together at midline, hold an object with two hands, or even to reach for and play with the feet while in the supine position. Sophisticated, mature motor development is characterized by controlled asymmetry where the extremities are dissociated from each other and from the trunk and head, evidenced by mature locomotion and upper extremity use. An examination of the development of movement patterns across the life span illustrates an overall evolution of asymmetry to symmetry and then a return to asymmetry.

▪ Relationship Between Weight Bearing and Weight Shifting

Stability in postures permits effective **weight bearing,** and weight-bearing experiences assist in the development of stability. Adequate weight bearing is made possible through stability around the proximal girdle, the scapula/shoulder for the upper extremity, and the pelvis for the lower extremity. To move with control, weight shifting must occur. **Weight shifting** occurs as one body part stabilizes simultaneously with the other body part being unweighted enough to move.

▪ Rotation/Dissociation

Rotation can be demonstrated because of a balanced control of both flexors and extensors and dissociation between body segments. Rotation through the trunk allows for such functional milestones as moving to sitting from prone, rotating within sitting, creeping, reaching on all fours, moving to stance through half kneel, and locomotion. Dissociation is the ability to move one body part or segment without an associated movement of another body part or segment, as seen in the breaking up of mass movement patterns, characterized by the ability to separate movement in one body part from associated movement in another (Cech & Martin, 1995). Examples of dissociation include the dissociation of the shoulders from the trunk and the hips from the pelvis, as seen in mature rolling; dissociation of the lower extremities from each other during gait; and dissociation of the upper extremities from the trunk during ball playing and reciprocal arm swinging during gait. Rotation and fluid dissociation also permit self-help skills such as independent dressing.

Developmental Sequence

Most developmental authorities recognize some type of developmental sequence. Current models suggest that development in childhood can be regarded as sequential but not necessarily linear. Rather than being made up of an unfolding of major components in sequence, there is a spiraling and flexibility in timing and mastery between individuals. The sequence is not a fixed and rigid order of motor behaviors. Areas of disagreement involve the exact composition of these sequential components and which specific skills are to be consid-

ered part of the sequence. It is also debated whether one skill in the sequence is a prerequisite for the next skill in the sequence. Movement development in the broadest sense is based on previously attained skills, but not as rigid building blocks. Each movement as it emerges and is practiced is slightly different from what was learned before. In this way, the mover participates in and influences the emergence, practice, and mastery of his or her own movement skills. Developmental change occurs because of active problem solving. The level of potential development that can occur is individually variable (Vygotsky, 1978).

Studying the acquisition of independent, functional movement as acquired during the first years of life offers an opportunity to observe and recognize key universal components of movement. An in-depth study of development during infancy and early childhood offers a model for understanding the process of the development of movement, from the acquisition of basic movement components during the first year through the attainment of fundamental movement skills by age 6. These observable "stages" of gross and fine motor development represent milestones of developmental progress toward achieving the goals of upright postural control, mobility and locomotion, and manipulation. As infants attain and perfect these developmental motor skills, they are incorporated into functional activities such as feeding, self-care, and play.

Despite the complexity of the contemporary view of development as being among multiple systems and along multiple processes, it is possible to summarize the development of mastery and use of various parts of the body in an overall schema of cephalocaudal direction (Campbell, 2000). In using the developmental sequence as a framework for study, it is important to recognize several limitations:

1. Motor milestones develop in overlapping sequence, with spurts and regressions common.
2. Development is characteristically variable, and therefore it is vital that the very term *sequence* not be construed to be rigid and fixed.
3. Although motor development during the first year certainly leads to the mastery of key movement components and skills, motor milestones should not be considered as an invariant sequence in lock-step order where one component is an absolute prerequisite for another movement or motor skill.
4. Development occurs simultaneously but perhaps at different rates within several domains: motor, social-emotion, language, and cognitive (Campbell, 2000).

It is more important to focus on the process than on product.

Developmental stages can be viewed as **"attractor" states,** whereby a complex set of biomechanical, neuromotor, cognitive, and environmental variables govern transition from one stage to the next. How many of us have heard parents comment about their son or daughter that he or she seems just about ready to roll over, stand alone, or take a first step? What is recognized is a somewhat intangible but instinctively strong feeling on the part of the observer that the skill being awaited is *just about* to happen. A state of readiness is perceived. This "attractor" state describes the coming together of all the vital variables allowing a transition to then occur.

Motor development is a continuous process of interaction between the individual and the environment. Throughout life, the individual and the environment form an interconnected system, and development itself has interactional causes and effects. Consider the infant: Once the young infant is motivated to do something (bat at an object, pick up a spoon, or move to the other side of the room), the infant's current development state physically and position in the particular environmental setting (positioned in an infant seat, in a crib, or prone on the floor) will offer opportunities and constraints that affect whether and how the goal will be achieved. Ultimately, a solution emerges as a result of trying out behaviors and retaining those that most effectively and efficiently accomplish the task. Rather than being solely in charge of this process, the developing nervous system is only part of it (Thelen, 1995).

Movement patterns change with age, each being qualitatively different but somewhat dependent on what came before. Movement patterns change because the different musculoskeletal and nervous subsystems change in their functional status, as detailed in the previous chapter (Woollacott & Shumway-Cook, 1990). Movement skill acquisition demonstrates a continuity and discontinuity. The developmental sequence, as observed during the first year of life, consists of the acquisition of motor milestones. The study of these milestones, which are often viewed as "stages," can act as a guide to the progression of movement control. Movement patterns continue to change throughout life, even after the pivotal gross motor milestone, walking, is achieved.

A study of the typical developmental sequence is a valuable way for the student or clinician to develop the observational skills required to be adept at not only assessing the patient/client with a movement disorder but also at designing effective intervention strategies for those patients/clients. Key accomplishments in the developmental sequence are typically the ability of the body to master antigravity control and strength, the ability to demonstrate proximal stability, and the ability to shift weight effectively to execute a movement or a transitional posture. Traditional texts often referred to this sequence as a progression from a starting posture of prone. Practical application of the typical developmental sequence to intervention application is summarized in Table 4–2. This text will use the developmental

sequence as only one aspect of a clinically useful model, rather proposing that the attainment of vital movement skills can be broadly defined as attempting to meet one of three main functional tasks: attainment of postural control; control of the lower extremity, including locomotor skills; and control of the upper extremity required for mature manipulation skills.

Milestones and the Acquisition of Motor Skill

▪ The Meaning of "Milestones"

A study of development often includes recognizing the observable milestones that represent progress toward the achievement of functional independence and mastery. During early development, motor skill acquisition is evidenced by the infant's increasing ability to problem solve ways in which to interact with the environment. These behavioral changes are demonstrated as milestones, actually a demonstration of skill development. Infants perform "age-appropriate" skills that are functional and meaningful *to them* in their limited experience with the world. Many of these behavioral activities are probably not meaningful or functional for an older child or adult (Bly, 1994).

Milestones are useful because they offer landmarks for recognizing the key skills that are typically mastered as increased independence and movement sophistication emerge. They are useful in charting progress toward the development of postural control, attainment of fundamental movement components and skills, mastery over the environment, and ultimately, independent function. Milestones also offer clinicians some guideposts along which to assess the attainment of functional movement independence or to identify a delay in motor skill development. The major gross motor milestones of the first 18 months include an upright head posture, functional head control during movement, development in the prone position, prone progression, rolling, sitting, quadruped movement, creeping, pulling to stand, and walking independently. As each position or skill is attained, further development requires the perfecting of postural control in these positions and the ability to make easy transitions from one position to another (Campbell, 2000). The major fine motor milestones of the first 18 months include the development of reaching, grasping, and manipulation abilities so vital for play, learning, and independence in self-care. As these major developmental gross and fine motor skills are attained, they are incorporated into functional activities of daily living, such as feeding, self-care, and play. Tables 4–3 and 4–4 list the main milestones commonly cited for gross and fine motor development.

TABLE 4-2
Intervention Application of Developmental Sequence Concepts

Position	Intervention Benefits
Supine	Facilitation of head and upper trunk forward flexion Can begin early weight bearing, knees bent, feet flat on surface For children, can foster visual and upper extremity (UE) development
Side lying	Neutral position of head and neck decreases effect of tonic reflexes, if problematic Promotes protraction of scapula and hip, important for functional use of UE and lower extremities (LEs) Achieves trunk elongation on weight-bearing side Excellent position to promote rolling, coming to sit, or as transitional posture
Prone on elbows or forearms	Improves upper trunk, neck, and head control Promotes weight bearing through UEs Increases co-contraction and proximal stability at shoulder girdle Increases range of motion at hip and knee extensors
Quadruped	Improves upper trunk, lower trunk, UE, LE, and head/neck control Improves co-contraction strength of abdominals and back extensors; trunk works against gravity Increases hip stabilizer strength Weight bearing to increase proximal stability at shoulder girdles and hips Weight bearing through extended arms Increases extensor range at wrists and fingers Wide base of support (BOS), lowered center of gravity (COG) Excellent opportunity for dissociation and reciprocal extremity movements
Sitting	Promotes active head and trunk control, trunk elongation, and rotation Excellent to facilitate head and trunk righting, equilibrium responses, UE protective reactions
Side sit with forearm or extended arm prop	Increases UE strength on weight-bearing side Improves trunk rotation and dissociation Offers opportunity for balanced sitting with narrowed base of support
Bridging in supine	Improve lower trunk and LE control Increase hip stabilizer strength Weight bearing through feet Activity to assist with bed mobility
Kneeling and half kneeling	Improve head/neck, upper trunk, lower trunk, and LE control Weight bearing through hips Increase hip stabilizer strength and control Improve balance reactions Weight bearing through foot in half kneel Narrow BOS, higher COG Encourages dissociation, good transitional postures
Standing	Improve head/neck, trunk, and LE control Weight bearing through LEs Improves balance reactions Narrow BOS, high COG Functional posture

Sources: Adapted from O'Sullivan, S. B. (2001). Assessment of motor function. In S. B. O'Sullivan & T. J. Schmitz (Eds.), *Physical rehabilitation: Assessment and Treatment* (4th ed.). Philadelphia: F. A. Davis with permission; and adapted from Martin, S., & Kessler, M. K. (2000). *Neurologic intervention for physical therapy assistants*, with permission from Elsevier.

Automatic Movements

Automatic movements are those movements that occur in response to a given stimulus, often without conscious, voluntary effort. Automatic movements include reflexes, postural reactions such as righting, equilibrium and protective reactions, and associated reactions.

▪ Significance of Automatic Movements as a Motor Response

Earlier reflex-based descriptions of development viewed the nervous system with a hierarchical emphasis, where increasingly complex motor responses could be observed as the brain developed at higher levels. According to this view, simple reflexes dominated the

TABLE 4–3

TABLE 4–3	
Gross Motor Milestones	
Age	Skill
Newborn	In prone, turns head to side to clear airway Vigorous rhythmical kicking in supine Reflexive standing and stepping Physiological flexion; full head lag Rolls partly to side in mass pattern
2 mo	Lifts head to 45 degrees in prone Prone on forearms with elbow behind shoulder but chest higher off floor Partial or full head lag Head bobs in supported sitting Appearance of more reciprocal kicking Spontaneous rolling side lying to supine Period of "astasia" (see text)
3–5 mo	Head control at 4 mo Active head lifting on pull to sit by 5 mo Prone prop onto forearms by 4 mo, onto extended arms by 5 mo Reaching in prone from forearm prop Increased symmetrical extensor and flexor antigravity control "Pivot prone" (see text) Landau reaction (see text) Plays with feet in supine Bridges in supine (5 mo) Scooting or pivoting on floor Rolls prone to supine (log roll) Sitting with support; momentary unsupported sitting Will stand with support; little control
6 mo	Belly crawling Rolls supine to prone Rolling becomes segmental Play in side lying Gets to sitting independently Sits with wide base independently Beginning reaching from sitting Stands with support; takes a stiff step or two with full support; bounces in standing
7–9 mo	Sitting in variety of postures with good control; independent sitting by 8 mo Trunk control well developed by 9 mo Pivots in sitting Assumes quadruped and rocks "Bear standing" (see text) Creeps Pulls self to stand; lowers to sitting from supported stand Cruising (see text)
10–12 mo	Creeping is primary locomotion mode Pulls to stand through half kneel Stands alone momentarily Walks with one or two hands held Climbs and creeps up stairs

TABLE 4–3	
Gross Motor Milestones (Continued)	
Age	Skill
18 mo	Rises to stand without pulling up Walks independently; walks backward Squats to pick up objects and squats in play Walks up stairs nonreciprocally, hand held
2–3 y (toddler)	Walks up stairs alternating feet Rides tricycle Climbs playground equipment Begins to run Jumps off step; short horizontal jump Can stand on one foot briefly Stands on low balance beam Hops on one foot; hand held or a few beats on preferred foot Kicks with leg straight
4–6 y (preschool)	Walks downstairs alternating feet Can stand on one foot 3–5 s Jumps increased distance; jumps over objects Hops a few feet Begins to skip Kicks and bounces large ball Runs fast, avoiding obstacles (mature run) Can walk a line 10 ft Walks balance beam alternating feet
6–10 y (school age)	Postural control is adultlike by 7–10 y Adult balance strategies developed by age 10 Masters adult forms of running, jumping Hops and skips skillfully by age 6
Adolescence	Development of specialized movement skills such as dodging, balancing, leaping, sliding, advanced climbing, volleying, and trapping permitting success in sports and recreational activities

Sources: Alexander, R., Boehme, R., & Cupps, B. (1993). *Normal development of functional motor skills.* Tucson, AZ: Therapy Skill Builders; Bly, L. (1994). *Motor skills acquisition in the first year.* Tucson, AZ: Therapy Skill Builders; Gallahue, D. L., & Ozmun, J. C. (2002). *Understanding motor development: Infants, children, adolescents, adults* (4th ed.). New York: McGraw-Hill; Miller Porr, S., & Berger Rainville, E. (1999). *Pediatric therapy: A systems approach.* Philadelphia: F. A. Davis; and Ratliffe, K. T. (1998). *Clinical pediatric physical therapy: A guide for the physical therapy team.* St. Louis, MO: Mosby.

movements seen in the newborn. These reflexes were thought to represent the functioning of subcortical primitive centers of the brain. In the normally maturing infant, early reflex responses were thought to diminish, integrated into more mature motor patterns. These changes were perceived to be reflective of maturation of a hierarchically organized nervous system: As the cortex increasingly assumed control of motor functions, the reflexes were thought to be inhibited or formed the basis for more functional movement (Kamm, Thelen, & Jensen, 1990). According to the early theorists, the

TABLE 4–4

Fine Motor Milestones

Age	Skill
Newborn	Grasp reflex Random upper extremity movements in supine
2 mo	Recognizes hands Primitive reaching behaviors Asymmetrical swiping at objects Grasp reflex dissipating; hands more open Palmar grasp
3–5 mo	Retains objects placed in hands Fingers hands in play at midline Mouths fingers Grasps and releases toys Primitive squeezing; raking Uses ulnar-palmar grasp
6 mo	Voluntary palmar grasp First sign of unilateral reach Rakes with fingers to pick up smaller objects Attempts to hold cup and spoon Finger feeds
7–9 mo	Radial palmar grasp (involving thumb) Radial digital grasp (beginning opposition) Strong grip against resistance Transfer objects hand to hand Develops active forearm supination Points and pokes with index finger Takes objects out of container
10–12 mo	Pincer grasp Three-jaw chuck Puts objects into container Stacks two cubes Increased bimanual dexterity Increased independence in feeding and undressing
18 mo	Can manipulate pencil or crayon with forearm supination, fisted hand Controlled grasp and release Turns container over to empty contents Stacks six cubes; strings large beads Hand preference begins to emerge
2–3 y (toddler)	Pencil or crayon held by fingers and thumb Emergence of mature grip onto pencil with thumb and two radial fingers (static tripod) Turns knob, unscrews jar Can use child-size scissors; unbuttons large buttons
4–6 y (preschool)	Mature dynamic tripod grip onto pencil Skilled hand use to manipulate utensils, tools, and self-care items Can use zipper and tie shoes by age 6 Bimanual coordination expands Demonstrates hand preference Develops printing skills Shows mature catching, throwing, and striking patterns (6 y)

TABLE 4–4

Fine Motor Milestones (*Continued*)

Age	Skill
6–10 y (school age)	Increased coordination for manipulating small objects and increased fine motor mastery Opportunity for development of task-specific prehensile skills May enjoy hobbies requiring complex fine motor skills, such as sewing or model building Handwriting and keyboarding skills Throws and catches with increased mastery
Adolescence	Skillful ball playing due to increased eye-hand coordination and improved reaction time Increased dexterity in tasks

Sources: Alexander, R., Boehme, R., & Cupps, B. (1993). *Normal development of functional motor skills.* Tucson, AZ: Therapy Skill Builders; Bly, L. (1994). *Motor skills acquisition in the first year.* Tucson, AZ: Therapy Skill Builders; Gallahue, D. L., & Ozmun, J. C. (2002). *Understanding motor development: Infants, children, adolescents, adults* (4th ed.). New York: McGraw-Hill; Miller Porr, S., & Berger Rainville, E. (1999). *Pediatric therapy: A systems approach.* Philadelphia: F. A. Davis; and Ratliffe, K. T. (1998). *Clinical pediatric physical therapy: A guide for the physical therapy team.* St. Louis, MO: Mosby.

appearance and disappearance of reflexes reflected the increasing maturity of cortical structures.

Contemporary motor theory has a more dynamic view of the role of automatic movements, including reflexes, and their role in motor control. It is now understood that although reflexes may provide a general framework or bias for movement, they do not address the dynamic and adaptive nature of early infant motor behavior. Dynamic systems theory does not deny the existence of reflexes but rather considers them as one of many influences on the control of posture and movement (Shumway-Cook & Woollacott, 2001). These motor responses may be in the form of expressed movement observed, given the capabilities, constraints, and self-organization of all the contributing subsystems.

Clinical Connection:

In some situations, a reflex motor response is simply the best motor response that the system can produce. For example, a reflex movement response (such as reaching using an asymmetrical tonic neck reflex [ATNR] pattern; see Table 4–5 for description) may simply be the only movement response available in the face of neurological damage and some of the impairments that accompany the damage, such as muscular weakness, impaired coordination, or the

TABLE 4–5

Primitive Reflexes (Early Preferred Movement Patterns)

Reflex	Stimulus	Movement Response	Age Typically Observable
Flexor withdrawal	Stimulus, usually noxious, to sole of foot	Entire lower extremity (LE) flexes, ankles dorsiflex, toes extend	28 wk gestation–1 mo
Crossed extension	Stimulus, usually noxious, to sole of foot	Opposite LE extends and adducts	28 wk gestation–1 mo
Rooting	Touch on cheek	Head turn to stimulus, mouth opens	28 wk gestation–3 mo
Stepping	Upright supported weight bearing onto firm surface on plantar surface foot	Reciprocal flexion and extension of legs "stepping"	38 wk gestation–2 mo
Positive support	Weight onto ball of foot in upright	Stiff extension of LE	35 wk gestation–2 mo
Moro	Sudden change in head position in relation to trunk	Mass extension and abduction, quickly followed by mass flexion and adduction	28 wk gestation–6 mo
Startle	Loud, sudden noise	Mass extension and abduction of arms	From birth on
Palmar grasp	Pressure on palm of hand, ulnar side	Strong flexion of fingers	Birth–4 mo
Asymmetrical tonic neck reflex	Rotation of head to one side	Extension of extremities on face side; flexion of extremities on skull side	Birth–6 mo
Symmetrical tonic neck reflex	Flexion or extension of the neck	With neck flexion: flexion of the upper extremities (UEs) and extension of LEs; with neck extension, extension of UEs and flexion of LEs	4–12 mo
Tonic labyrinthine reflex, supine or prone	Supine or prone position	With supine positioning, extension of the neck, trunk and extremities; with prone positioning, flexion of the neck, trunk, and extremities	Birth–6 mo

Source: Information compiled from multiple sources. See text and reference list.

secondary impairment of limited range of motion. In another example, a belly flop into a swimming pool off a diving board may be the motor outcome of a novel diver's movement response resembling an early reflex pattern (symmetrical tonic neck reflex [STNR]; see Table 4–5 for description). ▪

All automatic reactions, including reflexes, can be modified by the brain to produce the most appropriate and efficient movement for the task and the environment. As a motor expression, reflexes and other automatic movements are often observed during times of great developmental change, such as during the first year of life, as well as during or following periods of damage to the nervous system. As such, it is valuable to discuss and list the reflexes seen as part of the dynamic unfolding of continually developing postural control.

▪ Primitive Reflexes

A **reflex** is a largely automatic, somewhat stereotypical, consistent, and predictable motor response to a specific stimulus, usually sensory (Leonard, 1998). In its broadest sense, a reflex can be defined as a complex motor response pattern, not limited to activation by external stimuli, which, although relatively invariable, is nonetheless responsive to context or environment (Crutchfield & Barnes, 1993; Pimentel, 1996). Primitive reflexes are those movement responses where the neural circuitry is either at the spinal cord or the brainstem level. Some of these reflexes can be described as "phasic" in nature, of very short duration, or "tonic," with a longer duration. The simplest reflexes occur at the spinal cord level. Rather than being inflexibly paired to a sensory input, there is increasing evidence that if the sensory stimulus is applied during the course of an ongoing movement, the motor output associated with the stimulus will vary depending on its environmental context and the status of all the movement subsystems (Field-Fote, 2000). This view is in agreement with a dynamically responsive set of systems contributing to movement.

Consistent with a dynamic systems approach, primitive reflexes are not so much "hardwired" but are readily observed at certain ages, because at that period of

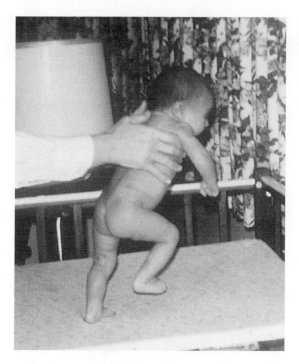

Figure 4–2. A newborn baby will exhibit a primitive stepping reflex, whereby weight-bearing pressure of the foot onto a surface will elicit a reflexive extension of the weight-bearing leg and flexion (or stepping) of the opposite leg.

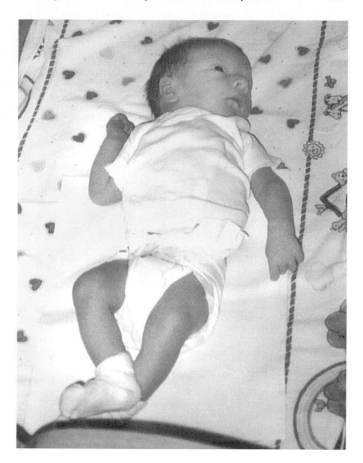

Figure 4–3. Asymmetrical tonic neck reflex, whereby turning of the head and neck will elicit extension of the arm and leg on the face side and flexion of the arm and leg on the skull side.

development, the infant's movement will "under certain circumstances, have a propensity [inclination or predisposition] to exhibit a particular motor response" (Kamm et al., 1990). Primitive reflexes always serve some sort of movement purpose. Early in development, they allow for muscle activation and joint excursion or even provide a primitive survival response. Functionally, primitive reflex responses are thought to contribute to the development of emerging mobility and stability in the developing child (McCormack & Perrin, 1997). Following a neurological insult, primitive reflexes are sometimes observed in the older individual, as the preferred movement pattern expressed by that individual at that time, within the capabilities and constraints of his or her movement system. Primitive reflexes are listed in Table 4–5. Examples of some of these reflexes are pictured in Figures 4–2 and 4–3.

▪ Postural Responses

Every movement involves a weight shift, and weight shifts, in turn stimulating vestibular and proprioceptive receptors, are the stimulus for righting and equilibrium reactions. Righting and equilibrium are complex postural responses that continue to be present throughout adulthood. Righting behaviors are thought to be mediated at a midbrain level in response to signaling from several different sensory receptors: proprioceptors and cutaneous receptors, the eyes, and the labyrinths of the ears. **Righting** is the act of realigning the head or trunk with each other or with an outside stimulus. Applied to movement, righting responses are demonstrated by the head or trunk when balance is disturbed, whereby the head and trunk realign themselves with each other or with the downward pull of gravity. Righting responses assist in keeping the head oriented in relation to the body or to gravity. They are named in a very descriptive fashion, the name telling exactly what body part is responsible for the realignment or righting action and often the mechanism for sending this signal. Examples of righting responses include head righting, neck righting, and trunk righting. They can be further described by adding a phrase to the nomenclature, such as labyrinthine head righting or optical head righting, where the stimulus that elicits the righting response is the effect of gravity or the position of the eyes regarding gravity, respectively.

Equilibrium is the act of reestablishing balance once one's balance is disturbed. **Equilibrium reactions** adjust for a change in the body's orientation in space. Equilibrium reactions are composed of righting responses of the head and trunk and protective extension responses of the extremities. An equilibrium

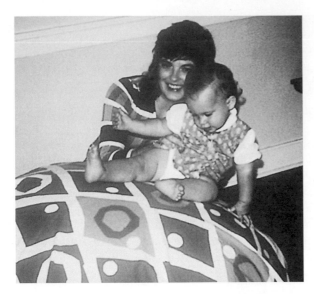

Figure 4–4. Equilibrium response, seen here in sitting, is characterized by lateral head and trunk righting away from the floor, abduction of the limbs in an effort to maintain balance, and protective extension of the upper extremity in the direction of gravity.

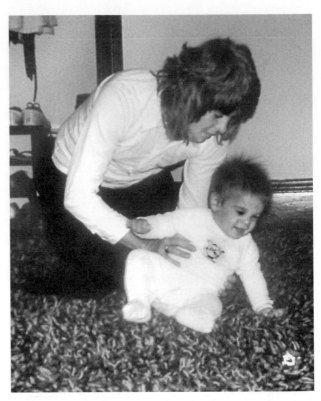

Figure 4–5. Example of protective extension in sitting, in this case of the left upper extremity to the side.

response is composed of head and trunk lateral righting and wide abduction of the upper extremity (UE) and lower extremity (LE) in the direction away from gravity and a protective extension of the UE and LE toward gravity (Fig. 4–4). The lateral righting and abduction of the head, trunk, and uppermost extremities are the body's attempt to right, realign, or reestablish balance in the face of the center of gravity moving outside the base of support. The **protective extension** motions of the lowermost extremities are in preparation for catching oneself from a fall.

Equilibrium reactions develop in increasingly more upright antigravity positions as postural control develops. Therefore, they are seen first in the child in prone, supine, sitting, quadruped, kneeling, and finally standing, continuing to mature throughout early childhood as postural control develops (Fisher & Bundy, 1982; Izraelevitz, Fisher, & Bundy, 1985). Protective extension also develops as movement control develops, seen as part of an equilibrium response or demonstrated first in sitting with the UEs extending when the infant is displaced forward, to the side, and then to the rear (Fig. 4–5). Functionally, righting and equilibrium reaction responses are thought to contribute to the development of combined mobility and stability in the developing child (McCormack & Perrin, 1997).

▪ Associated Reactions

Associated reactions are movements that occur involuntarily in accompaniment to another movement. Associated reactions are part of the normal movement repertoire, often observed during a heavily resisted movement or during periods of fatigue or stress. They are common through middle childhood, when postural control and fundamental movement skills are developing and being refined. They are common again whenever the movement system is stressed, such as during recovery from a pathological incident.

Clinical Connection:

We all have experienced associated reactions: Picture the kindergarten child unconsciously biting his tongue while concentrating on a new writing skill, the unconscious shoulder elevation and posturing of your neck and upper extremities while driving across an icy patch of roadway, or the involuntary movement of the unengaged upper extremity in an arm-wrestler. In an individual with a neurological disorder, associated movements often accompany attempts at new tasks or occur when experiencing fatigue or stress. ▪

Functional Movement

Function defines mastery and competence over the environment (Guccione, 1993). Throughout life, an individual demonstrates varying abilities and levels of mastery over the environment. Functional movements are the movement patterns that are used for or adapted to a function or a group of similar functions. In daily life, we use functional movement to accomplish our tasks and goals and to produce the desired occupational behaviors in a safe, efficient, and appropriate manner (Ryerson & Levit, 1997). The movement patterns used to perform daily activities are relatively consistent and uniform, although certainly it is the potential for variability that characterizes normalcy (Ryerson & Levit, 1997; VanSant, 1990). Typical functional movements use the patterns of muscle action and joint motion that are most suited to the biomechanical and kinesiological systems of the human body. Typical functional movements use the simplest strategy to accomplish the task, conserving power and energy while protecting the body from undue stress, injury, and loss of balance.

Operational Definition

The word **function** means the act of carrying out or performing an activity, referring to a specific role or occupation. **Functional movements** are the movement patterns that are used for or adapted to a function or group of similar functions (Ryerson & Levit, 1997). Functional movements are those movements used to meet basic needs, perform daily tasks, accomplish goals, and engage in purposeful activity and occupations. The movement patterns that we use to perform daily activities are relatively consistent and uniform. Most people stand up, walk, dress themselves, and eat or drink using movement patterns that are very similar. Although movements such as rolling may differ between people of different ages, body types, and fitness level, most people accomplish these functions with one of several common variants (Ryerson & Levit, 1997).

Functional Movement: Main Tasks and Components

Functional movement is made up of coordinated movements of trunk, upper extremities, and lower extremities. Functional movement is able to develop and be maintained as long as several key elements are present: adequate mobility and range of motion, appropriate muscle tone and strength, evidence of variability and isolation of movements, postural stability and central control, antigravity control, proximal stability, mature weight-bearing and weight-shifting capabilities, and the ability to make postural adjustments. The reader is invited to observe the lifelong development of functional movement, with an eye trained to detect the presence or absence of these key elements. In this text, the lifelong development of functional movement is divided into the accomplishment of three main tasks:

postural control of the head and trunk, upper extremity control, and lower extremity control.

■ Postural Control of the Head and Trunk

The emergence of postural control can be characterized by the development of rules that relate sensory inputs about the body's position with respect to the environment to motor actions controlling the body's position (Shumway-Cook & Woollacott, 2001). Control of the head and trunk are central to successful functional movement. The head must maintain alignment to center the visual field and receive vestibular input. **Head control** is defined as the ability to maintain a stable position (cocontraction), as well as move the head automatically (righting) or voluntarily (concentrically or eccentrically). Because the head serves as the base of support for the visual and vestibular systems, it is crucial that head position be accurate for the required task so that these receptors can receive and transmit information accurately. The development of postural control begins at the head.

The trunk, as the center of the body mass, must maintain the body in a balanced, erect position against gravity and must adapt to the moving extremities. This task can be defined as the **postural control of the trunk.** The trunk functions not only as a stable base from which other movements operate but also functions dynamically when movements are used to move the center of body mass over its base or to change to a new posture. In this dynamic fashion, trunk movements contribute to or increase the functional abilities of the upper and lower extremities (O' Sullivan, 2001; Ryerson & Levit, 2001).

Both the postural and the dynamic aspects of trunk control are based on the ability of the trunk to move in anterior, posterior, and lateral directions. To accomplish these movements, the muscles of the trunk must be able to work isometrically (to stabilize), concentrically (against gravity), and eccentrically (where the body moves with control toward the supporting surface). When the trunk is not stable and cannot move without loss of balance, the upper and lower extremities must be used to stabilize the body; thus they are not free for function. For this reason, trunk control is a precursor to all functional movement (Ryerson & Levit, 1997).

Postural control can be subdivided into several main tasks: the ability to maintain postural orientation, reactive control, proactive or anticipatory control, and adaptive postural control (O'Sullivan, 2001). The ability to maintain postural orientation involves controlling the relative positions of body parts by skeletal muscles with respect to gravity and to each other. This includes the ability to maintain equilibrium both during periods of stability and during function. Reactive control occurs in response to outside forces, such as perturbations, displacing the center of gravity or moving the base of support. Proactive or anticipatory control occurs in anticipation of internally generated, destabilizing forces, such as the intent to move. Anticipatory control provides a supportive framework for skilled movements (O' Sullivan, 2001). An individual's prior experiences allow the various elements of the postural control system to be readied for the intended movement. Adaptive postural control allows the individual to modify the sensory and motor systems in response to the changing environment or the task (Shumway-Cook & Woollacott, 2001). These different aspects of postural control will be expanded on in Chapter 8.

The emergence of postural control is ascribed to complex interactions between neural and musculoskeletal mechanisms. According to Shumway-Cook and Woollacott (2001), it includes the following:

1. Changes in the musculoskeletal system, including development of adequate muscle strength and changes in relative mass of body segment.
2. Development of the coordinative structures or neuromuscular response synergies used in maintaining balance.
3. Development of individual sensory systems including somatosensory, visual, and vestibular systems and the sensory strategies for organizing these multiple inputs.
4. Development of internal representations important in the mapping or connection of perception to action.
5. Development of adaptive and anticipatory mechanisms that allow developing children to modify the way they sense and move for postural control (Shumway-Cook & Woollacott, 2001; Woollacott, Shumway-Cook, & Williams, 1989).

▪ Upper and Lower Extremity Control

Functional movements of the extremities rely on the specific task-related movements required. It is helpful to divide extremity movement into two broad categories: weight-bearing or closed-chain activities and non–weight-bearing or open-chain activities. Skillful use of both the upper and lower extremities requires the ability to be functional in both weight bearing and non–weight bearing. Functionally, however, the main task of the lower extremities is concerned with weight bearing, stability, and mobility, including all the gross motor activities that accomplish the task of **locomotion** through space: rolling, crawling and creeping, and walking. The upper extremity is concerned with the task of **manipulation,** including all the aspects of reaching, grasping, and releasing. Although the primary task of the upper extremity is non–weight bearing, upper extremity weight bearing has important functional uses in increasing postural stability in upright positions.

▪ Upper Extremity Control, Including Manipulation

The major movement components of upper extremity function comprise either those required for movement in space or weight-bearing movements. Upper extremity function is most closely associated with the ability to move the arm in space and to manipulate objects (Ryerson & Levit, 1997). Ryerson and Levit offer a succinct method for assessing for the presence or absence of key movement components necessary for upper extremity functional performance. Those key components are the ability to reach forward, reach into abduction away from the body, reach backward, reach away from midline, reach across midline, and position the elbow and hand. Refer to the text *Functional Movement Reeducation* (1997) for details. A mastery of basic biomechanics and kinesiology by the reader is assumed by this author and is beyond the purpose of this text.

Although support of body weight is a function most commonly associated with the lower extremities, weight bearing is an important function of the upper extremity. Weight bearing on the upper extremity is used to support the weight of the trunk and upper body, to lift or move the body through transitional movements (such as sitting to side lying or pushing up to stand) and to stabilize against a surface for optimal task performance. All these functions require activity in the arm muscles to maintain the arm on the supporting surface and to support the weight of the body.

▪ Lower Extremity Control, Including Locomotion

Lower extremity control requires the ability to support body weight on both legs, to transfer weight from one to the other, to bear weight on one leg and then move the other, and to constantly adapt to movements of the trunk and upper extremities. We use lower extremity control with trunk control for safety and balance in all the possible position options. Lower extremity capabilities allow for all the functions of moving the body through space, including all the locomotor skills of rolling, crawling and creeping, walking, running, skipping, and hopping. The lower extremity is commonly associated with the function of weight bearing. The part of the leg that is supporting weight and the amount and type of muscle activation used during weight support vary according to body position and functional activity (Ryerson & Levit, 1997). Ryerson and Levit (1997) give detailed descriptions of key movement components necessary for lower extremity functional performance. Refer to that excellent text for specifics and details.

Control of the lower extremity is typically associated with locomotor abilities. The three major requirements for successful locomotion are progression, defined as the ability to generate a basic pattern that can move the body in the desired direction; stability, defined as the ability to support and control the body against gravity; and adaptability, defined as the ability to adapt the locomotion to meet the individual's goals and the demands of the environment (Shumway-Cook & Woollacott, 2001).

Life Span Development of Functional Movement

The remainder of this chapter will describe the development of postural control, upper extremity control, and lower extremity control during infancy, childhood, adolescence, adulthood, and aging. Several sources, in addition to the author's clinical experience, have been used to compile this information (Alexander et al., 1993; Bly, 1994; Campbell, 2000; Cech & Martin, 1995; Martin & Kessler, 2001; O'Sullivan, 2001; Ryerson & Levit, 1997; Shumway-Cook & Woollacott, 2001).The first year contains more detail than the later age stages, because it is during this first year that the basic movement components are developing, which will serve the individual for a lifetime. Never in the life span does an individual undergo such a rapid rate of change as during that incredible first year. The developmental process that is observed during the first year serves as a good model for studying the unfolding process of movement component acquisition and motor development (Alexander et al., 1993; Bly, 1994). When looking carefully at motor development during infancy, close attention should be paid to the emergence of key functional movement components: antigravity control (flexor and extensor), stability, mobility, the ability to demonstrate proximal stability (weight bearing), the emergence of smooth weight shifting, and rotation and dissociation. The focus should not be so much on the ages themselves but rather on the spiraling process that unfolds as the newborn transforms from a dependent being to an independent mover by the end of only 12 short months, then developing into an active toddler, adolescent, and productive adult.

Newborn

Anatomical differences between the newborn and the adult human being impact on the development of posture and movement. One anatomical variable is the relative size of one body part to another. For example, the newborn's head is proportionally larger than the rest of the body and the lower extremities are quite short in comparison to the trunk or upper extremities. The contour of the skeleton in the newborn is absent the effects of mature modeling and curvature seen in the older child secondary to the effects of gravity, weight

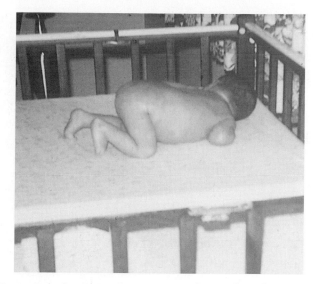

Figure 4–6. In prone on a support surface, a flexed posture is predominant whereby the limbs are held in symmetry and close to the body.

bearing, and muscle pull. The newborn vertebral column is kyphotic. Range of motion differences are also typical for the newborn, with some joints demonstrating hypermobility and others hypomobility. The newborn's ankles are typically excessively dorsiflexed (example of hypermobility), whereas the hips and knees demonstrate 30-degree flexion contractures (example of hypomobility). Both these differences are present secondary to the predominant flexed positioning of the baby within the confines of the womb.

■ Postural Control

The newborn baby is very much at the mercy of gravity, encountering it for the first time. At rest, newborn posture is typically flexed with the head usually positioned to either side. Held suspended in a prone position, there is obviously no ability to extend against gravitational pull (see Fig. 4–1). Prone on a support surface, the baby's hips are flexed, the spine is kyphotic, and weight is therefore borne on the upper trunk, shoulders, and head, making it difficult to raise the head or move about in this position. The limbs are typically postured in flexed symmetry and held close to the body (Fig. 4–6). The baby can lift the head and turn it from side to side to clear the airway for breathing. This ability to independently rotate the head, already available to the neonate, is life sustaining. Reflexive righting responses are seen, including neck righting and the beginning of labyrinthine righting. In supine, the head is usually positioned to the side and random movements of the extremities into mass extension and flexion are seen. The physiological flexion of the newborn provides the necessary stability at this age for posture and to permit random movements. When pulling to a sitting position, the newborn is not able to assist and a

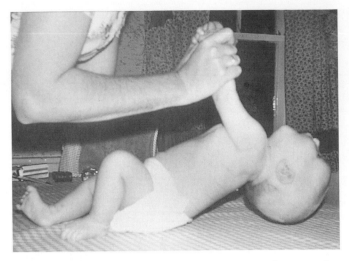

Figure 4–7. A full head lag is seen on pull to sit because the neck flexors have not yet developed voluntary antigravity strength and control.

full **head lag** is evident (Fig. 4–7). Sitting is not a functional position for the newborn because of the inability to maintain alignment or control in this position.

▪ Upper Extremity Control

Upper extremity movements are random, limited within a 90-degree plane, with the motion originating from the shoulder. Hands will open as the arm abducts, and hand movements are usually related to arm movements. Arm and hand movements are synergistically coupled (working together) (Von Hofsten, 1990). When the arms are held close to the body, the fingers usually are flexed and adducted; with shoulder abduction and elbow extension, the fingers abduct and extension increases. The **grasp reflex** is strong, where strong finger flexion accompanies tactile stimulation to the palm of the hand, especially the ulnar side. Newborns demonstrate reflexive hand-to-mouth and hand-to-hand contact, usually accomplished in a side-lying position.

In the prone position, the upper extremities are usually flexed and adducted underneath, with weight shifted forward onto the hands (see Fig. 4–6). Already, however, by 2 weeks after birth, the small rotator cuff muscles begin to activate by adducting the humerus into the glenoid fossa, thereby increasing joint stability so that the shoulders can begin to accept weight without collapsing. These small muscles provide an important base of stability for random movements, such as early swiping, and future shoulder girdle development in weight bearing (Alexander et al., 1993).

▪ Lower Extremity Control

Newborn babies are not passive, but are usually moving when awake. In the newborn, the available range of motion limits the expressed movements. The neonate has soft tissue tightness, which holds the hips in flexion, abduction, and external rotation, the knees in flexion, the ankles dorsiflexed, and the upper extremities flexed close to the body (Bleck, 1987). During active periods, the newborn kicks vigorously in a rhythmical, **reciprocal** pattern. Movement can be described as random and undifferentiated. There are total body movements into flexion or extension, accompanied by rhythmical alternating wide-ranged movements of the limbs. Movements are reflexive in nature, triggered by a specific stimulus with a stereotypical response. Newborn babies demonstrate an automatic standing reaction, as well as automatic stepping (see Fig. 4–2), accepting weight when held in standing with a straightening of the lower limbs, trunk, and neck.

One to Two Months

Many changes occur during the first 2 months of life. Physiological flexion decreases and active postural control is beginning. Increases in spinal extension and resolution of the soft tissue tightness are initially seen at the hips and knees.

▪ Postural Control

By 2 months of age, posture at rest is less flexed and beginning antigravity control is evident. Random movements continue but are less jerky. Supine posture is generally more extended but predominantly still asymmetrical. Functional activity in the supine position is still quite limited, characterized by active head turning and random, semi-controlled extremity movements

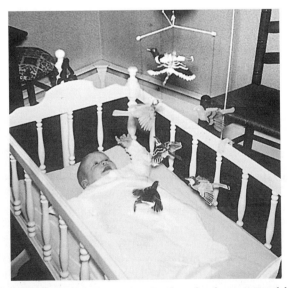

Figure 4–8. Posture in supine is already characterized by a more midline orientation of the head, and sweeping arm movements are seen.

(Bly, 1994) (Fig. 4–8). The head and extremities appear to move more freely in the supported position of supine, as they begin to dissociate from the trunk. The physiological flexor tone begins to be reduced by gravity and by the beginning development of antigravity extensor strength and control. Extensor muscle activation enables the flexor muscles to be systematically elongated. This elongation puts the muscles at optimal length for the development of voluntary control. The physiological flexor tone has been reduced by gravity and by increased extensor activity, but active antigravity flexor activity has yet to emerge. When pulled to sitting, asymmetrical antigravity flexion of the neck may be seen with a partial or even full head lag demonstrated. The baby can now hold the head momentarily when supported in sitting. When tipped forward or backward, the baby attempts to hold the head upright but is unable to maintain it as flexor and extensor control are not yet working together. Until this balance occurs, the head bobs and lateral control cannot develop.

In the prone position, increased cervical and thoracic extension permits more success against gravity and the head and neck muscles are the first to exhibit antigravity activation. Head and neck hyperextension are therefore the first components of antigravity postural control. This head extension in turn causes a posterior weight shift, freeing the upper trunk from the supporting surface. Prone positioning is crucial in decreasing the hip and knee flexion through elongation of the hip flexors and the hamstrings. The head can be lifted to 45 degrees in the prone position by the end of the second month. This baby is able to maintain a posture of prone on elbows, although the elbows are positioned behind the shoulders in an effort to increase stability (Fig. 4–9). The trunk is used actively against the supporting surface to gain the needed stability.

▪ Upper Extremity Control

Random motion in wider ranges is seen. In the supine position, gravity has succeeded in pulling the arms into

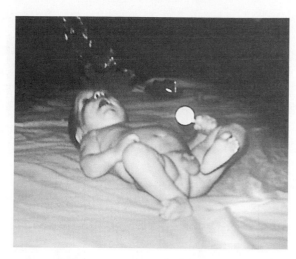

Figure 4–10. Baby can now hold on to an object placed in the hand.

increased external rotation, elongating the anterior chest and arm muscles. Asymmetrical swiping at an object occurs by the end of the second month. The grasp reflex is dissipating, and the infant can now briefly voluntarily retain an object placed in the hand (Fig. 4–10). Shoulder girdle muscles may provide the synergistic stability required to allow for early head lifting.

The 2-month-old baby is beginning to use the arms to push up in prone. However, limited shoulder girdle stability makes this a difficult, less than functional position for this young infant. In the prone position, the baby can bring the head and mouth to the hand rather than the hand to the mouth. The prone on elbows posture is typically seen with the elbows behind the shoulder, allowing the humerus to assume a position of abduction, extension, and internal rotation to ensure maximum positional stability. Bilateral scapular retraction and spinal extension seem to provide synergistic stability for head lifting. The baby's weight can now be shifted caudally, but the upper chest is still pressed onto the surface, serving as the pivot point for head lifting. Because the hands are bearing some of the weight in the prone position, head lifting will facilitate proprioceptive feedback to the upper extremities and trunk. This weight bearing and proprioceptive feedback are important precursors for future forearm stability and weight shifting (Alexander et al., 1993; Bly, 1994).

▪ Lower Extremity Control

The increased range of motion into spinal extension and hip and knee extension allows for greater antigravity movement in many positions. Movement and kicking patterns are usually quite variable. This variability is an important characteristic of normal motor development. Reciprocal kicking may be interspersed with bilateral symmetrical kicking. Kicking usually occurs with the legs in the air, due to continued hip flexor tightness.

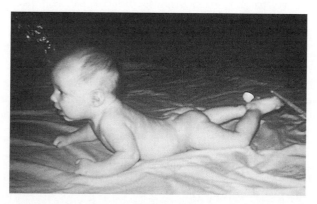

Figure 4–9. Early forearm propping in prone is characterized by flexion of the elbows behind the shoulders.

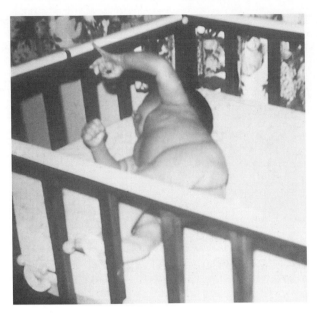

Figure 4–11. Rolling is first seen as a spontaneous motor pattern.

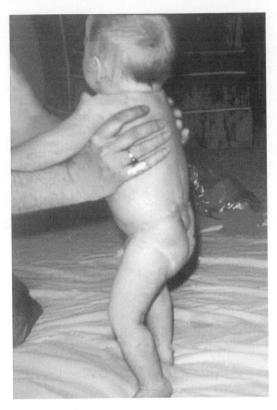

Figure 4–12. A period of astasia ("without stance") is demonstrated by no assumption of weight bearing when placed on feet; automatic stepping has also disappeared.

Thelen suggests that the infant's kicking is not completely random, but rather occurs as a result of linked muscle synergies, linkages that are necessary for the first walking patterns (Thelen, 1985).

Rolling, defined as the earliest form of locomotion, is seen as a spontaneous motor pattern as early as 1 to 2 months of age (Fig. 4–11). The first pattern seen is from side lying back into supine and is largely simply a matter of gravity succeeding in moving the infant as a unit, returning onto the back from a side-lying position.

The infant demonstrates little or no weight bearing when placed on the feet, and automatic stepping is no longer elicited. This time is called a period of **astasia,** which literally means "without stance," gradually giving way to a more voluntary assumption of stance later on (Fig. 4–12).

Three to Five Months

Head and trunk symmetry and midline orientation are the hallmarks of the third through fifth month. The 3 month old demonstrates a marked increase in bilateral symmetrical activities and antigravity flexor control, with the head well controlled in midline. Around the fourth month, posture and movement change from being typically asymmetrical to typically symmetrical. Motions of the head and cervical spine become almost complete and are used in functional movement. As a result of weight shifting and rotational movements, thoracic motion increases. The first secondary lordotic curve is developing in the cervical region as a response to mastery in the prone and the vertical positions, with the ability by 4 months to hold the head erect and

steady against gravity. In addition to spinal extension, hip and knee extension are increasing and the muscle bulk of the spinal extensors is easily seen. The hamstrings elongate, and ankle plantar flexion increases (Alexander et al., 1993; Bly, 1994).

▪ Postural Control

Antigravity flexor and extensor muscle activity develop in supine and prone positions. Functional head control is attained in all positions. In supine, the infant tucks the chin when pulled to sitting by 3 months and lifts the head completely by 5 months. Head-righting reactions are developed and the trunk rights when tipped forward and backward in space. Lateral trunk righting begins to be seen during the fifth month (Fig. 4–13). The infant can now hold symmetrical postures and begins to demonstrate postural anticipatory activity in preparation for volitional movements. The infant can shift weight laterally through the head, shoulders, and upper trunk.

In the prone position, the baby can lift and hold the head in the erect position with good control, propping on forearms by 4 months and pushing up onto extended arms by 5 months (Fig. 4–14). The elbows are in line with the shoulders already by 3 months and in front of

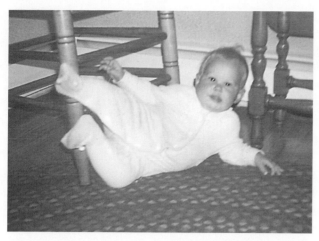

Figure 4–13. Lateral trunk righting and beginning control in side lying is seen at 5 months. Note the elongation of the trunk on the weight-bearing side in combination with the lateral flexion on the non–weight-bearing side of the trunk.

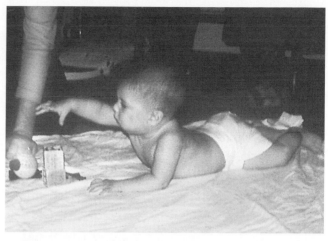

Figure 4–15. Early reaching from the prone position. Note that the reaching pattern of the lower upper extremity (LUE) is in shoulder internal rotation.

the shoulders shortly after, permitting the opportunity for weight shifting and reach in prone (Fig. 4–15). Increasing proximal stability at the shoulder girdle allows for reaching in prone. Forearm propping causes a marked posterior weight shift so that the weight-bearing fulcrum then moves caudally. The chest is now elevated off the support surface, which is reflective of increasing upper trunk control. Gradually, spinal extension proceeds from the cervical and thoracic area into the lumbar area, a hallmark of normal postural development as the infant gradually acquires a more upright posture. Rood described the prone extension pattern as the "pivot prone" position, which serves to increase spinal extension and thoracic expansion dramatically (Stockmeyer, 1966) (Fig. 4–16). Symmetry and increased

extension are dominant in the prone position. Strong, active antigravity trunk extension is demonstrated by the ability to maintain trunk extension when held horizontally in the air (**Landau reaction**).

Sitting can be maintained for brief periods with first upper trunk and then lower trunk support. To first stabilize in this position, posture is typically characterized by increased cervical spine and upper back extension and the arms are initially held in a **high on-guard position** of abduction and external rotation. Sitting can be maintained independently for brief periods with minimal or intermittent support. Although spinal extensors are the primary postural muscles used in sitting, the baby at this early age reinforces this stability with scapular retraction, which in turn limits upper extrem-

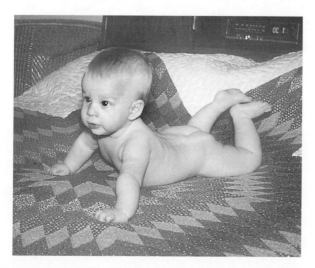

Figure 4–14. Early pushing up onto extended arms is characterized by a broadened UE base and some hyperextension of the elbows because of still-emergent muscular strength and control.

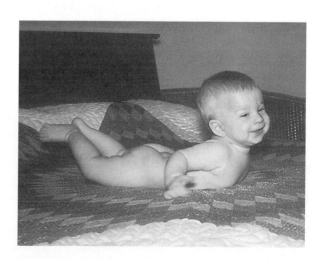

Figure 4–16. "Pivot prone" is a position that serves to increase spinal extension and thoracic expansion as the baby continues to master gravity.

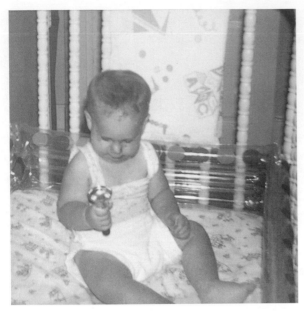

Figure 4–17. Tactile awareness develops in the hand as the hand accommodates to the shape of an object.

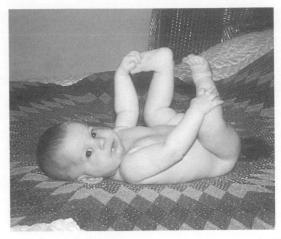

Figure 4–18. Antigravity flexion strength and continued laxity of the pelvic soft tissue allow for hand-to-foot play in supine, as the baby explores his or her own boundaries.

ity function in unsupported positions (Alexander et al., 1993). Sitting in seats with a safety strap is functionally important at this age.

■ Upper Extremity Control

The range of **reach** varies with the position and the degree of support, but the following abilities are seen: voluntary swiping and reaching, reaching forward, bilateral reach patterns, and strong hand-to-mouth preferences. Elbow extension has increased, taking the hands farther away from the body. Eye-hand coordination improves. The baby can actively adduct and internally rotate the shoulders to bring the hands closer to the body. Active control of the shoulders in many positions and within all three planes is increasing.

Sustained voluntary **grasp** has now replaced the grasp reflex. Grasp is now completely visually and tactually controlled. The baby now enjoys increasing opportunities to learn body awareness as play includes exploration of his or her own hands and body parts, as well as tactile exploration of a greater variety of objects. The weight-shifting experiences in prone have now opened the hand and contributed to dissociation of the thumb from the rest of the fingers (see Fig. 4–15). The infant is able to use the fingers in a grasp without thumb involvement by 3 months and progresses to a symmetrical palmar grasp by 5 months of age. The hand then starts to accommodate to the shape of an object, and tactile awareness develops in the hand (Fig. 4–17). Objects can be transferred from hand to hand by 5 months, another skill that contributes to an emergent body awareness (Alexander et al., 1993; Bly, 1994).

■ Lower Extremity Control

In the supine position, the infant demonstrates increasing mastery over gravity, as evidenced by the ability to bring hands to knees (4 months) and hands to feet (5 months) (Fig. 4–18). The infant can bridge by 5 months and begins to move about in the supine position. This lower extremity pushing against the floor will increase spinal extension and lateral weight shifting, eventually stretching the tight hip flexors and allowing for increased hip extension (Fig. 4–19). Alternating movements of the trunk and lower extremity flexors and extensors allow for anterior and posterior tilting of the

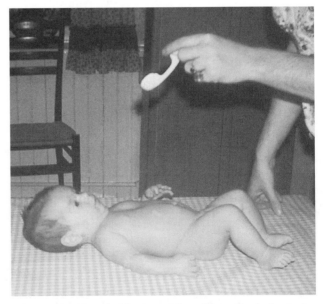

Figure 4–19. This "bridge" position allows the baby to bear weight through the feet and eventually push up, activating the hip extensors and abdominals.

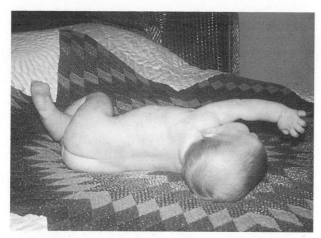

Figure 4–20. Log rolling means that the baby first rolls as a unit, without segmental rotation.

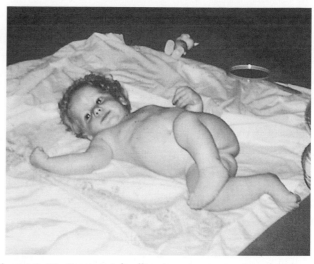

Figure 4–21. Segmental rolling is seen as rotation develops.

pelvis, providing a basis for further development of lower extremity movements. The change from lower extremity symmetry to the beginning of lower extremity dissociation is a major step, usually emerging at around 5 months. Lower extremity weight shifting begins.

Rolling is actively initiated by 4 to 6 months of age. Rolling to the side is accomplished by 4 months and rolling prone to supine emerges typically by the end of the fifth month. Initially, rolling is a loss of control rather than an act of control. These earliest active rolling movements are initially performed with the body moving as a unit, described as "log-rolling," without segmental rotation (Fig. 4–20).

The baby will stand with arms or hands held with a wide base of support and may begin to bilaterally flex and extend knees in a supported stance at this time. Isolated knee flexion and extension have both increased, but there is not yet smooth alternation between the two. It is important to remember that the infant is still unable to move into sitting or standing independently, but the ability to right the body or move into a more upright posture is beginning to evolve. The seeds of this ability are in initial rolling movements and in the actions that lift the pelvis and chest up off the support surface in the prone position (Campbell, 2000).

Six Months

The sixth month is characterized by increased antigravity control, more trunk control, and evidence of a greater variety of both upper and lower extremity positions, creating the opportunity for more movement options in supine, prone, and side-lying positions. The baby further develops voluntary asymmetrical, dissociated, and reciprocal movements, coordinating and integrating previously developed movement components

(Bly, 1994). This is the time when segmental rotation is first seen. The baby is much more active, especially in prone and supine positions, requiring less positional stability. The instinctive need to be upright becomes obvious at this age.

■ Postural Control

By 6 months of age, the baby has sufficient postural control to maintain a variety of postures against gravity. Antigravity control is strong enough now that the baby has an equal ability to either fully flex in supine or fully extend in prone position. The baby sits for long periods and actively holds a variety of other postures in supine, prone, and side-lying positions. There is greater postural activity of the lower trunk, pelvic girdle, and lower extremities than in previous months. The baby can now shift the weight from the lower part of the body in prone, supine, and side-lying positions, working off the supporting surface. This provides more lateral control and allows for greater dissociation of one side of the body from the other. These postural responses are used to accompany reach or for the first transitions in space, such as segmental rolling (Fig. 4–21) and belly **crawling.** Eventually, these increased transitions in space offer opportunity for broader exploration of the child's world (Fig. 4–22). There is greater control for unilateral movements and asymmetrical postures.

In concert with increased trunk control, head control is fully developed by this age. Trunk righting is present when the baby is tipped in space, and equilibrium reactions are evident first in prone, then in supine positions. There is more evidence of rotation through the trunk. The infant demonstrates protective extension of the arms when displaced forward. The infant sits well in a highchair and begins to sit independently with arm

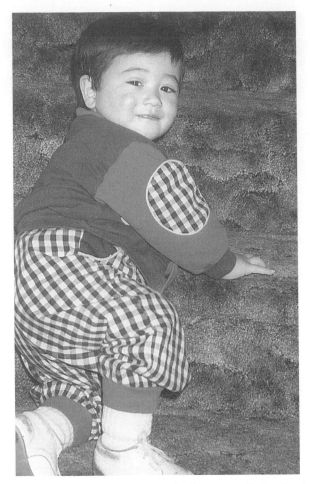

Figure 4–22. Locomotion on the floor in the form of either crawling or creeping soon offers the young child an opportunity to further explore the world (such as crawling up those steps!).

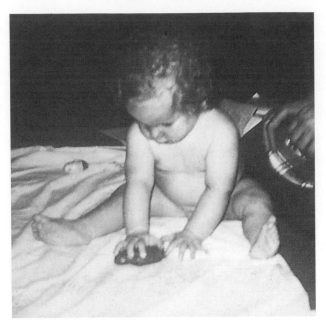

Figure 4–23. Early independent floor sitting is seen with a very wide base, arms propped forward onto the floor.

■ Upper Extremity Control

Shoulder girdle muscles can now move and stabilize the humerus through a greater range of motions. Weight shift through the upper extremities is now smooth and controlled in prone. Reaching forward from prone is now functional. The baby can prop onto an extended arm or a forearm and stretch forward with the other arm. Fine motor control at this age varies with the degree of proximal stability that is provided. For example, when sitting, the baby's reach and grasp control is better when the trunk is supported than when the baby attempts to use the upper extremities while in independent sitting. In the supine position, where the entire trunk is stabilized by the supporting surface, the child has optimal control of the upper extremity (Alexander et al., 1993). In sitting, supine, and side-lying positions, the baby continues to primarily use a bilateral reach but the first signs of unilateral reach are seen. This ability accompanies increased pelvic control, allowing for a stable base on which to move.

Reach is consistently visually directed and quite accurate by this time. Reach in upright positions is typically accomplished with forearm pronation and internal rotation at the shoulder (see Fig. 4–15). Forearm supination accompanies external rotation at the shoulder, seen when the baby is fully stabilized in the supine position, such as when reaching forward to engage in foot play. A consistent palmar grasp is demonstrated, followed by a radial palmar grasp, as the thumb begins to emerge as a separate prehensile tool. Functionally, attempts are made at holding a cup and spoon; finger feeding is successful (Fig. 4–24) (Alexander et al., 1993; Bly, 1994).

support. Characteristic floor sitting is with a very wide base, arms propped forward onto the floor (Fig. 4–23). Postural synergies that are vital to maintaining the sitting position include the erector spinae, abdominals, hip extensors and hip flexors. Reaching from sitting with one arm while propped with the other begins to be seen (Alexander et al., 1993).

In the prone position, lateral weight shifting through the lower trunk and pelvis is now seen. Play in prone is now very functional, with a variety of forearm and extended arm positions. The baby experiments with how far weight can be shifted and starts to gain control of moving through space, between prone and side-lying positions. The baby can also pivot in a circle while prone. There is obvious trunk elongation and a lower extremity extension pattern on one side, with lateral trunk flexion and slight flexion of the lower extremity on the other side. This pattern of one leg extended and the other flexed signifies dissociation and preparation for the reciprocal pattern required for belly crawling.

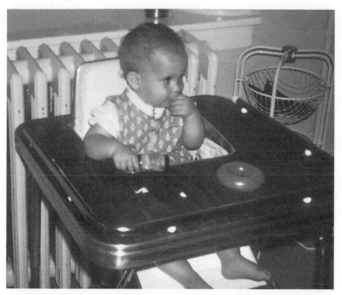

Figure 4–24. Finger feeding becomes possible as the fingers separate from the thumb and the hand develops increasing prehensile skill.

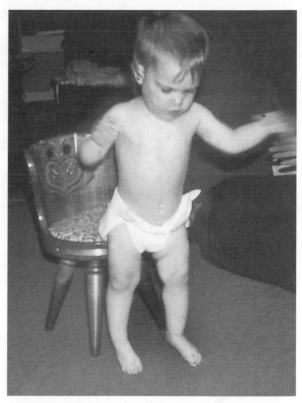

Figure 4–25. Early supported stance is precarious, as evidenced by fixed hip extension with a narrow base and scapular retraction.

▪ Lower Extremity Control

The baby now demonstrates increased antigravity control in all positions, with increased strength, endurance, and coordination of muscle patterns. This is the age when babies often play with their feet, arching and twisting about in a supine position, sometimes making diaper changes a real challenge for parents. Increased postural activity of the lower extremities is seen, both to maintain postures and to accompany voluntary movements. The baby frequently uses the side-lying position for play, often weight bearing onto one foot. This weight bearing on the plantar surface of the foot, rolling onto the medial and lateral surfaces, may be important for setting up the postural activity of the foot needed for later development. Play in this now-controlled side-lying position helps to develop strength in the abdominal oblique muscles on the shortened (upper) side and to elongate the weight-bearing (lower) side of the trunk (see Fig. 4–13). The desire to get upright can be observed as the baby tries to sit up from side lying but lacks the strength and rotational control of the trunk necessary to be successful.

The baby rolls from between supine, side-lying, and prone positions with control, able to stop at any point within the roll. Rolling is now used for locomotion to move about the environment, as the baby consecutively rolls across the floor. As with all movement patterns, practice is required and individual variations exist. Some babies may push off of one foot from supine to initiate the roll, followed by extension and then flexion until the weight is shifted into the prone position. Others may initiate the roll from supine by flexing the

lower extremities and then initiating the momentum with horizontal adduction of the arm and trunk rotation until the weight is shifted sufficiently to roll.

Supported stance posture is characterized by a narrower base and increased hip extension, accomplished with less support (Fig. 4–25). The infant readily bounces up and down in a supported stance. This bouncing increases the strength of the lower extremities and provides important sensory information.

Seven to Nine Months

This third trimester after birth is marked by less time spent in the prone or supine position and a great deal of time spent in sitting, assuming **quadruped** (all fours) positions, and pulling to stand (Fig. 4–26). Sitting is the most favorite and preferred position for the 8 month old. The change now occurs to assumption of more upright positions, requiring a great deal more postural stability. Babies at this time are extremely active against gravity. In particular, pelvic and hip stability increases from 7 to 9 months and is coordinated with head, shoulder girdle, and trunk control in a variety of positions. The baby at this age is capable of many functional motor skills and uses movement to interact with the environment (Alexander et al., 1993). It is important to

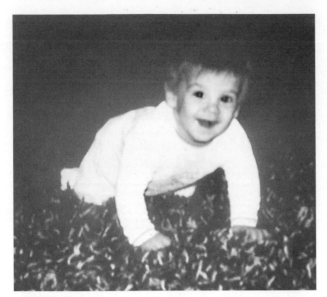

Figure 4–26. The assumption of all fours (quadruped) quickly leads to creeping as a locomotor skill.

realize that the components used by the 7- to 9-month-old baby are a continuation of those initiated by the 5 and 6 month old: proximal stability and weight bearing, weight shifting and lateral righting, dissociation and rotation, and increased antigravity strength. One important aspect of normal motor development is the variety of patterns available to accomplish a motor skill. This age is also characterized by a fairly large number of transitional postures assumed during the process of moving from one position to another, a feature that decreases in later development. Prone and quadruped are the preferred positions for the 7 month old, with occasional play in supine with a lightweight toy. By 9 months, the more upright the position, the happier the baby (Alexander et al., 1993; Bly, 1994).

▪ Postural Control

There is now increased postural activity to maintain upright positions and to engage in the transition among sitting, quadruped, and supported standing. More postural stability is required to accompany functional movements within these more upright positions. Postural activity must provide stability and control the weight shifts during all these movements. There is an increased ability to adapt the posture before a movement to allow for more efficient movement execution. The baby may change posture before a movement so that it is mechanically more efficient to support a movement or move over the base of support. These postural adjustments are vital for the emergence of sophisticated, mature motor control. Synergistic activity of all proximal areas is crucial for function in and transition from one position to another (Bly, 1994).

Feedback-based postural reactions continue to develop over these months. Postural reactions occur when an outside force challenges balance or when the baby loses control of the center of gravity over the base of support. Equilibrium reactions are fully developed in prone and supine by 7 months, in sitting by 8 months, and emerging in quadruped during the eighth month. The arms will now extend in protective extension when the baby is displaced to either side in sitting.

The baby can now sit on the floor with an erect trunk without support and move the upper body over the base of support to play. Independent sitting is typically achieved by 8 months of age. Trunk control is well developed by 9 months of age. Sitting becomes much more dynamic as the baby is able to shift weight in wider ranges without falling. Moving the trunk over the lower extremities, the baby learns to efficiently reach out and move into the surrounding space (Fig. 4–27). Upper trunk rotation is demonstrated during play, and the arms dissociate from the trunk, allowing the arms to move across and away from the body. The base in sitting has now narrowed, and greater varieties of floor-sitting positions become observable, including side sitting (Fig. 4–28) or half-ring sitting (Fig. 4–29). **Transitions** can now be made between sitting and prone or quadruped (Fig. 4–30).

▪ Upper Extremity Control

The baby uses the upper extremities at this time for two very divergent tasks: to reach and manipulate and to pull with in order to move the body into increasingly upright positions. Control of arm function continues to improve as the child gains control of the upper extremity in weight bearing. Scapulohumeral muscles become stronger, allowing the child to utilize humeral rotation

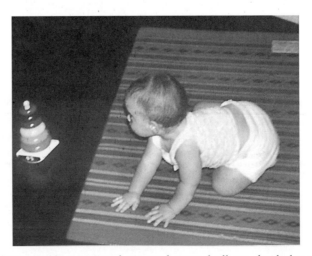

Figure 4–27. Increased postural control allows the baby to move the trunk over the lower extremities and move out farther into the surrounding world.

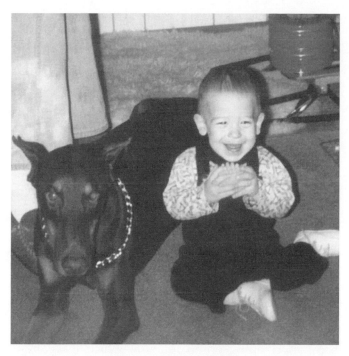

Figure 4–28. Side sitting.

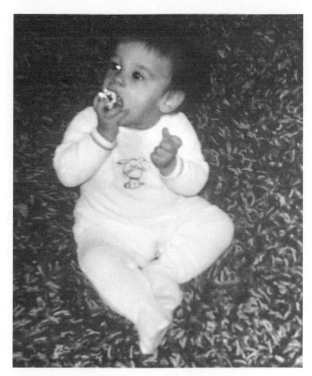

Figure 4–29. Half-ring sitting.

smoothly during function. Dynamic scapular stability improves in many positions. The increased trunk and pelvic control frees the arms from the postural system and enables the baby to use a variety of shoulder and forearm movements (Bly, 1994) (Fig. 4–31). The infant can now reach farther in all directions due to increasing

postural control, and the upper extremities are often freed from their support role in sitting so that they can engage in play, exploration, and manipulation.

Grasp is typically radial palmar, and a radial digital grasp is developing. The baby can isolate a finger to point and is developing a pincer grasp. Grip is quite strong and can maintain an object against resistance,

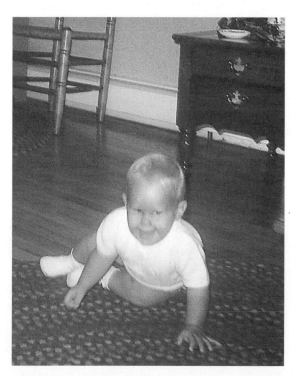

Figure 4–30. Floor movement is characterized by the ability to make transitions between sitting and prone or quadruped.

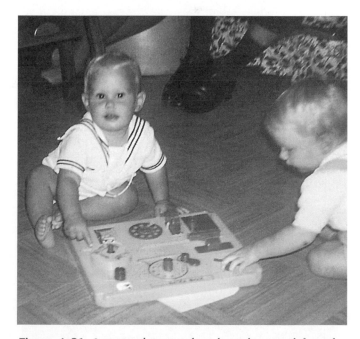

Figure 4–31. Increased postural and trunk control free the arms and enable the body to practice an increased variety of fine motor skills.

requiring not only upper extremity strength but also trunk control. The amount of upper extremity weight bearing and the rocking seen in the quadruped position serve to lengthen the muscles and soft tissue of the palm and fingers. The palmar arches are strengthened and reinforced (Boehme, 1988). The increased space visible between the thumb and fingers indicates that the palmar arches are active. By 9 months of age, reaching is accomplished in supination or pronation with good shoulder control and the wrist in extension. **Release** is precisely accurate. The emergence of grasp, reach, and release will be expanded on in Chapter 9.

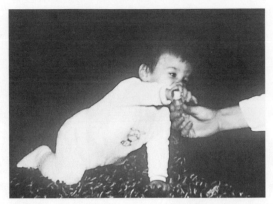

Figure 4–33. Reaching from a quadruped position.

■ Lower Extremity Control

The greater control and mobility within sitting allows for sitting to be a transitional position between prone, sitting, and eventually quadruped. The baby can easily independently achieve sitting. Play in prone is in a laterally shifted, asymmetrical posture, where the baby simply uses the prone position as a departure point for moving around the floor and transitioning to another position. Rolling during this third trimester after birth assumes a relatively common pattern among infants of similar age, of trunk rotation with predominant flexion patterns of the extremities.

The baby can maintain a quadruped position, rocking back and forth to gain proximal stability and proprioceptive awareness. The quadruped position can also be modified by weight bearing on one or both feet rather than the knees, a position often described as a "bear-standing" position (Fig. 4–32). The infant is stable

enough in quadruped to reach from it and to use it as a common transitional position to sitting (Figs. 4–33 and 4–34), side lying, and finally, kneeling at a support. Belly crawling and pivoting continue to be seen in prone, but the primary locomotion mode quickly becomes **creeping** on all fours, at which the baby is proficient by 9 months (see Fig. 4–26). This locomotion is possible because weight can be shifted from one set of supporting limbs to the other, requiring trunk control, proximal stability, dissociation, and rotation. Creeping is demonstrated in a reciprocal pattern on hands and knees, using a lateral flexion and elongation pattern through the trunk.

By the end of this period, the infant can kneel at a supporting surface, often with incomplete hip extension at first, using this position as both a play position and as a transition to standing (Fig. 4–35). Pulling to stand at a support surface is accomplished with a great deal of effort from the arms and upper trunk at first. Transition

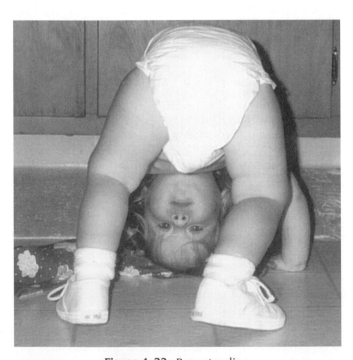

Figure 4–32. Bear standing.

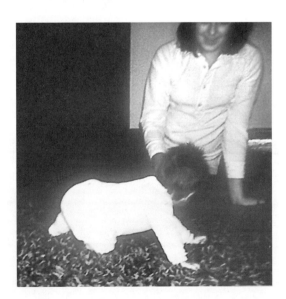

Figure 4–34. Use of a quadruped position as a transition to sitting.

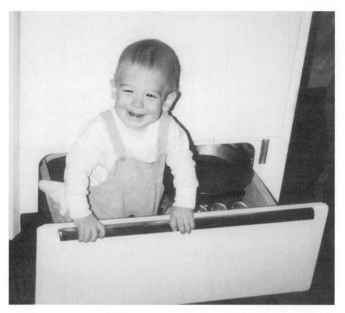

Figure 4–35. Kneeling at support (also allows for exploration of some unique aspects of the environment).

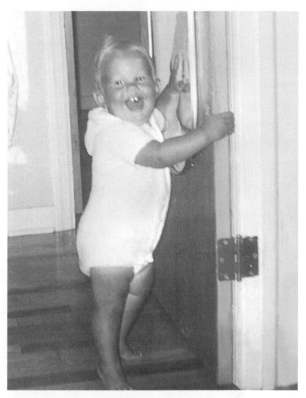

Figure 4–36. Early standing and cruising require that the baby lean against support.

to standing at support typically occurs in a straight movement from sitting or kneeling, occasionally using a half kneel. Half kneeling requires a great deal of lower extremity dissociation, usually emerging later. Once in standing, the baby experiments with pelvic and lower extremity weight shifting. The baby first needs to lean against the support surface and then eventually demonstrates adequate trunk control and postural stability to pull away from the surface (Fig. 4–36). The baby can lower himself or herself to the floor, with increasing control after a great deal of practice. **Cruising** along furniture is the next accomplishment, allowing experience in stepping. The baby initially steps sideways and then experiments with turning diagonally to step forward (Fig. 4–37). Rotation is being practiced in standing, initiated by head rotation, as it first was in supine, prone, and sitting. With one hand held, the 9-month-old baby can often stand alone, and he or she can venture a few steps with bilateral hand support. The baby's urge to explore the environment at this age is not limited to movement on the floor. This is the age when climbing begins as well (Fig. 4–38).

Ten to Twelve Months

At 10 to 12 months, the baby is more efficient in the upright position than ever before. The second secondary lordotic curve is developing in the lumbar spine as it becomes more extended, allowing the upper body to be vertically aligned with the pelvis in kneeling and standing. The curves of the vertebral column are now in their adult configuration, providing not only muscular

but also skeletal stability, needed for postural alignment. A great deal of time is spent pulling to stand, cruising, and lowering the body back down to the floor. Climbing becomes a favorite activity, much to the parent's chagrin. By the end of the first year, the baby is

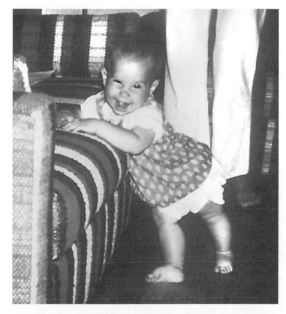

Figure 4–37. Cruising along furniture allows the baby to practice standing with support with increasing amounts of rotation and dissociation. Notice the weight shifting over the bare feet.

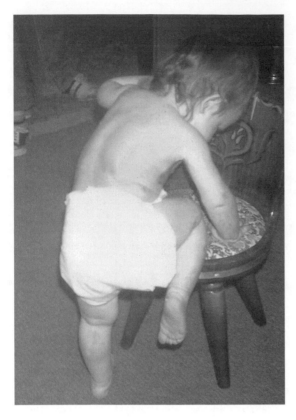

Figure 4–38. Climbing begins, allowing for increased practice in balance and weight shifting.

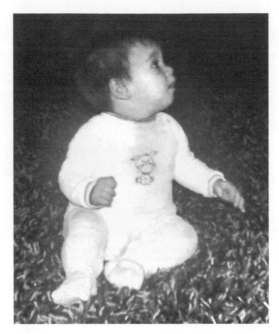

Figure 4–39. Stable sitting with rotation, arms free.

in sitting and quadruped positions and beginning to develop in kneeling and standing. The newly assumed standing position is the infant's preferred posture for developing balance. Hanging onto furniture or with

able to sequence many different movement patterns and begins upright locomotion. Creeping, however, is still the main mode of fast, efficient locomotion. Babies at this time are very busy, actively exploring the environment and practicing all their motor skills.

▪ Postural Control

Postural stability of the lower body develops rapidly during this time as the baby gains more efficiency and functional control of more upright positions. The baby is now totally stable in sitting, able to demonstrate protective extension with the upper extremities when displaced to the rear. Sitting is very dynamic, with a great variety of positions and transitions available and the ability to reach and play accomplished with ease (Fig. 4–39). Transitions from the floor are efficiently accomplished from sitting and a quadruped position, including the ability to sit up independently from side lying. The baby has enough postural control to sit on a small stool, perhaps having climbed up onto it (Fig. 4–40). The child can now creep up stairs independently.

The pelvis and lower extremities are increasingly engaged in postural activity, initiating and controlling weight shifts from the pelvic girdle in sitting and during movement transitions. Equilibrium reactions are refined

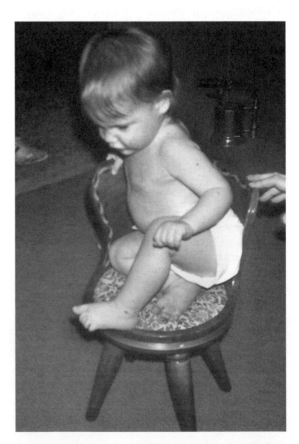

Figure 4–40. Baby now has sufficient postural control to sit on a small stool, having climbed up onto it.

parental support, the child begins to exercise stepping movements that challenge dynamic balance development in the upright position (Cech & Martin, 1995). Postural reactions to an unexpected movement of the center of gravity continue to develop. Spontaneous postural reactions occur less often in sitting and quadruped positions because postural changes are more adequately coordinated with movement in these now stable positions. However, postural adjustments are seen often in the newer positions of standing and beginning walking.

■ Upper Extremity Control

Increased lumbar extension stabilizes the trunk and frees the upper extremities for exploration and play. The upper extremities are now freed from the previous tasks of weight-bearing and pushing activities and are able to develop more refined prehensile skill. In kneeling and standing, the arms are used only as a distal point of stability for balance, whereas in sitting, they are completely free to reach and play. Because of this increased trunk control, scapular retraction is no longer needed in sitting to ensure stability.

Increased trunk control and rotation in sitting allows the child to reach across midline. The child enjoys manipulating objects of many different sizes, textures, and shapes. The child masters the three-jaw chuck, the pincer grasp, and finally the finger-to-tip prehension ability (see Figs. 9–1 through 9–5). Increased dissociation enables isolation of the fingers from the thumb and from each other. Finger control is more refined for grasp than for release initially, but release is being practiced by putting objects of varying sizes into containers. Bimanual dexterity is evident with a great deal of pushing, pulling, squeezing, and rotating of objects as the baby explores and learns. Functionally, this increased upper extremity control allows for increased independence in feeding and undressing (Alexander et al., 1993; Bly, 1994).

■ Lower Extremity Control

The increased lumbar extension frees the lower extremities from positions such as hip abduction and external rotation that previously had served to increase stability by widening the base of support. Any variety of floor sitting is now seen, including positions that require rotation to play, such as side sitting and half-ring sitting, as well as long sitting, available because of elongated hamstrings and full pelvic control. The baby at this age is able to sit, kneel, stand with or without support, and perhaps begin a few steps. Some precocious infants begin independent walking at this time. The child has

sufficient control and strength to pull to stand using less upper body strength and less physical support; more of the strength is coming from the lower extremities. The child can now lower himself backward off of furniture. Most children at this age can either stand independently momentarily or stand with minimal support, even reaching and playing from supported stance. Children can attain upright stance independently at a support and lower to the floor through a squat, indicative of eccentric control of the hip and knee extensors. Pulling to stand using a half-kneel position in transition is seen more frequently (Fig. 4–41). Postural stability and reaching while standing at support is developing, with reach from upright accompanied by a great deal of trunk rotation and dissociation. In cruising, the timing and coordination of the steps and the movement of the center of gravity become smoother and less choppy. Independent standing and walking still require positional stability of the lower extremities, especially external rotation. A wide base, lordosis, protruding abdomen, and high on-guard position of the upper extremities, combining to offer increased positional stability, characterize the initial independent stance posture (Fig. 4–42).

Pelvic and lower extremity activity not only contribute to the maintenance of more upright postures but also play an important role in the coordination of posture with movement. In sitting and quadruped positions, the baby begins to displace the center of gravity by moving the pelvis over the femurs during weight shifts. In sitting, the baby can move the pelvis in all planes to shift the center of gravity in wider ranges for reaching and transitional movement. The range of hip internal rotation increases, allowing for greater ranges

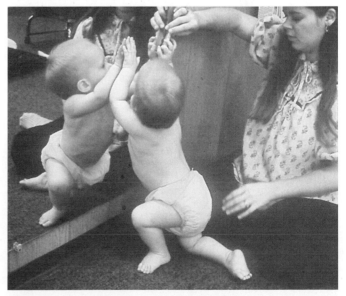

Figure 4–41. Pulling to stand using half kneel as a transitional position.

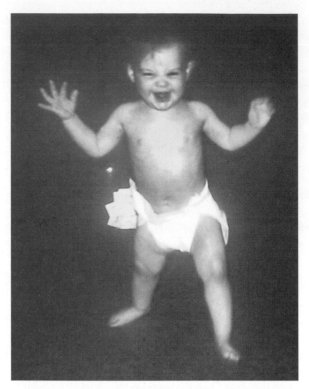

Figure 4–42. Early walking is characterized by high on-guard position of upper extremities, lumbar lordosis and protruding abdomen, and a wide base of support of the lower extremities.

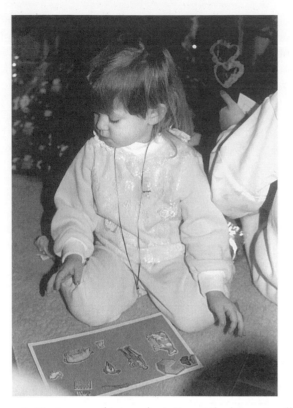

Figure 4–43. Increased internal rotation at the hips may allow the child to use w sitting as one of a variety of sitting position options.

of motion of the pelvis over the lower extremities. This increased degree of internal rotation may allow the child to w sit, often seen as just one of a variety of sitting position options (Fig. 4–43).

The musculature of the lower extremities is very active throughout play and movement transitions. The ankle and foot muscles are intensely active during play in floor sitting, providing distal stability. Also, the weight-bearing foot is more active against the surface in both sitting and standing. The toes, in particular, demonstrate an increased level of participation, flexing, extending, and abducting to stabilize the foot and leg. In weight bearing, the toes grasp the surface or extend to push against the floor (Alexander et al., 1993; Bly, 1994; Martin & Kessler, 2000).

Twelve to Eighteen Months

The infant becomes a toddler at 12 months. By 18 months of age, the toddler can efficiently coordinate postural control and movement for ambulation on a smooth surface without falling; has made significant gains in fine motor control, allowing for beginning independence in feeding; and is rather capable of some level of functional independence. When ready to walk, the child rather quickly develops the coordination of

postures and movement needed for upright function. The child walks to objects, squats, and picks them up. Push-and-pull toys give tremendous enjoyment as the baby practices this new skill. The child can now walk to drawers and cupboards, quickly learning to balance while not only opening and closing them but also emptying the contents onto the floor. The amount of environmental exploration available is now expanded, offering increased opportunity for continued development. This next age stage describes the increased postural control, stability, and functional independence achieved by the typical child between 12 and 18 months of age. Major occurrences will be described, again focusing on the *process* of the attainment of functional movement rather than the specific age or stage.

■ Postural Control

The child now practices and perfects many of the movement skills attained during the first action-packed year. Although the movement patterns for walking are generated by a central pattern of neural control evidenced by the earliest signs of automatic stepping, this basic program requires maturation and modification as the motor development and learning occur that accompany the refinement of postural control and balance. The beginning walker demonstrates patterns that reflect the immature level of postural control. In order to step, weight must be transferred to one leg. The toddler shifts this weight through a lateral displacement of the head, shoulder, and upper body. The child frees the un-weighted leg to move it forward, quickly followed by a rapid step forward of the trailing leg. The timing is usually off, and these first steps are often jerky and without rhythm. Postural reactions may be seen if the child shifts the weight too far laterally. The arms abduct and a righting action can be seen in the trunk, which may realign the trunk over the center of gravity. Because postural reactions are controlled through central processing and feedback, the reaction may happen too late and the baby falls (Alexander et al., 1993; Bly, 1994; Campbell, 2000). Falling is a common occurrence. As postural control develops and postural adjustments are coordinated with the walking pattern, the pattern becomes more rhythmical and the child falls less often.

Trunk rotation is smoothly used during transitions around the floor and to and from standing. The trunk initiates the direction of rotation and is under good control. Dissociation of the lower extremities from each other and from the trunk continues to develop.

■ Upper Extremity Control

During early walking, the upper extremities are postured into a stabilizing high on-guard pattern, unavailable for any other functional purpose (see Fig. 4-42). Changing these postural patterns may result in what seems to be a regression in upper extremity and fine motor skills. This apparent regression is transient and is related to the new postural challenges (Campbell, 2000). As the baby experiments with new postural muscles and patterns in the lower extremities, the degrees of freedom in the upper trunk and arms are limited. This produces a stabilization or "fixing" maneuver of the upper extremities and perhaps a dete-rioration in the accomplishment of new fine motor skills. As the baby practices the new synergistic postural control and develops postural synergies, the control and available degrees of freedom will again be manifested in the upper trunk and arms (Bly, 1994). As the baby develops stability in walking, less posturing of the arm is seen. A reciprocal arm swing usually develops by 18 months of age.

During play, positioning and movement of the hand are done primarily from the elbow, utilizing graded elbow flexion, extension, and forearm rotation. The shoulders are now fairly quiet. During these months, the hands begin to develop more coordinated asymmet-rical roles. One hand may be active, while the other hand is more passive, providing stability. Hand prefer-ence may begin to emerge. The hands are often now engaged in complementary asymmetrical roles, such as

when one hand stabilizes a container so that the other hand can unscrew the lid (Bly, 1994; Fagard, 1990). Smooth rotation of the trunk occurs when the child reaches across midline.

The synergistic relationship between wrist exten-sion and finger flexion is mature. The palmar arches are fully developed. Release becomes smooth and graded for large objects but may still be clumsy for smaller objects.

■ Lower Extremity Control

The age at which a child begins to walk is highly vari-able, with some babies walking as early as 9 months, others as late as 16 months. The average age for inde-pendent walking in the United States is 12 to 14 months (Caplan, 1971). During initial attempts at independent walking, the baby's movement components tend to return to those used during the first days of independ-ent stance. Hip abduction, external rotation, and a wide base of support with the arms high on-guard character-ize early walking. The posture of scapular retraction and lumbar extension increases the trunk stability required by the child during these first attempts. The lower extremity movements return to the steppagelike gait used in initial handheld walking. Early walking is characterized by co-activation of agonist and antago-nist, preceding the establishment of a reciprocal pattern (see Fig. 4-42).

The child develops the ability to rise to stand with-out pulling up. This initial form of rising typically involves rolling into prone and pushing up with both arms and elevating the pelvis by extending both legs; walking forward onto the hands, a squat is assumed, and then the child rises from the squat position. This transition requires tremendous antigravity strength. Reaching for objects from standing may be seen accom-panied by a return to upper extremity asymmetry during play in a squat position (Fig. 4-44).

Early Childhood

Early childhood, the developmental stage between 2 and 6 years of age, is the period when children acquire increased independence and gain a sense of their own effectiveness in the world. Healthy children experience physical growth, coordination of motor skills, and an energetic zest for play and activity (Vander Zanden, 2000).

By the end of the second year, children have devel-oped the basic movement components of antigravity flexor and extensor strength and control, proximal stability and weight bearing, smooth weight shift, and rotation/dissociation. These movement components

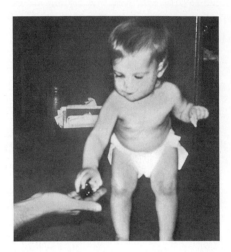

Figure 4–44. The early stander's squat will be characterized by asymmetrical posturing of the upper extremities as stability is challenged while engaged in a functional task.

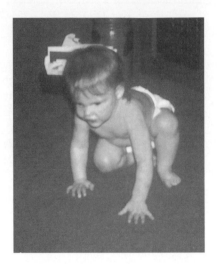

Figure 4–45. Rising to stand midfloor emerges in a more mature fashion as half-kneeling to stand without support.

form the basis on which the child develops and refines the fundamental movement patterns of early childhood and then the specialized movement skills of adolescence (Gallahue & Ozmun, 2002). Fundamental movement pattern development is concerned with developing acceptable levels of proficiency and efficient body mechanics in a variety of movement situations. Motor development during early childhood leads to the attainment of new skills and refinement of movement, but not necessarily with the emergence of any new movement components. In keeping with this chapter's organization, functional tasks will be grouped into the development and refinement of postural control or stability, locomotion, and manipulation.

It is important to remember that while new movement skills are developing, each body segment has its own developmental time line within the overall system; one part may be at a different level of development and skill than another, although all parts are at first at an immature level and then able to function at an advanced level. Therapists and assistants need to be aware that the emergence of these more sophisticated movement patterns is not always a neat and tidy sight. When demands of the task change, for example, or when fatigue sets in, one body part may regress in its action while another continues to perform at an advanced skill level. The task requirements and the constraints of the contributing subsystems are very influential in determining the characteristics of the motor response (Campbell, 2000). Movement patterns

of normal children are characterized by variability, very much in contrast with the limited movement patterns seen in the atypically developing child (Marsala & VanSant, 1998; Miller & Roid, 1993).

▪ Postural Control

Posture and postural control develop, change, and are refined during these preschool years. Research shows that postural responses in children between the ages of 4 and 6 are very variable. This variability is possibly due to the fact that there are several periods of critical change in growth and body dimensions, requiring adaptation and change. This developmental period is marked by periods of stability and time for practice and refinement, interspersed with periods of change or transition, requiring the development of newly adapted postural strategies (Shumway-Cook & Woollacott, 2001). The system remains in a state of stability until dimensional changes reach a point where previous motor programs are no longer the most effective. At that point, the system undergoes a period of transition marked by variability and instability, followed again by a plateau of stability. These years are also a time when there is a decrease in transitional postures with the emergence of the ability to stand from supine in a more mature fashion (Fig. 4–45). Reciprocal actions begin to be mastered, which is reflected in the ability to ride a tricycle and climb playground equipment (Figs. 4–46 and 4–47).

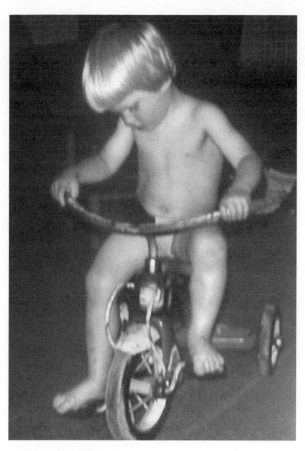

Figure 4–46. Riding a tricycle requires mastery of reciprocal and dissociated extremity use.

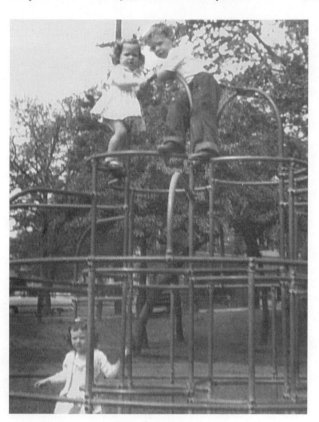

Figure 4–47. Although a dated photo, the author couldn't resist including this picture of herself and her brother climbing the monkey bars.

Skilled movement has both postural and voluntary components: The postural component establishes the stabilizing framework that supports the action or voluntary component, the primary movement. Increased postural control allows for independence in many life skills, including dressing (Fig. 4–48). Postural control and stability develop and refine with improvements in the demonstration of fundamental movement patterns requiring dynamic balance and static balance. Balance improves, as indicated in the ability to stand on one foot and walk on a balance beam. Dynamic balance, allowing the maintenance of equilibrium as the center of gravity shifts, is reflected in the ability to first walk a straight line, then a balance beam in tandem. Reciprocal descent from stairs is evidence of increasing balance and postural control (Fig. 4–49). Static balance, involving the ability to maintain one's equilibrium while the center of gravity remains stationary, permits the ability to balance on one foot. The developing skills of running, hopping, skipping, and jumping require increasing degrees of balance and successful control of force production (Fig. 4–50). Contrasted with older adults, children under the age of 7 have difficulty balancing efficiently when both somatosensory and visual cues are removed. Children under 7 also have a reduced abil-

ity to adapt their senses for postural control when receiving conflicting information (Campbell, 2000; Gallahue & Ozmun, 2002; Shumway-Cook & Woollacott, 2001).

▪ Upper Extremity Control

As a fundamental movement skill, manipulation involves an individual's relationship to objects and is characterized by giving force to objects and receiving force from them (Gallahue & Ozmun, 2002). The fundamental movement patterns of throwing, catching, and striking develop during early childhood. Sequences of change in movement patterns can be seen in the developmental mastery of these skills. Throwing actually begins with an accidental letting go of an object at about 18 months of age. Throwing styles are variable between 2 and 4 years, as the child experiments with underhand and overhand styles. By about 4 years, the child can throw a ball a measurable distance, secondary to several variables, including height, strength, and of course the size and type of ball. Development of mature throwing is related to changes in height and the ability to use body force in combination with integration of shoulder

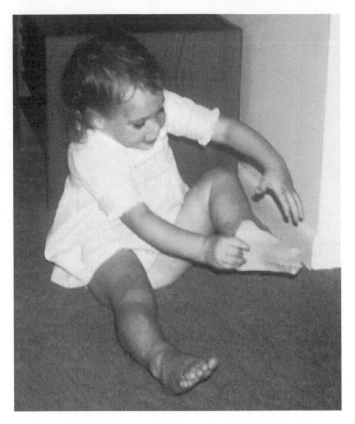

Figure 4–48. Increased postural control, dissociation, and weight shift allow for the emergence of many life skills, including independence in dressing.

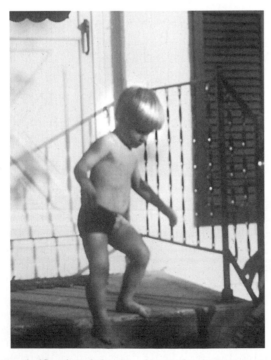

Figure 4–49. The ability to descend stairs reciprocally is made possible by maturing balance and postural control.

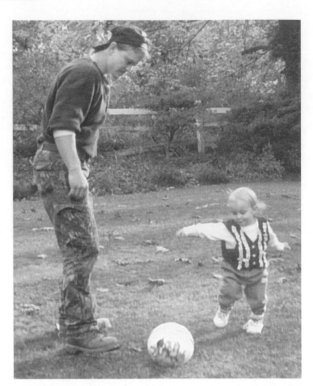

Figure 4–50. Early attempts to kick may be characterized by increased posturing of the upper extremity, a sign of instability and postural challenge.

and trunk movements. Across childhood, the distance of the throw becomes greater. Catching also depends on many variables, including ball size, speed, arm position of the catcher, and several age-related sensory and perceptual factors. Some of these perceptual factors involve the use of visual cues, depth perception, eye-hand coordination, experience, and practice (Martin & Kessler, 2000). Striking, the act of swinging and hitting an object, is equally complex. The earliest form of striking is accomplished usually with an ungraded extension motion, causing the object to be literally struck down. Eventually, at around age 5 to 6, the child will begin to strike more horizontally, just in time for Little League.

During early childhood, prehensile patterns and eye-hand coordination are refined and practiced. Skilled hand function and use of implements, such as crayons, markers, utensils, self-care items, and scissors, develop rapidly during this time. Implement use requires many forms of manipulation: sustained pinch, in-hand manipulations, and bimanual coordination of bilateral hand use (see Chapter 9). Strength of the hand intrinsic muscles increases, and distal control becomes more refined. Motor planning plays a major role in the acquisition of new fine motor tasks. By 4 to 6 years of age, hand preference is well established (Levine, 1987). Chapter 9 of this text will include more detail on manipulation and prehensile skill development.

▪ Lower Extremity Control

Lower extremity strength and stability increase; a child younger than 6 may still push off from the seat of the chair to rise to standing, but by the end of this phase, the arms are rarely engaged in this transfer. The standing position has become more erect, and squatting can be maintained for long periods. Gradually the wide-based stance of the toddler narrows, the abdomen protrudes less, and the feet develop a longitudinal arch, allowing for a mature lower extremity weight-bearing pattern.

As a fundamental movement skill, locomotion is the aspect of learning to move effectively and efficiently within one's own environment (Gallahue & Ozmun, 2002). The locomotor pattern of walking is refined, and new locomotor skills are added, including running, hopping, jumping, and skipping. Mature gait is established by 3 or 4 years of age and is characterized by reciprocal movement of the lower extremities, reduced out-toeing, the appearance of pelvic rotation, and initial contact onto the heel (Sutherland, Olshan, Biden, & Wyatt, 1988). Chapter 10 will describe in detail the development of mature gait and the age-related gait changes that accompany maturation.

An examination of jumping offers a good illustration of the developmental changes that occur as movement patterns mature. The child will first jump off a step or box about 1 foot in height at about 22 months of age. This skill at first resembles a quick stepping-down pattern rather than an actual jump with two feet off the ground simultaneously. With time, the ability to jump for distance emerges, and across childhood, the height and distance jumped increase. Early jumping is characterized by a very shallow preparatory crouch, whereas advanced jumpers demonstrate deep crouches (VanSant & Goldberg, 1999). Initially, the arms move into a high on-guard position, whereas later the arms are used to create momentum, being thrust up and overhead to assist in jump propulsion. Young jumpers hold their head and trunk flexed, whereas older jumpers utilize full head and trunk extension (Fig. 4–51).

Running differs principally from walking in that there is a brief flight phase during each step, when the body is out of contact with the supporting surface (Fig. 4–52) (Martin & Kessler, 2000). Many children begin to run before mastering a mature walking pattern. Kicking develops and matures from an initial pattern of kicking with the leg extended and very little body movement (2 to 3 years) to flexing the knee (3 to 4 years) and finally to a mature pattern of forcefully kicking the ball through (5 to 6 years). Hopping seems to be an extension of the ability to balance on one leg and is not performed well until the child is approximately 6 years old. Skipping is a complex motor pattern that involves a step and a hop on one leg, followed by a step and hop on the other leg; this also is not achieved until age 6 (Gallahue & Ozmun, 2002; Martin & Kessler, 2000).

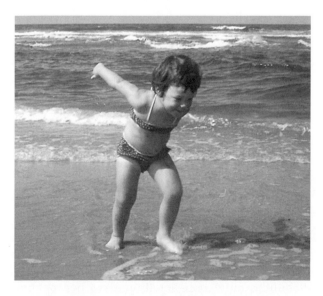

Figure 4–51. A young jumper holds her head and trunk flexed and readies herself by gaining some momentum by hyperextending her arms.

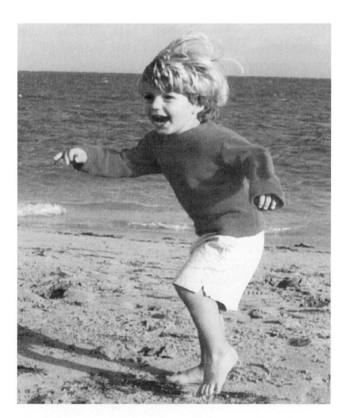

Figure 4–52. The gleeful expression of a running child is a beautiful sight!

Middle Through Late Childhood

Later childhood is the period from age 6 through the onset of puberty at age 10. Postural control is essentially adultlike by 7 to 10 years of age. Symmetry tends to become more frequent during the middle childhood years in the process of rising to stand from a supine position. The lower limbs are more likely to demonstrate asymmetry than the trunk or upper extremities. By 7 years of age, the child depends primarily on proprioceptors to maintain balance in standing. Adult balance strategies are demonstrated by age 10.

Later childhood is a time of slow but steady physical growth that allows gradual mastery of movement skills. Skills are being stabilized before adolescence. During this time, the child is engaged in a great deal of experimentation and practice, seeking the most efficient form of movement within skills that have already been attained. Between 6 and 10 years, children master the adult forms of running, throwing, and catching (Porter, 1989). Common patterns of striking that emerge are overhand, sidearm, and underhand. As the child progresses to striking in an increasingly horizontal pattern, increased trunk rotation is seen as the swing matures (Robertson & Halverson, 1977). The greatest changes in reaction time occur until 8 or 9 years of age, beginning to become increasingly more accurate and responsive. These middle to late childhood years are years of continued development of fine motor mastery. This school-aged child has increased demand for writing skills, allowing for task-specific development of complex prehensile skills.

Adolescence

Adolescence is a time of *tremendous* change: accelerated change in the dimensions of physical growth, sexual maturation, and concomitant social-emotional development. In the area of movement development, the now mature fundamental movement patterns in the areas of stability or postural control, locomotion, and manipulation become further developed. Mature fundamental movement development is a prerequisite for the successful incorporation of corresponding specialized movement skills into one's movement repertoire. The development of specialized movement skills occurs during this time and is highly dependent on opportunities for practice, encouragement, and skilled instruction. Refinement and greater skill occur during this time. Reaction times are at adult level by 16 to 17 years of age. Examples of specialized movement skills are as follows:

- In stability/postural control: swinging, twisting, dodging, and balancing

- In upper extremity control/manipulation: volleying, bouncing, punting, catching, and trapping, commonly applied to success in sports, dance, and tumbling
- In lower extremity control/locomotion: running and leaping, as well as combinations of two or more elements, such as in galloping, sliding, and advanced climbing

The postural alignments of childhood disappear and an adult ideal posture is achieved during adolescence. Postural individuality, however, also becomes apparent during later adolescence. Teens exhibit a refined competence in simultaneously controlling the upper extremities, lower extremities, and trunk. Control of the force and direction of movement is impressive at this age (Cech & Martin, 1995). Symmetrical movement patterns during transitions are the norm.

The prehensile demands on the adolescent resemble those of the school-aged child, except that the skill level is often higher, with less time spent in trial and error and more time spent in task-specific practice. Skills performed with the dominant hand continue to advance beyond those of the nondominant hand. Bilateral hand skills, such as using a computer keyboard or engaging in sports-related activities, play a major role at this age (Duff, 1995).

Adulthood

The healthy adult is highly flexible in choosing postural patterns most appropriate for a functional task. Symmetrical performance is still seen, but asymmetry in transitional movement becomes more commonplace. Compared with adolescence, adulthood offers less formalized opportunities to participate in physical activity. Occupational choice will be a major determining factor in further development or refinement of prehensile skills.

Activity level is very much related to performance in transitional movement tasks. More active adults use more symmetrical patterns (Cohen et al., 1998). Body size is another variable. A study by VanSant showed that taller and thinner women are more likely to demonstrate a symmetrical pattern than shorter and heavier women (VanSant, Cromwell, and Deo, 1989). More active adults demonstrate more developmentally advanced movement patterns as compared with their inactive counterparts. Lifestyle patterns of regular, moderate physical activity appear to influence how a person integrates a smooth, coordinated use of righting and equilibrium responses within his or her movement patterns (Green & Williams, 1992). Throughout adulthood, changes in the body's physiological systems may influence movement performance. Variability in movement patterns continues to be characteristic for healthy, active adults (VanSant, 1988). Variability in motor performance increases with each decade of life (Gallahue and Ozmun, 2002).

Aging

Before continuing this section, it must be stressed that the most important fact to remember about aging is that it is highly variable from one person to the next. The continuum of function among older adults has been described well by Spirduso (1995), who points out that at one end of the continuum are the physically elite, then the physically fit, physically active, physically independent, physically dependent, and finally those older adults with a disability. Age-related differences in movement patterns seem to be a function of developmental changes in the movement subsystems, most predominantly by decreases in muscular strength (Gross, Stevenson, Charette, Pyka, & Marcus, 1998). As with every other life stage, generalizations can be made but must be kept in perspective.

■ Postural Control

Postural sway in standing increases with age (Cech & Martin, 1995). Many factors can contribute to declining balance control in older adults, putting them at risk for imbalance and falls. Researchers have documented impairments in all the systems contributing to balance control. With increased age comes the increased probability that pathology may cause a loss in postural control and balance. No predictable pattern is characteristic. Any one of or a combination of the age-related changes described in Chapter 3 could contribute to a decrease in postural control for the older adult. It has been demonstrated that when the stability of an older adult is disturbed, the restoration process is different and often ineffective compared with the process used by younger persons (Woollacott & Shumway-Cook, 1990). Differences in muscle activation patterns are typical, as is co-activation of agonist and antagonist, a pattern reminiscent of that seen in young children (Forssberg & Nashner, 1982; Woollacott, Shumway-Cook, & Nashner, 1986). Exercise can aid in the maintenance of good balance and reduce the likelihood of falls as people age.

With aging, movement patterns again become increasingly asymmetrical. Transitional movements return to the asymmetry previously seen in childhood. Transitions are also characterized by a tendency to return to the use of several intermediate transitional postures (Fig. 4–53). Generally, transitions become less efficient and require more energy. The effect of inactiv-

ity and poor physical fitness is very noticeable. A typical transition for an 80 year old is to turn from supine to side lying, rise up into a side-sitting position, then go into quadruped to half kneel, often with support, and then stand. As seen in younger children, transitions are typically characterized by asymmetry in movement patterns, pausing at each transition, and less smoothness.

■ Upper Extremity Control

The system changes that occur in elderly adults (see Chapter 3) will affect hand function. Hand strength, performance time, and the frequency with which varying prehension patterns are used are affected by age (Shiffman, 1992). Manual dexterity is decreased, which is noticeable in activities of daily living such as tying shoelaces or fastening buttons. The time required to manipulate a small object increases by 25 to 40 percent by 70 years of age (Cole, 1991). It is known that tactile sensation is decreased in older adults, which may also affect their ability to gauge their grip strength accurately. Interestingly, Cole and colleagues (Cole, 1991; Cole, Rotella, & Harper, 1999) have demonstrated that older adults tend to use grasp forces that are on average twice as large as those of younger adults. It is important for clinicians to include training in energy conservation when working with older adults; often they expend more energy and force than required by the task.

Older adults demonstrate slowness of reach, probably due to a delay in central processing. This slowness is directly related to the complexity of the task, with more complex tasks characterized by marked slowness (Shumway-Cook & Woollacott, 2001). Reaction time across the board is longer for older adults. On the other hand, elderly persons manage to adapt and remain quite functional. Many studies indicate that with practice, response time can be decreased and hand function made optimal (Falduto & Baron, 1985). Task-specific practice may be a valuable way to maintain eye-hand coordination well into old age.

■ Lower Extremity Control

Postural changes affecting stance posture seen with aging can include a forward head, thoracic kyphosis, and an increase in hip and knee flexion. With aging, the two secondary curves decrease, with a return to a primarily kyphotic posture. Decreased activity definitely increases these age-related changes. Studies investigating the relationship of age, activity level, and movement patterns used to rise to standing from either a supine position or from the floor indicate that symmetrical patterns, which typically require more strength, are seen predominantly in younger adults.

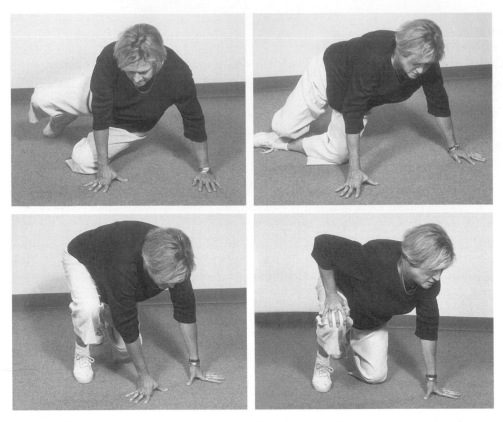

Figure 4–53. With aging, movement patterns become increasingly asymmetrical and transitions are characterized by the return to use of several intermediate transitional postures.

Older adults, on the other hand, may need to employ asymmetrical standing strategies in the face of extensor weakness and limited ankle range of motion (Thomas, Williams, & Lundy-Ekman, 1998; VanSant, 1990).

Gait characteristics common to older adults include a wider base of support, decreased reciprocal arm swing, and slower cadence. Stride length decreases and time in double support increases. These gait changes are due to a combination of musculoskeletal age-related changes, as well as to a decline in the sensory systems. Most research indicates that the changes seen in locomotor patterns of aging adults are due to a decline in muscular strength, reflected most commonly by a decreased step length and increased time spent in double support (Wilder, 1992). The strength declines apparently most responsible for these changes in gait characteristics are losses in strength at the hip and ankle. In older adults there is also evidence of a return to agonist and antagonist co-activation patterns, as originally seen in the toddler. This co-activation pattern may be an adaptive strategy to compensate for decreased postural control and balance deficits (Woollacott, 1989). Walking requires more energy for most older adults.

The gait changes that accompany aging will be expanded on in Chapter 10. For the purposes of this chapter, gait changes in the older adult can be summarized as follows, as presented by Shumway-Cook and Woollacott (2001):

Temporal and Spatial Factors

- Decreased velocity
- Decreased step length
- Decreased stride length
- Increased stride width
- Increased time in stance phase
- Increased time in double support
- Decreased time in swing phase

Kinematic Changes

- Decreased vertical movement of the center of gravity
- Decreased arm swing
- Decreased hip, knee, and ankle flexion
- Increased incidence of foot flat on initial contact
- Decreased dynamic stability during stance

Summary

This chapter has presented a life span perspective on development, most specifically motor development. The contributions of main developmental theorists, including Piaget, Erikson, and Gesell, are presented, highlighting clinical implications to be gained from these theorists for occupational and physical therapy professionals. A contemporary view on motor development, from a dynamic system perspective, is explained and clarified. Key concepts and terminology useful to the student of motor development are summarized, so that the language used is universal and standardized.

Functional movement is presented as accomplishments within three broad movement tasks: postural control, upper extremity control and function, and lower extremity control and function. The development of functional movement within these three task areas is traced through the life span: infancy and early childhood, middle to late childhood, adolescence,

adulthood, and the aging adult. The first year of life is used as a model for describing the emergence of the fundamental movement components: antigravity control, proximal stability and the ability to bear weight, smooth weight shift, mobility, and rotation and dissociation. Current knowledge indicates that therapists should consider a patient's age when selecting movement patterns to teach (Ford-Smith & VanSant, 1993). In addition to age, it is vital to consider body size, body shape, gender, and activity level, because all these variables will affect the selection of the most optimal movement pattern (VanSant, 1990). If clinicians are sensitive to the development phase within which the patient/client is functioning, effective assessment and intervention strategies can then be designed.

References

Alexander, R., Boehme, R., & Cupps, B. (1993). *Normal development of functional motor skills.* Tucson, AZ: Therapy Skill Builders.

Baltes, P. (1987). Theoretical propositions of life-span developmental psychology: On the dynamics between growth and decline. *Developmental Psychology, 23,* 611–626.

Bertoti, D. B, & Stanger, M. (1994). Pediatric musculoskeletal assessment: The impact of developmental factors. *Orthopedic Physical Therapy Clinics of North America, 3,* 31–43.

Bleck, E. E. (1987). *Orthopedic management in cerebral palsy. Clinics in developmental medicine.* Philadelphia: J. B. Lippincott.

Bly, L. (1994). *Motor skills acquisition in the first year.* Tucson, AZ: Therapy Skill Builders.

Boehme, R. (1988). *Improving upper body control.* Tucson, AZ: Therapy Skill Builders.

Campbell, S. K. (2000). The child's development of functional movement. In S. K. Campbell, D. W. Vander Linden, & R. J. Palisano (Eds.), *Physical therapy for children.* Philadelphia: W. B. Saunders.

Caplan, F. (1971). *The first twelve months of life.* New York: Grosset and Dunlap.

Case-Smith, J., Fisher, A. G., & Bauer, D. (1989). Analysis of the relationship between proximal and distal motor control. *American Journal of Occupational Therapy 43,* 657–662.

Cech, D., & Martin, S. (1995). *Functional movement development across the life span.* Philadelphia: W. B. Saunders.

Cohen, B. G., Cardillo, E. R., Lugg, D., Schwartz, D. N., Mount, J., VanSant, A., & Cornman-Levy, D. (1998). Description of movement patterns of young adults moving supine from the foot to the head of the bed. *Physical Therapy, 78,* 999–1006.

Cole, K. J. (1991). Grasp force control in older adults. *Journal of Motor Behavior, 23,* 251–258.

Cole, K. J., Rotella, D. L., & Harper, J. G. (1999). Mechanisms for age-related changes of fingertip forces during precision gripping and lifting in adults. *Journal of Neuroscience, 19,* 3228–3247.

Crutchfield, C. A., & Barnes, M. R. (1993). *Motor control and motor learning in rehabilitation.* Atlanta: Stokesville Publishing.

Duff, S. V. (1995). Prehension. In D. Cech & S. Martin (Eds.), *Functional movement development across the life span.* Philadelphia: W. B. Saunders.

Falduto, L., & Baron, A. (1985). Age-related changes and effects of practice and task complexity on card sorting. *Journal of Gerontology, 41,* 659–661.

Fagard, J. (1990). The development of bimanual coordination. In C.

Bard, M. Fleury, & H. Hay (Eds.), *Development of eye-hand coordination across the life span.* Columbia, SC: University of South Carolina Press.

Field-Fote, E. C. (2000). Spinal cord control of movement: implications for locomotor rehabilitation following spinal cord injury. *Physical Therapy, 80,* 477–482.

Fisher, A. G., & Bundy, A. C. (1982). Equilibrium reactions in normal children and boys with sensory integration dysfunction. *Occupational Therapy Journal of Research, 2,* 171–183.

Ford-Smith, C. D., & VanSant, A. (1993). Age differences in movement patterns used to rise from a bed in subjects in the third through fifth decades of age. *Physical Therapy, 73,* 300–309.

Forssberg, H., & Nashner, L. (1982). Ontogenetic development of posture control in man: adaptation to altered support and visual conditions during stance. *Journal of Neuroscience 2,* 545–552.

Gallahue, D. L., & Ozmun, J. C. (2002). *Understanding motor development: infants, children, adolescents, adults* (5th ed). New York: McGraw-Hill.

Gesell, A. (1954). The ontogenesis of human behavior. In L. Carmichael (Ed.), *Manual of child psychology.* New York: Wiley.

Green, L. N., & Williams, K. (1992). Differences in developmental movement patterns used by active versus sedentary middle-aged adults coming from a supine position to erect stance. *Physical Therapy, 72,* 560–568.

Gross, M. M., Stevenson, P. J., Charette, S. L., Pyka, G., & Marcus, R. (1998). Effect of muscle strength and movement speed on the biomechanics of rising from a chair in healthy elderly and young women. *Gait and Posture, 8,*175–185.

Guccione, A. A. (1993). Health status: A conceptual framework and terminology for assessment. In A. A. Guccione (Ed.), *Geriatric physical therapy* (pp. 101–111). St. Louis, MO: Mosby.

Heriza, C. (1991). Motor development: Traditional and contemporary theories. In M. J. Lister (Ed.), *Contemporary management of motor control problems: Proceedings of the II-Step Conference* (pp. 99–126). Alexandria, VA: Foundation for Physical Therapy.

Higgins, S. (1985). Movement as an emergent form: Its structural limits. *Human Movement Science, 4,* 119–148.

Izraelevitz, T. A., Fisher, A. G., & Bundy, A. C. (1985). Equilibrium reactions in preschoolers. *The Occupational Therapy Journal of Research, 5,* 154–169.

Kamm, K., Thelen, E., & Jensen, J. L. (1990). A dynamical systems approach to motor development. *Physical Therapy 70,* 763–775.

Leonard, C. T. (1998). *The neuroscience of human movement*. St. Louis, MO: Mosby.

Levine, M. D. (1987). *Developmental variation and learning disabilities*. Toronto: Educators Publishing Service.

Marsala, G., & VanSant, A. (1998). Age-related differences in movement patterns used by toddlers to rise from a supine position to erect stance. *Physical Therapy, 78*, 149–158.

Martin, S., & Kessler, M. (2000). *Neurologic intervention for physical therapist assistants*. Philadelphia: W. B. Saunders.

McCormack, D. B., & Perrin, K. R. (1997). *Spatial, temporal, and physical analysis of motor control: A comprehensive guide to reflexes and reactions*. San Antonio, TX: Therapy Skill Builders.

Miller, L. J., & Roid, G. H. (1993). Sequence comparison methodology for the analysis of movement patterns in infants and toddlers with and without motor delays. *American Journal of Occupational Therapy, 47*, 339–347.

Miller Porr, S., & Berger Rainville, E. (1999). *Pediatric therapy: A systems approach*. Philadelphia: F. A. Davis.

O'Sullivan, S. B. (2001). Assessment of motor function. In S. B. O'Sullivan & T. J. Schmitz (Eds.), *Physical rehabilitation: Assessment and treatment* (4th ed). Philadelphia: F. A. Davis.

Papalia, D. E., Olds, S. W., & Feldman, R. D. (2001). *Human development* (8th ed). New York: McGraw-Hill.

Piaget J. (1952). *The origins of intelligence*. New York: W. W. Norton.

Pimentel, E. D. (1996). The disappearing reflex: A reevaluation of its role in normal and abnormal development. *Physical and Occupational Therapy in Pediatrics, 16*, 19–41.

Porter, R. E. (1989). Normal development of movement and function: Child and adolescent. In R. M. Scully & M. L. Barnes (Eds.), *Physical therapy*. Philadelphia: J. B. Lippincott.

Rainville, E. B. (1999). The special vulnerabilities of children and families. In S. M. Porr & E. B. Rainville, *Pediatric therapy: A systems approach*. Philadelphia: F. A. Davis.

Ratliffe, K. T. (1998). *Clinical pediatric physical therapy: A guide for the physical therapy team*. St. Louis, MO: Mosby.

Robertson, M., & Halverson, L. (1977). The developing child: His changing movement. In B. J. Logsdon (Ed.), *Physical education for children: A focus on the teaching process*. Philadelphia: Lea & Febiger.

Ryerson, S., & Levit, K. (1997). *Functional movement reeducation*. Philadelphia: Churchill Livingstone.

Scholz, J. (1990). Dynamic pattern theory: Some implications for therapeutics. *Physical Therapy, 70*, 827–843.

Sellers, J. S. (1988). Relationship between antigravity control and postural control found in young children. *Physical Therapy, 68*, 486–490.

Shiffman, L. M. (1992). Effects of aging on adult hand function. *American Journal of Occupational Therapy, 44*, 893–900.

Shumway-Cook, A., & Woollacott, M. H. (2001). *Motor control: Theory and practical application* (2nd ed.). Philadelphia: Lippincott Williams & Wilkins.

Spirduso, W. (1995). *Physical dimensions of aging*. Champaign, IL: Human Kinetics.

Stockmeyer, S. A. (1966). An interpretation of the approach of Rood to the treatment of neuromuscular dysfunction. *American Journal of Physical Medicine, 46*, 900–946.

Sutherland, D. H., Olshen, R. A., Biden, E. N., & Wyatt, M. P. (1988). *The development of mature walking*. London: MacKeith Press.

Taber's Cyclopedic Medical Dictionary (19th ed.). (2001). Philadelphia: F. A. Davis.

Thelen, E. (1985). Developmental origins of motor coordination: Leg movements in human infants. *Developmental Psychobiology, 18,*1–22.

Thelen, E. (1995). Motor development: A new synthesis. *American Psychologist, 50*, 79–95.

Thelen, E., & Corbetta, D. (1994). Exploration and selection in the early acquisition of skill. *International Review of Neurobiology, 37*, 75–102.

Thelen, E., & Fogel, A. (1987). Toward an action-based theory of infant development. In J. Lockman & N. Hazen (Eds.), *Action in social context*. New York: Plenum Press.

Thomas, R. L., Williams, A. K., & Lundy-Ekman, L. (1998). Supine to stand in elderly persons: Relationship to age, activity level, strength, and range of motion. *Issues Aging, 21*, 9–18.

Vander Zanden, J. W. (2000). *Human development* (7th ed.). New York: McGraw-Hill.

VanSant, A. F. (1988). Rising from a supine position to erect stance: Description of adult movement and a developmental hypothesis. *Physical Therapy, 68*, 185–192.

VanSant, A. F. (1990). Life-span development in functional tasks. *Physical Therapy, 70*, 788–798.

VanSant, A. F., Cromwell, S., & Deo, A. (1989). *Relationships among body dimensions, age, gender, and movement patterns in a righting task*. Poster presentation at 64th annual conference of American Physical Therapy Association, Nashville, TN.

VanSant, A. F., & Goldberg, C. (1999). Normal motor development. In J. S. Tecklin (Ed.), *Pediatric physical therapy* (3rd ed.). Philadelphia: Lippincott Williams & Wilkins.

Vygotsky, L. S. (1978). *Mind in society: The development of higher psychological processes*. Cambridge, MA: Harvard University Press.

Von Hofsten, C. (1990). A perception-action perspective of the development of manual movement. In M. Jeannerod (Ed.), *Attention and performance, Vol. 13* (pp. 739–762). Hillsdale, NJ: Lawrence Erlbaum Associates.

Wilder, P. A. (1992). Developmental changes in the gait patterns of women: A search for control parameters. Ph.D. Thesis, University of Wisconsin.

Woollacott, M. H. (1989). Aging, postural control, and movement preparation. In M. H. Woollacott & A. Shumway-Cook (Eds.), *Development of posture and gait across the life span* (pp. 155–175). Columbia: University of South Carolina.

Woollacott, M. H., & Shumway-Cook, A. (1990). Changes in posture control across the life span: A systems approach. *Physical Therapy, 70*, 799–807.

Woollacott, M. H., Shumway-Cook, A., & Nashner, L. M. (1986). Aging and postural control: Changes in sensory organization and muscular coordination. *International Journal of Aging and Human Development, 23*, 97–114.

Woollacott, M.H., Shumway-Cook, A., & Williams, H. (1989). The development of posture and balance control (pp. 77–96). In M. H. Woollacott & A. Shumway-Cook (Eds.), *Development of posture and gait across the life span*. Columbia: University of South Carolina.

Part 2

An Integrated Clinical Approach to the Management of Common Clinical Problems

Motor Learning Through the Life Span

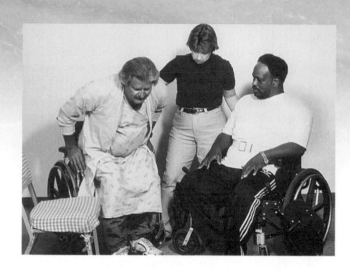

The best therapist is a lifelong learner who can in turn then be a gifted teacher. To teach is to empower and to help ignite someone else's possibilities and help bring a dream into being.

Cornerstone Concepts

- Motor learning defined and differentiated from motor control
- Types of learning including clinical examples
- Motor learning theories: Adams', Schmidt's, and ecological theory
- Key elements of learning and therapeutic considerations including the environment, arousal, attention, motivation, meaning, instruction, guidance, feedback, practice, and skill acquisition versus transfer
- Stages of motor learning: Fitts model and Gentile model
- The therapist's role in acquisition and transfer and the importance of purposeful activity
- Life span issues related to motor learning
- Learning during childhood
- Adult learners
- Learning changes related to aging
- Learning as affected by common neurological disorders
- Learning for individuals with cognitive impairment
- Learning after brain injury
- Learning after a cerebrovascular accident
- Learning challenges for individuals with Parkinson's disease

Introduction

Effective therapists think of themselves as teachers or facilitators of human movement education or reeducation. Patients/clients are learners and therefore are our students. It is imperative that physical and occupational therapists and assistants utilize effective teaching and learning strategies when working with patients/clients. This chapter is the first chapter in Part 2 of this text, devoted to application of theory to patient/client intervention. This chapter will discuss learning, specifically motor learning, offering concrete suggestions on how the clinician can effectively approach the client as a teacher approaches a student. Issues of life span learning and learning as it is challenged by commonly encountered pathological conditions will also be explored. A pediatric and an adult neurorehabilitation case study offer examples on the useful application of these principles.

Definition

It is important to differentiate among the processes of learning a skill, being trained in a skill, and performance. There is a distinction between temporary changes in performance and the relatively permanent changes that are associated with learning. **Training** occurs when the performer is provided with solutions to problems, such as when a therapist encourages a patient to memorize a specific set of exercise instructions or when a teacher provides a student with the correct answer to a specific question. Training often results in short-term **performance** capabilities. Performance is defined as a temporary change in behavior readily observable during practice sessions. Learning, on the other hand, occurs when the performer is encouraged to develop solutions to encountered problems (Fredericks & Saladin, 1996). When learning has occurred, the learner demonstrates the ability to actively problem solve and derive the solution in a variety of circumstances. Although training is appropriate in many therapeutic intervention situations, most therapeutic intervention should focus on learning.

Learning is defined as a relatively permanent change in the capability for responding that occurs as a result of practice or experience (Schmidt & Lee, 1999). To clarify, Schmidt and Lee (1999) offer the following analogy: When water freezes, it changes and becomes ice; however, this change is reversible. When the temperature increases, the ice thaws and becomes water again. On the other hand, when an egg is cooked, it also changes form, but, in contrast with the water, under no circumstance can the egg return to its previously uncooked state. This change therefore is permanent, as compared with the reversible change observed of the water. Learning is a *permanent* change (the egg), whereas often training is a *temporary* one (the water). Although this example is quite easy to visualize, learning is not always so directly observable.

Motor Learning Versus Motor Control

It is important to differentiate between motor control and motor learning and to clarify these definitions. Because the terms sound so similar, they are often incor-

rectly interchanged, although they are two distinct areas of study, each offering unique clinical insights.

Motor control is the study of the nature and cause of movement, focusing on both the control and coordination of the movement and posture. The field of motor control has grown primarily from the specialized study of neurophysiology, looking closely at models of neural function and evolution of the nervous system. Because movement arises from the interaction of multiple processes, motor control also involves a study of all the interactive processes, including perception and cognition (Shumway-Cook & Woollacott, 2001). Movements or actions are performed always within the context of an environment, and the sensory-perceptual systems provide information about the body within this environment. Because movement is not usually performed in the absence of intent, cognitive processes, such as attention, motivation, and the emotional aspects of movement control, are also essential to motor control. Motor control emerges from an interaction between the individual (the patient), the task, and the environment. There are many different theories and models of motor control, summarized in previous chapters of this text. Some of the theories stress peripheral influences; others may stress central influences, and still others may stress the role of information from the environment in controlling behavior. All the theories offer some unique slant and should be viewed by the inquisitive student and clinician as offering different insights and clinical suggestions.

Motor learning is concerned typically with how "motor skills" are acquired. An understanding of motor learning has grown largely from the fields of psychology and physical education. Motor learning is a process that brings about a relatively permanent change in the capacity for motor performance as a result of experience or practice. Three major factors that affect motor learning are environmental conditions, cognitive processes, and movement organization (Jarus, 1994). Occupational and physical therapy intervention involves all the fundamental characteristics of motor learning: Clinicians provide instruction, feedback, opportunities to practice, and encouragement to patients. Therapists and assistants utilize teaching strategies such as instruction, practice, and feedback to guide patients/clients through skill mastery. An understanding of motor learning will enhance the clinician's ability to view the patient as the learner and therefore enable the clinician to be most effective in maximizing functional rehabilitation for the patient. Patients/clients will achieve maximal progress when therapy is guided by principles of motor learning.

Theories on motor learning emphasize the role of feedback and practice during learning. It is helpful for the student of motor learning to view learning, or patient progress, as occurring in stages from the initial fumbling attempts to mastery of a skill. Sensitive utilization of teaching strategies throughout these phases is the mark of a master clinician. Motor learning involves two distinct phases: an acquisition or practice stage, in which skills are learned or relearned, and a retention and transfer phase, in which information is stored for retrieval and application to novel situations. The acquisition phase may indicate performance, but the retention and transfer phases indicate learning (Magill, 1989; Sage, 1984; Schmidt, 1988, 1999).

In summary, motor control processes involve neural circuitry and neurophysiological interactions. Motor control processes occur within very small intervals, typically fractions of seconds. Motor learning is a process that occurs across hours, days, and weeks (Shumway-Cook & Woollacott, 2001). A skillful clinician must incorporate key concepts from both motor control and motor learning into patient/client intervention. Motor control theory was integrated into Chapters 2, 3, and 4 of this text; this chapter will present motor learning.

How Do We Learn?

Learning is a fascinating capability that almost always is taken for granted until this ability is challenged. How does the brain code, store, and then retrieve information on command and often without conscious attention? For example, if a student learns a muscle's name with origin, insertion, and action, how is that student's brain changed and different from immediately before he or she learned that information?

Learning is defined as the *acquisition* of knowledge or ability; memory is the *retention and storage* of that knowledge or ability (Kupfermann, 1991). Learning reflects the actual process by which we acquire knowledge, whereas memory is the product of that process. In a discussion on the neurobiology of learning, it is important to discuss both.

Memory storage is divided into short-term and long-term components. **Short-term memory** is actually working memory, which lasts only for a few minutes. Short-term memory is used to remember a series of numbers, like a phone number, for a brief period. **Long-term memory** is actually stored in the brain and available for later retrieval and is therefore intimately related to the process of learning. True learning, therefore, is accomplished by the establishment of long-term memory. Once structurally encoded, long-term memories are less susceptible to disruption (Shumway-Cook & Woollacott, 2001).

There appear to be at least two types of modifications that occur in the brain with learning and memory. The first involves a change in the internal structure of neurons, and the second modification involves an increase in the number of synapses. Even in the initial stages, long-term memory formation reflects functional changes in the efficiency of brain synapses. In later stages, it is accompanied by actual structural changes in these synaptic connections. These changes associated with learning and memory are not localized in a specific brain structure but rather occur in all parts of the brain. Learning and memory storage involve both parallel and hierarchical processing within the central nervous system (CNS), and multiple parallel information channels are used. Information can literally be stored in many different areas of the brain. Current knowledge suggests that a memory consists of a pattern of changes in synaptic connections among networks of neurons distributed throughout the brain. Loss of memory abilities is related not to the site of the lesion but to the amount of cortex damaged (Lashley, 1929, 1950).

Clinical Connection:

This explains why memory deficits and difficulties with learning accompany so many different types of neurological damage. Memory and learning processing are not limited to a discrete area of the brain. Patients with a head injury often present with significant memory and learning difficulties because of diffuse brain damage. On the other hand, patients with a brain tumor or a focal cerebrovascular accident (CVA) may present with very minimal memory loss.

Motor memory is specifically stored as sensory information in association with a motor activity, so that a person is reminded what a specific movement should feel like. Memory traces are created for movements that are performed frequently and skillfully (Sabari, 1991; Smyth, 1984; Stelmach, 1982). Research has demonstrated that individuals can recall a movement most efficiently when they have had an opportunity to control all aspects of the initial movement. This includes the preliminary planning of the movement, initiation, execution, and termination (Smyth, 1984). This active planning, execution, and termination of a movement sequence apparently enables a person to code the movement-related kinesthetic, visual, and motor information most efficiently. It has also been demonstrated that the environmental context is an important factor. If a movement sequence is performed as part of a specific task within a natural environment, it is encoded more efficiently than if the movement was learned outside a naturally occurring environmental context.

Repeated practice of a motor skill results in improved synaptic efficiency and long-term potentiation (LTP) of the pathways between the sensory and motor cortexes (Asanuma & Keller, 1991). With even more practice, changes in these sensory-motor cortical pathways also increase the efficiency of the pathways between the thalamus (remember the importance of this relay center from Chapter 2) and the cortex. These findings suggest that the somatosensory cortex participates in the learning of new skills through long-term potentiation (see Chapter 2) and that after learning, other areas, such as the thalamus, take over, contributing to the automaticity of well-learned movements (Asanuma & Keller, 1991).

Types of Learning and Clinical Correlates

Learning occurs through a set of processes involving complex CNS phenomena whereby sensory and motor information are organized and integrated. These processes are not functions of specific CNS structures but may involve broad neural network development. Therapies directed toward facilitating the acquisition or relearning of functional skills must take into account the processes underlying learning. As succinctly described by Shumway-Cook and Woollacott (2001), there are two general types of learning: nonassociative and associative. These names imply whether or not the learning occurs due to a process whereby stimuli and outcomes are linked or associated with each other.

■ Nonassociative Learning

Nonassociative learning occurs when a single stimulus is given repeatedly, so that the nervous system learns about the characteristics of the stimulus (Kupfermann, 1991). Nonassociative learning does not involve any temporal relationship between the two stimuli. The simplest types of nonassociative learning are habituation and sensitization (Shumway-Cook & Woollacott, 2001).

Habituation causes a decrease in a behavior due to repeated exposure to a nonpainful stimulus. A simple example in everyday life is how the ticking of a clock is ignored or how the feeling of a clothing tag against the skin receives no conscious attention. Clinical examples of habituation include activities to decrease dizziness in a patient with vestibular dysfunction or procedures used to decrease tactile defensiveness in a child with neurological disorganization. The physiological basis underlying habituation is thought to be related to a decrease in synaptic activity between sensory neurons following continual stimulation, whereby the amplitude of the excitatory postsynaptic potential (EPSP) at the sensory motor synapse is decreased, resulting in synaptic depression (Cohen, 1999; Shumway-Cook & Woollacott, 2001).

Sensitization, on the other hand, results in an increased responsiveness to a threatening or noxious stimulus, following a period of ongoing stimulation. An example in everyday life would be the feeling of being "jumpy" following an unexpected explosion or crash, resulting in an increased level of arousal. Clinical examples of sensitization include increasing a patient's awareness of stimuli to improve patient safety or stimulating activities used to arouse a comatose patient. The physiological basis underlying sensitization is thought to be related to strengthened synaptic efficiency, possibly improving mobilization of neurotransmitters. Short-term sensitization is thought to involve changes in pre-existing protein structures, whereas long-term sensitization may involve the synthesis of new protein, resulting in an actual structural change (Shumway-Cook & Woollacott, 2001).

A more complex example of nonassociative learning is perceptual or sensory learning. **Perceptual learning** results in the formation of sensory memories via circuitry that perhaps serves as a spontaneous rehearsal mechanism. The physiological basis is hypothesized to be the creation and storage of coded representations within the brain, which then have serial and parallel connections to other neural areas and pathways. A clinical example of perceptual learning is the visual demonstration of a new skill to a patient, which is thought to activate the process of reactivating stored, interconnected sensory memories of that skill or a similar skill (Shumway-Cook & Woollacott, 2001).

■ Associative Learning

Associative learning involves the association of ideas to help the learner (patient) to detect and establish causal relationships in the environment. In associative learning, two events or stimuli are temporarily paired, allowing for conclusions to be drawn about causal relationships in the environment, allowing a person to predict relationships. Recognizing key relationships between events is an essential part of the ability to adapt behavior to novel situations. Associative learning probably results from long-term potentiation (LTP), where a sustained increase in synaptic strength is elicited by brief but frequent stimulation of excitatory afferent neurons (see Chapter 2). Examples of associative learning are classical conditioning, operant conditioning, procedural learning, and declarative learning.

Classical conditioning involves learning to pair stimuli in a process whereby an initially weak stimulus becomes highly effective in producing a response when it is associated with another stronger stimulus. Classical conditioning was originally described by Pavlov (1927) in his well-known description about a conditioning procedure used to cause salivation in dogs (Pavlov,

1927). For example, babies often learn to fear the doctor or nurse in a white coat within the intervention room because the setting and the individuals in white coats become quickly associated with a painful event, such as receiving a shot. It is important to remember clinically that learning in patients/clients is most likely to occur in tasks and environments that are relevant and meaningful because of this predisposition to associate meaningful events and stimuli. Therapy situations should be supportive environments so that patients/clients of all ages associate therapy with a positive event. The physiological basis behind classical conditioning is thought to be an extension of the synaptic strengthening processes involved in sensitization. Increases in synaptic efficiency are caused by growth or metabolic changes that take place in the presynaptic and postsynaptic cells (Shumway-Cook & Woollacott, 2001).

Operant conditioning involves trial and error learning whereby the learner associates a certain response from among many that have been made, with a consequence. Behaviors that are rewarded tend to be repeated. A clinical example of using classical conditioning is employed by clinicians whereby as a patient gains skills, the patient is progressed along a continuum of levels of assistance. The new behavior is shaped (formed) by the therapist as the learner (patient) acquires new skills. Operant conditioning offers an effective tool for clinical intervention: verbal praise, biofeedback, or setting up a therapy session so that a particular movement is rewarded by the successful accomplishment of a task important to the patient. The physiological basis underlying operant conditioning is the same cellular mechanism as for classical conditioning.

Procedural learning is the process whereby a task is learned by forming movement habits. This type of learning develops slowly over time through the repetition of an action over many trials. Repetition of the movement continuously under varying circumstances will enable learning of the rules for that movement, or "movement schema" (Shumway-Cook & Woollacott, 2001). Movement can then be performed automatically without conscious thought. A clinical application of this type of learning is in the provision of many opportunities for a patient to practice safe and effective transfers in a variety of settings and contexts, such as different chair or bed heights and different setup positions. This allows the patient to learn "the rules of transfer" (Shumway-Cook & Woollacott, 2001) for use in a variety of situations, preparing the patient to safely and effectively perform a transfer in unfamiliar circumstances. The physiological basis behind procedural learning appears to involve the cerebellum, whose unique circuitry is perfect for the refinement and long-term modification of motor responses.

Declarative learning results in knowledge that can be continuously recalled and thus requires processes such as awareness and attention. A skill learned in this way can be demonstrated in contexts other than that within which it was learned. This type of learning can be demonstrated in other situations. Mental practice is a classic example of declarative learning. Used so often clinically, the clinician verbally explains a procedure to a patient and allows the patient to mentally practice the movement before or between practice sessions. This is a great energy-conserving technique. The physiological basis of declarative learning is thought to involve circuitry in the temporal lobe of the cortex and the hippocampus, contributing to the creation of spatial memory (Shumway-Cook & Woollacott, 2001).

Theoretical Background/ Motor Learning Theories

The evolution of motor learning theories has taken place largely over the past four decades. As with all theories, each one offers insights and limitations. The key elements and clinical insights from each of these theories are presented in Table 5–1. Theories are also expected to be expanded on and continue in evolution as understanding of the brain expands.

Adams' Closed-Loop Theory

In 1971, Adams, a researcher in the field of physical education, offered the first comprehensive theory on motor learning. Adams proposed that sensory feedback from ongoing movement is compared with the stored memory of the intended movement, providing the CNS with a reference for correctness and an ability to detect error (Adams, 1971; Ivry, 1997). This process was described as a closed-loop process between the sensory feedback and the production of skilled movement. This closed-loop theory proposed that two very distinct types of memory were important for this process to occur. The brain used a memory trace in the selection and initiation of movement, and a perceptual trace was built up over a period of practice, supplying an internal reference of correctness. Adams proposed that after movement is initiated by the memory trace, the perceptual trace takes over to execute the movement and detect error (Shumway-Cook & Woollacott, 2001). This theory is credited with introducing therapists and assistants to the importance of practice and the value of retraining in motor re-education, but it is limited in its ability to explain how novel movements can be learned or how movements can be executed in the absence of sensory feedback.

TABLE 5–1

Comparison of Motor Learning Theories: Contributions to Clinical Practice

Motor Learning Theory	Key Concepts	Limitations	Contributions to Current Clinical Practice
Adams' closed-loop theory	Sensory feedback is compared with stored movement memory, providing CNS with reference for correctness. Brain uses "memory traces" in selection and initiation of movement. "Perceptual trace" is built up over period of practice time.	Limited in ability to explain the execution of a novel movement. Limited in ability to explain how movement can occur in absence of sensory feedback.	Underscores the importance of practice.
Schmidt's schema theory	Schema, or abstract memory construct that represents the rules for a motor action, are stored in memory. Fast timing tasks are based on a set or rules, stored as a "motor program," whereas slow movements may be more feedback based.	Does not stress the value of feedback on movement. Suggestion that motor program is a generalized, prestructured plan is a limited, simplistic view.	Patients need to learn the rules of movement so that these can then be adapted to new situations or generalized within broad environments. Supports concept that practicing a variety of movement outcomes promotes learning through the development of expanded rules or schema. Promotes clinical value of feedback. Stresses importance of practice variation. Emphasizes importance of learning skills in open, changing environments.
Ecological theory	Motor learning increases coordination between perception and action as learner searches for effective strategies. Emphasizes value of perceptual cues. Emphasizes *dynamic* nature of movement exploration.	Rather inclusive of theories to date.	Emphasizes importance of viewing the mover as an active problem solver. Reinforces value of practice, feedback, and active processing learning. Transfer of learning depends on similarity of the two tasks. Stresses value of learning a task within specific constraints in a variable environment.

Source: Information compiled from multiple sources. See text and references for details.

Schmidt's Schema Theory

Schmidt proposed that schema, rather than detailed specific motor programs, were stored in memory. A **schema** is defined as an abstract memory construct that represents a rule or a generalization about a motor action, perception, or event (Schmidt, 1975). As such, this theory takes into account the execution of fast movements, theorizing that slow movement may be feedback based, but that fast movements are based more on a **motor program** or a set of movement rules

that may be generalized from. A "motor program is an abstract structure in memory that is prepared in advance of the movement; when it is executed, the result is the contraction and relaxation of muscles causing movement to occur without the involvement of feedback leading to corrections for errors in selection" (Schmidt & Lee, 1999, p. 189). Selecting another set of commands then involves a less automatic process (Duncan & Badke, 1987).

This theory suggested that a motor program is a generalized prestructured plan that can then be modified according to the specific task demands (Duncan &

Badke, 1987). Clinically, this theory supports the concept that practicing a variety of movement outcomes would improve learning through the development of expanded rules or schema (Schmidt, 1999). It is also supportive of the clinical value of feedback, the importance of practice variation, and the value of learning skills in open, changing environments.

Ecological Theory

Ecological theory suggests that motor learning is a process that increases the coordination between perception and action as the learner searches for optimal strategies consistent with the task and environment (Newell, 1991). Ecological theory emphasizes the importance of perceptual cues as the learner practices and searches for the most effective movement strategy. One central prediction of this theory is that the transfer of motor skills will depend on the similarity of the two tasks, including the optimal perceptual-motor strategies and the relatively independent set of muscles used. This approach emphasizes the *dynamic* nature of movement exploration and the problem solving actively engaged in while learning a task within specific constraints and in a variable environment.

Key Elements of Learning and Therapeutic Considerations

The Therapeutic Environment

The physical aspects of the learning environments are an important first consideration for optimizing patient/client learning. The rehabilitation environment should provide the opportunity for active participation so that the setting is a viable learning environment. The literature suggests that environmental factors specifically influence learning outcomes by affecting how people organize purposeful movement and how tasks are attempted (Sabari, 1991; Trombly & Radomski, 2001). Understanding the individual client's needs is paramount. In the early stages of learning, a closed or controlled environment may be most appropriate. Extraneous environmental stressors such as bright lights and noise may need to be minimized. The treating clinician should remember that he or she is a part of the patient's environment, so it is important to consider personal attributes such as voice quality and level, use of strong perfumes, and other extraneous stimuli, and how they may affect the patient.

Because learning is task specific within specific environments, tasks should be practiced in the environment in which they naturally occur. As soon as perform-

ance becomes consistent, the therapist or assistant should modify the environment, opening it up to increasing amounts of natural interference. Research has clearly demonstrated that both children and adults respond positively to a multicontext intervention approach, where the individual is required to apply the new skill in a variety of situations (Toglia, 1991). Among the theories of motor learning, the ecological theory emphasizes the interaction between the performer and the environment, proposing that motor behaviors emerge as a result of regulatory conditions in the environment. The environment directly impacts on successful goal attainment. Performing in a novel, unfamiliar environment may demand more ability than a person possesses, resulting in lowered functional performance. Therapists are advised that observation of a patient's performance in a clinic setting may not be representative of the patient's optimal performance (Park, Fisher, & Velozo, 1994). The familiarity of the natural environment enhances process skills, enabling a person to compensate for motor and cognitive deficits (Nygard, Bernspang, Fisher, & Winblad, 1994; Park et al., 1994). Natural contexts, rich with sources of sensory, visual, and auditory information, have been demonstrated to elicit optimal performance, both during initial skill acquisition and during the transfer and retention phase (Ma, Trombly, & Robinson-Podolski, 1998).

Arousal and Attention

Arousal and attention are basic processes required for cognitive functioning essential to any activity. The consciousness system of the body governs arousal and attention. **Arousal** refers to the overall level of alertness or excitement of the cerebral cortex. Low arousal is associated with sleep or feelings of drowsiness, whereas high arousal is associated with high energy or excitement. **Attention** is the capacity of the brain to process information from the environment or retrieve information from long-term memory (O'Sullivan, 2001). Attention includes the ability to be aware of and respond to stimuli, to focus on the desired information and ignore irrelevant information, to shift the focus to other information if necessary, and to sustain the focus (Ben-Yishay, Rattok, & Diller, 1987; Shimelmann & Hinojosa, 1995). Attention is believed to be regulated through the reticular formation, hypothalamus, hippocampus, amygdala, and frontal cortex (Ayres, 1972; Bracy, 1972).

Several factors can influence arousal, including medication, time of day, fatigue, and emotional status. A certain level of arousal is necessary for optimal motor performance and for learning to occur. High states of arousal cause deterioration in performance and interfere with learning, whereas low states fail to yield the necessary responsiveness required for effective performance (O'Sullivan, 2001). Patients with brain damage may demonstrate decreased arousal and alertness, as seen in comatose or semicomatose states. On the other hand, brain damage may also result in an agitated state. In both cases, the patient is unable to effectively process information and then attend selectively to a specific input.

Deficits in attention may be characterized by difficulties with selective attention, sustained attention, or divided attention. **Selective attention** is the ability to focus on a specific stimulus while screening out extraneous stimuli. A person with selective attention is able to screen and process information so that relevant information receives a focus and extraneous information is ignored. **Sustained attention** requires the ability to maintain attention for a task-appropriate length of time. **Divided attention** is the ability to perform several tasks at the same time. Effective assessment of attention deficits requires careful consideration by the therapist. General strategies for intervention include carefully structuring the environment to eliminate distractions and limiting the amount of information presented to the patient. Focus should be on key elements of the task and on the patient's previous knowledge to assist in retrieval of familiar motor actions. Therapy sessions should be scheduled to accommodate a patient's limited attention span, with shorter sessions or frequent rest periods (O'Sullivan, 2001).

In terms of attention to task, research has shown that directing learners' attention to the effects of their movements is more beneficial for learning than directing their attention to the details of their own actions (McNevin, Wulf, & Carlson, 2000). These researchers found that "nonawareness strategies," in which the learners were instructed to perform the task without consciously attending to the movement pattern, produced a more effective performance during acquisition and transfer than an "awareness strategy," which required learners to consciously attend to the movement. When learning, it is better to offer patients an external focus of attention around the movement goal rather than asking the patient to attend to the movement pattern itself. This is presumed to be true because there is evidence that directing the performer's attention to his or her own movements can disrupt the execution of automated skills and have a degrading influence on the learning of new skills.

Clinical Connection:

We have all experienced this phenomenon. How many of us have experienced the disintegration of a movement performance while watching ourselves moving, as compared with just letting the movement pattern take over? An internal focus of attention is a more appropriate strategy for therapists to use, especially during early intervention. ▪

Motivation and Meaning

Motivation is the internal state that tends to direct or energize a system toward the goal (Schmidt, 1999). Motivation can be described as a force that leads to task engagement or sustained involvement in a task. Motivated learning is a highly individual process. Emphasis must be place on the individual's goals within a person-based perspective. The learner needs to experience satisfaction from executing a movement and remain encouraged to attain higher but achievable goals. The patient must understand the goal and the meaningfulness of the task in order to be motivated to achieve that goal.

Clinical Connection:

The following clinical practices are important to keep in mind in an effort to maximize and maintain patient motivation:

- Involve the patient/client and caregivers in goal setting. Find out from the patient or caregiver what kinds of activities or tasks may be meaningful for that person, including becoming familiar with the patient's past experiences.
- Use positive reinforcement to maximize motivation.
- End every session with a success. ▪

Motivational theorists have argued that the meaning an individual attaches to a situation determines that individual's choices, effort, and persistence with respect to that situation; that is, a person will try harder because of the meaning a given situation holds for him or her (Lewthwaite, 1990). **Meaning** refers to the sense that is made or the personal implications that are drawn; it can exist at multiple levels, from the immediate and superficial to the enduring and fundamental (Baumeister, 1989). Meaning arises from a combination of social, personal, and cultural factors, but it is also dynamic and can change over time or even within a single encounter.

Clinical Connection:

Clinicians are also reminded of the influence that an audience may have on a patient's performance. We have all experienced the phenomenon whereby simply being observed influences a performance. This influence of an audience may have a positive effect on performance, such as in the well-known phenomenon that accompanies observation, whereby performance improves "under the lights." On the contrary, stage fright is also a reality for many of us, where the presence of an audience (perhaps only of one) impairs performance dramatically. Clinicians simply need to be alert to the individual patient's response to observation during learning or practicing a movement skill. ■

Motivation is directly related to the meaning and purpose of the task for that patient/client. For all of us, functional tasks are those that have meaning, whereby the use of these functional tasks promote health. Nelson (1994) defined meaning as an interpretative process that an individual experiences when perceiving something in the environment. This "something" is associated with purpose. Added purpose increases the meaningfulness of an activity. This added purpose is defined as purposefulness that is multidimensional. Embedding an exercise within an occupation, which has been the hallmark of the occupational therapy profession, adds purpose to the exercise situation (Ferguson & Trombly, 1996). "Once a person finds meaning in an occupational form, a sense of purposefulness is possible" (Nelson, 1994, p. 23). This feeling, or affective meaning, is the type of meaning thought to be important for enhancing performance and learning.

Instruction

The therapist's instructions before practice are crucial not only for motivational purposes but also for clarity of conveying the information to the learner about the task. Instructions can take on many forms, including verbal, demonstration, and modeling.

The therapist's verbal instructions have the potential to focus the patient's attention to different levels of information about the task. Verbal instructions about the motor activity should first be offered about the entire movement, describing the typical speed and accuracy required in the desired skill (Gentile, 1987). According to the patient's level of attention and capability to process information, the clinician has the option to break down the verbal instruction, with an emphasis on one or two essential elements. Brevity and clarity are key factors for consideration.

Demonstration or modeling may either replace or supplement verbal instruction. Modeling is effectively used both as an initial demonstration and throughout practice. Observational motor learning has clearly been demonstrated to promote learning (Weiss, Ebbeck, & Wiese-Bjornstal, 1993). Peer modeling has been shown to be more effective than instructor modeling in some instances (Schmidt & Lee, 1999). Researchers have clearly demonstrated that for a model to be effective, the model does not have to be an expert performer; the

observation of any other model can have a positive effect on learning (Adams, 1986; Lee & White, 1990). A suggested protocol is alternating between physical and observational practice, so that while the learner is resting, observational learning of the model can continue. This offers a rationale for the benefits of therapy in group settings (McNevin et al., 2000).

Guidance

Physical or verbal guidance, often called "facilitation" in the physical and occupational therapy fields, is a major strategy employed in neurorehabilitation. Physical and verbal guidance generally assist the learner, in varying degrees, through the execution of the movement task. Guidance has been found to be most effective in the following situations:

1. In early practice
2. In performing unfamiliar tasks
3. For slower rather than rapid tasks
4. In the prevention of injury
5. For the reduction of fear or anxiety (Schmidt & Lee, 1999)

Guidance has a positive impact on performance during the practice of a task during the skill acquisition stage but not on long-term learning.

As learning progresses, guidance, including therapeutic facilitation, needs to be graded and decreased as the learner masters the movement task. Guidance modifies the natural feel of the task, and if the learner relies too strongly on it, he or she can develop a dependency. Continuous guidance alters the task and greatly reduces its ability to be transferred and generalized (Salmoni, Schmidt, & Walter, 1984). The clinician should generally aim at reducing the use of guidance while increasing independent practice. When needed, the therapist or assistant should alternate between trial and error, independent movements, and guided movements. Trial and error, or discovery procedures, increase learning. Reduced guidance in therapy may progress from firm physical handling with verbal input to a lesser, modified physical contact, to minimal verbal input with supervision, to nonverbal, nonphysical guidance (Larin, 2000).

Feedback

■ Definition and Clinical Importance

Feedback is considered one of the most powerful variables affecting learning (Schmidt, 1982). **Feedback** refers to the use of sensory information for the control of action in the process of skill acquisition (Winstein &

Schmidt, 1989). Feedback is important because it provides guidance, a reference for correction, and motivation. The type of feedback employed should be patient specific, matching the abilities of the learner and enhancing the ability of that patient to learn.

▪ Types of Feedback

There are many different types of feedback, as depicted in Table 5–2. Feedback may be positive or negative, intrinsic or extrinsic. **Intrinsic feedback** is sensory information from within one's body that comes from the proprioceptors, skin, visual, vestibular, and auditory receptors either during or following movement production. It is "response-produced feedback" that normally occurs along with a movement. Intrinsic feedback is often distorted in the patient with a neurological impairment. In this case, the need for extrinsic feedback is greater. **Extrinsic feedback** is augmented (amplified or enhanced) information about movement provided to the mover from an external source. Verbal and tactile cuing from the therapist, biofeedback, the use of rhythm or music, and videotaped replays are common clinical applications of extrinsic feedback. Motor learning can occur with extrinsic feedback alone, in the absence of intrinsic feedback. This is an important fact for clinicians to remember when working with those with neurological dysfunction, who may have impaired intrinsic feedback systems (Rothwell et al., 1982).

The purpose of extrinsic feedback is to provide the person with **knowledge of the results (KR)** of the movement or **knowledge about the performance (KP)**. KR is defined as information, usually verbal and augmented, about the response outcome or the outcome of the movement (Duncan & Badke, 1987; Magill, 2001). KR is a post-response type of feedback that serves to guide error correction, motivate the learner, and reinforce optimal and correct performance (Magill, 1989; Schreiber et al., 2000). An example of KR is a therapist telling a patient, "Your shirt is on backward." On the other hand, KP is information about the movement pattern or characteristics that led to the performance outcome. KP typically represents the kind of extrinsic feedback most often given by clinicians to patients. KR differs from KP in terms of which aspect of the performance the information refers to. An example of KP feedback for the clinical example stated previously is, "You did not turn the shirt around first before putting your head though the neck opening."

Clinical Connection:

To further illustrate the difference between KP and KR, the following example is described. If a clinician were instructing a patient/client on reaching forward for a glass of water, the clinician might offer the patient feedback about the success of the reach in terms of how closely the patient met the goal or whether the glass was actually retrieved or perhaps was knocked over. This information would be described as KR, knowledge of the outcome of the movement attempt—in this case, successful retrieval of the glass or upsetting it. In addition, the therapist or assistant may give the patient feedback regarding the height of the extremity during the reach attempt, the employed range of motion, the muscular force used, or the observed ability to coordinate the extremity's movement in space—all performance, or KP, attributes. The patient could then be asked to focus on a specific performance variable that may have been faulty and produced a performance difficulty, perhaps resulting in knocking the glass of water over. Both types of information are valuable to the learner. KP draws the learner's attention to the specific individual performance attributes of the task, and KR draws attention to the overall result of the movement. ▪

Another clinical example: If the goal is to rise from a sitting to a standing position in a given amount of time, KR might be given in the amount of time needed to complete the task; KP might be the amount of trunk flexion used to lean forward, the beginning posture for initiating the task, or where the feet were on the floor at the beginning of the transfer attempt.

The most effective KP seems to be information about the critical components of the action and provides prescriptive information about how to correct the errors (Carr & Shepherd, 2000; Magill, 2001). Researchers have found that providing constant KR is not as effective in promoting motor learning as giving KR intermittently (Ho & Shea, 1978; Winstein & Schmidt, 1990). With a decrease in KR, the learner appears to increase the level of cognitive processing and rely on other cues in an effort to improve task performance. Learning through more elaborate encoding processes appears to result (Schmidt, 1988). Combinations of KR and KP are useful in most therapeutic interventions.

TABLE 5–2	
Types of Feedback	
Intrinsic	**Extrinsic**
Proprioceptive	Knowledge of results
Tactile	Knowledge of performance
Vestibular	Common clinical mechanisms
Visual	Verbal cues
Auditory	Tactile cues
	Videography
	Biofeedback

Learning involves trial and error. The experience a person has in correcting errors is especially important in skill learning (Carr & Shepherd, 2000; Magill, 2001).

Patients/clients need to be able to recognize error in order to use error knowledge as a learning reference or tool. When do clinicians give up "correctness" in order to allow learning, perhaps through error? "Error-free" therapy, where quality of movement is emphasized and only actions that can be performed "normally" are permitted, is currently being re-examined and is coming under great scrutiny. Although the importance of quality of movement is not being disputed, practice under more natural conditions, laden with trial and error, has been found to be superior (Singer, 1978).

■ Clinical Use of Feedback: Selection and Timing

Important clinical decisions surround choosing the kind of feedback that is most appropriate, as well as the quantity and timing of that feedback. The accuracy of feedback is extremely important because erroneous feedback will impair learning. Feedback should focus on only one or two movement components at a time and should be easily understood by the learner. Additional cuing can be nonverbal so as not to verbally bombard the learner.

Major clinical consideration needs to be given to the timing of the feedback: how often it is given and when it is offered. In the initial stages of learning, frequent feedback quickly guides the learner to the correct performance. Therapists and assistants, however, are warned that too much feedback fosters dependence. After the initial stages of learning, frequent feedback distracts the learner and interferes with the information processing activities required for skill learning. As learning increases, feedback should be "faded," or decreased in both frequency and quantity. During the later stages of learning, feedback should not only decrease, but needs to be more precise (Poole, 1991). Feedback can be given concurrently during the performance or after the performance is completed, called summary or terminal feedback. Research suggests that practice with concurrent feedback may result in improved performance, while summary feedback may be actually detrimental for immediate performance but beneficial for long-term retention (O'Sullivan, 2001 & Winstein, 1996). Research also shows that varying the type of feedback may slow the initial learning but improve retention. Additional consideration should be given to the amount of time that elapses between the performance and the feedback. A delay of seconds or even minutes is not of so much concern as is the importance of preventing competing input from interfering with the learner's attention to the task. Learning happens as long as competing events do not occur and interfere with the neural processing while it is occurring. Clinical choices by the therapist are vital in optimizing learning and must be individualized for the patient/client and re-evaluated constantly.

Practice

■ Definition and Clinical Importance

In addition to feedback, practice is one of the most powerful variables affecting learning. **Practice** is the continuing and repetitive effort to become proficient in a skill. Practice needs to be accurate so that desired movement patterns are repeated and learned. Faulty practice, or practice of incorrect movement patterns, may lead to habits and postures that may then need to be unlearned. Practice should be active, not passive, and it should be patient initiated. The amount of guidance or assistance during practice needs to be supportive of promoting optimal active learning on the part of the patient learner.

A consistent characteristic of theories of motor skill learning is their emphasis on learning benefits derived from varying the practice. *Practice variability* refers to the use of a variety of movement and context characteristics while the leaner is practicing a skill. It is a well-accepted prediction that successful future performance of a skill depends on the amount of variability the learner experiences during practice. Dynamic pattern theory is supportive of this position, emphasizing the importance of the learner's freedom to actively explore the perceptual motor workspace and to discover solutions to movement dilemmas. Practice must be task specific whenever possible. A functional task is the best choice because there is minimal transfer of skill between tasks when function is not the cornerstone concept. Clinical decisions about practice center around choosing the type of practice and the organization of the practice itself.

Types of Practice

Types of practice include physical, mental, and whole versus part training. Effective practice requires more than just movement repetition. The problem-solving operations undertaken by the learner, especially those involved in the development of an action plan, make important contributions to the acquisition, development, and refinement of a skill. Cognitive processing is a key component of practice, sometimes actually undermined by rote repetitive performances (Lee, Swanson, & Hall, 1991). Practice under conditions of trial and error, where active learning and problem solving are maximized, has been found to be superior with regard to transfer and generalizability of a skill (Singer, 1978).

Physical practice allows the learner to gain direct experience. Kinesthetic stimulation during practice and retention phases seems to enhance task acquisition because kinesthetic information appears to provide important feedback for learners that enables them then to make necessary adjustments during performance (Jarus & Loiter, 1995). It is crucial for the shaping of a motor program. It appears that such stimulation affects the motor memory processes and leaves a more stable cortical representation of the movement pattern. **Shaping,** a term borrowed from the education field, refers to a gradual process whereby a behavior is changed from an initial status to a desired terminal outcome. The use of physical practice is commonly employed in movement education, where the learner performs the movement over and over again in an effort to increase skill.

Mental practice, on the other hand, is the cognitive rehearsal of a motor task without any overt movement. The patient/client is instructed to visualize or remember a task and to then imagine it occurring. Mental practice is thought to form a kinesthetic image that allows for movement rehearsal without actual movement performance (Jarus & Ratzon, 2000). It has been found that mental practice activates many of the neural components in the brain that are responsible for actually directing the movement (Sage, 1984). There is convincing evidence that some of the motor units that are normally activated during movement execution are activated, though not mobilized, when a person mentally practices a movement (Decety & Ingvar, 1990). Mental practice also appears to allow the learner to gain cognitive-perceptual insights into the movement pattern, assisting the learner to consolidate strategies, as well as to correct errors (Magill, 1989; Sage, 1984). Studies measuring electromyographic (EMG) activity, cortical motor evoked potentials, and cerebral blood flow also have shown that the appropriate motor pathways imagined as being used are actually being used and that metabolic activity of neurons is increased during mental practice as if the activity is actually being performed (Livesay & Samras, 1998; Page, Levine, Sisto, & Johnston, 2001; Roth, Decety, & Raybaudi, 1996).

There has been a great deal of research validating the effectiveness of mental practice on both skill acquisition and movement re-education (Linden, Uhley, Smith, & Bush, 1989; Maring, 1990; Warner & McNeill, 1988). Most studies have concluded that physical practice was superior in performing tasks in which the motor component is dominant and that physical practice combined with mental practice facilitates skill performance in tasks whose cognitive component is significant (Annett, 1995; Jarus & Ratzon, 2000; Wrisberg & Ragsdale, 1979). Debate continues as to the importance of prior experience in the effectiveness of mental practice (Jarus & Ratzon, 2000). Mental practice is also a valuable energy conservation technique for patients/clients who fatigue easily.

Practicing the entire task or separate components, one at a time, can be different methods employed in learning. The clinical decision of "whole versus part" training is another way that the clinician can choose the best method for the particular situation. For rapid skills of short duration, practice of the whole task from the outset usually leads to the best results. If the learner has the prerequisite skills to master the whole skill in its entirety, or if the degree of cognitive processing is minimal, the "whole" method has been reported to be far superior to one based on parts (Croce & DePaepe, 1989). On the other hand, slower, serial skills of long duration are often best practiced by practicing the most troublesome parts first and then gradually integrating all the parts into the whole. It is essential, however, for therapists and assistants to remember that movement is usually smooth and unbroken in its natural manifestation. Breaking a movement into parts does take the movement components out of context and may actually interfere with skill mastery and the desired smoothness of movement. Skills can be broken into component parts, but these subtasks need to be functional. Practice of tasks needs to include the appropriate timing. Slowing down a movement that is typically performed at a higher speed changes the task requirements enough that it may impede task mastery. Within the constraints of safe practice, movement skills are best practiced at a speed that approximates the patient's self-chosen speed.

Careful task analysis is important, including recognition of the task requirements; deciding whether the task is simple or complex; familiar or novel; and choosing the best environmental interface for this task (O'Sullivan, 2001). Movement organization in part tasks is different from movement organization of the corresponding segments of the whole task. Functional whole tasks elicit better movement quality than practicing part tasks with less functional goals (Ma & Trombly, 2000). Tasks involving connected discrete movements are effectively practiced in discrete component parts, but whole-task practice generally results in more efficient, smoother movements. The clinical decision whether to have the patient practice the whole task or its parts is largely task dependent. Current research supports the premise that multistep functional tasks are best kept whole, because breaking down a functional task may in effect create a set of new tasks, each with different goals, thus changing the movement characteristics (Davis & Burton, 1991; Ma & Trombly, 2000).

According to Carr & Shepherd (1998), in general, intensive practice is required to accomplish the following:

1. Enable a movement pattern to be initially learned, refining the neural commands to the muscles (Gottlieb, Corcos, Jaric, & Agarwal, 1988)
2. Strengthen muscles specifically for similar actions
3. Allow for learning the rules of movement in specific contexts
4. Enable a stable pattern to be modified as necessary according to environmental and other demands—to develop flexibility of performance

Transfer of learning refers to the gain or loss of task performance as a result of practice or experience in some other task (Schmidt, 1999). Transfer of learning refers to the positive influence that a previously practiced skill has on the learning of a new skill or the performing of the same skill in a new environmental context (Magill, 1993). In the therapy setting, the most common application of this principle is practicing component parts of a motor activity to learn the whole activity. According to O'Sullivan (2001), the success of this strategy is dependent on the nature of the task and the learner. If the task is complex, with highly independent parts that can be naturally subdivided into units, or if a learner has a limited attention span, then learning can be enhanced with this practice method. On the other hand, if the task is highly integrated with dependent parts (such as gait), then practice of the integrated whole is much more successful (O'Sullivan, 2001). Discrete tasks may be effectively learned if practiced as a whole rather than broken down into component parts. Regardless of which method is used, it is important to practice both the components and the integrated whole within the same session. It is also important to work on accuracy and speed concurrently, which is best done within the natural context of the task. If coordination and sequencing are important between the parts, the whole task must be practiced as a unit. Delaying the practice of the integrated whole for days or weeks will interfere with the transfer effects and ultimately diminish learning.

▪ Organization of the Practice

Practice can be organized in several different ways as follows:

1. Practice can be organized around the repetition of one task repeatedly, as in **constant practice,** or several variations of the same or similar tasks can be performed, such as in **variable practice.** Although both methods allow for learning, variable practice has superior long-term effects in retention and generalizability of skills. For example, when practicing transfers, the types of transfers practiced can be varied rather than practicing the same transfer over and over again. Although it is true that constant practice of one type of transfer does improve initial performance, varying the same task improves long-term learning and the ability to generalize the skill outside the intervention environment.

2. Practice can also be organized by manipulating the frequency and duration of rest periods. **Massed practice** consists of a sequence of practice and rest times in which the rest time is much less than the practice time (Schmidt, 1999). Massed practice may improve initial performance, but issues of fatigue and injury need to be taken into account. **Distributed practice** is defined as organizing the practice so that rest periods either equal or exceed the practice periods. Although learning will occur with both massed and distributed methods, distributed is most widely acceptable in rehabilitation. Distributed practice is preferred whenever fatigue, poor attention span, limited motivation, or the risk of injury is noted. Evidence suggests that massed practice greatly improves motor performance but only weakly improves learning (Schmidt, 1988).

3. **Practice order,** or the sequence in which the tasks are practiced, is the final organization consideration for clinicians. Tasks can be practiced in a blocked order, where the sequence of tasks repeats in a very predictable way; in a serial order, where the tasks are predictable but the order is changed; or in a random order, where the order is unpredictable and out of sequence. Although skill acquisition occurs with all three methods of practice order, blocked order seems to improve early learning, whereas serial and random orders produce improved retention. Both serial and random order increase the probability of interference from outside stimuli interspersed during the practice session. Dealing with such episodes of interference increases the cognitive demand on the learner and thereby makes the learner a more active participant in the processing of learning. This increased depth of cognitive processing improves the learning quality. Presenting tasks in random order creates high **contextual interference,** defined as a practice situation where performance of one task results in a performance detriment of another task (Battig, 1979; Lee & Magill, 1983). High contextual interference forces the learner to use multiple cognitive processes to meet the challenges of the tasks, as opposed to a situation with low contextual interference, as in blocked practice. Random practice, rather than constant practice, is more effective for retention and transfer of motor skills (McCracken & Stelmach, 1977; Wrisberg & Ragsdale, 1979). On the other hand, because of the high contextual interference found in random practice, the rate of skill acquisition is slower than that during blocked prac-

tice (Goode & Magill, 1986). Random practice has been demonstrated to be more effective than blocked practice with respect to retention over time in learners attempting to relearn functional skills (Hanlon, 1996). Block practice appears to enhance performance rather than learning, whereas random practice seems to enhance learning (Tse & Spaulding, 1998).

Skill Acquisition and Retention/Transfer

Transfer of learning refers to the gain or loss of task performance as a result of practice or experience on some other task (Schmidt, 1999). The ability to *transfer* refers to the positive influence that a previously practiced skill has on the learning of a new skill or performing or generalizing of the same skill within a new environmental context (Magill, 1993). Current motor learning research illustrates that differing conditions are optimal for initial skill acquisition than those that are optimal for retention and transfer. Table 5–3 summarizes the differences in conditions that are most effective for acquisition of skill as compared with those for retention and transfer of skills.

Stages of Learning

Three-Stage Model of Motor Learning

Fitts and Posner (1967) described motor learning as occurring in three distinct stages: cognitive, associative, and autonomous. These stages offer a very useful framework for therapists and assistants to conceptualize the learning process and to determine effective strategies for intervention with patients (O'Sullivan, 2001).

▪ Cognitive Stage

The cognitive stage requires the acquisition of factual knowledge, often before attempting any action. This is called the cognitive stage because it requires a great deal of conscious processing. According to O'Sullivan (2001), during the cognitive stage, the patient is attempting to answer the question *"What is it that must be done?"* The patient (learner) needs information about the goal of the action and some idea of how the goal is to be accomplished. The patient is facing the task of what to do, such as where to place the hands before attempting a sit-to-stand transfer.

This stage is characterized by a large number of errors, many of them inconsistent. The patient is engaged in repetitive efforts at skill performance, marked by successive approximations of the task, the discarding of unsuccessful strategies, and the retention of those that are successful (O'Sullivan, 2001). The patient may know that something is wrong with the attempted task execution but may not know what needs to be done to improve performance. This trial and error period usually results in observably uneven and inconsistent performance. Movement patterns are often disorganized as the patient relies on sensory and perceptual cues to eventually select a successful motor program. The patient learner engages predominantly in cognitive activity while listening to instruction, watching demonstration, and receiving initial feedback from the therapist or assistant, who acts very much like a coach at this stage.

It is important for therapists and assistants to remember that in order for the patient/client to learn, *active* participation must occur (Carr & Shepherd, 2000). The learner usually relies primarily on vision and tactile cues to guide learning. A stable, "closed" environment, free from distractions, optimizes learning during this initial stage. Clinically, this acquisition phase is a period during which a great deal of change and progress is readily observable.

Clinical Connection:

Effective clinical strategies during the cognitive stage of learning include the following summarized from O'Sullivan (2001):

1. Structure the environment, reduce stimuli, and minimize stress. Use visual demonstration, establishing a reference for correctness, and describe in simple terms the meaningfulness of the task. Refer to other tasks with similarities within the patient's past experience and use mental practice. Vision is extremely important at this time; have the patient watch your demonstration and his or her own attempts at movement execution. Refrain from verbally bombarding the patient with extraneous instruction. Direct attention only to critical elements of the task.
2. Organize the practice by breaking down tasks into parts, using manual guidance to assist if appropriate. Use blocked practice of the same task to increase skill acquisition, but offer a random practice order in an attempt to improve cognitive processing. Provide adequate periods of rest.
3. Select the appropriate use of feedback, perhaps frequently initially and fading later. Give feedback available from the intact and strongest sensory

TABLE 5-3

Summary of Conditions to Promote Acquisition (Initial Learning) Compared with Those That Promote Retention and Transfer (Long-Term Learning)

Key Learning Element	To Promote Acquisition (Initial Learning)	To Promote Retention and Transfer (Long-term Learning)
Extrinsic feedback	High quantity Frequent Concurrent with performance	Decrease quantity. Make less frequent, "faded." Offer summary feedback. Provide decreased or intermittent KR. Provide high contextual interference (delay).
Practice	Physical and mental practice Movement repetition Consistency Part practice to master components Blocked practice Correct only significant errors Give opportunities to fixate on closed skills Requires great deal of cognitive activity; problem solving	Promote production of entire movement pattern. Encourage problem solving, searching for active solutions. Practice within context of task. Provide random or variable practice. Differentiate movement. Ensure diversification of open skills.
Guidance	Manual Verbal cueing	Avoid manual guidance. Don't over cue. Allow error and refinement.

Sources: Reprinted from Craik, R. L., & Oatis, C. A. (1995). *Gait analysis: Theory and application,* with permission from Elsevier.

subsystems. Do not focus on random or inconsistent errors. Focus on success, and use praise as appropriate. ▪

▪ Associative Stage

During the associative or intermediate stage, the learner starts to distinguish between correct performance and errors. This stage is called associative because the patient is linking, or associating, the movement attempts and the feedback received (both intrinsic and extrinsic) to outcome. It is during this phase that the learner starts to diminish errors that are inherent in the performance of a new skill, or, as applied to rehabilitation, to the relearning of previously mastered skills. The patient learner is attempting to answer the question *"How to do?"* at this time (O'Sullivan, 2001). The need for cognitive attention and concentration decreases.

Performance improves, and errors become more consistent. This is a time of skill refinement as the movement becomes more organized into a coordinated pattern. The learner has less dependence on vision and touch, and a shift is made to internal proprioceptive cues. Refinement of the motor program occurs through a great deal of practice. This is often the longest stage in the rehabilitation process, with the learning process dependent on a variety of factors, including the health status, motivation level, prior experience, and resources available to the patient/client.

Clinical Connection:

Effective clinical strategies during this associative intermediate stage of learning include the following summarized from O'Sullivan (2001):

1. Continue to structure the environment, but progress to a more open one, stressing the importance of function and task meaningfulness.
2. Organize the practice to focus on a more variable practice order in an attempt to increase retention. Encourage performance to be consistent, and intervene only when errors are consistent and significant. Facilitation and manual guidance may be counterproductive at this stage.
3. Select the appropriate use of feedback, emphasizing proprioceptive awareness and the ability of the patient to self-assess. Avoid excessive guidance or feedback, including augmented feedback. ▪

▪ Autonomous Stage

During the final, or autonomous, stage of skill learning, the speed and efficiency of performance gradually improve and skill emerges. Performance is less dependent on cognitive control and less affected by interference. During this stage, the shift is made to performance becoming more automatic. According to O'Sullivan (2001), the learner is now able to concentrate on *"How to succeed?"*

Movements are largely error-free, with little interference from environmental distractions. Movement patterns become increasingly automatic. In the clinical setting, the environment can now be organized to incorporate distraction and the opportunity to perform more than one task simultaneously.

Clinical Connection:

Effective clinical strategies during the autonomous stage of learning include the following summarized from O'Sullivan (2001):

1. Open up and vary the environment, preparing the patient for multiple settings. Challenge the learner.
2. Vary the practice, stressing consistency of performance in variable environments with some task variation.
3. Provide only occasional feedback, and encourage the learner to develop increased self-evaluation skills. Give feedback when errors are evident and significant.

Gentile's Two-Stage Model of Motor Learning

Another popular model commonly referred to in motor learning is that proposed by Gentile (1972, 2000). This model proposes that, in contrast to three stages, motor learning progresses through two stages, the stages presented from the perspective of the learner and the learner's goal. In the initial stage, the goal of the learner is to develop an understanding of the task and the requirements of the movement. This refers to the need for the learner to "get the idea of the movement" (Magill, 2001, p. 185), whereby the learner needs to establish an appropriate movement coordination pattern to accomplish the goal. For example, if a patient is relearning the ability to independently don a shirt, the person's focus in this first stage would be on acquiring the appropriate postural control and extremity strength and coordination that will lead to successful completion of this task. The focus would be on learning the required task dynamics, including establishing the required amount of muscular strength, range of motion, and coordination necessary to don the shirt.

In this first stage, to establish the basic movement pattern, the person must not only understand the goal but must also learn to understand the environmental features critical to organization of the movement. This requires the need to discriminate between environmental features that are critical to the task, called **regulatory conditions**, and those that are irrelevant, called **nonregulatory conditions**. Regulatory conditions are characteristics of the performance environment that influence (regulate) the characteristics of the movement used to perform the skill. In the example of learning to put on a shirt, the regulatory conditions would include information about the characteristics of the shirt, such as whether it is a pullover or button style, the opening size for the arms and neck on the shirt, and so on. On the other hand, there are characteristics of the performance environment that do not influence the movement characteristics of the skill. In the same example, such nonregulatory characteristics would include the color of the shirt or the material that the shirt is made of.

In this first stage, the learner explores a variety of movement possibilities. Through trial and error, the patient experiences movement characteristics that are successful and unsuccessful and begins to focus on practice that yields successful results. The learner is engaged in active problem solving, often requiring a great deal of cognitive activity. When the learner reaches the end of this first stage, according to Gentile (1987), the learner has "a framework for organizing effective movement," but this achievement is not consistent or efficient.

In the second, or later, stage of learning, the learner's goal is to improve and refine the movement skill. In this stage, the learner has three main tasks:

1. The person must develop the capability to adapt the movement pattern he or she has acquired in the first stage to the specific demands of different environmental contexts or performance situations.
2. Consistency of performance must improve.
3. The person must learn to perform the skill with efficiency (Magill, 2001).

During this second stage, the learner's goals are largely dependent on the type of skill. Gentile divides skills into two classifications: closed or open. **Closed skills** require what Gentile terms "fixation," meaning that the learner works toward developing the capability to perform the pattern automatically and efficiently. The learner is given the opportunity to "fixate" the required movement coordination pattern so that it can be performed consistently. These types of tasks have features that are somewhat stationary. In a therapy setting, the therapist may offer the patient opportunity for blocked practice with high repetition with little variety introduced into the task. For example, gait practice would be limited to walking on similar surfaces in similar environments. On the other hand, **open skills** require "diversification" of the basic movement pattern acquired during the first stage of learning, so that the learner is required to adapt to continuously changing regulatory conditions. These types of tasks have features (objects or people) that are not stationary. In the example described earlier, the gait practice would be expanded to an environment with contextual interference, walking in different directions, at various speeds, with varied hallway parameters.

Gentile has proposed two concurrent processes that mediate skilled learning (Gentile, 1998). **Explicit learning** is a process that develops an initial mapping between the performer's body and environmental conditions. During practice, explicit learning requires active processing of information and effort. The learner selectively attends to features in the environment that determine the configuration of body segments, as well as the intermediate and endpoints within the task sequence. These markers assist in understanding how to achieve the task goal. General movement solutions then are able to emerge and, with repeated practice, become more finely tuned. **Implicit learning** occurs with subsequent tries as the learner then attempts to anticipate more precisely what is needed to be more efficient. Implicit learning involves predicting the impact of forces, such as the effects of gravity and momentum and active muscular force, on the emergent and intended movement. Implicit learning is thought to occur when changes in performance occur as the practice conditions are changed, requiring a somewhat automatic change in response behavior. Recent research has demonstrated that implicit learning can and does occur without awareness of what is being learned, a vitally important fact for clinicians working with individuals with neurological dysfunction (Pohl, McDowd, Filion, Richards, & Stiers, 2001). This implicit process is important because it allows the learner to learn how to estimate movement characteristics and anticipate the appropriate force requirements. Both these processes are important aspects of motor learning. Learners, our patients, need to be offered opportunities to move actively, engage in problem solving, make errors, and self-correct (Lesensky & Kaplan, 2000).

The Therapist's or Assistant's Role in Facilitating Skill Acquisition

The models presented by Fitts and Posner (1967) and Gentile (1972) both offer clinicians a framework within which to view the patient as a learner. Skill development is enhanced by appropriate instruction, including appropriate goal selection, structuring of the environment, and manipulation of the variables of practice and feedback. Therapeutic interventions must be creatively designed based on the characteristics of the performer, the task, and the phase of learning. Practicing the task in its most appropriate environment best facilitates learning a task. Therapists and assistants, as instructors, must remember to think of the patient as a learner and therapy as a learning process. Figure 5–1, adapted from Watts' *Handbook of Clinical Teaching* (1990), is a representation of the process of learning and the functions of teaching. The learner, or patient, is represented in the center of the diagram, and the activities of the teacher, or clinician, are represented as having an impact from the outside on the learner's process. *Effective therapy complements the learner.* Box 5–1 summarizes the practitioner's role in instruction and practice.

The initial learning phase for a patient with a neurological insult may be very long. Learning abilities may be altered by damage to any or all of the subsystems involved in movement production. During the initial phase, the first responsibility of the clinician is to select a functional task and avoid goal confusion. The second responsibility is to engage the patient/client by promoting self-confidence and motivation by creating opportunities for some degree of success. The environment

---

BOX 5–1

Practitioner's Role in Instruction and Practice

Provide a nurturing, safe, supportive, and facilitating environment for bringing about change in functional movements.
Facilitate the development of the motor skill, recognizing where the learner is within his or her developmental life span process.
Analyze tasks; be cognizant of simple versus complex tasks.
Identify prerequisite skills required of a task and allow for compensation of identified deficits.
Clarify the goal and minimize goal confusion. Establish appropriate conditions for understanding the goal, the task, and the task conditions.
Allow for observation, demonstration, and functional and active problem solving.
Clarify relevant (regulatory) environmental features.
Identify the critical features of the movement for both observation and for instruction and practice.
Select tasks that require a variety of strategies and incorporate variable environmental conditions.
Employ appropriate motivational strategies.
Provide feedback appropriate to not only the task but to the skill level of the learner.
Capitalize on the learner's successes. Use failure and error as a positive learning opportunity.

Source: Craik, R. L., & Oatis, C. A. (1995). *Gait analysis: Theory and application.* Philadelphia: Mosby, with permission from Elsevier.

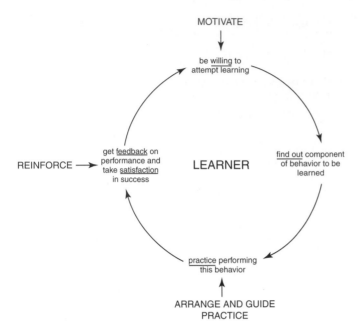

Figure 5–1. The therapeutic relationship is aptly pictured as a process of learning and the functions of teaching. (Reprinted from Watts, N. T. [1990]. The events of learning and the functions of teaching [p. 7]. In *Handbook of clinical teaching*. New York: Churchill Livingstone, with permission from Elsevier.)

should be structured to promote acquisition of the specific skill, eliminating unnecessary environmental variables. Choice of feedback type and timing and the organization of practice are important considerations in promoting learning.

During the intermediate and later phases of learning, the therapeutic focus is on the learner's further development, improvement, and refinement of the skill. The main goals are consistency across environmental contexts and efficiency. The environment can be structured to introduce interference and to increase opportunities for practicing efficiency. Feedback is reduced to encourage more independent learning by the performer (Gentile, 2000). The learner must develop flexibility and a repertoire of strategies to match changing and often novel conditions.

Goal-Directed and Purposeful Activity

Current knowledge in the field of motor learning research lends compelling support to the importance of task-related intervention for the improvement of motor control (Sabari, 1991). The motor learning approach should be task oriented, centered around the accomplishment of everyday activities. The main concern of learning movement depends on a person's ability to solve movement problems in order to accomplish

everyday, functional tasks. Active participation in such purposeful activity is the key to improving or maintaining function and independence (Kaplan, 1994). **Purposeful activity,** according to the American Occupational Therapy Association (AOTA) position statement, is defined as goal-directed behaviors of tasks that comprise occupations (Hinojosa, Sabari, & Pedretti, 1993). An activity is *purposeful* if the individual is an active, voluntary participant and if the activity is directed toward a goal that the individual considers meaningful (Evans, 1987; Gilfoyle, 1984; Mosey, 1986; Nelson, 1988).

A return to the task approach has been advocated by researchers and clinicians in the fields of physical and occupational therapy. Developmentally, an infant first develops coordinated and controlled movement by *actively* exploring the environment and matching his or her body characteristics to the environment in the context of accomplishing a task, rather than by doing a movement unrelated to the task (Thelen et al., 1993). Through this experience, the infant develops some motor programs and general rules from movement that can then later be retrieved from memory when needed. The importance of this "discovery learning" in goal-directed natural environments continues to be valuable throughout the life span.

Research continues to accumulate to support that active participation in purposeful activity is the key to improving or maintaining function and independence (Gilner, 1985; Kaplan, 1994; VanderWeel, VanderMeer, & Lee, 1991). When an individual is interested in the activity, the nervous system is activated and engaged. Goal-directed activity has clearly been demonstrated to elicit more coordinated movement than rote exercise (Flinn, 1999; Mathiowetz & Wade, 1995; Trombly & Wu, 1999). Goal-directed occupation can have a powerful influence on motor behavior. Interestingly, it may be the converse of this statement that has the greatest impact—not using goal-directed activity may produce motor performance that is different from the individual's actual ability in tasks that *are* goal-directed (Flinn, 1999). This disconnect between the individual's true performance and performance during a less effectively designed therapy session has important implications for practitioners.

Embedding movement education or re-education into an occupation is very effective in adding purpose to activity and thereby positively impacting on learning and performance (Ferguson & Trombly, 1996; DeKuiper, Nelson, & White, 1993; Hsieh, Nelson, Smith, & Peterson, 1994). The term **occupationally embedded** was coined by the occupational therapy profession to describe occupations that have greater meaning and purpose to a given individual. Research is indicating that contextually relevant occupationally embedded tasks can enhance occupational performance.

Intervention in natural environments aids not only in the reacquisition of skills but in the generalization of learned motor skills. The more relevant the context, the more improved the occupational performance (Rice, Alaimo, & Cook, 1999). Choosing an environment and task that have the greatest meaning to the individual can be instrumental in attaining the best outcome.

Life Span Issues Related to Motor Learning

The brain is clearly a dynamic organ. We are constantly learning new information that then is converted into functional and structural changes, so that the actual architecture of the brain is changing at all times. Learning continues over the course of the life span. Problem-solving techniques can be learned throughout one's lifetime (Drubach, 2000).

Our ability to learn information and therefore to modify the brain is limitless, although many factors, such as age and presence or absence of pathological changes, limit the speed and degree of learning. Indeed, the ability of the brain to change its structure and function (plasticity; see Chapter 2) decreases with age. Brain plasticity continues throughout the lifetime of an individual, although the type and degree of that plasticity may change over time.

Learners of all ages benefit from careful selection of key learning elements, as discussed previously in this chapter: environmental considerations, motivation, attention, guidance and instruction, and selection of feedback and practice. Additionally, learners (patients) at different age stages offer teachers (therapists and assistants) some unique challenges and opportunities. There certainly are some commonalities for learning across the life span. For example, learners of motor skills of all ages appear to benefit from the effects of positive verbal reinforcement, documented from the preschool child (Terrell & Kennedy, 1957) to the young adult in college (Kirschenbaum & Smith, 1983) to the older adult (Burgio, Burgio, Engel, & Tice, 1986). Motivation is crucially important for intentional learning regardless of the age of the learner. On the other hand, there are some learning styles and issues unique to the different phases of the life span. For a therapist or assistant to be an effective teacher for patients/clients of any age, familiarity with age-related learning issues is paramount.

Learning During Childhood

Throughout infancy and childhood, play is a child's work. Play has been linked to work because the child learns skills and develops interests through play that later affect choices in both work and leisure (Knox, 1998). Play is a mechanism for an elaboration on experience, for exploration, for social development, for the development of coordination skills, and to further cognitive processing. In infancy and early childhood, most time is spent in play. As children mature, time is divided between school and free time, and play/leisure takes on different forms.

Physical and occupational therapy intervention is a teaching and learning relationship. Familiarity with developmental theory (see Chapter 4) and learning theory can help clinicians to assimilate key developmental and teaching concepts into the intervention setting and interaction with children. Readers are reminded to use the concept of developmental stages as a loose guideline, not as a rigid rule. Most recent research has shown that cognitive skills and processing can bridge different stages, but still, in a broad sense, children do learn on a continuum. In a broad sense, children of different ages or levels of experience or ability have different developmental tasks, skills, and strategies for play.

During infancy, play activities assist the infant in developing skills through engagement with objects and through interaction with caregivers and family members. The infant practices and develops mastery of skills in motor planning and problem-solving, developing form and space perception, equilibrium, and postural adaptability to the environment. Activities during infancy stimulate and serve to foster integration between the tactile, vestibular, visual, auditory, musculoskeletal, nervous, and proprioceptive systems. Cognitive development during this time is fostered through repetition and combining of sensory and motor experiences. Movement and play that stimulate sensorimotor functioning and interaction are vital at this time (Knox, 1998).

During early childhood, movement activities are focused on continual exploration and investigation of the environment. Engagement in repetitive activity and imitative behavior characterize most of the activities during these years. Practice and exploratory play gradually shift into more constructive play, as children become more interested in the outcome of an activity. Mental practice has been demonstrated to be a highly effective strategy for motor learning in childhood, possibly due to the spontaneous mental rehearsal opportunities that then become available (Jarus & Ratzon, 2000). Children at this age start to learn about social systems, character roles, and functional roles. Self-absorption gives way to cooperative group play, as the capacities to follow directions, take turns, and concentrate for longer periods unfold. Sensory and motor development continue to mature and culminate by age 6 in the acquisition of most fundamental movement patterns and refinement of the tactile, vestibular, visual, auditory, musculoskeletal, nervous, and proprioceptive systems. Children at this age are focusing on achieving a balance between holding on and letting go, as they develop independence and autonomy and begin to comprehend the effects of making decisions and choices. Thinking and reasoning are developing, as self-absorption gives way to increased social skills. Experts agree that with maturation, there is an increase in the capacity to process information and to process it more rapidly and with greater efficiency (Goodgold-Edwards, 1991; Klein, 1978). Children are thought to have more decision-making requirements during a task than adults, because adults rule out actions as a result of experience (Kay, 1970).

Clinical Connection:

It is theorized that learning throughout childhood actually promotes and fosters further development and continued learning. An essential feature of childhood learning processes has been termed the creation of a zone of proximal development. This concept means that learning awakens a variety of internal developmental processes that are able to operate only when the child is interacting with people within the environment, and usually in cooperation with peers. From this perspective, organized learning actually results in mental development and sets into motion a variety of developmental processes that would be impossible apart from the learning experience itself (Vygotsky, 1978). Current research supports the contemporary practice premise that children's development occurs when they experience development-enhancing learning opportunities (Bronfenbrenner, 1992). Many of these opportunities occur within natural environments as part of the everyday activities of childhood, as part of daily living; on the playground; within the home and day care setting; and during family, community, and social activities (Dunst, Bruder, Trivette, & McLean, 2001). Clinicians are reminded that the learning of motor skills and subsequent performance improvements are only seen when the use of these skills is generalized by the child to tasks encountered within daily living (Coster, 1995). ▪

Middle to late childhood is a time of refinement in perceptual skills and the emergence of higher levels of mastery in all domains. In children without a motor impairment, physical capabilities expand and efficiency is gained in this area. Interpersonal skills expand, and a main focus is on group activities, team membership, and the importance of peers. During adolescence, these roles further expand and are refined, with increased levels of mastery, independence, and the importance of recognition and acceptance (Llorens, 1991). Some useful strategies for teaching children are summarized as follows.

▪ The Importance of Context

Context is defined as the setting within which an activity or task is placed or the circumstances that surround an event. During therapeutic intervention, the overall context must be set and remain adequate and conducive to the child's learning. This includes consideration of the physical aspects of the setting so that the environment is safe, stimulating but not stressful, and aesthetically pleasing. Understanding of the child's attentional abilities and level of sensory processing and organization, as well as the influence of the environment on movement production, is crucial in enabling the therapist or assistant to modify and adapt the environment appropriately and individually for each child (Cook-Merrill, Slavik, Holloway, Richter, & David, 1990). Natural environments, within the interaction settings of home, school, and community, are the most functional contexts where practice and learning for transfer are most likely to occur.

In addition to environmental context, effective learning contexts are those that promote initiation by the learner, reciprocity, shared control, and the provision of responsive feedback. With attention to the quality of instructor (therapist) and learner (child) interaction, children may gain some control over their own learning and become more functionally independent (Glynn, 1985).

▪ Importance of Motivation

Motivation is crucially important for intentional learning regardless of the age of the learner. To facilitate motivation for learning in children, emphasis should be placed on keeping the goals important and meaningful to the child, involving the child in the anticipatory and planning phases of the activity, offering opportunity for repetition and explorative learning, and giving reinforcement. Encouraging creative behaviors has been demonstrated to be a powerful way of enhancing motivation in children. Such creative behaviors include offering opportunities for movement variability, originality, and elaboration. Promoting some degree of flexibility in therapy could entail allowing and acknowledging a child's independent thinking and ability to generate a creative movement response. The therapist or assistant can support the child's attempts to express movements, allowing some originality in demonstration, so that movement exploration is an active process with a perceptual, cognitive, and motor aspect (Larin, 2000). Instructional strategies that go beyond the command style and promote process-oriented rather than product-oriented approaches constitute in themselves sources of motivation and enhance the desired, perceived internal control of the child (Ritson, 1987).

Setting appropriate and meaningful goals is another major motivating force available to therapists and assistants. The uses of functional activities that provide opportunities to explore and dynamically interact with the environment are of unquestionable value (Goodgold-Edward, 1991). If at all possible, involve the child in setting the goal. Movements preselected by the child result in greater goal clarity, increased energy production, increased success, and superior performance as compared with movements selected solely by the therapist (Larin, 2000). Goals need to be specific, consistent, attainable, and short in duration. The standard needs to be high enough to foster interest and promote improved performance but not so high as to provide discouragement with consequent loss of interest. It is important to include error awareness as a necessary element of the learning process, so that the child can make comparisons and systematic improvements in performance. Gentile (1972) offers these helpful guidelines:

- If a goal and a movement are successful, use repetition.
- If a goal is unsuccessful in spite of an apparent good movement attempt, help the learner identify relevant conditions that may have affected the performance.
- If a goal is successful but the movement actually produced a surprised success, describe the movement to the learner.
- If both the goal and the movement were unsuccessful, encourage the learner but analyze further the task at hand.

▪ Instructions and Modeling

Instructions are important not only for informational purposes but for motivational purposes as well. The therapist's or assistant's instructions have the potential to bring the child's attention into focus and either engage or distance the learner. Nonverbal prompting can also be used to assist in processing and attention facilitation. Modeling is an extremely powerful teaching tool for use with children. Children tend to be more visually dependent than adults, who rely more on a combination of visual and proprioceptive input (Shumway-Cook & Woollacott, 1985). Observational motor learning is an effective strategy for developing the perceptual skills necessary for children to attend to appropriate environmental cues, improve performance, and develop self-confidence (Weiss et al., 1993). Peer modeling and instructor modeling are both known to be effective.

Adult Learners

Adults learn throughout their lifetime. Adults tend to have a problem-solving orientation to learning. Real-life situations and problems are the main motivator for an adult learner. Most adult learners value the immediate application of learned information. The field of study concerned with understanding the instructional processes for adults is called **andragogy,** as compared with **pedagogy,** the correlate term for children learners. The following principles, developed by Darkenwald & Merriam (1982), summarize the tenets applicable to teaching the adult learner in all situations, including physical and occupational therapy intervention settings:

- An adult's readiness to learn depends on his or her previous learning.
- Intrinsic motivation produces more pervasive and permanent learning.
- Positive reinforcement is highly effective and preferred by adult learners.
- Material to be learned needs be presented in an organized fashion.
- Learning is enhanced by repetition.
- Tasks that are more meaningful are more fully and easily learned.
- Active participation in learning improves retention.
- Environmental factors affect learning.
- Adults exhibit learning styles that illustrate various learning theories, such as:
  1. Having personal strategies for coding information ("I need to process and remember this *my* way")
  2. Perceiving in different ways
  3. Perceiving learning activities to be problem centered and relevant to life
  4. Desiring some immediate appreciation
  5. Having a concept of themselves as learners
  6. Being self-directed

Therapists and assistants are encouraged to engage in a dialogue with an adult learner (patient) and, through discussion, discern that individual adult's unique learning style. **Learning style** refers to how information is processed and is unique to an individual (Kolb, 1999; Dunn, Dunn, & Price, 1981). Readers are encouraged to learn more about learning styles and how an individual's learning style can and will influence patient/client learning in the therapeutic environment. Therapeutic interaction that attempts to complement that learning style will be more effective (Avers & Gardner, 2000). An active learning experience in the companion workbook will assist the reader in assessing his or her own learning style in an attempt to become sensitized to recognizing differences in styles between different patients/clients.

Learning Changes Related to Aging

Aging is a normal developmental process of change. Longitudinal studies (studying the same people over a long period) have demonstrated that intellectual abilities of healthy people grow over the years, not lessen (Davis, 1996). Level of intelligence, however, does not automatically predict the quality of performance. In fact, these studies specifically show that although verbal abilities decline very little, if at all, over the life span, psychomotor skills do decline, beginning as early as in the late 20s. Performance skills that are time related and influenced by a decrease in reaction time tend to demonstrate the most noticeable decline (Avers & Gardner, 2000).

Learning new tasks is an essential component of geriatric rehabilitation. Mental practice has been demonstrated to be a highly effective strategy for teaching older adults, probably due to a combination of mental rehearsal effects and energy conservation having a positive impact on performance (Jarus & Ratzon, 2000). A person's ability to learn a new task is dependent on intelligence, learning skills acquired over the years, and flexibility of learning style, as well as noncognitive factors such as visual and auditory acuity, health status, motivation to learn, level of anxiety, the speed at which the learning is paced, and the meaningfulness of the material to be learned (Peterson & Orgen, 1983). Peterson and Orgen (1983) suggest attention to the following noncognitive factors when teaching a new skill to an older adult:

- Pain and poor physical health affect performance. Concentration, stamina, and endurance are then reduced.
- Individuals with visual or auditory impairments are not likely to perform at an acceptable level. Be prepared to repeat directions, use additional cues, and allow longer response time.
- Older people often benefit when new material is presented on a continuum with what they already know. Proceed in a slow and careful manner.
- Older people may need more time to integrate new learning and to rehearse it before it becomes assimilated into memory. Concentrate on one task at a time initially, avoiding contextual interference. Space new learning experiences apart.
- Reduce the potential for distraction in an attempt to increase concentration. Background noise, room conditions, and personal anxiety can be sources of distraction.
- Allow the individual to set the learning pace. This may mean reducing content in a given time period to offer greater clarity, specificity, and depth. Allow time for questions. Frame questions so they are specific and directed. Allow adequate time.

- Initially, provide a brief overview of the entire learning session so the individual can self-organize and anticipate the sequence. This overview will also decrease anticipation anxiety.
- Learning is facilitated for older adults when they can see and hear the material presented at the same time. Be sure, however, that the presentation of seen and heard material is consistent. Inconsistency creates confusion and interferes with learning.

If neurologically intact, older adult performers seem to benefit greatly from cognitive learning strategies, especially when learning closed motor skills (Greenwood, Meeuwsen, & French, 1993).

Clinical Connection:

The following strategy, known as the Singer five-step strategy, is thought to be particularly appropriate for older adults when learning self-paced gross motor skills (Avers & Gardner, 2000). The five sequential strategies are as follows:

1. Readying: allows the learner to prepare mentally and physically for task execution.
2. Imaging: assists the learner in creating a visual picture of the task, thereby developing a positive mindset.
3. Focusing: allows the learner to ignore irrelevant cues and concentrate on the few most meaningful cues related to the task.
4. Executing: assists the learner in initiating the task, *without* considering the performance outcome.
5. Evaluation: allows the learner to analyze performance outcomes, as well as the effectiveness of each of the sequential substrategies employed during the entire cognitive performance process (Singer, 1986).

This 5-step process can be easily applied to teaching within a therapeutic setting, when the learner is able to use cognitive processing. ■

The processing of information in the cognitive and emotional areas of the CNS cannot be ignored when considering the normal nervous system changes that accompany aging (Chapter 3), with or without pathology. All health care providers need to remember that in the older nervous system, processing will take longer. If processing of cognitive materials becomes a consistent problem, that avenue for assistance in motor learning may be lost as a teaching strategy. Without cognitive assistance, procedural learning of motor programs may become the only available avenue for regaining functional control over movement. The principles of motor learning, including adapting and varying those principles for the unique needs of the individual learner, become paramount in optimizing the therapeutic environment for patient/client improvement (Umphred & Lewis, 1999).

Learning as Affected by Common Neurological Disorders

Learning, including motor learning, is affected by any pathological condition affecting the brain, thereby impacting on cognitive processing. Strategies used by clinicians in applying motor learning principles to patients must accommodate the differences encountered by these patients in their learning capabilities as affected by the pathological condition. All individuals with neurological dysfunction present with impaired neural processing, some degree of disturbed intrinsic feedback, and some decrease in the amount of new learning that can occur.

There has been some beginning research on the impact of various pathologies on learning. A search of the literature in both physical and occupational therapy reveals research information available on learning differences encountered by patients with the following commonly encountered pathological conditions: cognitive impairment such as in mental retardation (MR), traumatic brain injury, post-cerebrovascular accident (CVA), and Parkinson's disease. These findings are summarized in the following section because this information can offer valuable insights to the treating therapist or assistant encountering these and similar clinical situations.

Learning in Individuals with Mental Retardation and Cognitive Impairment

About three percent of the population of the United States has mental retardation. As defined by the American Association on Mental Retardation (AAMR, 1992), mental retardation is characterized by significantly subaverage intellectual functioning, existing concurrently with related limitations in two or more of the following applicable adaptive skill areas, manifesting before age 18: communication, self-care, home living, social skills, community use, self-direction, health and safety, functional academics, leisure, and work. The key elements within this definition are *capabilities, environment,* and *function.* Mental retardation is not a *trait,* although it is influenced by certain characteristics or capabilities of the individual; rather, mental retardation is a *state* in which functioning is impaired. Therapists and assistants should be aware of the cogni-

tive challenges faced by an individual with mental retardation.

The primary neuropathology causing CNS disorder in individuals with mental retardation can be attributed to any combination of several well-documented brain abnormalities. Some of these differences may include a lower brain weight, microcephaly, a paucity of small neurons, a migrational defect involving small neurons, decreased synaptogenesis due to altered synaptic morphology, abnormalities in the dendritic spines, and delay of and lack of myelination (Marin-Padilla, 1976; Penrose & Smith, 1966; Scott, Becker, & Petit, 1983; Wisniewski & Schmidt-Sidor, 1989). Any one or a combination of these pathological changes will have an impact on neural processing, affecting the ability to learn.

Learning is impaired in individuals with mental retardation. The levels of cognitive impairment seen in individuals with mental retardation vary, from profoundly to mildly impaired, with a mild to moderate impairment being most common. Physical and occupational therapists must be able to adapt assessment and intervention approaches to accommodate this co-impairment of deficient intellectual functioning. Clearly, the range of cognitive deficit and ability found in individuals with mental retardation is indicative of variant levels of performance, functioning, and potential (Horvat & Croce, 1995). It is the task and the challenge of the therapist or assistant to assist the individual to maximize his or her potential for optimal functioning across environments.

Most of the research on learning differences among persons with mental retardation has been done on children with Down syndrome. As the most common cause of mental retardation, these differences can be generalized as characteristic of those for individuals with mental retardation. The research has also been done on children but can be extrapolated to adults with mental retardation. Generally, individuals with mental retardation have been found:

1. To be capable of learning a fewer number of things.
2. To need a greater number of repetitions to learn.
3. To have greater difficulty generalizing skills.
4. To have greater difficulty maintaining skills that are not practiced regularly.
5. To have slower response times.
6. To have a more limited repertoire of responses (Brown, 1979; Orelove & Sobsey, 1996).

As with any individual with coexistent visual or hearing deficits, therapists and assistants must adapt interaction, assessment, and teaching to accommodate these additional co-impairments. Individuals with mental retardation typically demonstrate attentional difficulties and difficulties with information processing (Petit-Markus, 1987). Individuals with mental retardation demonstrate an impaired ability to handle advanced cognitive processes, simultaneous demands, and organization of information, with subsequent effects on task performance, as well as task mastery (Hartley, 1986).

Research also shows myriad specific cognitive problems encountered, including difficulties in sequential verbal processing, auditory memory, and motor planning (Edwards, Elliott, & Lee, 1986; Elliott & Weeks, 1993; Hartley, 1981; Horvat & Croce, 1995; Marcel & Armstrong, 1982). It is important, therefore, for clinicians to utilize frequent visual demonstration, practice, rehearsal, and multimodal sensory avenues to teach individuals with mental retardation. Patients/clients with mental retardation are more likely to remember the rules and patterns of a new activity if presented with input over many modalities—visual and kinesthetic, as well as verbal (Bertoti, 1999). Individuals with mental retardation are less able to grasp abstract concepts than concrete concepts, so it is important for therapeutic activities and instructions to be concrete and meaningful, based on purposeful activity. Box 5–2 lists suggestions for accommodating the cognitive impairment typically presented by an individual with mental retardation or other cognitive deficits.

Clinically, mental retardation is highly correlated with developmental delay, including delay in attainment of gross motor and fine motor milestones, as well as with delay in other areas of development, such as speech acquisition and cognitive development. Additional studies have also demonstrated difficulties in postural control and antigravity control and deficits in postural response synergies when balance perturbations were introduced. Consequently, the development of compensatory movement strategies as children with developmental delay attempt to learn to move and stabilize themselves is delayed and possibly impaired (Haley, 1986; Hartley, 1986; Lydic & Steele, 1979; Rast & Harris, 1985; Shumway-Cook & Woollacott, 1985). Therapists and assistants working with individuals with mental retardation should expect that attainment of fundamental movement skills will be delayed. It is also reasonable to expect that additional practice time in each developmental phase may be required to attain a functional level of proficiency. Some individuals with mental retardation may not be able to achieve a level of skillful mastery, but individual levels of functional performance should be welcomed and applauded.

Learning After Brain Injury

The recovery and learning potential of a person with an injured brain is dependent on several factors: genetics, age, general physical and mental health, severity of the brain injury, and quality of environmental stimuli. Learning after brain injury is associated with neural plasticity. Some of the mechanisms involved in plastic-

---

BOX 5–2

Suggestions for Working with Individuals with Cognitive Impairments

Simplify information. Reduce the amount of information given at any one time. Give simple, concise instructions. Avoid verbal bombardment.

Reduce distraction. Remove irrelevant, distracting material from the intervention area.

Seek a moderate level of sensory arousal to optimize learning.

Be sure the goal of the task is clear to the patient/client. To improve motivation, work on tasks that are relevant and meaningful to the patient/client.

Begin with simple tasks and progress to more difficult ones.

If using part practice, present each component of the task clearly and separately. If using whole practice, present the entire task clearly and without unnecessary verbal "window dressing."

Make sure the information is understood; for example, ask the individual to repeat the instructions to you in his or her own words. Explain your expectations clearly.

Encourage the learner to link or associate information with material already known or familiar.

Encourage the individual to ask questions, because this will promote active processing.

Repeat directions as often as necessary, but only when necessary.

Be specific with task choice and offer opportunity for repetition.

Check for accuracy frequently and chose an appropriate quantity, frequency, and timing of feedback for the learner and the task.

Ensure that learning occurs in different contexts to promote generalization. Give the learner knowledge of his or her results and offer an opportunity to practice the skill independently.

Recognize that progress may be slower when working with patients/clients who have cognitive impairments.

Sources: Bertoti, D. B. (1999). Mental retardation: focus on Down syndrome. In J. S. Tecklin (Ed.), *Pediatric physical therapy* (3rd ed.). Philadelphia: Lippincott Williams & Wilkins; Carr, J., & Shepherd, R (1998). *Neurological rehabilitation: Organizing motor performance.* Oxford, UK: Butterworth-Heinemann; Shumway-Cook, A., & Woollacott, M. H. (2001). *Motor control: Theory and practical application* (2nd ed.). Philadelphia: Lippincott Williams & Wilkins; Wilson, B. A. (1989). *Memory problems after head injury.* Nottingham: National Head Injuries Association.

ity and recovery after brain damage were presented in Chapter 2; refer to that chapter for review.

Many traumatic brain injuries are diffuse rather than focal in nature, resulting in processing, memory, and learning deficits that can vary from fairly insignificant to disabling. Memory, as previously discussed, is required for the learning of new skills. The fact that memory is not a unitary system also means that different deficit profiles can ensue. Thus, evidence of good performance in one area, during one intervention session, or in one setting does not imply a fully functioning system or significant recovery. For example, although some aspects of motor learning, such as immediate recall or repetition, may be evident, this does not mean that the individual who demonstrates progress within an intervention session will be able to generalize that knowledge or recall the performance results accurately (Campbell, 2000). The assessment of memory loss is a complex process, beyond the scope of this text. Refer to other sources for additional information.

Lesion-specific deficits in information processing and subsequent learning capabilities are likely to change over the course of the initial weeks following the injury. As this change occurs, it is important that therapeutic intervention and teaching style accurately match the informational processing capabilities of the patient/client. Some demands should be made at or just beyond the limits of the patient's capabilities to stimulate and facilitate the physical, biochemical, and electrical neural changes that underlie recovery and learning. On the other hand, constant demands for information processing beyond the individual's abilities can cause undue stress and frustration, which in turn can inhibit learning (Neistadt, 1988, 1993).

Learning After Cerebrovascular Accident

A CVA can contribute to a long list of impairments, dependent on the nature and extent of the vascular insult and subsequent damage to brain tissue. Sometimes, major deficits in perception, communication, and cognition accompany a CVA. All these impairments impact on the ability of the patient/client to attend, to learn, and to retain the information. A major task in stroke rehabilitation involves teaching patients to perform functional tasks by maximizing use of spared motor functions. As a result, the individual's capacity to learn to perform functional tasks in ways that differ from the way the tasks were performed before the stroke is a crucial part of clinical rehabilitation (Hanlon, 1996). Neurorehabilitation typically includes training in the use of the hemiparetic limbs and compensation for the dysfunctional side by the motori-

cally preserved side. These and other intervention approaches will be explored in the next chapter.

Clinical Connection:

Based on research done on stroke survivors, the following findings can be applied to motor learning strategies employed by physical and occupational therapists and their assistants working in CVA rehabilitation (Hanlon, 1996; Hsieh et al., 1994; Magill & Hall, 1990; Page et al., 2001):

1. Active participation clearly promotes learning.
2. Contextual interference promotes retention and transfer of the skill.
3. Random practice, because it requires that the learner regenerate solutions, is more effective for retention and is generally considered to be more effective in hemiparetic motor learning.
4. Some stroke patients demonstrate difficulty mastering tasks during the acquisition phase of learning if random practice is the sole method. Blocked and random practice should be alternated, probably due to difficulty regenerating the components of the motor program (body position, amount of force, speed, postural adjustments).
5. Mental practice can be employed as a vital complement to improve motor function.
6. Added purpose occupation enhances motor performance by promoting motivation and meaningfulness.

Learning Challenges for Individuals with Parkinson's Disease

Parkinson's disease affects 1 percent of the population over the age of 60. One of the main symptoms affecting motor learning in Parkinson's disease is akinesia (defined in Chapter 2). Parkinson himself (1817) defined akinesia as an inability to convert a potential for movement into actual motion. A discussion of akinesia and some strategies used to promote motor learning in the face of akinesia appropriately illustrate the importance of creative clinical teaching.

Functionally, akinesia produces difficulty with initiation (seen as hesitancy or "freezing"), absence or reduction in the amount of movement, difficulty stopping movement especially once momentum has taken over, and difficulty monitoring posture and making postural adjustments. All the processes involved in learning, such as continual repetition and transferring a motor skill, are challenged by this very impairment so typical of individuals with Parkinson's disease.

The presence of akinesia requires that therapists and assistants be creative in providing means for patients with Parkinson's disease to be engaged in motor learning. Specific suggestions for clinical success in teaching movement skills to individuals with akinesia include imitation, verbal and tactile cues, the use of rhythm, and visualization or imagination. Observing and copying the performance of another person may serve to "unfreeze" the body part when the individual encounters initiation or hesitancy difficulties. Verbal and tactile cues can also assist in the release of akinesia. A light touch or a verbal cue may assist the patient/client in the initiation, initial weight shift, or weight transfer during a movement. Rhythm can be a very useful movement initiator and maintainer of movement. Visualizing a movement or an object doing the moving may help the patient overcome hesitancy or difficulties with hesitancy (Quintyn & Cross, 1986).

In many patients with Parkinson's disease, training alternative movement strategies for functional tasks may be more realistic than retraining for exact re-emergence of original movement patterns. Perhaps motor learning needs to focus on the training of new rules and relationships for movement programs. Current research suggests teaching alternative movement strategies that involve simple movement patterns reorganized and arranged sequentially and consciously, executed without time constraints (Kamsma, Brouwer, & Lakke, 1995).

Case Studies

The following case studies describe the teaching and learning strategies used in a typical therapeutic interaction—one in pediatric rehabilitation and the other in the rehabilitation of an adult patient/client. Consistent with the holistic approach to rehabilitation as advocated by this author, the teaching and learning strategies used draw from all the available motor learning and motor control theories.

Case Study: Child

Trudy: Child Learning to Propel a Power Wheelchair

Trudy is a 4-year-old girl who is being trained in the use of a power chair. She lives in a farmhouse where most of the common rooms and Trudy's bedroom are on the first floor. She is presently attending a preschool and will be starting kindergarten next year. The school district will provide transportation to and from school.

Trudy is seated comfortably in the power chair, adapted with modifications to assist with trunk control. The drive mechanism for the power chair has been mounted at a location most accessible for Trudy. This chair has the ability to allow Trudy to adjust the height and depth of her seat so that she can be raised or lowered to enjoy greater accessibility. Vision is normal. Trudy has had some experience with using a computer mouse while playing computer games with her older brother.

The following describes a sample of the teaching and learning strategies employed by the therapist.

Initial Training Sessions

Environment. Because Trudy is served through the county preschool services, therapy appointments could be scheduled at the home or school, at the choice of the therapist and family. Initial sessions were scheduled at the home, within a natural, familiar environment. For the first teaching session at home, a large, uncluttered room was selected, devoid of extraneous distractions. The pet dog was left outside and the television was turned off. Lighting was adequate and scatter rugs were removed. Sessions were also scheduled in the school center, where quiet space was available.
Instruction and Guidance. The importance of safe driving and the benefits of self-propelling a chair were discussed, so that Trudy understood the meaning and value of the tasks. The therapist familiarized Trudy with the power mechanism on the chair by first pointing out the similarities between the drive mechanism and Trudy's prior experiences with a computer mouse while playing computer games. The therapist and Trudy explored salient features of the power drive mechanism, including allowing Trudy to experience the sensitivity of the mechanism, where a small movement could elicit a larger movement from the chair. Her older brother, an important model in Trudy's life, was included in the teaching as needed. Mental practice was used to allow Trudy to visualize handling the mechanism and imagining "steering" herself initially through the middle of a large open space. The therapist then used manual guidance, hand over Trudy's hand, on the drive mechanism to explore the very first attempts at propulsion (Fig. 5–2). Vision was used to direct Trudy's attention to key elements of the task.
Practice. During these initial sessions, part practice was chosen as a strategy, breaking the task of propelling the chair into components of that whole task. Practice was blocked with the opportunity given to fixate on the individual skills and repeat the same movement component over and over again. Rest was offered as needed. Some limited opportunity was given for discovery, or trial and error learning, so that Trudy could have an opportunity to experience, within safe practice, a sampling of the consequences of erroneous task execution (such as jerking the control and having the chair lurch).

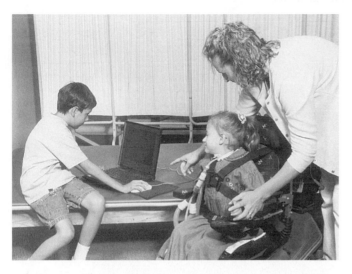

Figure 5–2. The therapist uses peer modeling (brother), past experience (computer mouse), and manual guidance during initial training sessions.

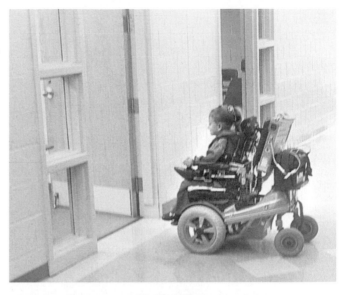

Figure 5–3. After some skill mastery becomes evident, practice opportunity is offered in new environments including school.

Feedback. During the initial sessions, feedback was given often but in a very concise manner. The therapist avoided too much talk, so that Trudy could concentrate and maintain attention to the task. Feedback was verbal and primarily positive. Trudy was given knowledge of her performance, such as whether her arm or head position appeared to be accurate, as well as knowledge of the results, whereby she was told about the outcome of her attempt. Feedback was offered concurrent with task execution, as well as at the end. Following the performance, the therapist discussed the performance with Trudy and Trudy was encouraged to critique her own attempts.

Intermediate Training Sessions

Environment. After some skill mastery became evident, the environment was opened up a bit, allowing some interference from furniture and even the family dog, as long as he was quiet. Additionally, Trudy was able to practice in a variety of settings, including sessions scheduled at school (Fig. 5–3). Different environmental conditions allowed for Trudy to generalize and diversify her newly acquired skill to different areas, driving through doorway openings, up and down slight inclines, and practicing using her control to access features such as a water fountain (Figs. 5–4 and 5–5). Instructions and Guidance. Instructions were given at the beginning of the session, with decreased concurrent input from the therapist. Physical guidance was almost completely withdrawn. Mental practice continued to be used, inviting Trudy to mentally rehearse driving within the novel situations, so that she could begin to anticipate and engage in active problem solving.

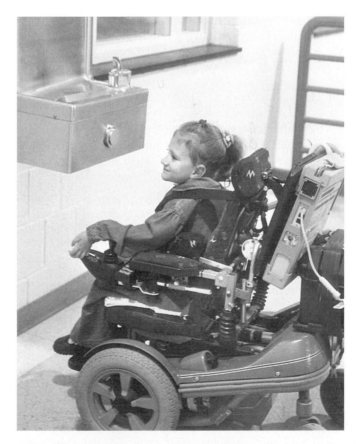

Figure 5–4. Typically, a power chair will not allow access to a standard water fountain.

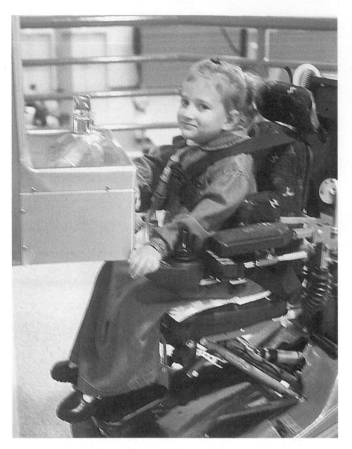

Figure 5–5. Permobil Kaola power chair allows for raising of seat height and changing of depth to access many features of the environment.

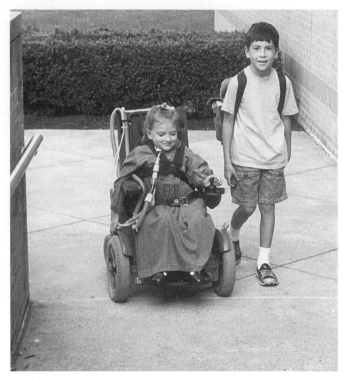

Figure 5–6. Power mobility allows for a world of accessibility.

Practice. Practice was almost totally whole practice, returning to part practice only when a consistent error or difficulty was encountered. Practice was varied, with opportunities for sampling of random propulsion and driving tasks. Contextual interference was increased during the practice sessions. The opportunity for trial and error learning was increased.

Feedback. Concurrent feedback was faded, with more emphasis on summary feedback, offered as knowledge of the results of Trudy's performance. Extraneous errors were ignored but consistent ones were pointed out and corrected. Trudy was actively engaged in analyzing her performance and discovering adjustments to her performance attempts.

Final Stages of Skill Mastery

Environment. The environment was completely open, with opportunity to drive the chair in a large variety of settings. Full contextual interference was permitted, with Trudy experiencing propelling her chair up the driveway from the bus, into a building alongside peers, and through a crowded mall or school cafeteria (Fig. 5–6). Changes in terrain, including those resulting from

adverse weather conditions, were presented. Trudy was challenged with new and changing conditions.

Instruction and Guidance. Very little instruction was given, with attention to the entire task and not the components. Instructions were limited to giving whole, novel assignments, such as "Drive through the doorway into the hall, find the elevator, and prepare to enter it." Mental rehearsal and active problem solving continued to be vital.

Practice. Practice was consistently whole, not part practice. Practice was variable and randomized among several different tasks. Contextual interference was high.

Feedback. Consistent performance was encouraged, with propulsion of the chair happening automatically while Trudy attended to other aspects of daily life. Only consistent significant errors were corrected. Trudy was continually asked to assess her own performance, especially when solving a novel task or a variation of the familiar.

Case Study: Adult

James: Adult Learning to Perform Wheelchair Transfers

James is a 58-year-old man who was in a motor vehicle accident, sustaining a brain injury, which has resulted in generalized muscular weakness, incoordination, and a mild cognitive deficit affecting selective attention. Vision and hearing are within normal limits. He is seen by a therapist first while an inpatient and then in follow-up outpatient sessions after discharge to home. This particular case study focuses on the specific task of transfer training. The following describes a sample of the teaching and learning strategies employed by the therapist or assistant.

Initial Training Sessions

Environment. Initial sessions were scheduled while James was an inpatient, where therapy services were delivered on the patient's floor either in the room or at a small intervention room located in the sunroom. For the first teaching session, the therapist saw James in his own room, because James appeared to be comfortable in that setting (Fig. 5–7). Closing the door to the hallway, ensuring that James's roommate was at another appointment, turning off the television, and avoiding visiting hours minimized the chance for extraneous distractions. The initial sessions were also scheduled at a time when James was rested and alert. Lighting was adequate, and the room temperature was comfortable. Instruction and Guidance. The importance of being able to safely transfer out of bed and from his wheelchair was discussed with James, highlighting the benefits of independent mobility, so that James understood the meaning and value of the tasks. The therapist included James in the selection of the first specific transfer task goal. The therapist then familiarized James with some of the key elements of transferring, by physically demonstrating the first transfer to be taught. The safety mechanisms on the wheelchair were visually pointed out, with simple highlights offered. The therapist invited James to recall and imagine prior similar experiences by mentally rehearsing with him the simple but familiar act of standing up from the seated

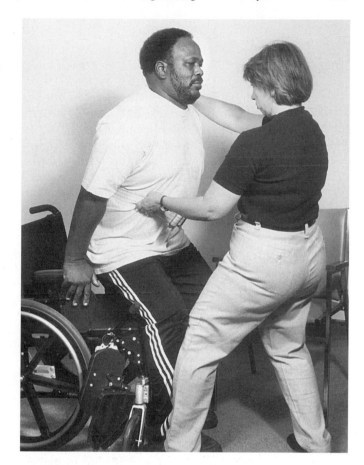

Figure 5–8. The therapist uses physical guidance to assist with early transfer attempts.

position, sitting down into his favorite chair, and even switching from one chair to another while seated in a living space, pointing out the similarities between those familiar prior experiences with the current situation. Vision was used to direct James's attention to key elements of the task. The therapist continually assessed James's level of arousal and attention to task. Verbal bombardment and too much activity on the part of the therapist were avoided. The therapist used physical guidance to assist with the first attempts (Fig. 5–8).

Practice. During these initial sessions, part practice was chosen as a strategy, breaking the task of transferring into components of that whole task. Practice was blocked, with opportunity given to fixate on the individual skills and repeat the same portion of the movement over and over again. Rest was offered as needed. Some limited opportunity was given for trial and error learning so that James could have an opportunity to experience, within safe practice, a sampling of the consequences of erroneous task execution (such as not locking the wheelchair or incorrect foot placement).

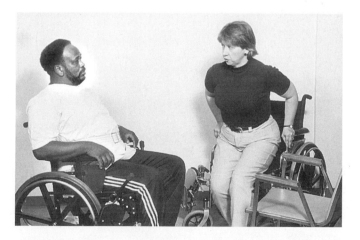

Figure 5–7. The therapist demonstrates transfer, highlighting the key elements of the task.

Feedback. During the initial sessions, brief verbal feedback was given often but in a very concise manner. The therapist avoided too much talk, so that James could concentrate and maintain attention to the task. Feedback was primarily positive, with mention only of significant errors that compromised safety. James was given knowledge of his performance, such as whether the chair was placed correctly or his postural set appeared stable to execute the transfer. Summary knowledge of the results was also given, so he learned about the outcome of his attempt. Feedback was offered concurrent with task execution, as well as at the end, but careful attention was given to the timing of the concurrent feedback so that it did not interfere with attention to the task. Following the performance, the therapist discussed the performance with James. James was encouraged to critique his own attempts.

Intermediate Training Sessions

Environment. After some skill mastery became evident, the environment opportunities were expanded, allowing some interference. The door to the hallway from James's room was left open and other persons were permitted within the learning space. Practice was done in additional settings, including in James's bathroom and in the sunroom on the floor. Different environmental conditions allowed for James to generalize and diversify his newly acquired skill to different areas and different transfer situations, such as transferring to bed, to toilet, and to different types and heights of chairs (Figs. 5–9 and 5–10). Emphasis was placed on procedural learning, focusing on learning the rules of transfer rather than on splinter skills isolated to limited contexts.

Instructions and Guidance. Instructions were given at the beginning of the session, with decreased concurrent input from the therapist. Physical guidance was given only when necessary to ensure safety. Visual demonstration continued to be used as a valuable observational learning tool. Peer modeling was included, offering James opportunities to observe other patients practicing transfers (Fig. 5–11).

Practice. Practice was almost totally whole practice, returning to part practice only when a consistent error or difficulty was encountered. Practice was varied, with opportunities for practice of different transfer tasks and observational and mental practice opportunities encouraged in between therapy teaching sessions. Mental practice continued to be used, inviting James to mentally rehearse transferring within his home situation, so that he could begin to anticipate and engage in active problem solving. Contextual interference was increased during the practice sessions. The opportunity for trial and error learning was increased.

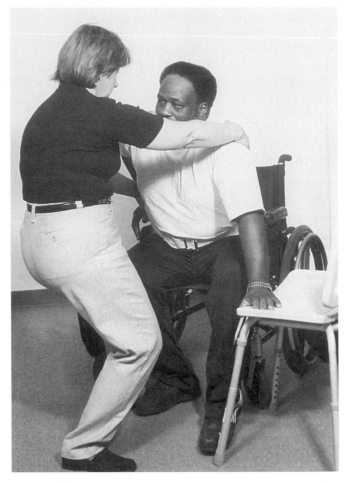

Figure 5–9. Practicing new skill to new situations, such as a bath seat.

Feedback. Concurrent feedback was faded, with more emphasis on summary feedback, offered as knowledge of the results of James's performance. Extraneous errors were ignored but consistent ones were pointed

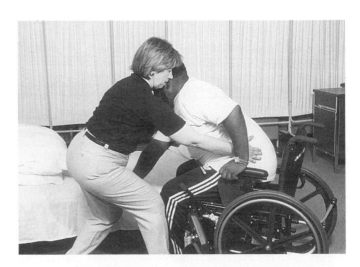

Figure 5–10. Practicing transfer to a bed.

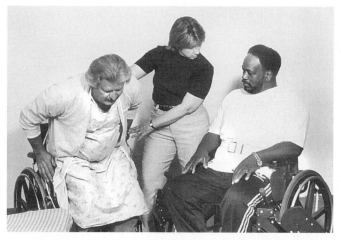

Figure 5–11. Peer modeling is an effective training technique.

out and corrected. James was actively engaged in analyzing his performance and discovering adjustments to his performance attempts.

Final Stages of Skill Mastery

Environment. The environment was completely open, with opportunity to transfer in a large variety of settings. Full contextual interference was permitted, with James experiencing transferring as integrated into his daily round. James was challenged with new and changing conditions. James was either being seen at home or being prepared for discharge home.

Instruction and Guidance. Very little instruction was given, with attention to the entire task and not components. Instruction was limited to giving whole, novel assignments, such as wheeling up to the car or minivan and executing that transfer. Mental rehearsal and active problem solving continued to be vital.

Practice. Practice was consistently whole, not part practice. Practice was variable and randomized among several different tasks. Contextual interference was high.

Feedback. Consistent performance was encouraged, with a variety of transfers happening automatically while James acquires full wheelchair independence and attends to other aspects of daily life. Only consistent significant errors were corrected. James was continually asked to assess his own performance, especially when solving a novel task or variation of the familiar.

Summary

This chapter is the beginning of Part 2 of this text, focusing on intervention application. As the first of six chapters in the practical application section of the book, this chapter attempts to create a teacher of the therapist or assistant. Effective clinicians are great teachers who are able to actively engage the patient/client as a learner in the task of motor learning.

This chapter defines learning, specifically motor learning, and differentiates between learning, training, and performance, as well as between motor learning and motor control. Motor learning theory is summarized, and current models of motor learning are described in detail. A brief overview of the neurobiology of learning and a practical description of the different ways individuals learn attempt to engage the reader in thinking about all the possible learning strategies that can be applied to therapeutic intervention. The key elements of learning for therapeutic consideration are defined and elaborated on. Learning as it changes over the life span, and how it may be challenged by commonly encountered neuropathological conditions, is discussed so that therapists and assistants can effectively "teach" anyone of any age and any capability. Case studies are offered to help the reader assimilate and integrate learning theory into daily practice.

References

Adams, J. A. (1971). A closed-loop theory of motor learning. *Journal of Motor Behavior 3*, 111–150.

Adams, J. A. (1986). Use of the model's knowledge of results to increase the observer's performance. *Journal of Human Movement Studies, 12,* 89–98.

American Association on Mental Retardation (1992). *Mental retardation: Definition, classification, and system of supports* (9th ed.). Washington, DC: American Association on Mental Retardation.

Annett, J. (1995). Imagery and motor processes. *British Journal of Psychology, 86,* 161–167.

Asanuma, H., & Keller, A. (1991). Neuronal mechanisms of motor learning in mammals. *NeuroReport, 2,* 217–224.

Avers, D. L., & Gardner, D. L. (2000). Patient education as a treatment modality. In A. A. Guccione (Ed.), *Geriatric physical therapy* (2nd ed.). St. Louis, MO: Mosby.

Ayres, A. J. (1972). *Sensory integration and learning disorders.* Los Angeles: Western Psychological Services.

Battig, W. F. (1979). The flexibility of human memory. In L. S. Cermak & F. I. Craik (Eds.), *Levels of processing and human memory.* Hillsdale, NJ: Erlbaum Associates.

Baumeister, R. F. (1989). Social intelligence and the construction of the meaning of life. In R. S. Wyer & T. K. Srull (Eds.), *Advances in social cognition.* Hillsdale, NJ: Erlbaum Associates.

Ben-Yishay, Y., Rattok, J., & Diller, L. (1987). A clinical strategy for the systematic amelioration of attentional disturbances in severe head trauma patients. In *Working approaches to remediation of cognitive deficits in brain damage persons: Supplement to 7th Annual Workshop for Rehabilitation Professionals*. New York: New York University Medical Center.

Bertoti, D. B. (1999). Mental retardation: focus on Down syndrome. In J. S. Tecklin (Ed.), *Pediatric physical therapy* (3rd ed.). Philadelphia: Lippincott Williams & Wilkins.

Bracy, O. L. (1972). Cognitive rehabilitation: A process approach. *Cognitive Rehabilitation, 4*, 10–17.

Bronfenbrenner, U. (1992). Ecological systems theory. In R. Vasta (Ed.), *Six theories of child development: Revised formulations and current issues*. Philadelphia: Jessica Kingsley.

Brown, L. (1979). A strategy for developing chronological age appropriate and functional curricular content for severely handicapped adolescents and young adults. *Journal of Special Education, 12*, 81–90.

Burgio, L. D., Burgio, K. L., Engel, B. T., & Tice, L. M. (1986). Increasing distance and independence of ambulation in elderly nursing home residents. *Journal of Applied Behavior Analysis, 19*, 357–366.

Campbell, M. (2000). *Rehabilitation for traumatic brain injury: Physical therapy practice in context*. Edinburgh, UK: Churchill Livingstone.

Campbell, S. K., Vander Linden, D. W., & Palisano, R. J. (Eds.). (2000). *Physical therapy for children* (2nd ed.). Philadelphia: W. B. Saunders.

Carr, J., & Shepherd, R. (1998). *Neurological rehabilitation: Organizing motor performance*. Oxford, UK: Butterworth-Heinemann.

Carr, J., & Shepherd, R. (2000). *Movement science: Foundations for physical therapy in rehabilitation* (2nd ed.). Gaithersburg, MD: Aspen Publishers.

Cohen, H. (1999). *Neuroscience for rehabilitation* (2nd ed.). Philadelphia: Lippincott Williams & Wilkins.

Cook-Merrill, S., Slavik, B., Holloway, E., Richter, E., & David, S. (1990). *Environment: Implications for occupational therapy practice*. Rockville, MD: American Occupational Therapy Association.

Coster, W. (1995). Clinical interpretation of "the relationships among sensorimotor components, fine motor skill, and functional performance in preschool children." *American Journal of Occupational Therapy, 49*, 653–654.

Croce, R., & DePaepe, J. A. (1989). A critique of therapeutic intervention programming with reference to an alternative approach based on motor learning theory. *Physical and Occupational Therapy in Pediatrics, 9*, 5–33.

Darkenwald, G., & Merriam, S. (1982). *Adult education: Foundations of practice*. New York: Harper and Row.

Davis, C. M. (1996). The Psychosocial aspects of aging. In C. Bernstein-Lewis (Ed.), *Aging: The health care challenge*. Philadelphia: F. A. Davis.

Davis, W. E., & Burton, A. W. (1991). Ecological task analysis: Translating movement behavior theory into practice. *Adapted Physical Activity Quarterly, 8*, 154–177.

Decety, J., & Ingvar, D. H. (1990). Brain structures participating in mental stimulation of motor behavior: A neuropsychological interpretation. *Acta Psychologica, 73*, 13–34.

DeKuiper, W. P., Nelson, D. L., & White, B. E. (1993). Materials-based occupation versus imagery-based occupation versus rote exercise: A replication and extension. *Occupational Therapy Journal of Research, 13*, 183–197.

Drubach, D. (2000). *The brain explained*. Upper Saddle River, NJ: Prentice-Hall.

Duncan, P. W., & Badke, M. B. (1987). *Stroke rehabilitation: The recovery of motor control*. Chicago: Year Book.

Dunn, R., Dunn, K., & Price, G. E. (1981). *Learning style inventory*. Lawrence, KS: Price Systems.

Dunst, C. J., Bruder, M. B., Trivette, C. M., & McLean, M. (2001). Natural learning opportunities for infants, toddlers, and preschoolers. *Young Exceptional Children, 4*, 18–25.

Edwards, J. M., Elliott, D., & Lee, T. D. (1986). Contextual interference effects during skill acquisition and transfer in Down's syndrome adolescents. *Adapted Physical Activity Quarterly 3, 250*.

Elliott, D., & Weeks, D. J. (1993). A functional systems approach to movement pathology. *Adapted Physical Activity Quarterly, 10*, 312–323.

Evans, A. K. (1987). Nationally speaking: Definition of occupation as the core concept of occupational therapy. *American Journal of Occupational Therapy, 41*, 627–628.

Ferguson, J. M., & Trombley, C. A. (1996). The effect of added purpose and meaningful occupation on motor learning. *American Journal of Occupational Therapy, 51*, 508–515.

Fitts, P., & Posner, M. (1967). *Human performance*. Belmont, CA: Brooks/Cole.

Flinn, N. A. (1999). Clinical interpretation of "effect of rehabilitation tasks on organization of movement after stroke." *American Journal of Occupational Therapy, 53*, 345–347.

Fredericks, C. M., & Saladin, L. K. (1996). *Pathophysiology of the motor systems: Principles and clinical presentations*. Philadelphia: F. A. Davis.

Fry-Welch, D. (1996). Neurology education in transition: Balancing the traditional and contemporary models of motor control and motor learning. *Neurology Report, 20*, 14–33.

Gentile, A. M. (1972). A working model of skill acquisition with application to teaching. *Quest Monograph, 17*, 3–23.

Gentile, A. M. (1987). Skill acquisition: action, movement, and neuromotor processes. In J. Carr & R. Shepherd (Eds.), *Movement science: Foundations for physical therapy in rehabilitation* (2nd ed.). Gaithersburg, MD: Aspen Publishers.

Gentile, A. M. (1998). Implicit and explicit processes during acquisition of functional skills. *Scandinavian Journal of Occupational Therapy, 5*, 7–16.

Gentile, A. M. (2000). Skill acquisition: action, movement, and neuromotor processes. In J. Carr & R. Shepherd (Eds.), *Movement science: Foundations for physical therapy in rehabilitation* (2nd ed.). Gaithersburg, MD: Aspen Publishers.

Gilfoyle, E. (1984). Eleanor Clark Slagle Lectureship, 1984: Transformation of a profession. *American Journal of Occupational Therapy, 38*, 575–584.

Gilner, J. (1985). Purposeful activity in motor learning theory: An event approach to motor skill acquisition. *American Journal of Occupational Therapy, 39*, 28–34.

Glynn, T. (1985). Contexts for learning: implications for mildly and moderately handicapped children. *Australian and New Zealand Journal of Developmental Disabilities, 10*, 257–263.

Goode, S., & Magill, R. A. (1986). Contextual interference effects in learning three badminton serves. *Research Quarterly on Exercise and Sport, 57*, 308–314.

Goodgold-Edwards, S. A. (1991). Cognitive strategies during coincident timing tasks. *Physical Therapy 71*, 236–243.

Gottlieb, G. L., Corcos, D. M., Jaric, S., & Agarwal, G. C. (1988). Practice improves even the simplest movements. *Experimental Brain Research, 73*, 436–440.

Greenwood, M., Meeuwsen, H., & French, R. (1993). Effects of cognitive learning strategies, verbal reinforcement, and gender on the performance of closed motor skills in older adults. *Activities, Adaptation, and Aging, 17*, 39–53.

Ferguson, J. M., & Trombley, C. A. (1996). The effect of added-purpose and meaningful occupation on motor learning. *American Journal of Occupational Therapy, 51*, 508–515.

Hanlon, R. E. (1996). Motor learning following unilateral stroke. *Archives of Physical and Medical Rehabilitation, 77*, 811–815.

Haley, S. M. (1986). Postural reactions in children with Down syndrome. *Physical Therapy, 66,1*, 17–31.

Hanlon, R. R. (1996). Motor learning following unilateral stroke. *Archives of Physical and Medical Rehabilitation, 77*, 811–815.

Hartley, X. Y. (1981). Lateralization of speech stimuli in young Down's syndrome children. *Cortex, 17,* 241.

Hartley, X. Y. (1986). A summary of recent research into the development of children with Down's syndrome. *Journal of Mental Deficiency Research, 30,* 1–14.

Hinojosa, J., Sabari, J., & Pedretti, L. (1993). Purposeful activity: Position paper of AOTA. *American Journal of Occupational Therapy, 47,* 1081–1082.

Ho, L., & Shea, J. B. (1978). Effects of relative frequency of knowledge of results on retention of a motor skill. *Perceptual and Motor Skills, 46,* 859–866.

Horvat, M., & Croce, R. (1995). Physical rehabilitation of individuals with mental retardation: Physical fitness and information processing. *Critical Review of Physical Rehabilitation Medicine, 7,* 233–252.

Hsieh, C-L., Nelson, D. L., Smith, D. A., & Peterson, C. Q. (1994). A comparison of performance in added-purpose occupations and rote exercise for dynamic standing in persons with hemiplegia. *American Journal of Occupational Therapy, 50,* 10–16.

Ivry, R. (1997). Representational issues in motor learning: phenomena and theory. In S. Keele & H. Heurer (Eds.), *Handbook of perception and action: Motor skills.* New York: Academic Press.

Jarus, T. (1994). Motor learning and occupational therapy: The organization of practice. *American Journal of Occupational Therapy, 48,* 810–816.

Jarus, T., & Loiter, Y. (1995). The effect of kinesthetic stimulation on acquisition and retention of a gross motor skill. *Canadian Journal of Occupational Therapy, 62,* 23–29.

Jarus, T., & Ratzon, N. Z. (2000). Can you imagine? The effect of mental practice on the acquisition and retention of a motor skill as a function of age. *Occupational Therapy Journal of Research, 20,* 163–178.

Kaplan, M. (1994). Motor learning: implications for occupational therapy and neurodevelopmental treatment. *Developmental Disabilities Special Interest Section Newsletter, 17,* 1–4.

Kamsma, Y., Brouwer, W., & Lakke, J. (1995). Training of compensational strategies for impaired gross motor skills in Parkinson's disease. *Physiotherapy Theory and Practice, 11,* 209–229.

Kay, H. (1970). Analyzing motor skill performance. In K. J. Connolly (Ed.), *Mechanisms of motor skill development.* New York: Academic Press.

Kirschenbaum, D. S., & Smith, R. J. (1983). A preliminary study of sequencing effects in simulated feedback. *Journal of Sport Psychology, 5,* 332–342.

Klein, R. M. (1978). Automatic and strategic processes in skilled performance. In C. G. Roberts & K. M. Newell (Eds.), *Psychology of motor behavior and sport.* Champaign, IL: Human Kinetics Publishers.

Knox, S. H. (1998). Treatment through play and leisure. In H. L. Hopkins & H. D. Smith (Eds.), *Willard and Spackman's occupational therapy* (9th ed.). Philadelphia: J. B. Lippincott.

Kolb, D. A. (1999). *Learning style inventory* (3rd ed.). Boston, MA: Experience Based Learning Systems.

Kupfermann, I. (1991). Learning and memory. In E. R. Kandel, J. H. Schwartz, & T. M. Jessell (Eds.), *Principles of neuroscience* (3rd ed.). New York: Elsevier.

Larin, H. M. (2000). In S. K. Campbell, D. W. Vander Linden, & R. J. Palisano (Eds.), *Physical therapy for children* (2nd ed.). Philadelphia: W. B. Saunders.

Lashley, K. S. (1929). *Brain mechanism and intelligence.* Chicago: University of Chicago.

Lashley, K. S. (1950). In search of the engram. *Symposia of the Society for Experimental Biology, 4,* 454–482.

Lee, T. D., & Magill, R. A. (1983). The locus of contextual interference in motor skill acquisition. *Journal of Experimental Psychology: Learning, Memory and Cognition, 9,* 730–746.

Lee, T. D., Swanson, L. R., & Hall, A. L. (1991). What is repeated in a repetition? Effects of practice conditions on motor skill acquisition. *Physical Therapy, 71,* 150–156.

Lee, T. D., & White, M. A. (1990). Influence of an unskilled model's practice schedule on observational motor learning. *Human Movement Science, 9,* 349–367.

Lesensky, S., & Kaplan, L. (2000). Occupational therapy and motor learning. *Occupational Therapy Practice, September 25,* 13–16.

Lewthwaite, R. (1990). Motivational considerations in physical therapy involvement. *Physical Therapy, 70,* 808–819.

Linden, C. A., Uhley, J. E., Smith, D., & Bush, M. A. (1989). The effects of mental practice on walking balance in an elderly population. *Occupational Therapy Journal of Research, 9,* 155–169.

Livesay, J. R., & Samras, M. R. (1998). Covert neuromuscular activity of the dominant forearm during visualization of a motor task. *Perception and Motor Skills, 86,* 371–374.

Llorens, L. (1991). Performance task and roles throughout the life span. In C. Christiansen & C. Baum (Eds.), *Occupational therapy: Overcoming human performance deficits.* Thorofare, NJ: Slack.

Lydic, J. S. & Steele, C. (1979). Assessment of the quality of sitting and gait patterns in children with Down's syndrome. *Physical Therapy, 59,* 1489–1494.

Ma, H., & Trombley, C. A. (2000). The comparison of motor performance between part and whole tasks in elderly persons. *American Journal of Occupational Therapy, 55,* 62–67.

Ma, H., Trombley, C. A., & Robinson-Podolski, C. (1998). The effect of context on skill acquisition and transfer. *American Journal of Occupational Therapy, 53,* 138–144.

Magill, R. A. (1989). *Motor learning: Concepts and applications* (3rd ed.). Dubuque, IA: Wm. V. Brown.

Magill, R. A. (1993). *Motor learning: Concepts and applications* (4th ed.). Madison, WI: Brown & Benchmark.

Magill, R. A. (2001). *Motor learning: Concepts and applications* (6th ed.). New York: McGraw-Hill.

Magill, R. A., & Hall, K. (1990). A review of the contextual interference effect in motor skill acquisition. *Human Movement Science, 9,* 241–289.

Marcel, M. M. & Armstrong, V. (1982). Auditory and visual sequential memory of Down syndrome and nonretarded children. *American Journal of Mental Deficiency, 87,* 86–95.

Marin-Padilla, M. (1976). Pyramidal cell abnormalities in the motor cortex of a child with Down's syndrome. *Journal of Comparative Neurology, 67,* 63–81.

Maring, J. (1990). Effects of mental practice on rate of skill acquisition. *Physical Therapy, 70,* 165–172.

Mathiowetz, V., & Wade, M. G. (1995). Task constraints and functional motor performance of individuals with and without multiple sclerosis. *American Journal of Occupational Therapy, 48,* 733–745.

McCracken, H. D., & Stelmach, G. E. (1977). A test of the schema theory of discrete motor learning. *Journal of Motor Behavior, 9,* 193–201.

McNevin, N. H., Wulf, G., & Carlson, C. (2000). Effects of attentional focus, self-control, and dyad training on motor learning: Implications for physical rehabilitation. *Physical Therapy, 80,* 373–389.

Mosey, A. C. (1986). *Psychosocial components of occupational therapy.* New York: Raven Press.

Neistadt, M. E. (1988). Stress management. In H. I. Hopkins & H. D. Smith (Eds.), *Willard and Spackman's occupational therapy* (7th ed.). Philadelphia: J. B. Lippincott.

Neistadt, M. E. (1993). The neurobiology of learning: Implications for treatment of adults with brain injury. *American Journal of Occupational Therapy, 48,* 421–430.

Nelson, D. L. (1988). Occupation: Form and performance. *American Journal of Occupational Therapy, 42,* 633–641.

Nelson, D. L. (1994). Occupational form, occupational performance, and therapeutic occupation. In C. B. Royeen (Ed.), *AOTA self-*

study series. The practice of the future: Putting occupation back into therapy. Rockville, MD: AOTA.

Newell, K. M. (1991). Motor skill acquisition. *Annual Review of Psychology, 42,* 213–237.

Nygard, L., Berspang, B., Fisher, A. G., & Winblad, B. (1994). Comparing motor and process ability of persons with suspected dementia in home and clinic sittings. *American Journal of Occupational Therapy, 48,* 689–696.

Orelove, F. P., & Sobsey, D. (1996). Designing transdisciplinary services. In F. P. Orelove & D. Sobsey (Eds.), *Educating children with multiple disabilities: A transdisciplinary approach* (3rd ed.). Baltimore: Paul H. Brooks.

O'Sullivan, S. B. (2001). Strategies to improve motor learning. In S. B. O'Sullivan & T. J. Schmitz (Eds.), *Physical rehabilitation: Assessment and treatment.* Philadelphia: F. A. Davis.

Page, S. J., Levine, P., Sisto, S. A., & Johnston, M. V. (2001). Mental practice combined with physical practice for upper-limb motor deficits in subacute stroke. *Physical Therapy, 81,* 1455–1462.

Park, S., Fisher, A. G., & Velozo, L. A. (1994). Using the assessment of motor and process skills to compare occupational performance between clinic and home settings. *American Journal of Occupational Therapy, 48,* 697–709.

Parkinson, J. (1817). *An essay on the shaking palsy.* London: Whittingham and Rowland.

Pavlov, I. P. (1927). *Conditioned reflexes: An investigation of the physiological activity of the cerebral cortex.* London: Oxford University Press.

Penrose, L. S., & Smith, G. F. (1966). *Down's anomaly.* London: Churchill Livingstone.

Peterson, D. A., & Orgen, R. A. (1983). Older adult learning. In O. Jackson (Ed.), *Physical therapy of the geriatric patient.* New York: Churchill Livingstone.

Petit, T. L., & Markus, E. J. (1987). The cellular basis of learning and memory: The anatomical sequel to neuronal use. In N. W. Milgram, C. M. MacLeod, & T. L. Petit (Eds.), *Neuroplasticity, learning, and memory.* New York: Alan R. Liss.

Pohl, P. S., McDowd, J. M., Filion, D. L., Richards, L. G., & Stiers, W. (2001). Implicit learning of a perceptual-motor skill after a stroke. *Physical Therapy, 81,* 1780–1789.

Poole, J. L. (1991). Application of motor learning principles in occupational therapy. *American Journal of Occupational Therapy, 45,* 531–537.

Quintyn, M., & Cross, E. (1986). Factors affecting the ability to initiate movement in Parkinson's diseases. *Physical and Occupational Therapy in Geriatrics, 4,* 51–60.

Rast, M. M., & Harris, S. R. (1985). Motor control in infants with Down syndrome. *Developmental Medicine and Child Neurology, 27,* 682–685.

Rice, M. S., Alaimo, A. J., & Cook, J. A. (1999). Movement dynamics and occupational embeddedness in a grasping and placing task. *Occupational Therapy International, 6,* 298–310.

Ritson, R. J. (1987). Psychomotor skill teaching: Beyond the command style. *Journal of Physical Education, Recreation, and Dance, 58,* 36–37.

Roth, M., Decety, J., Raybaudi, M, Massarelli, R, Delon-Martin, C., Segebarth, C., Morand, S., Gemignani, A., Decorps, M., & Jeannerod, M. (1996). Possible involvement of the primary motor cortex in mentally simulated movement: A functional magnetic resonance imaging study. *NeuroReport, 17,* 1280–1284.

Rothwell, J. C., Traub, M. M., Day, B. L., Obeso, J. A., Thomas, P. K., & Marsden, D. (1982). Manual motor performance in a deafferented man. *Brain, 105,* 515–542.

Sabari, J. S. (1991). Motor learning concepts applied to activity-based intervention with adults with hemiplegia. *American Journal of Occupational Therapy 45,* 5, 523–530.

Sage, G. H. (1984). *Motor learning and control: A new neuropsychological approach.* Dubuque, IA: Wm. V. Brown.

Salmoni, A. W., Schmidt, R. A., & Walter, C. B. (1984). Knowledge of results and motor learning: A review and critical reappraisal. *Psychological Bulletin, 95,* 355–386.

Schmidt, R. A. (1975). A schema theory of discrete motor skill learning. *Psychological Review, 82,* 225–260.

Schmidt, R. A. (1982). More on motor programs. In J. A. S. Kelso (Ed.), *Human motor behavior: An introduction.* Hillsdale, NJ: Lawrence Erlbaum Associates Publishing.

Schmidt, R. A. (1988). *Motor control and learning* (2nd ed.). Champaign, IL: Human Kinetics.

Schmidt, R. A. (1999). *Motor control and learning* (3rd ed.). Champaign, IL: Human Kinetics.

Schmidt, R. A., & Lee, T. D. (1999). *Motor control and learning: A behavioral emphasis* (6th ed.). Champaign, IL: Human Kinetics.

Schreiber, J., Sober, L., Banta, L., Glassbrenner, L., Haman, J., Mistry, N., & Olesinski, K. (2000). Application of motor learning principles with stroke survivors. *Occupational Therapy in Health Care, 13,* 23–44.

Scott, B. S., Becker, L. E., &. Petit, T. L. (1983). Neurobiology of Down's syndrome. *Progress in Neurobiology, 21,* 199–237.

Shimelmann, A., & Hinojosa, J. (1995). Gross motor activity and attention in three adults with brain injury. *American Journal of Occupational Therapy, 49,* 973–979.

Shumway-Cook, A., & Woollacott, M. (1985). Dynamics of postural control in the child with Down syndrome. *Physical Therapy, 65,* 1315–1322.

Shumway-Cook, A., & Woollacott, M. H. (2001). *Motor control: Theory and practical application* (2nd ed.). Philadelphia: Lippincott Williams & Wilkins.

Singer, R. N. (1978). Motor skills and learning strategies. In H. L. O'Neil (Ed.), *Learning strategies.* New York: Academic Press.

Singer, R. N. (1986). Sports performance: A five-step mental approach. *Journal of Physical Education, Recreation, and Dance, 57,* 2, 82–84.

Smyth, M. M. (1984). Memory for movements. In M. M. Smyth & A. M. Wing (Eds.), *The psychology of movement* (pp. 83–117). San Diego, CA: Academic Press.

Stelmach, G. E. (1982). Information processing framework for understanding human motor behavior. In J. A. S. Kelso (Ed.), *Human motor behavior: An introduction.* Hillsdale, NJ: Erlbaum Press.

Terrell, G., & Kennedy, W. A. (1957). Discrimination learning and transportation as a function of the nature of the reward. *Journal of Experimental Psychology, 53,* 257–260.

Thelen, E., Corbetta, D., Kamm, K., Spencer, J. P., Schneider, K., & Zernicke, R. F. (1993). The transition to reaching: mapping intention and intrinsic dynamics. *Child Development, 64,* 1058–1098.

Toglia, J. P. (1991). Generalization of treatment: A multicontext approach to cognitive perceptual impairment in adults with brain injury. *American Journal of Occupational Therapy, 45,* 505–516.

Trombly, C. A., & Radomski, M. V. (Eds.). (2001). *Occupational therapy in physical dysfunction* (5th ed.). Philadelphia: Lippincott Williams & Wilkins.

Trombly, C. A., & Wu, C-Y. (1999). Effect of rehabilitation tasks on organization of movement after stroke. *American Journal of Occupational Therapy, 53,* 333–344.

Tse, D. W., & Spaulding, S. J. (1998). Review of motor control and motor learning: implications for occupational therapy with individuals with Parkinson's disease. *Physical and Occupational Therapy in Geriatrics, 15,* 19–38.

Umphred, D., & Lewis, R. W. (1999). Aging and the central nervous system. In T. L. Kauffman (Ed.), *Geriatric rehabilitation manual.* New York: Churchill Livingstone.

VanderWeel, F. R., VanderMeer, A. L., & Lee, D. N. (1991). Effect of task on movement control on cerebral palsy: Implications for assessment and therapy. *Developmental Medicine and Child Neurology, 33,* 419–426.

Vygotsky, L. S. (1978). *Mind in society: The development of higher psychological processes.* Cambridge, MA: Harvard University Press.

Warner, L., & McNeill, M. (1988). Mental imagery and its potential for physical therapy. *Physical Therapy, 68,* 516–521.

Watts, N. T. (1990). *Handbook of clinical teaching.* New York: Churchill Livingstone, Inc.

Weiss, M. R., Ebbeck, V., & Wiese-Bjornstal, D. M. (1993). Developmental and psychological factors related to children's observational learning of physical skills. *Pediatric Exercise Science, 5,* 301–317.

Wilson, B. A. (1989). *Memory problems after head injury.* Nottingham: National Head Injuries Association.

Winstein, C. J., & Schmidt, R. A. (1989). Sensorimotor feedback. In D. H. Holding (Ed.), *Human skills.* Chichester, UK: John Wiley and Sons.

Winstein, C. J., & Schmidt, R. A. (1990). Reduced frequency of knowledge of result enhances motor skill learning. *Journal of Experimental Psychology: Learning, Memory and Cognition, 16,* 677–691.

Winstein, C. (1996). Learning a partial-weight-bearing skill: Effectiveness of two forms of feedback. *Physical Therapy, 76,* 985–993.

Wisniewski, K. E., & Schmidt-Sidor, B. (1989). Postnatal delay of myelin formation in brains from Down's syndrome. *Clinical Neuropathology, 6,* 55–62.

Wrisberg, C. A., & Ragsdale, M. R. (1979). Further tests of Schmidt's schema theory: Development of a schema rule for a coincident timing task. *Journal of Motor Behavior, 11,* 159–166.

6

Neurorehabilitation Intervention Approaches

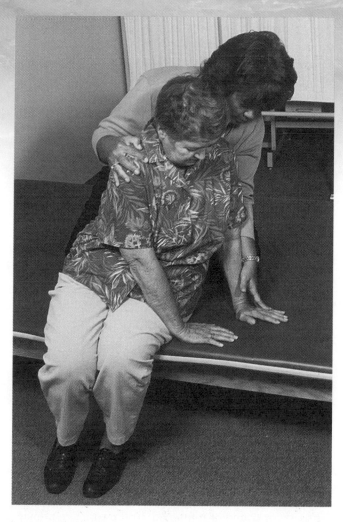

Approaches to intervention continually emerge as a result of the interface between theory and clinical problem solving. Creativity in intervention is the hallmark of the effective, dynamic clinician, who matches the client's capabilities and needs to a management approach that will foster optimal quality of life and well-being. Although therapeutic intervention might include any combination of intervention approaches, therapeutic touch is one of a master therapist's greatest gifts to a patient.

- Sensorimotor approaches: PNF, NDT, SI neurophysiological approach, contributions from Brunnstrom

- Task-oriented models: strategies used to perform functional tasks, age-related strategy changes, functional training approach (strategies to improve mobility, stability, controlled mobility, and skill)

- Importance of person-centered functional goals

- Integrated approach to intervention with patients with neurological dysfunction at any age

Cornerstone Concepts

- Evolution of practice from theory
- Historical roots viewed within the current perspective: reflex theory, hierarchical model, and dynamic systems approach
- Approaches to intervention/frames of reference

Introduction

This text has presented first an overview of how the nervous system functions and how the systems that contribute to the production of human movement develop over the life span. The text further presented how movement control develops and changes over the life span and how motor learning is a dynamic process, giving human beings a unique ability to adapt to changing conditions, including not only normal age-related changes but also to the challenges presented by a neuropathological incident. This theoretical knowledge is essential for clinicians who are engaged in the very real and very dynamic business of helping to create a bridge between theoretical knowledge and available intervention options, as they engage in the practice of working with children and adults who are neurologically challenged.

Therapeutic approaches to intervention with individuals with neurological disorders have evolved over the past several decades since the birth of the professions of occupational therapy and physical therapy. These patient-centered rehabilitation professions of physical therapy and occupational therapy are dynamic, constantly building on an ever-growing body of neuroscience knowledge. Approaches to patient intervention or frames of reference naturally emerge and develop as the base of knowledge broadens. It is crucial that the treating clinician (therapist or therapist assistant) develop an ability to make sound clinical decisions in selecting from among these sometimes diverse approaches and interventions to offer the patient/client the best intervention approach possible. Furthermore, it is reasonable to expect that therapeutic approaches to intervention will continue to emerge, develop, and become refined. Critical thinking is a must for the contemporary clinician, who is charged with staying abreast of new knowledge and therefore innovative intervention opportunities, as they continually unfold.

Intervention approaches emerge as a result of the interface between theory and clinical problem solving. Therapists and assistants are encouraged to study the contributions from each approach and become eclectic in an approach to patient care. It is rarely best for the patient that a clinician be proficient in only one intervention approach. Although current scientific knowledge undoubtedly encourages therapists to prioritize a dynamic systems approach and the importance of functional movement, new knowledge will continue to emerge. Any current theory of motor control with an accompanying clinical intervention model is in a sense unfinished, because there must always be room to revise and incorporate new information, knowledge, and insights.

This chapter will present and summarize the salient features of the most popular intervention approaches available for intervention with the individual with a neurological disorder. Although many of the original tenets of some earlier intervention approaches have now been abandoned, there is value in some of their insights. No one approach offers all the answers or is the best choice for all patients/clients of any age who present with the plethora of clinical dilemmas encountered. The remainder of this text, therefore, is far from a "cookbook." Rather, it is an attempt to present the most common approaches so that the clinician can assimilate that information and choose the relevant concepts from each of the frames of reference to solve commonly encountered individual clinical problems. Many practicing therapists choose from among different approaches frequently and equally. The most effective clinicians are problem solving, informed, and perhaps eclectic, constantly searching for the closest match between the presenting patient's main movement problem and the tools that are available to help the patient optimize functional performance, independence, and well-being. The best approach to a patient/client is most often an integrated one, assimilating the information available and deriving an individual, patient-centered custom approach. The choice of interventions must be function based and have the greatest chance of promoting successful motor function for the unique individual person.

History

The Evolution of Practice from Theory

Therapeutic approaches are always intertwined with the state of the scientific knowledge base. Rehabilitation practices reflect the prevailing theories about the nature of function and dysfunction (Shepard, 1991). Any theoretical approach aimed at the rehabilitation of patients with neurological disorders is based on assumptions regarding how the central nervous system (CNS) controls movement. From these assumptions, a theoretical model is developed, guiding a particular theoretical approach or frame of reference. In the practice arena, it is when current approaches are perceived as inadequate, both practically and theoretically, that optimal conditions exist for therapeutic innovation. It is important to remember that clinical frustration often forces new levels of insight. New ideas are born from theoretical advances, such as in the neurosciences, and practical experimentation, in the clinic (Carr & Shepherd, 2000). This phenomenon illustrates the inseparable nature of basic science and clinical practice. As knowledge in the basic sciences increases, there is a natural evolution of advanced therapeutic approaches as practitioners attempt to apply this new neuroscience knowledge to application in patient care. Concurrently, experienced practitioners demand innovative answers and new ideas from the basic scientists.

Clinical Connection:

One of the reasons that I still love being a therapist after 28 years is because the field is so interesting and dynamic, constantly unfolding literally before my eyes. I often tell my students, "The text from which we are currently teaching is a work in progress; the last chapters are not yet written. It will be up to you to continue adding to this unfinished book!"

Historical Roots Viewed Within Current Perspective

In the early years of physical and occupational therapy as professions, most therapists served persons with musculoskeletal disorders, reflected by the early name "reconstruction aide," which was given to those therapists providing service to injured soldiers. This historical fact is true for both physical and occupational therapists. Margaret Rood, a well-known name in early neurorehabilitation, was an occupational and physical therapist who first served during World War I (Low, 2001).

A tremendous increase in therapy services occurred as a direct result of the polio epidemic in the 1920s, with this tremendous need continuing until the discovery of the polio vaccine in 1955. With medical advances also ensuring that children and adults with neurological impairment, such as spinal cord injury or stroke, could survive their actual injury and acute phases of rehabilitation, therapists became increasingly involved in the rehabilitation of children and adults with neurological impairment. During the 1940s and 1950s, an interest in treating children with neurological problems led to the development of several still well-accepted neurophysiological and developmental approaches to intervention, such as neurodevelopmental treatment (NDT) and sensory integration (SI).

Most recently, an appreciation of motor control and motor learning has become a driving force behind intervention. Occupational therapists are clarifying their professional focus with emphasis on occupational science and purposeful activity (AOTA, 1999). As an example, a review of recent literature in the occupational therapy field uncovers the coining of a new term, **neuro-occupation,** in the occupational therapy literature, indicative of that profession's belief in the inexorable link that exists between the neurosciences, an individual's nervous system, and the way in which that individual engages in **occupation** (Padilla & Peyton,

1999). Physical therapists, identifying themselves as movement scientists, are ensuring that prevention and minimizing functional limitation is a cornerstone to intervention. Both professions currently have a Guide to Practice, offering practitioners a concrete method for moving through the clinical decision making necessary to most efficiently optimize a *functional outcome* for the patient/client. Most physical and occupational therapists currently subscribe to an eclectic approach to intervention, selecting aspects from several different intervention approaches or frames of reference to meet the individual needs of the patient. The main emphasis in both physical and occupational therapy is now on a functional approach to assessment and intervention.

▪ Reflex Theory

The earliest theoretical insights into the way the human nervous system produces movement were offered by Sherrington, based on his experiments in 1906 (Sherrington, 1906). Sherrington's work formed the foundation of the reflex theory, which proposed that movement was peripherally driven, meaning that the sensory system literally drove motor output. Once a stimulus is provided, a chain of responses is created throughout the nervous system, resulting in movement. Sherrington theorized that reflexes were the basic building blocks of complex movement and that reflexes work together or in sequence as a chain of movements to achieve a movement purpose. The reflex model suggested that sensory input regulates motor output, leading to a core assumption but also to the main limitation of that theory—*that sensation was necessary for movement to take place.* According to the early theorists, the appearance and disappearance of reflexes reflected the increasing maturity of cortical structures.

Clinical Connection:

An example of how the reflex model conceptualized movement production can be illustrated with a manual intervention technique still used, called tapping. In this technique, the therapist or assistant taps on the muscle to elicit a muscle contraction. Tapping on the muscle belly facilitates muscle activation by eliciting quick stretches of muscle spindles that contribute to the activation of alpha motor neurons innervating that same muscle. This very simple but phasic (short-lived) response can be used to initiate a muscle contraction, activate a muscle response, or increase kinesthetic awareness. This *sensorimotor* technique is most effective for patients with limited voluntary muscle control in the very early phases of rehabilitation. Obviously, however, unless that elicited muscle contraction is strengthened and integrated into a functional use of the muscle, this technique in isolation is of limited value. Later in this chapter, we will discuss how this and similar sensorimotor techniques can be useful as assimilated into a functional, holistic intervention plan. ▪

Because Sherrington looked primarily at reflexes and reflex chaining as an explanation of motor control, his work was understandably skewed, limited by the level of theoretical knowledge at that time. The limitations of the reflex theory on motor control center largely around the inability to explain movements that happen in the absence of a sensory stimulus, inability to explain the generation of fast movements or movements expressed for the first time, and most importantly, the fact that a single stimulus may produce varying responses depending on the unique movement context (Shumway-Cook & Woollacott, 2001). We now know that voluntary movement is not limited to responses from incoming peripheral stimuli.

The contributions from this early theory are still of value, as now assimilated into a much broader perspective. Contemporary motor theory has a more dynamic view of the role of automatic movements (including reflexes) and their role in motor control. It is appreciated that although reflexes may provide a general framework or bias for movement, they do not solely address the dynamic and adaptive nature of early infant motor behavior. Contemporary dynamic systems theory does not deny the existence of reflexes, but rather considers them as one of *many* influences on the control of posture and movement (Shumway-Cook & Woollacott, 2001). These motor responses may be the form of expressed movement observed, given the capabilities, constraints (limitations), and self-organization of all the contributing subsystems.

As a motor expression, reflexes and other automatic movements are often observed during times of great developmental change, such as during the first year of life, and during or following periods of damage to the nervous system. There was a time in practice history that physical therapists (PTs) and occupational therapists (OTs) thought that reflexes were "bad," an example of aberrant or exaggerated primitive motor behavior that needed to be inhibited or lessened as a goal in and of itself before more "normal" motor behavior could be developed. Today, reflexes are recognized as one of several choices of movement patterns that may or may not be dominant, depending on the composite of that individual person's state of movement control. Reflexes may be more accurately conceptualized as one of several choices of functional movement patterns, as opposed to how they were previously viewed, as "culprits" preventing more mature patterns of movement from emerging (Fetter, 1991).

Reflex theory continues to give therapists and assistants important clinical insights. Despite the limitations, the work of Sherrington has influenced clinical practice. Assessment of reflexes is still used to recognize the controlling or obligatory nature of reflex patterns when they are the preferred movement patterns in individuals with impaired motor control (see Chapter 4). There are examples of how sensory-driven activation of motor responses are generated in response to peripheral stimulation of the receptor, such as stimulation of the labyrinth to activate trunk extension as part of a righting response. Later in this chapter, use of some simple facilitation techniques will be described (Table 6–1), many of these techniques having their roots in the reflex theory.

▪ Hierarchical Model

The work of Hughlings Jackson contributed to the view of the nervous system as a **hierarchical** organization, where the nervous system had higher, middle, and lower levels of control (Walsche, 1961). This model has been described as a "top-down" approach with each successive, anatomically higher level of the nervous system exerting control over the levels below. The hierarchical model is based on the premise that there are central control mechanisms that separate reflex from voluntary control patterns (Kohl & Sheal, 1992). According to this model, the control of movement is organized hierarchically, with the spinal cord providing reflex motor patterns, the brainstem providing static or tonic reflex control and integration, and the cerebral cortex superseding all lower structures with voluntary control mechanisms. Its limitation was based on its cornerstone presumption that one system, the CNS, was thought to be the primary source of movement (Shumway-Cook & Woollacott, 2001).

As with the reflex model, the hierarchical model held that stereotypical movements are governed by sensory input. The hierarchical model allowed for many levels of control, but the emphasis remained on the spinal cord level being predominantly reflexive and higher cortical levels being less automatic, more voluntary, and superior in function. Using the hierarchical model, sensorimotor intervention approaches developed, directed at helping patients to progress from automatic control mechanisms to higher levels of voluntary control. The work by Gesell (1954), known as the neuromaturational theory of development, described the maturation of the developing child (see Chapter 4) in a hierarchical fashion. As discussed in Chapter 4, this theory of development had originally proposed that the CNS was the primary agent for change during development and maturation. We now appreciate that multiple subsystems develop and change over the course of a life

TABLE 6–1

Manual Facilitation and Inhibition Techniques

Technique	Receptor	Stimulus	Response	Comments
Quick stretch	Muscle spindle Ia endings detecting length and velocity changes	Quick stretch or tapping over a muscle belly or tendon	Activates agonist to contract; reciprocal innervation effect will inhibit the antagonist; activates synergists	Response is very temporary; can add resistance to augment response; not appropriate to use in muscles where increased muscle tone limits function
Prolonged stretch	Muscle spindle Ia and II endings Golgi tendon organs (GTO)	Maintained stretch in a lengthened range	Dampens (inhibits) muscle contraction	Rationale for serial casting and splinting; to increase the effect, activate the antagonist
Resistance	Muscle spindles	Resistance given manually or with body weight or gravity; mechanical weights	Enhances muscle contraction through recruitment; facilitates synergists; enhances kinesthetic awareness	Resistance needs to be graded dependent on patient response and goal; additional recruitment and overflow may be counterproductive to movement goal
Approximation	Joint receptors	Compression of joint surfaces: manual or mechanical; bouncing; applied in weight bearing	Enhances muscular co-contraction, proximal stability and postural extension; increases kinesthetic awareness and postural stability	Effective in combination with rhythmic stabilization (see PNF) Contraindicated in inflamed joints
Traction	Joint receptors	Joint surfaces distracted, usually manually and at the beginning of movement	Facilitates muscle activation to improve mobility and movement initiation	Useful to activate initial mobility; also used by qualified practitioners as part of mobilization
Inhibitory pressure	GTO, muscle spindles, tactile receptors	Firm pressure manually or with body weight over muscle belly or tendon	Inhibits muscle activity; dampening effect	Equipment can be used to achieve effect: casts and splints, placing cones in hands, positional use of wheelchair lap tray; weight-bearing activities can provide inhibitory pressure, for example, onto open hand to inhibit finger flexors
Light touch	Rapidly adapting tactile receptors, autonomic nervous system (ANS) (sympathetic division)	Brief, light contact to skin	Increased arousal, withdrawal response	Effective in initiating a generalized movement response, to elicit arousal; contraindicated with agitated patients or where ANS is unstable
Maintained touch	Slowly adapting tactile receptors, ANS (para-sympathetic division)	Maintained contact or pressure	Calming effect, desensitizes skin, provides general inhibition	Useful for patients with high level of arousal or hypersensitivity

(Continued on following page)

TABLE 6–1

Manual Facilitation and Inhibition Techniques (Continued)

Technique	Receptor	Stimulus	Response	Comments
Manual contacts	Tactile receptors, muscle proprioceptors	Firm, deep pressure of hands over body area	Facilitates contraction of muscle underneath hands	Activates muscle response; enhances sensory and kinesthetic awareness; provides security and support
Slow stroking	Tactile receptors ANS (parasympathetic division)	Slow, firm stroking with flat hand over neck or trunk extensors	Produces calming effect, general inhibition; induces feeling of security	Appropriate for overly aroused patients
Neutral warmth	Thermo receptors ANS (parasympathetic division)	Towel or elastic wrap of body or body parts (warm)	Provides general relaxation and inhibition; decreased muscle tone; decreased agitation or pain	Use for 10–15 min; avoid overheating; appropriate for highly agitated patients or individuals with increased sympathetic response
Slow vestibular stimulation	Tonic vestibular receptors	Slow rocking, slow movement on ball, in hammock, in rocking chair	Produces calming effect, decreased arousal, generalized inhibition	Useful for patients who are defensive to sensory stimulation, hyperreactive to stimulation, hypertonic, or agitated
Fast vestibular stimulation	Semicircular canals	Fast or irregular movement with an acceleration and deceleration component, such as spinning, use of a scooter board, fast rolling	Facilitates general muscle tone and promotes postural responses to movement	Used with patients with hypotonia (CP, Down syndrome); used to promote sensory integration (requires specialized training and certification)

Source: Adapted from O'Sullivan, S. B., & Schmitz, T. J. (Eds.). (2001). *Physical rehabilitation: Assessment and treatment* (4th ed.). Philadelphia: F. A. Davis.

span, in a spiraling, ongoing developmental change process (see Chapter 3).

Contemporary theories assert the importance of multiple factors in the lifelong development of human movement control. Modern neuroscientists have confirmed the importance of some elements of the hierarchical model of motor control, although the concept of a strict hierarchy has been modified. Current concepts recognize the fact that each level of the nervous system can act on other levels, depending on the task. Reflexive patterns of movement are not considered to be the sole determinant of motor control, but they are one of many processes important to the generation and control of movement.

■ Dynamic Systems Approach and Contemporary Ideas

Today, clinicians use an integrated approach to assessment and intervention with the patient with neurological dysfunction. The evolution of the systems model of motor control has brought many of the assumptions of the sensorimotor models into question. However, rather than thinking of these theories or models as mutually exclusive, they can be viewed as a continuum in which the earlier models presumed that movement relied heavily on sensory input and feedback, whereas the dynamic systems model relies *not only* on sensory information but also heavily on information from nonsensory sources (McCormack & Feuchter, 1996). Contemporary motor theory does not negate the value of the sensory-motor connection. Sensorimotor approaches can be used in the context of the systems model, with sensory input as one of many critical elements necessary for the achievement of motor control and motor learning.

Clinical Connection:

It would be difficult to totally abandon our roots as reflected within the early sensorimotor theories. Physical and occupational therapy are unique professions because of the importance that the practitioner places on the value of touch and the therapeutic use of the self. Although both professions certainly now recognize that human movement control is optimized by *actively* engaging the patient in creating and demonstrating a movement solution, no therapist would underestimate the power of our "hands" as we effect the patient's responses. When a therapist or assistant touches a patient, that clinician becomes an intimate part of that individual's environment, a fact to be respected and honored. ■

Contemporary models of motor control view the movement system as a **heteroarchical** organization involving the interaction of many subsystems, resulting in movement that is influenced by development, training, and changing environmental conditions. The systems involved include the parts of the CNS working together, the various components of the musculoskeletal system, the goal of the task, and relevant conditions in the environment. Dynamic systems theory views motor control as an emergent phenomenon arising out of the dynamics of all these components that interact. This view emphasizes that the parts of the movement system cooperate together to achieve performance so that all the contributing systems come together in a functionally related and context-dependent way, not in a fixed or centrally instructed way (Kamm, Thelen, & Jensen, 1990; Kielhofner, 1997). According to the dynamic systems view, development is a variable process of learning to uncover individual optimal solutions to motor problems, such as movement challenges encountered by patients/clients. These contemporary views stress the importance of learning the entire task, or occupation, rather than discrete, splintered parts. Individuals are encouraged to find their own optimal solutions to motor problems. The goals of intervention in this approach can be summarized as follows:

- Accomplishment of necessary and desired task selection, goal-directed activity, and occupational forms in the most meaningful and efficient way, given the individual's unique characteristics.
- Allowing the individual to practice in varying and natural contexts so that the learned behaviors become more stable.
- Maximizing the personal and environmental characteristics that enhance performance.
- Enhancing the problem-solving abilities of individuals so that they will more readily find solutions to challenges encountered in new environments beyond the intervention setting.

Therapists now recognize that motor output is dependent on the interaction of many intrinsic and extrinsic factors. The contemporary motor control approach, based on dynamic systems theory, has largely replaced the more mechanistic explanations of movement with a more dynamic, individualized, and holistic

viewpoint. The dynamic systems model is in concert with a holistic view of functional human performance, motor learning principles, emphasis on environment, and the evolving knowledge of neuroscience. As a theoretical basis for intervention, the following guiding principles, as summarized by Newell and Valvano, are offered by this approach (Newell and Valvano, 1998):

- Individuals with movement difficulties caused by neurological dysfunction are faced with constraints (limitations) to movement.
- There are many sources of constraints to action, some within the environment, the individual, or the task itself. Constraints are an important consideration because they literally provide boundary conditions to the action and the organization of the movement. Within the individual, constraints to action exist at various levels: neurological, biomechanical, musculoskeletal, and behavioral/cognitive. Some of these constraints can be changed, others not.
- Individuals with neurological disorders may present with a problem with the appropriate number of degrees of freedom necessary for unimpaired task execution. In some cases, the individual may need to control (decrease) the degrees of freedom by learning to stabilize a body part or practice postural control; in other instances, when encountering limited range of motion or decreased strength, the degrees of freedom are insufficient to execute the desired movement. Clinicians can interface with patients/clients to help offer solutions for problems with controlling the required degrees of freedom.
- Therapeutic intervention strategies are offered by the therapist as an action that interacts with the boundary conditions already present within the individual, the environment, or the attempted task. The role of the therapist is to select a physical or informational input that induces an efficient and effective search strategy on the part of the individual, enabling the individual to identify task-relevant changes so that the functional movement outcome is more successful. Intervention strategies are chosen to induce change in the movement dynamics of the patient/client.
- In practice, most therapeutic intervention is directed to manipulations of the environment or the task, with some success in changing the constraints presented by the individual.
- The therapist is thus viewed as a *change agent*, working on behalf of and in concert with the individual patient/client to generate a movement solution. The role of therapists as change agents is to systematically adjust the confluence (influence together) of all the constraints on the individual as he or she attempts to move so that a new set of conditions enables the individual to search for a stable and adaptive coordination solution to the task demands.
- Therapists can physically manipulate the environment (altering the physical environment or the

specific physical demands of the task), provide augmented information (by offering instruction and feedback), or physically manipulate the individual (through therapeutic exercise or manual guidance).

- Therapists also can use motor learning as a search strategy, facilitating the learner to discover and develop new movement strategies as a solution to a movement problem.

To arrive at present-day practice, many approaches to intervention or therapeutic frames of reference have been developed. The remainder of this chapter doesn't only summarize these approaches, but presents key concepts that continue to be of value from each. The salient contributions from each frame of reference can then be at the disposal of the contemporary physical or occupational therapy practitioner, available for application to patient intervention.

Approaches to Intervention/Frames of Reference

Sensorimotor Approaches

Sensorimotor approaches are also known in the literature as **neurofacilitation** or **neurophysiological approaches**. These approaches were the first proposed for intervention with the neurologically impaired person, growing out of the research performed by Sherrington (1906) and Hughlings Jackson (Walsche, 1961). As applied to patient/client intervention, the contributions from the reflex and hierarchical models have similarities but also a striking dissimilarity. The reflex model proposed that movement and motor control were predominantly peripherally driven and peripheral-based, whereas the hierarchical model proposed that movement production and control were central-based. However, they both shared important assumptions:

1. The brain controls movements, not muscles.
2. The CNS is organized in such a way that higher centers normally are in command of lower centers, in turn controlling more automatic behaviors.
3. An individual's movement pattern can be altered (facilitated) by applying sensory stimulation or promoting a progression of movement control (Gordon, 2000).

The sensorimotor approaches to intervention had their foundations in the reflex and hierarchical models of motor control. These models assumed the following:

1. Motor control and motor skill development were dependent on reflexes that are organized in a hierarchical fashion.
2. Motor output was dependent on sensory input.

These assumptions are now recognized not so much as faulty but limited in perspective. Nonetheless, the sensorimotor or neurofacilitation intervention approaches, including proprioceptive neuromuscular facilitation, NDT, and SI, and the work of Signe Brunnstrom, which arose from these theories, offer tremendous clinical tools as updated today. The neurofacilitation/sensorimotor approaches still dominate the way clinicians examine and intervene with patients who have CNS pathology (Shumway-Cook & Woollacott, 2001). Currently, within these approaches, there is greater emphasis on explicitly training function and less emphasis on retraining for "normal" patterns of movement. There is more consideration of motor learning principles when developing intervention plans and strategies. The boundaries between approaches, as currently used, have become less distinct as each approach integrates into its theoretical base new concepts related to motor control. The following will describe, in historical order, the evolution and continuing contributions offered by these intervention approaches. There are salient concepts and applicable intervention insights available from each. All these intervention approaches offer today's clinician some useful tools and insights for application within an integrated approach to the patient/client with neurological dysfunction.

▪ Proprioceptive Neuromuscular Facilitation

Herman Kabat, a neurophysiologist, and Maggie Knott, a physical therapist, developed the method of **proprioceptive neuromuscular facilitation (PNF)** between 1946 and 1951, later expanded upon by Voss (a PT) and Meyers (an OT). By correlating the works of scientists in the fields of motor learning, motor development, and neurophysiology, Kabat and Knott considered that PNF was the ideal tool to treat paralysis, which was quite prevalent at the time. In the development of this approach to intervention, Kabat and Knott relied heavily on the work of Sherrington and Gesell, recognizing the capability of neuromuscular mechanisms to promote movement (Kabat & Knott, 1953). Knott and Voss define **facilitation** as "the promotion of any natural process; specifically, the effect produced in nerve tissue by the passage of an impulse" (Knott & Voss, 1968, p. 4). The term *proprioceptive* (see Chapter 2) means sensory stimulation that is received from the receptors within the body's own muscles, tendons, and joints. *Neuromuscular* clearly means that this technique applies to the nerves and muscles. PNF is therefore defined as an approach that includes methods of promoting or hastening the response of the neuromuscular mechanism through stimulation of the proprioceptors.

The basic tenets of this approach are that the body's movements are predominantly rotational and that each major body part has two basic diagonal (rotational) movement patterns, with each diagonal consisting of two antagonistic patterns, one predominantly into flexion and the other into extension. These patterns allow a series of muscles to contract from their completely lengthened range to their completely shortened range, with rotation being an important consideration. Inherent to these patterns of muscle contraction is the concept of "timing," whereby normal timing is considered to be the typical sequence of muscular activity resulting in coordinated movement. It was also found that touch, resistance, pressure, stretch, and verbal commands could be used to heighten the excitability of the motor neurons, creating more activity in the production of volitional movements (Burke, Culligan, & Holt, 2000; Morris & Sharpe, 1993).

The basic philosophy, as proposed by the early proponents of these techniques, is still applicable today. "The philosophy of treatment using techniques of PNF is … a philosophy based upon the ideas that … movements must be specific and directed toward a goal, that activity is necessary to the best development of coordination, strength, and endurance, and that the stronger body parts [can] strengthen weaker parts through cooperation leading toward a goal of optimum function" (Knott & Voss, 1968, p. 3). Knott and Voss (1968) elaborated by saying that "purposeful movements are basic to a successful life; they are coordinated and directed toward an ultimate goal. Ability, strength, and endurance are developed by active participation in life, and repetition of an activity is important to the learning process. Movement responses may be developed in accordance with environmental influences and voluntary decisions, within the limits of anatomical structure and developmental level, and inherent in previously learned responses" (Knott & Voss, 1968, p. 3). These direct citations clearly demonstrate that the earliest leaders in the field of neurorehabilitation recognized and prioritized the importance of purposeful movement, goal-directed activity, motor learning, and environmental influences—a familiar and contemporary message!

PNF proposes the following main tenets central to application of its techniques:

- The brain knows nothing of individual muscle action, but rather recognizes movement as mass movement patterns (known as Beevor's axiom).
- In normal functional motor activity, muscles shorten and lengthen in varying degrees. Normal movement

depends on a balance between flexors and extensors and between different types of muscle contractions.
- All the facilitated movements are performed in a diagonal fashion, resembling naturally occurring movements seen in sports and work activities. There are two diagonal patterns of motion for each of the major parts of the body: head and neck, upper trunk, lower trunk, and extremities. Each pattern has a major component of flexion and extension, with rotation ensuring a spiral nature to the motion and integration of both body sides.
- Motor learning requires repetition and the integration of multisensory information. Auditory, visual, tactile, and proprioceptive information combine in the learning or relearning of movement.
- When performed against resistance, patterns of facilitated movement produce selective irradiation, whereby muscle contraction is then induced throughout the muscle and into synergists. By stimulating the stronger muscle groups first, contraction can be induced in the weaker synergistic muscles.

A variety of specific techniques have been developed to facilitate movement. Examples of the application of the most commonly used upper and lower extremity diagonals are depicted in Figures 6–1 and 6–2. Manual stimulation techniques, which can be used during the performance of the diagonal movement patterns, including the use of manual contacts, resistance, stretch, traction, approximation, timing, and rhythmic stabilization, are described in Table 6–2. These manual techniques are selected by the clinician to increase muscle activation during the performance of the movement pattern. PNF incorporates motor learning strategies into its application: instruction, guidance, repetition, practice, and feedback. As a therapeutic exercise approach, PNF continues to be very appropriate and has widespread use still today (Burke et al., 2000; Morris & Sharpe, 1993). A more in-depth discussion of PNF is beyond the scope of this text; readers are encouraged to become familiar with the summarized basic tenets and techniques and to incorporate the salient concepts as appropriate into patient intervention. For additional information and details on PNF, refer to available resources, including texts and continuing education workshops.

Clinical Connection:

Applicable insights and tools from PNF still relevant for today's clinician include the incorporation of motor learning strategies into intervention, the use of multisensory input, and the modeling of the diagonal patterns on functional movement patterns. The manual

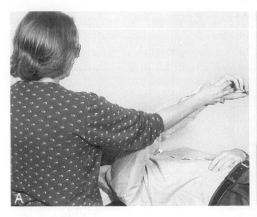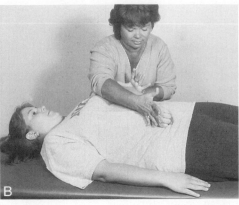

Figure 6–1. PNF diagonal emphasizing (A) upper extremity rotation and elbow extension and (B) the importance of therapist's hand placement to emphasize wrist and elbow extension.

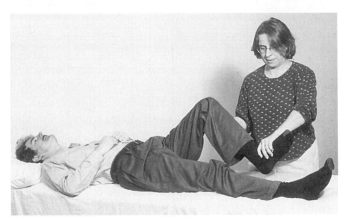

Figure 6–2. PNF diagonal emphasizing lower extremity dorsiflexion and inversion.

facilitation techniques are highly effective in eliciting muscular activation within fundamental movement patterns. Interestingly, this sensorimotor approach is the earliest among the frames of reference (being developed as early as the 1940s and 1950s), but these earliest writings could have been written today: "Purposeful movements are basic to a successful life; they are coordinated and directed toward an ultimate goal" (Knott & Voss, 1968, p. 3). ■

■ Neurodevelopmental Treatment

Neurodevelopmental treatment, as an intervention approach, was initially developed by Drs. Karl and Berta Bobath during the 1950s, as they studied the movement difficulties commonly experienced by children with cerebral palsy (CP) (Bobath, 1965, 1969). The approach was then quickly expanded to intervention with the adult with hemiplegia (Bobath, 1970). Originally, NDT concentrated on the effects of the disturbed postural control mechanism on movement. The Bobaths identified the essential problems of the patient with neurological dysfunction to be abnormal muscle tone, disordered control due to abnormally strong primitive and postural reflex activity, and an inability to demonstrate mature motor responses, including equilibrium, due to brain damage. The neurodevelopmental framework assumed that the role of the CNS is to provide the organization necessary to perform highly skilled activities while maintaining posture and equilibrium (Valvano & Long, 1991). In the original applications of NDT, therapists facilitated movement control by using the developmental sequence to design intervention activities that would promote the acquisition of normal motor milestones. Each activity had the emergence of postural control, including demonstration of automatic postural reactions, as one of its main goals. The therapist, through the use of manual guidance, originally termed therapeutic **handling,** attempted to use this physical guidance to facilitate the demonstration of automatic postural movements from the patient. The therapist typically used the pelvis or the shoulder girdle as a **key point of control** to encourage the emergence of normal movement components, such as flexor and extensor control, weight shifting, and the smooth use of rotation and dissociation. The overall goal of therapy was to encourage voluntary control, believing that once an individual could control a movement pattern voluntarily, it could then be integrated into functional activity.

NDT theory and intervention application have gone through many changes since their inception, continuing to evolve as knowledge of movement and motor control expands. Contemporary proponents of NDT have integrated current motor control and motor learning theory into its approach. Although certain points of emphasis have changed, the basic rationale that motor function can be improved by modifying abnormal movement patterns has basically remained unchanged. Intrinsic to this rationale is that movement is a changeable, dynamic phenomenon that can be affected by external sensory inputs (Bobath & Bobath, 1984; Valvano & Long, 1991). However, the importance of functional independence is currently stressed more emphatically than in the earlier writings.

Using selective guidance and instruction, the therapist attempts to help an individual experience active

TABLE 6–2
Summary of Stimulation Techniques Used During PNF and Application to Intervention

Stimulation Technique	Application	Goal and Presumed Benefit
Manual contacts	Pressure is given to the skin over the muscle being facilitated.	Manually contacting the patient utilizes sensory cues to direct the patient's attention to the desired movement. Pressure activates mechanoreceptors.
Vision	Patient/client is asked to watch the movement and to participate in giving the movement direction.	Visually directed movement is used as reinforcement and to offer extrinsic feedback to the patient as he or she learns the movement.
Verbal commands	Tone of voice and specific commands are used selectively to prepare the patient for movement, direct the movement, and motivate the patient/client.	Voice is used to affect the quality of the patient's response. Tone and timing of commands are used as teaching aids.
Stretch	Quick stretch is given to the muscle being facilitated. Stretch can be applied at the beginning of the motion or intermittently throughout the range of motion to activate or reinforce muscle activation/contraction.	Quick stretch activates the muscle spindle and excites the agonist muscle through activation of the monosynaptic reflex arc.
Traction	Separation of the joint surfaces to activate joint receptors.	A traction stimulus activates proprioceptive joint receptors, theorized to promote movement.
Approximation	Compression of joint surfaces together, usually done with the body part in a weight-bearing position.	Approximation is used to activate proprioceptive joint receptors to promote muscular co-contraction, joint stability, and weight bearing.
Resistance	Resistance given to an active contraction; resistance can be graded or maximal, depending on the movement goal.	Resistance is used to increase muscular strength, reinforce a contraction, or induce irradiation (spread) of the contraction to synergists.
Timing	Timing is selectively used by the therapist to either facilitate motor learning as the patient recognizes the familiarity of a frequently used movement pattern (normal timing) or to emphasize a specific portion of the movement pattern (timing for emphasis).	The movement patterns used in PNF are based on typically occurring patterns of normal movement, used in work and sports. Timing is an important component of learning a movement pattern.
Rhythmic stabilization	Rhythmic, alternating isometric contractions of agonist and antagonist without intermittent relaxation; resistance is carefully graded to achieve co-contraction.	Used to promote weight bearing and holding and improve postural stability, strength, and proximal control.

Source: Information compiled from multiple sources. See text and references for details.

movement with correct alignment and more efficient movement patterns, as well as to anticipate changes in posture. By experiencing active, appropriate movement repeatedly in several positions, the individual may learn to move more effectively. The goal of intervention is to prepare the individual for independent, active functional performance (Kielhofner, 1997). Intervention in functional environmental contexts is encouraged. Current NDT theory adheres to the following key concepts (Styer-Acevedo, 1998; Whiteside, 1997):

• During the acquisition of functional motor skills, the therapist or assistant encourages the individual to focus on the goal rather than the specific movement

components of the task. Movement is composed of many subsystems that are interactive and independent but also plastic and adaptive to both internal and external changes.

• A standard of reference for proficient human motor function is based on a study of motor control, motor development, and motor learning. Learning and adaptation of motor skills involves repetition, practice, and experience.

• Individuals with motor control problems associated with CNS pathophysiology, such as CP or adult hemiplegia, present with predictable primary and secondary impairments. It is these impairments that limit function.

- Intervention begins with assessment of the individual's functional performance. Intervention focuses on increasing function by building on the individual's strengths while addressing the limiting impairments. Therapeutic handling or facilitation using NDT principles is one strategy that can be utilized.
- Facilitation techniques are methods used to assist the individual in attaining his or her own functional movement goals. Through facilitation, the therapist/assistant communicates with the individual using somatosensory cues to foster any one of the following movement responses:
  - A gain in stability or mobility
  - Synergistic recruitment and timing of muscular activation
  - Improved muscular timing
  - Grading of a movement
  - Variability of movement when solving a functional task

Currently, an NDT approach to intervention is a sequenced approach involving facilitation of movement control and management of the impairments that limit motor performance. Intervention can be viewed as divided into two overlapping phases: preparatory activities and facilitation of active, voluntary, automatic movement (Schoen & Anderson, 1993). Preparatory activities are directed at increasing mobility and facilitating postural alignment as a postural set for active movement. Following preparatory activities, the therapist or assistant facilitates active movement by providing graded sensory inputs and physical guidance as needed at key points of control (Fig. 6–3). The therapist or assistant may use any of the following techniques: handling, inhibition and facilitation, weight bearing and weight shifting, integration of functional tasks, and positioning and adaptive equipment to promote voluntary movement control (Breslin, 1996; DeGangi & Royeen, 1994) (Fig. 6–4).

Clinical Connection:

The following tips are useful to guide today's clinician in the effective application of physical guidance (handling), integrated into a holistic approach to assist the patient/client with a neurological impairment in establishing or reestablishing voluntary movement control.

Handling Tips for Patients/Clients with Neurological Dysfunction

1. Handle the person slowly. Give physical support where necessary and wait to give the individual time to make his or her own adjustments and assist with active movement.
2. When assisting someone with a movement, always

let the person see what is happening, talk about the movement goal, and encourage active participation, however limited. Anxiety about the uncertain can make the movement more difficult.

3. Helpful hints include the following:
   - Side lying is useful for positioning or during transition with movement patterns that are predominated by tonic reflex patterns.
   - Head and neck flexion can decrease the effect of extensor hypertonus on the trunk and extremities (Fig. 6–5).
   - Approach a seated individual at eye level if at all possible to prevent the individual from needing to hyperextend the neck and trunk to look at you (see Fig. 6–5).
   - Slow rocking and rotational movement can dampen the effect of high muscle tone.
   - Try to attain and maintain symmetrical body alignment, promoting head and trunk in midline and arms forward in front of the person.
   - Dissociating the extremities from each other and the upper body from the lower body can decrease the influence of uncontrolled total patterns of flexion or extension.
4. Remember the motor learning principles of repetition, feedback, practice, and active problem solving. ▪

Intervention using this approach proposes that motor skills develop from an interaction among many systems, including the sensory systems, and that postural control and alignment provide a foundation for complex functional skill development. Intervention targets proximal and distal control, active movement, and graded facilitation through judicious use of positioning, handling, and sensory input (Breslin, 1996). It emphasizes consistency of handling, maximization of the therapist's sensory feedback through manual contacts, participation of the mover, creation of a motivating environment, use of ongoing assessment, incorporation of movement into functional activities, and use of preventative strategies such as adaptive equipment and orthotic devices (Schoen & Anderson, 1993). NDT theory and motor learning theory are highly complementary.

Clinical Connection:

Although the name neurodevelopmental is reflective of its early years, when the concept of development was hierarchical, this approach currently advocates the use of selective guidance as the therapist attempts to help

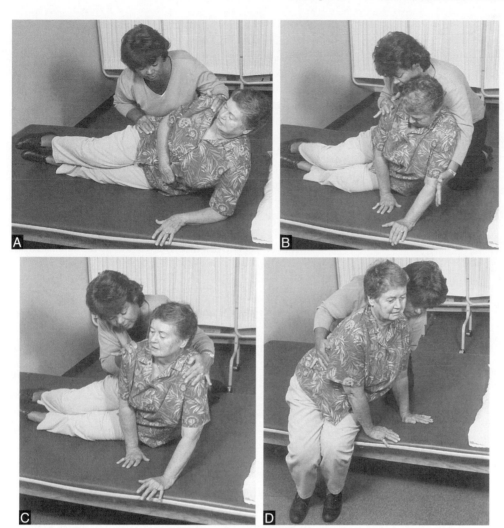

Figure 6–3. Therapist uses graded sensory input and physical guidance as key points of control. (A) through (D) show sequence of movement. Notice how the therapist's use of her hands changes throughout the transition and supports but does not replace or block the movement attempts of the patient/client.

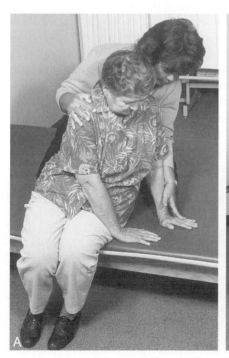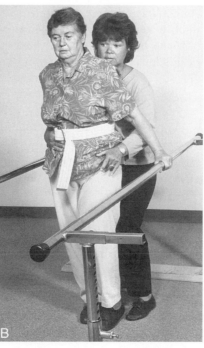

Figure 6–4. (A) Therapist uses facilitation to encourage weight bearing and weight shifting during performance of a functional task, shown with an upper extremity activity. (B) Therapist uses approximation and mild resistance on right and gentle tapping on left to cue patient's effective functional use of lower extremities. Notice purposeful hand placement by the therapist to encourage active control from the patient/client.

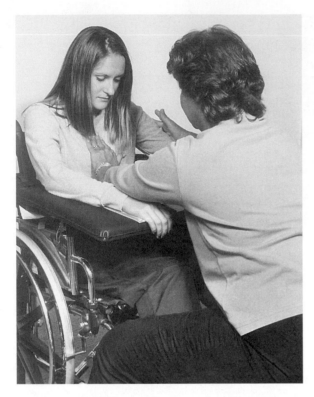

Figure 6–5. Head and neck flexion and midline symmetry of head, trunk, and upper extremities is encouraged by therapist's use of not only her hands but her own body position.

an individual experience active movement with more efficient movement patterns. The goal of intervention is to prepare the individual for independent, active functional performance. Through experiencing active, appropriate movement repeatedly in several positions, the individual may learn to move more effectively. During intervention, integration of the valuable key concepts gleaned from NDT into intervention can be ensured by the clinician asking the following questions:

• Was the individual able to do the selected task?
• How did this individual perform or attempt to perform this task?
• Which components of this individual's movements appeared to be "normal"?
• Which components of this individual's movements appeared to be atypical and either ineffective or undesirable?

The sensory systems are crucial for the acquisition, monitoring, and regulation of movement. Individuals with neurological impairments often have sensory processing difficulties, as well as decreased proprioception and kinesthetic awareness secondary to diminished or altered movement experiences. During movement facilitation, the therapist monitors the individual's use

of sensory systems through his or her responses to sensory feedback and encourages the use of feedback to initiate and refine movements. Support is given judiciously so that the individual has the opportunity to experiment with and experience increased levels of independence in movement. Handling by the therapist or assistant is dynamic, assisting with smoothly graded transitions as active movement provides opportunities for voluntary control. Carryover is promoted, with a strong emphasis on not only the individual patient but also the family, caregivers, and others involved in the care of the individual. Caregivers may include nursing personnel for the adult or educational personnel if the patient is a child. Key intervention techniques, clinical use, intervention application, and examples are summarized in Table 6–3.

▪ Neurophysiological Approach

The neurophysiological approach was the name given to the concepts gathered and synthesized by an occupational and physical therapist, Margaret Rood (1962), as its foundation. This approach was first developed as an approach for individuals with CP but has been expanded for application to a variety of motor control problems.

Rood conceptualized that different types of muscles had different responsibilities in the body, that they performed different types of work. She divided movement into fulfilling one of two main tasks: weight bearing and stabilization, therefore considered a type of heavy work, and mobility tasks as seen in skilled movement, accomplished in non–weight bearing and therefore a light type of work. Rood envisioned motor development as progressing from a state of mobility to stability to heavy work movement combining mobility and stability in weight bearing, and then finally to skill, which combines mobility and stability in non–weight bearing (Farber, 1982, p. 122).

This early intervention approach was built on that time's understanding of neurophysiology. It theorized that these movement capabilities of mobility, stability, controlled mobility, and then skill occurred in this developmental order, because reciprocal innervation developmentally preceded co-innervation within the nervous system. Reciprocal innervation, which causes activation of the agonist and simultaneous relaxation of the antagonist, was thought to be primarily responsible for allowing for mobility. Co-innervation, which resulted in muscular co-contraction and therefore stability, followed. Figure 6–6 gives a diagrammatic representation of the developmental sequence and how the key components of stability and mobility were taught to evolve into functional movement control (Farber, 1982,

TABLE 6-3

Summary of NDT Techniques and Application to Intervention

Technique	Clinical Use	Intervention Application	Example
Handling	Hands are used to support and assist movement (active or passive) from one position to another; active assisted movement is always encouraged.	Use of hands: light touch, intermittent touch, or firm manual contacts to guide and assist with movement; also taught to caregivers.	Caregivers taught to pick up, carry, and move individual from one position to next by incorporating encouragement of key movement components into motion: midline control, symmetry, weight shift, rotation, and dissociation.
Positioning	Used to provide alignment, comfort, support, prevent deformity, and provide readiness to support or enhance independent movement.	Positioning for support is used to provide stability and alignment and prevent deformity. Positioning is also used to promote optimal independent function or position from which movement can most likely occur.	Positioning of persons with hemiplegia is with trunk and head in midline, both extremities forward and resting on tabletop. Positioning of child may be on floor in side-sit to encourage and assist in acquisition of transition to all fours for creeping.
Use of adaptive equipment	Used to provide postural support, prevent deformity, promote alignment, enhance function, and offer mobility; a common adjunct to intervention for children with neurological impairment.	In addition to positional uses, equipment can be used dynamically to assist in movement control. Common uses include using the equipment to place the individual in a set position to enhance the opportunity for movement, to increase the possibility of desirable responses, to decrease the possibility of undesirable responses, or to control the instability and thereby limit the degrees of freedom of a given movement.	Can range from the simple towel roll under the scapula to promote scapular protraction for reaching, to the very complex, such as powered mobility. Examples include adapted tricycles, switch toys, seating inserts, toilet adaptations, standers, strollers, and wide ranges of pediatric wheelchairs. Equipment commonly used during dynamic movement, such as during therapy, includes wedges, rolls, bolsters, benches, and gymnastic balls.
Key points of control	Parts of the body are chosen by the therapist as optimal from which to guide the person's movement.	Proximal key points of control include trunk, shoulders, and pelvis; distal points are hands and feet (less frequently used).	Guide from the scapula or the pelvis to protract the extremity in preparation for a movement. The more proximal the therapist's guiding hands, the more control the therapist has and the less is given to the mover; more distal key points of control give more control to the mover.
Facilitating transitional movement	Facilitates key movement components during active transitional movement.	Provides facilitation of antigravity control, weight bearing, weight shifting, responses to movement such as automatic postural responses, rotation, and dissociation.	Used clinically most often to assist with weight shift in preparation for movement; movement is guided once the weight-bearing body part is stable, allowing for the weight shift to be followed by movement of the body segment.

(Continued on following page)

TABLE 6-3
Summary of NDT Techniques and Application to Intervention (*Continued*)

Technique	Clinical Use	Intervention Application	Example
Use of sensory input	Voluntary movement control is facilitated through use of proprioceptive inputs, exteroceptive inputs, visual, vestibular, and verbal inputs.	Proprioceptive inputs include weight bearing, approximation, stretching and traction, or tapping. Exteroceptive inputs include manual guidance and therapeutic use of hands. Movement stimulates vestibular system and vision and verbal inputs are used for motor learning.	Handling, guided movements, visual demonstration and verbal feedback; movements are used to stimulate the vestibular system (with and without equipment).
Motor learning strategies	Active movement is encouraged through practice, repetition, feedback, and use of functional activities.	Use of variable practice and problem solving in natural environments promotes motor learning.	Intervention takes place within environmental context: home, school, and community.

Source: Information compiled from multiple sources. See text and references for details.

p. 122). Although this neurophysiology is outdated, the concept of viewing movement development as requiring these four key aspects of mobility, stability, and combinations of mobility and stability is still insightful, offering valuable clinical guideposts of use today. The importance of mobility, stability, controlled mobility, and skill will be expanded on as currently updated in a later section of this chapter, describing a functional training approach to neurorehabilitation.

The incorporation of sensory stimulation techniques into remediation approaches is based largely on the work of Margaret Rood (Rood, 1962; O'Sullivan, 2001; Stockmeyer, 1967, 1972). Stimuli were organized into phasic and tonic categories based on the goal of the

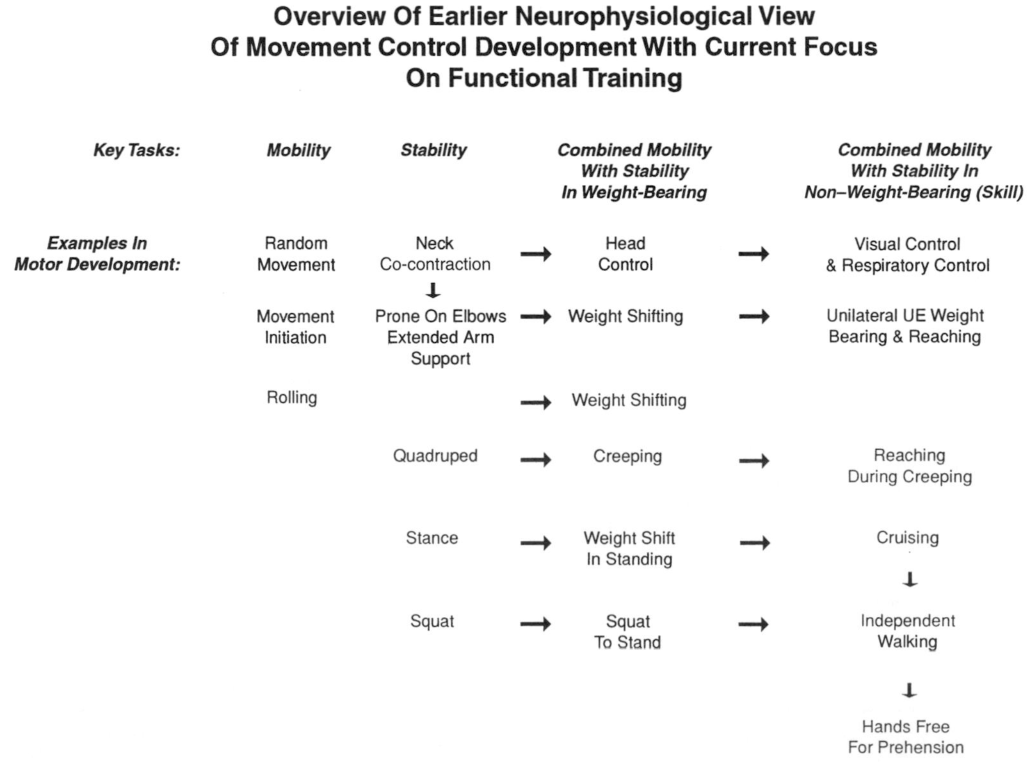

Overview Of Earlier Neurophysiological View Of Movement Control Development With Current Focus On Functional Training

Figure 6-6. Overview of earlier neurophysiological view of movement control development adapted with current focus on motor components required in functional task training. (Adapted from Farber, S. (1982). *Neurorehabilitation: A multisensory approach.* Philadelphia: W. B. Saunders.)

stimulation and the stage of motor control the patient exhibited. **Tonic stimuli,** such as approximation or resistance, were used to assist in the development of control in a stability activity such as holding in a sitting position. **Phasic stimuli**—for example, quick stretch and vibration—were used to facilitate a mobility response, such as initiating a movement or activating a muscular response. Rood used the terms **inhibitory** or **facilitory** to describe the use of stimulation to either activate or suppress a patient response.

The primacy of this neurophysiological explanation for motor control problems following brain damage was limited in its scope, resulting in inattention to other systems and important parameters of movement control, as is currently recognized. Many of the intervention techniques, however, continue to be appropriate to use within a functional framework for patients who require a more "hands-on" approach, to assist in early movement attempts. In these cases and situations, manual facilitation or inhibition techniques can be useful, as described in Table 6–1.

Clinical Connection:

Margaret Rood was undoubtedly a pioneer in the field of sensory stimulation. Although current research warrants a new look at sensory stimulation as a therapeutic modality, some useful principles can be extracted for integration into a holistic approach to a patient/client. Therapists and assistants use touch as one of the most important intervention methods available to us. The concept of therapeutic use of self (AOTA, 1994) is synonymous in intent with the use of therapeutic touch. Touch as sensory stimulation focuses on neuromuscular and physiological responses but certainly can have powerful psychosocial effects. It is commonly agreed that touch can promote bonds, attachment, and emotional well-being (McCormacke, 1996). Current research demonstrates that touch has an integrating effect on many organ systems and on homeostatic mechanisms throughout the body (Rose, 1984; Weiss, 1986). The value of touch as a therapeutic tool can never be overemphasized.

■ Brunnstrom's Movement Therapy in Hemiplegia

Movement therapy in hemiplegia, developed by Signe Brunnstrom in 1970, was designed to promote recovery in individuals who had suffered a stroke (Brunnstrom, 1970). Although the actual approach to intervention is considered outdated and inappropriate today, Brunnstrom is credited with two main contributions that are still valuable: a description of the stereotypical synergy patterns and the recovery stages of patients seen following a cerebrovascular accident (CVA). Brunnstrom carefully observed thousands of stroke survivors and meticulously recorded her observations of their movement patterns in the weeks and months following the stroke. An appreciation of this detailed observational knowledge left to us by Brunnstrom is extremely helpful to clinicians and patients today. Those observations on movement highlight the importance of the current emphasis on working toward the goal of voluntary functional control and the functional limitations experienced by patients as they work toward recovery.

A concept basic to Brunnstrom's approach is that of synergies, the linkage of muscles into functional units. Synergies, or motor patterns, are fundamental to contemporary neurological rehabilitation medicine. The concept of synergy has expanded in concert with evolving neuroscience theory, beyond Brunnstrom's early belief that synergies were organized at a spinal cord level. Neuroscientists have proven that synergistic movement patterns can result from influences both within and outside the CNS, although Brunnstrom is credited with recognizing synergies as reflective of the organizational status of the damaged CNS (VanSant, 1990). **Synergies** (Table 6–4) are patterned, recognizable flexion or extension movements of the entire limb, evoked by attempts to move or by sensory stimuli, characteristically seen during the period of recovery following a neurological incident such as a CVA (Fig. 6–7). The flexion synergy is typically stronger in the upper extremity and the extensor synergy more predominant in the lower. Repeated use of the synergies, which makes isolated motor control more difficult, is viewed now as inappropriate and undesirable. However, it is important that clinicians recognize the presence of a synergy if it dominates movement and interferes with voluntary movement attempts. Recognition of the pattern, including an understanding of the strongest components of that pattern, can offer useful information to the treating clinician and the patient, as they together attempt to solve a patient's movement dilemma. Practical training activities to stimulate out-of-synergy isolated movements are encouraged. Concepts of motor learning such as positive reinforcement and repetition are stressed (Sawner & LaVigne, 1992; Smith & Sharpe, 1994).

The stages of recovery (Table 6–5) are still used as an overall framework from which to view the patient's progression toward recovery of voluntary motor control (Martin & Kessler, 2000). There have also been attempts to correlate the stage of recovery with outcome following a stroke (Shah, Harasymiw, & Stahl, 1986). Regardless of the specific use, viewing the patient's/client's progress along a continuum of recovery guides therapists in selecting activities that can be adapted to promote the return of voluntary control.

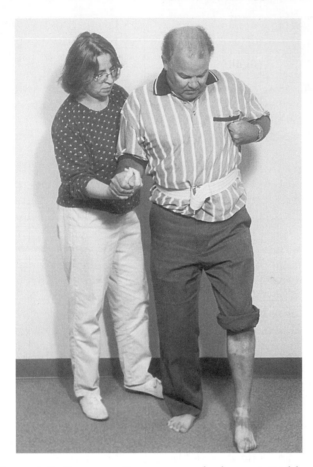

Figure 6–7. Synergy patterns commonly demonstrated by a patient after CVA, affecting both the upper and lower extremity on the left involved body side. Note predominant flexion of upper extremity and extension of lower extremity.

Clinical Connection:

Brunnstrom's observations of motor recovery and motor behaviors that accompany recovery from a CVA are valid, offering therapists an insightful tool for recognizing progression toward recovery. Some of the activities for upper and lower extremity training continue to be useful, although our current knowledge of motor control has made many of Brunnstrom's intervention ideas not only outdated but also controversial and possibly contraindicated. No one, however, minimizes her contribution to rehabilitation by her careful observational descriptions of the synergy patterns and recovery stages so universally recognized in a patient following a stroke. ■

■ *Sensory Integration*

Sensory integration, a theory founded and popularized in 1973 by Jean Ayres, is based on three main assumptions:

- Individuals receive information from their bodies and the environment, process and interpret the information within their CNS, and use the information in a functional manner.
- Individuals with difficulties in sensory processing will demonstrate problems in the planning and execution of adaptive responses.
- Individuals who receive sensory stimulation within a meaningful context will have the opportunity to integrate the sensory information, demonstrating more efficient motor skills and adaptive behaviors (Long & Toscano, 2002).

Sensory integration is a theoretical intervention frame of reference that is built around the relationship between the brain and behavior. The three main postulates of sensory integration theory are as follows:

1. Learning is dependent on the ability to take in and process sensation from movement and the environment and use it to plan and organize behavior.
2. Individuals who have a decreased ability to process sensation may also have difficulty producing appropriate actions, which in turn may interfere with learning and behavior.
3. Enhanced sensation, as a part of meaningful activity that yields an adaptive interaction, improves the ability to process sensation, thereby enhancing learning behavior (Bundy, Lane, and Murray, 2002).

When incorporating sensory integration into an intervention program, controlled sensory input may be used to help individuals to experience sensation, explore the environment, and process the sensations within a movement or learning task. Sensory stimulation activities emphasizing the tactile, proprioceptive, and vestibular systems are selected to engage the individual in a meaningful, self-directed context (Ayres, 1973; Bundy et al., 2002). Intervention activities are often directed at promoting antigravity flexion or extension, increasing proprioception and a sense of gravitational security, promoting equilibrium responses and balance, and enhancing tolerance of and integration of vestibular stimulation. In pediatrics, varying kinds of equipment, such as hammock swings, bolster swings, scooter boards, large barrels, and balls, are used to encourage antigravity postural responses, proximal stability and co-contraction strength, and balance (Figs. 6–8 and 6–9). For integration into intervention with adults, functional activities are selected that allow the individual to practice the development of sensory processing needed for successful purposeful activity. In Chapter 8, some suggested activities to improve vestibular processing and balance will be described.

Adaptive behaviors or responses are purposeful actions directed toward a goal. As such, adaptive responses are thought to be inherently organizing to the

TABLE 6-4

Synergy Patterns Seen Commonly in Patients Following Stroke

Synergy	Description	Significance in Clinical Presentation
Upper extremity (UE) flexion	Scapula retraction and/or elevation, shoulder external rotation, shoulder abduction (90°), elbow flexion, forearm supination, wrist and finger flexion	Most prevalent synergy pattern seen in the UE Strongest components are scapula retraction and elbow flexion
UE extension	Scapula protraction, shoulder internal rotation, shoulder adduction, elbow extension, forearm pronation, wrist and finger flexion	Not as common a pattern in the UE Shoulder internal rotation and adduction, forearm pronation most common components
Lower extremity (LE) flexion	Hip flexion, abduction, and external rotation; knee flexion, ankle dorsiflexion with inversion, toe extension	Prevalent pattern when the patient is in a non–weight-bearing position Strongest component is hip flexion
LE extension	Hip extension, adduction, and internal rotation; knee extension, ankle plantar flexion with inversion, toe flexion	Prevalent pattern when the patient is in upright or weight-bearing position Strongest components are knee extension and plantar flexion with inversion

Sources: Data from Brunnstrom, S. (1970). *Movement therapy in hemiplegia: A neurophysiological approach*. New York: Harper & Row; Martin, S., & Kessler, M. (2000). *Neurological intervention for physical therapist assistants*. Philadelphia: W. B. Saunders; O' Sullivan, S. B., & Schmitz, T. J. (Eds.). (2000). *Physical rehabilitation: Assessment and treatment* (4th ed.). Philadelphia: F. A. Davis; and Sawner, K., & LaVigne, J. (1992). *Brunnstrom's movement therapy in hemiplegia* (2nd ed.). New York: J. B. Lippincott.

TABLE 6-5

Stages of Recovery Following a CVA: Intervention Application

Stage	Description of Motor Control	Intervention Priority
1. Flaccid Stage	Muscle tone is flaccid; absent deep tendon reflex (DTR); no muscular contraction seen.	Ensure safe positioning of flaccid extremity. Facilitation techniques to activate muscle contraction can be effective.
2. Beginning development of spasticity	Spasticity is first evident in the strongest components of the synergy patterns, often expressed as associated reactions.	Activities and movements to encourage the re-emergence of voluntary motor control, especially shoulder stability, elbow extension with wrist and finger extension; lower extremity stability with extensor control in stance.
3. Spasticity	Passive posturing and voluntary movements predominated by synergy patterns; limited voluntary movement out of the synergy pattern.	Increase voluntary movements, focusing on movement components essential to present functional needs: elbow extension to assist with transferring, scapular protraction to assist with forward reach; lower extremity protraction and extension to support upright mobility.
4. Spasticity begins to decline; voluntary control begins to emerge	Some isolated voluntary movement out of synergy patterns begins to emerge. Some limited combinations of movement may be evident.	Expand on voluntary movement, including strengthening of functional movements.
5. Spasticity continues to decrease and voluntary control improves	Voluntary movement is returning with less dominance from synergy patterns. Combinations of movements become increasingly evident.	As motor control improves, isolated voluntary control and muscle strength increase.
6. Minimal spasticity, good voluntary control	Isolated movements are evident. Difficulties with coordination and timing errors may accompany rapid movements, stress, and fatigue.	Focus on advanced functional retraining.
7. Normal muscle tone	Return of fine motor skills, coordination, and dexterity.	Full return to premorbid motor activities.

Sources: Data from Brunnstrom, S. (1970). *Movement therapy in hemiplegia: A neurophysiological approach*. New York: Harper & Row; Martin, S., & Kessler, M. (2000). *Neurological intervention for physical therapist assistants*. Philadelphia: W. B. Saunders; O' Sullivan, S. B., & Schmitz, T. J. (Eds.). (2000). *Physical rehabilitation: Assessment and treatment* (4th ed.). Philadelphia: F. A. Davis; and Sawner, K., & LaVigne, J. (1992). *Brunnstrom's movement therapy in hemiplegia* (2nd ed.). New York: J. B. Lippincott.

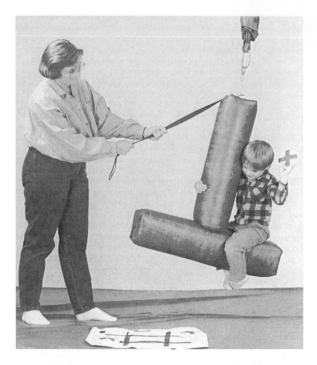

Figure 6–8. Use of т swing in sensory integration therapy approach, integrated into a playful activity. (From Bundy, A. C., Lane, S. J., & Murray, E. A. [2002]. *Sensory integration: Theory and practice* [2nd ed., p. 254]. Philadelphia: F. A. Davis.)

brain (Reeves, 2001). Ayres always advocated for active participation of the individual and emphasized that the patient/client and not the therapist should initiate the "doing." SI is not an approach by which practitioners do something to the patient; rather, the clinician observes how the individual responds to cues, interacts with people and the environment, and adapts to the environment as the demands change (Ayres, 1973; Bundy et al., 2002; Reeves, 2001). The person's involvement in the task is paramount to success. According to an article in a recent *Sensory Integration* newsletter, published by the AOTA, "The therapist or assistant

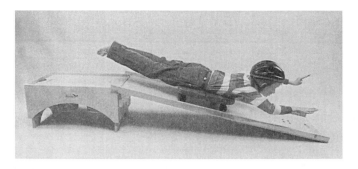

Figure 6–9. Use of scooter board and ramp in sensory integration therapy approach. (From Fisher, A. G., Murray, E. A., & Bundy, A. C. [1991]. *Sensory integration: Theory and practice* [1st ed., p. 260]. Philadelphia: F. A. Davis.)

structures the materials, the setting, and the task to facilitate specific adaptive responses. Therapists who employ a sensory integrative approach create an environment that entices clients to attempt new challenges, adapting in new ways, and building more sophisticated skills" (Reeves, 2001, p. 3).

Task-Oriented Models

▪ Background

A more contemporary frame of reference for intervention is described in a task-oriented model or intervention approach. Because movement is normally goal directed, functional tasks are thought to be a natural way to achieve or promote motor control. The task-oriented model is based on the idea that the movement system must solve problems to accomplish motor tasks (Horak, 1991). This model assumes that movement control is organized around goal-directed functional behaviors rather than specific muscles or movement patterns. Recognizing that tasks can be accomplished in more than one way, individuals are encouraged to actively problem solve and to learn alternative movement patterns that can then be used in a variety of environments. The clinician's role is to provide feedback while manipulating environmental and musculoskeletal demands to help promote the emergence of smooth and efficient functional behaviors (Horak, 1991; Poole, 1997). As discussed previously when describing degrees of freedom, movement execution can be accomplished or modified by controlling the degrees of freedom, sometimes as offered by the underlying impairment (limited range of motion) or as offered by a support (thorough postural support, manual support, or equipment). Assumptions underlying a task-oriented approach can be summarized as follows:

- Normal, functional movement emerges as an interaction among many systems, each contributing its own aspect of control.
- Movement is organized around a behavioral goal, constrained by the environment.
- Movement problems, as demonstrated in abnormal motor control, result from impairments within one or more of the systems controlling movement. The movement that is observed in the individual with neurological dysfunction emerges from the best mix of the systems remaining and able to participate in movement production. This means that the movement patterns that are observed are not just a result of the lesion itself, but also are the result of the efforts of the remaining systems to compensate for the damage and continue to be functional. The compensatory strategy developed by the individual may or

may not be optimal and efficient (Shumway-Cook & Woollacott, 2001).

These assumptions suggest that when training movement control, it is essential to work on identifiable functional tasks rather than on movement patterns for movement's sake alone. A task-oriented approach to intervention assumes that individuals learn by attempting to solve the problems inherent in a functional task rather than by repetitively practicing "normal" patterns of movement. Individuals are then guided in learning a variety of ways to solve the task goal so that the carry-over between different environmental contexts can occur (Flinn, 1995).

■ Task Analysis

A task-oriented approach uses a multifaceted approach to the clinical management of the individual with movement control problems. To apply this approach, a method for task analysis is necessary. What is the best way to analyze movement behavior? Gentile (1992) has suggested that goal-directed functional behavior can be analyzed at three levels: action, movements, and the neuromotor process.

Analysis at the Action Level. An analysis at the action level simply examines the behavioral outcome that results from the interaction of the individual, the task, and the environment. At this level, motor learning may be suggested by the accomplishment of a new task, the accomplishment of a task through an increased variety of movement patterns or strategies, or the performance of a task in a more efficient or consistent fashion (Majsak, 1996). Motor learning at the action level is reflected not only in the motor production and movement patterns of the performer but also in the ability of the performer to execute specific tasks in distinct and varied environments. For example, analysis of the functional behavior of getting out of bed at the action level answers the outcome question, "Was the patient able to get out of bed?"

Analysis at the Movement Level. This second level of analysis focuses on analyzing the movements used to perform the functional task. At this level, motor learning may be evident by the performance of new patterns of movement or changes in the kinematics of a movement. In the same example, the movement strategy and pattern used by the individual to get out of bed would be described.

Analysis at the Neuromotor Level. Finally, the functional task is analyzed from the perspective of the underlying processes that contribute to the movement being performed. Remembering that functional movement emerges through the interaction of many sub-systems, the contributions from each need to be recognized and described. At the neuromotor level, motor learning may be suggested by increased responsiveness of a cell to fire or changes in motor unit activation following repetition of motor acts (Majsak, 1996). The contributions from the individual's sensory systems, perceptual and cognitive systems, musculoskeletal system, and nervous system would all be examined in terms of their contribution to the execution of the functional task—in this case, getting out of bed.

The relationship between these three levels of analysis is not one to one. Instead, many movements can be used to achieve an action goal. Similarly, neuromotor processes can be organized in many ways to have a particular movement emerge. Changes at the neuromotor processes and movement levels may not necessarily be reflected in changes in behavior at the action level. The relationship among these three levels of analysis can rather be pictured as many to one. This relationship between movement patterns and the action goal has been referred to as **movement equivalence** (Gentile, 2000). For example, consider the many movements you could use to throw an object at a target: underhand, overhand, or sidearm. Any one of those movement patterns could produce the same outcome of hitting the target. You, however, probably prefer one, if you are free of constraints and have all the choices available to you. In a similar fashion, one particular movement pattern is not reduced to a fixed mode of organization within the CNS. Neuromotor processes are organized dynamically, in flexible ways, to yield similar movement patterns (Gentile, 2000).

Clinical Connection:

It is important to remember the individual nature of functional task solution. In the example of getting out of bed, there are multiple solutions and strategies that could be effectively used to get out of bed. Try this by observing different individuals within different environments, with different types of beds, and see how many different styles of getting out of bed are observable. It is important to remember that skilled movement behavior is defined by the ability to *adapt* the movements used to achieve the goal of the task consistently and efficiently across a variety of environments. You certainly wouldn't be considered functionally independent if you could only get out of one type of bed or out of a bed oriented in only one way in a room! ■

Shumway-Cook and Woollacott (2001) have adapted Gentile's method for task analysis to an approach readily applicable to physical and occupational therapy intervention. The goal of retraining at the functional task level focuses on having patients successfully practice the performance of a wide collection of functional tasks in a variety of contexts. For example, the ability to perform postural tasks in a natural environment requires that the patient modify strategies to changing task and environment demands. This could include the following:

1. Maintaining balance with a reduced base of support
2. Maintaining balance while changing the orientation of the head and trunk (i.e., leaning over, turning around, maintaining balance while performing a variety of upper extremity tasks)

All tasks require postural control; however, the stability and orientation requirements will vary with the task and the environment. As applied to ambulation, retraining at the functional task level focuses on having patients practice walking in a variety of contexts, which includes different environments and while executing simultaneous demands. Yes, it *is* functional to be able to walk and chew gum at the same time!

A task-oriented approach to establishing a comprehensive plan of care includes intervention strategies designed to achieve the following goals derived from assessment along a model of disablement view: to resolve or prevent impairments, to develop effective task-specific strategies and remediate within that framework, and to retrain functional goal-oriented tasks. These goals and the intervention of the patient/client to achieve these goals are not approached in a set sequence, but rather in parallel. Thus, a clinician may utilize techniques designed to focus on one or more of the aforementioned goals within the same therapy session in whatever order is most appropriate. Choosing a meaningful functional task for the individual is crucial to the success of this approach.

Clinical Connection:

When selecting a functional activity, ask the following questions:
- Is the activity meaningful to this individual?
- Does this person see the purpose of the activity?
- Does this activity require active participation and problem solving? ▪

This task-oriented approach looks at and treats motor behavior by focusing on three levels: functional abilities, a description of the strategies used to accomplish functional skills, and recognition of the underlying impairments that constrain the functional movement. Intervention can be targeted at all three levels. This approach can integrate within it the use of functional training, sensorimotor techniques when appropriate, and motor learning. Table 6–6 offers a helpful, concise worksheet for clinicians to use during task analysis. The specifics within that table are elaborated on in the following section.

▪ Functional Abilities According to a Task-Oriented Approach

Analysis of patient performance on the functional level focuses on the ability of the individual to perform essential tasks and activities. Functional status can be examined and evaluated using a number of assessment tools. It is beyond the scope of this text to discuss the various occupational therapy and physical therapy evaluation procedures and tools. Evaluation and assessment guidelines for practitioners in both disciplines are detailed in other sources. As part of any rehabilitation plan, assessment and documentation of the individual's functional status is an important starting point.

▪ Strategies Used to Perform Functional Tasks

Examination at the strategy level is actually a qualitative approach to measuring function. The term **strategy** refers not only to a description of the movement pattern used to accomplish the task, but also includes how an individual appears to organize the motor, sensory, and perceptual information necessary to performing a task in different environments. The strategies employed by the individual are a large determinant of the level of performance. The strategies that are used relate the demands of the task to the individual's capacity to perform the task.

Clinical Connection:

For example, if we choose poor strategies and the task is difficult, we may reach the limits of our capacities well before we have met the demands of the task. On the other hand, if the task is simple and less demanding, inefficient strategies may be sufficient to meeting the demand. Imagine attempting to use a potter's wheel for the first time. Imagine using a precarious sitting posture, in a poorly lit room, with excessively long fingernails interfering with manipulation skills. With such poor strategy choices in your attempt of such a difficult task, it would not be long before you would meet the limit of your capabilities and fail miserably. You would become exhausted because of the inefficiency of your movements. On the other hand, if you are engaged in the easy and familiar task of drying dishes (for the hundredth time!), you would still be successful sitting precariously on a stool, in a dark room, and even with those fingernails. ▪

TABLE 6–6

A Clinical Strategy for Using Task Analysis in Patient Instruction and Observation

Step	Main Decision/Action	Key Aspects
Step 1	Identify task.	Specify goal and subgoals. Gather critical information about: • Environment • Individual mover • Prerequisite skills needed • Expectations of outcome
Step 2	Develop a strategy to teach or observe task.	Develop strategy to make up for deficits identified in previous step. Plan any intervention strategy to optimize the individual-task-environment interaction.
Step 3	Effect the strategy and analyze the task.	Observe the performance of the individual. Make any appropriate comparison. Analyze. Record what happened: • What was the outcome of the attempt? • What was the approach? • What was the effect of the movement solution?
Step 4	Practice.	Identify missing components: • Explanation: clear goal identification • Instruction • Feedback • Manual guidance • Ongoing re-evaluation Encourage flexibility.
Step 5	Evaluate observations.	Compare expectations with outcome. Provide feedback and assist learner in generating plan for next attempt.
Step 6	Transfer training.	Give opportunity to practice in varying context. Offer consistency and variability of practice. Assist organization of self-monitored practice. Involve caregivers, relatives, and staff.

Sources: Adapted from Arend, S., & Higgins, J. R (1976). A strategy for the classification, subjective analysis, and observation of human movement. *Journal of Human Movement Studies,* 2, 36–52; Craik, R. L., & Oatis, C. A. (1995). *Gait analysis: Theory and application.* Philadelphia: Mosby; and Bennett, S. E., & Karnes, J. L. (1998). *Neurological disabilities: Assessment and treatment.* Philadelphia: Lippincott-Raven.

For the patient/client with neurological dysfunction, as capacity to perform a task declines, the demands may not be able to be met without the development of alternative strategies. Thus, in the individual with a neurological deficit, maintaining functional independence depends on the capacity of the individual to meet the demands of a task in a particular environment. When impairments limit the capacity to use well-learned and familiar strategies, the patient must learn new ways (strategies) to accomplish functional tasks despite these limitations.

The goal of treating at the strategy level involves helping patients to recover or develop sensory and motor strategies that are effective in meeting the functional demands of the task. There is limited information available defining the sensory, motor, and cognitive strategies used by individuals who are neurologically intact, and even less available on the compensatory strategies that develop as a result of neurological impairment. Today's clinicians are literally at the cutting edge of such practice-centered knowledge. The following sections summarize the current level of knowledge available from leaders in the field regarding how individuals use common strategies during the execution of functional movement (Carr & Shepherd, 1998; O'Sullivan & Schmitz, 2001; Palmer & Toms, 1992; Ryerson & Levit, 1997; Shumway-Cook & Woollacott, 2001).

▪ Typical Movement Performance Strategies

Some recognized movement performance strategies observed in the execution of functional tasks include, but are not limited to, the following. Examples of how a clinician would treat at the strategy level are also provided.

- Alignment: The goal when retraining alignment is to help the patient develop an initial position that:
  1. Is appropriate for the task.
  2. Is efficient with respect to gravity—that is, with minimal muscle activity for maintaining the position.
  3. Maximizes stability.
- A number of approaches and therapeutic tools are available, including verbal feedback, mirrors, biofeedback, and manual cues (Fig. 6–10).
- Movement strategies: The goal when retraining movement strategies involves helping the patient develop multijoint coordinated movements that are effective in meeting the demands of the specific task. Optimal function is characterized by strategies that are efficient in accomplishing a task goal in a relevant environment. Retraining strategies involve both the recovery of motor strategies and the development of compensatory strategies. Examples of retraining movement strategies include helping the patient develop appropriate muscular activation strategies and the intervention with timing, coordination, or force production problems that interfere with movement.
- Sensory strategies: The goal when retraining sensory strategies is to help the patient/client to learn to effectively use sensory information to meet task demands. This necessitates correctly interpreting the position and movements of the body in space. Intervention strategies generally require the patient to maintain balance during progressively more difficult static and dynamic movement tasks while the clinician varies the availability and accuracy of one or more of the senses. Balance training is a form of treating at a sensory strategy level, to be expanded on in Chapter 8.
- Phase-by-phase gait training: The goal of retraining gait at the strategy level is to assist the patient in developing movement strategies that are effective in meeting the inherent demands of the stance and swing phases of gait. This enables the patient/client to develop strategies necessary for stability, progression, and adaptation. A task-oriented approach to gait analysis, focusing on the functional demands of gait, will assist the clinician in developing effective, meaningful intervention ideas, to be expanded on in Chapter 10. Within a task-oriented approach, pre-ambulation skills would include functional mobility tasks that directly affect specific portions of locomotor strategies (Fig. 6–11). The use of an assistive device is a common clinical example of a compensatory gait-training strategy, used to contribute to a patient's stability by widening the base of support and providing additional support against gravity (Fig. 6–12).

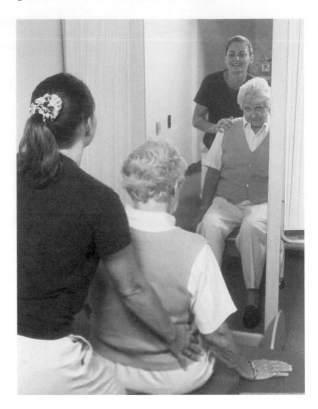

Figure 6–10. Use of verbal feedback, physical guidance, and visual cues in retraining alignment.

▪ Compensatory Strategies

Compensation is defined as a behavioral substitution where alternative behavioral strategies are adopted to accomplish a task. It is important to differentiate between recovery and compensation. **Recovery** is the achievement of function through original processes, whereas compensation is achieving function through alternative processes. Function returns, but not in its original premorbid form (Ryerson & Levit, 1997).

Compensatory strategies are alternative movement strategies that replace typical movement patterns when age-related changes or impairment prevent the use of the typical patterns of coordination. The contemporary perspective is that compensatory strategies are developed by the individual in an attempt to control all the elements that are free to vary and use the remaining systems to compensate to achieve functional goals. These patterns may or may not be optimal for a given task in its context given the individual's capabilities and limitations.

Ryerson and Levit (1997) differentiate between two categories of compensation: appropriate compensations and undesirable compensations. **Appropriate compensations** use movement patterns that resemble normal movements and incorporate the involved and uninvolved body segments into the movement pattern. The

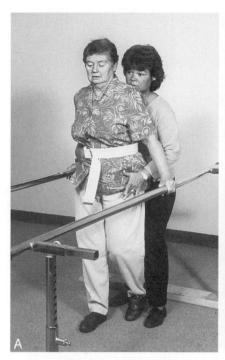

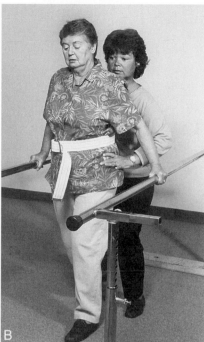

Figure 6–11. Pre-ambulation skill training. For example, focus can be directed (A) at activating hip flexion at the initiation of swing phase or (B) to acceptance of weight shift onto the forward limb on initial contact.

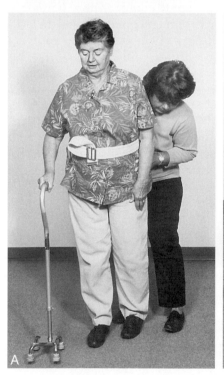

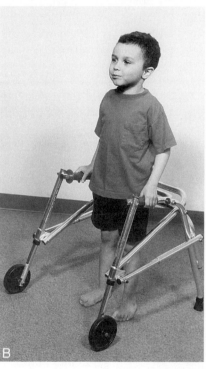

Figure 6–12. An assistive device can increase a patient's stability by widening the base of support and providing assistance against gravity, shown here (A) for an adult and (B) for a child.

purpose of these compensations is to decrease postural asymmetries and neglect while using the potential for unimpaired movement from the intact body segments. Appropriate compensations may also include the changes in strategy that necessarily accompany age-related changes in any of the movement subsystems, such as a change in the way an older adult rises from the floor as compared with an infant, a child, or a younger adult. Appropriate compensations incorporate the indi-vidual's active movement patterns into functional performance (Fig. 6–13). **Undesirable compensations** promote asymmetries and poor alignment in the trunk and limbs, decreased weight acceptance, and lead to inefficient or unsafe movement production. Undesirable compensations often lead to secondary impairments, such as range-of-motion limitations or joint instability. They do not utilize the individual's available movement patterns and work in opposition to

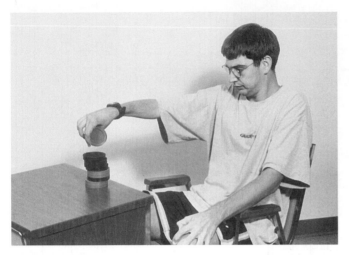

Figure 6–13. Patient effectively increases his postural stability and task execution using an appropriate compensation stabilization holding pattern of the left upper extremity.

the overall goal of optimal independent functional movement (Fig. 6–14).

Most individuals with CNS dysfunction will not fully recover from their impairments and will not attain or regain completely normal movement patterns. Most

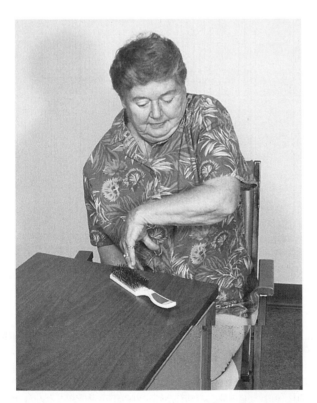

Figure 6–14. Patient demonstrating undesirable compensation such as scapular elevator on left, which further impairs reach, and lateral trunk flexion and shortening on right, which impairs postural stability, with subsequent difficulty in task execution.

individuals with residual movement system deficits must learn compensatory strategies to accomplish the tasks of daily living. The focus of a compensatory training approach is on the early resumption of functional independence using the preserved movement abilities for function. Central to this approach is the concept of substitution. The patient/client is first assisted to develop a cognitive awareness of the movement deficiencies. Changes are then made in the individual's overall approach to functional tasks. This type of compensatory training is the counterpart to movement re-education, which seeks to restore what used to be. Compensatory training attempts to allow the individual to regain independence using strategies that make use of existing patterns of muscle control but that substitute for movement deficits. There are great differences in the quality of movement, functional independence, and feelings of well-being and self-efficacy between individuals who are taught to compensate for their impairments by using only their uninvolved body segments and individuals who learn to move and function with the best remaining capabilities of *all* body segments. A second cornerstone concept to compensatory training is modification of the environment, or adaptation, to facilitate relearning of skills, ease of movement, and optimal performance.

Clinical Connection:

Examples of compensatory training are prevalent throughout rehabilitation experiences: the individual with a right hemiplegia learning to eat or write with the left hand, a patient with spinal cord injury regaining independent mobility through the achievement of wheelchair independence, or the child with cerebral palsy playing independently in an adapted playground using unimpaired upper extremities to self-propel an adapted swing. ▪

There are two main criticisms to the use of the compensatory training approach. Focus on the uninvolved body segments may suppress recovery and contribute to learned unuse of the impaired body segments (Taub, 1976). Focus on task-specific learning may also lead to the development of **splinter skills,** skills that cannot be generalized to other environments or to variations of the same task. However, a compensatory training approach may be the most appropriate strategy chosen by a therapist when an individual presents with severe impairments and functional limitations with little expectation of further recovery. Clinicians are encouraged to combine approaches and offer clients multiple opportunities for practice in natural, varying environments.

▪ Age-Related Strategy Changes

Age-related changes to movement strategies in healthy adults may contribute to slowed movement and changes in the pattern of the movement, due to some of the musculoskeletal changes that accompany normal aging. For example, an older adult may not only roll slower but may demonstrate more of a log roll rather than a segmental roll, due to back pain or reduced range of motion (ROM) limiting the ability to segmentalize the rolling pattern. Transitions from a supine position to sitting and sitting to standing may also be characterized by increased reliance on upper extremities and a return to asymmetrical movement patterns secondary to trunk and lower extremity weakness and proprioceptive loss experienced by older adults (Fig. 6–15). Changes in gait patterns in the older adult are well described (see Chapters 3, 4, and 10).

Clinical Connection:

An individual may present in a rehabilitation setting with a combination of compensatory strategies. An individual who is 82 years old may have developed compensatory strategies related to the normal developmental aging process of the musculoskeletal system before he suffered a stroke. The therapist and assistant must distinguish between the age-related appropriate compensatory changes that are a result of the aging process and those that have been caused by the neurological insult.

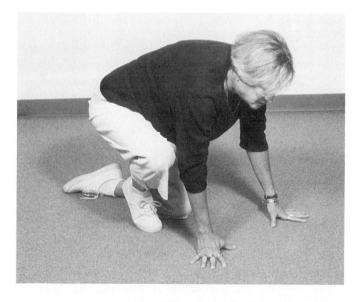

Figure 6–15. Older adult demonstrating increased reliance on upper extremities and asymmetrical movement pattern.

▪ Constraining Impairments

Intervention efforts can also be directed to reduce or eliminate the effect of impairments. The goal of interventions aimed at the impairment level is to identify those impairments that potentially constrain functional movement skills, correct those impairments that can be changed, and prevent the development of secondary impairments. Contributing constraining impairments can present from any one or combinations of limitations in any one of the systems contributing to movement production, as well as multisystem impairments of posture, balance, and gait. The motor system may be confounded by neuromuscular or musculoskeletal impairments. Numerous neuromuscular limitations lead to instability in the patient with a neurological deficit. Sensory and perceptual capabilities and limitations also need to be recognized. Because task-specific movement is performed within the context of intention and motivation, cognitive aspects of motor control, including mental status, attention, motivation, and emotional considerations, must be examined and included in the clinical picture. Impaired cognitive status or a perceptual deficit such as a visual spatial disorder can offer significant constraints to either initiating or planning a movement or movement execution (Shumway-Cook & Woollacott, 2001). Examples of commonly encountered impairments seen in neurological rehabilitation are described in Chapter 2 and listed in Table 6–7. Clinical management of these commonly encountered impairments and their functional limitations are described in detail in Chapters 7 through 10.

▪ Clinical Application of Task-Oriented Model

The following intervention principles summarize an application of the task-oriented approach (Davis & Burton, 1991; Duncan & Badke, 1987; Montgomery & Connolly, 1991; Haugen & Mathiowetz, 1995):

- Collaborate with the individual in identifying problematic tasks of interest and importance.
- An important focus of intervention is prioritizing meaningful occupation, as selected by the individual patient/client.
- Encourage an active learning process by allowing the person to discover and experiment with various movements that can be used to optimally perform a task.
- Analyze the preferred movements for task performance and outcome.
- Perturb (disturb) dysfunctional movement patterns by manipulating a critical element of the movement—a personal or environmental factor.

TABLE 6-7

Summary of Common Neurological Impairments

Motor System Primary Impairments	Sensory Impairments	Cognitive/Perceptual Impairments
Muscle weakness	Somatosensory deficits	Perceptual impairments 1. Disorders of body image/scheme 2. Apraxia 3. Spatial relation disorders

Abnormalities of muscle tone
1. Hypertonicity
   Spasticity
   Rigidity
2. Hypotonia
	Visual deficits	Cognitive impairments
		1. Attention deficits
		2. Difficulty with arousal/level of consciousness
		3. Problems with orientation
		4. Memory deficits
		5. Difficulty with problem solving

Coordination problems 1. Activation/sequencing problems 2. Timing problems 3. Problems with scaling forces	Vestibular dysfunction	
Involuntary movements 1. Dystonia 2. Associated movements 3. Tremor 4. Athetoid and choreiform movements		

Sources: From Shumway-Cook, A., & Wollacott, M. J. (2001). *Motor control: Theory and practical applications* (2nd ed.). Baltimore: Lippincott Williams & Wilkins.

- Record the observed changes in the preferred movements for task performance and outcomes.
- Grade the therapist's manipulations of critical elements until the movements approximate an efficient and effective pattern.
- Vary the practice conditions to facilitate learning and flexible task performance.

The goals of a therapist or assistant who uses the task-oriented approach are to assist the individual to do the following (Davis & Burton, 1991; Duncan & Badke, 1987; Haugen & Mathiowetz, 1995; Montgomery & Connolly, 1991):

- Discover the optimal movement patterns for performing a task.
- Achieve flexibility in task performance by providing practice opportunities with varying contexts.
- Maximize the use of personal characteristics and environmental factors that make efficient and effective task performance possible.
- Facilitate problem solving by the individual so that the individual can identify his or her solutions to motor problems in home and community activities.

Functional Training Approach

■ Definition, Evolution, and Description

Functional training, as an intervention approach, has developed from a practical application of motor control and motor learning knowledge, therapeutic exercise application, motor development, and a task-oriented approach to movement re-education. **Functional training** in the purest sense is a method of retraining the movement system using repetitive practice of functional tasks in an attempt to establish or re-establish the individual's ability to perform activities of daily living (Umphred, Byl, Lazaro, & Roller, 2001). Functional training focuses on using a variety of different motor skills necessary for everyday life, including transitions between and within postures; skills needed for activities of daily living, such as reaching, lifting, and turning; skills necessary for instrumental activities of daily living, such as performing simple home repair; and skills needed for engaging in meaningful hobbies and valuable work. It also focuses on showing each individual how to adapt different movements in order to respond to changing environmental demands (O'Sullivan, 2001). Functional training can be implemented once the clinician has identified the individual's functional limitations. Guided by the question "What tasks, of value to the patient/client, can he or she do and not do?" identified functional tasks can be performed and practiced. It is essential that the choice of functional task goals be centered on the activities that are meaningful and valuable to the individual patient/client. Occupation in meaningful activity is the cornerstone of wellness.

The main focus on functional training is the correction of functional limitations. A **functional limitation** is a restriction of the ability to perform, at the level of the whole person, a physical action, activity, or task in an efficient, typically expected, or competent manner (AOTA, 1994, 1999; APTA, 2001). The clinician identifies and emphasizes the patient's strengths, building on what the individual can already do. These strengths and capabilities are used to efficiently and effectively achieve functional change. A crucial next step is the prioritizing of what systems or activities the patient really needs to change and choosing the activities to emphasize during functional training. Although several skills may be learned by training the skills simultaneously, it is important to concentrate on the safe performance of a few carefully selected functional tasks. In an attempt to help individuals achieve their potential for movement and function, intervention is directed toward the primary and secondary impairments, movement problems, and the functional limitations that contribute to disability.

For patients with neurological disorders, this intervention process is threefold: movement re-education, elimination or reduction of impairments, and functional training (Ryerson & Levit, 1997). The goal of movement re-education is to increase the individual's ability to move independently in normal or typical patterns and to use those movement patterns in functional activities. Movement re-education is the part of intervention that is directed toward the primary impairments of muscular weakness, changes in muscle tone and patterns of muscle activation, perceptual impairments, and impairments of the sensory systems. This part of therapy is designed to minimize movement deficits and train patterns of movement that will be used to decrease functional limitations and compensations. The individual is directed toward using existing strength and coordination and funneling those capabilities into sequences of muscle activation. The therapist builds on the component building blocks of strength and coordination, teaching the individual to develop coordinated patterns of movement sequences. This approach also encourages that whenever possible, movement should be trained in the position where it will be used for function

(Fig. 6–16). Movement re-education includes sensory education, assisted practice, independent movement, and functional movement re-education including practice (Ryerson & Levit, 1997). Impairments are addressed using standard physical therapy and occupational therapy intervention approaches.

Activities incorporating task-oriented training are more motivating and goal directed for the individual. The most contemporary approach combines functional activities into task-oriented training. This approach integrates dynamic systems theory with motor learning theory. It is based on the theory that the systems within the CNS are organized primarily to control function (Reed, 1982). Its central theme is that the interacting subsystems contributing to the production of movement are organized around essential functional movement tasks and the environment within which the task is performed. Its emphasis is on the use of functional tasks and contexts in intervention, drawing from a systems model of motor control.

To understand the salient concepts from this approach, it is essential to understand tasks, the essential elements of a task, and the contribution of environment to task execution. This approach selects several basic functional tasks, including sitting up and sitting down, balanced sitting, rolling, standing up, balanced

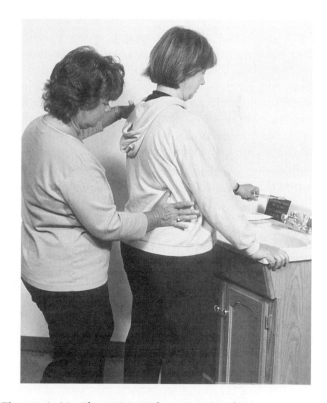

Figure 6–16. Therapist and patient working on postural control, trunk strength, and weight shifting through the upper extremities while engaging in a functional task.

standing, walking, and upper limb activities such as reach and grasp. The practice of these tasks may involve task-specific training or compensatory training. Task-specific training includes either part or whole practice, depending on the complexity of the task and the individual's capabilities.

There are several texts available that describe this approach to functional retraining for persons with a neurological impairment (Carr & Shepherd, 1987, 1998; Palmer & Toms, 1992; Ryerson & Levit, 1997). In its original form, Carr and Shepherd presented functional training to the clinical community in 1987, calling this approach the motor relearning program (MRP). At its inception, it attempted to address the limitations of the NDT approach in response to the new ideas available in motor learning and behavioral literature (Mathiowetz & Haugen, 1994). According to the MRP approach, movements should be goal directed and related to the environment to maximize recovery of function. The four steps universally accepted as central to MRP are as follows (Carr & Shepherd, 1987, 1998; Palmer & Toms, 1992; Ryerson & Levit, 1997):

1. Analysis of the task and individual performance
2. Practice of difficult or poorly performed components
3. Practice of the entire task
4. Transfer of the training into varied environmental situations

The clinician is a facilitator, keeping physically guided movements to a minimum, so that the individual is encouraged and supported to be an active participant in solving his or her unique movement problems. This approach offers an insightful perspective on motor education and re-education, offering specific suggestions on how to break down common functional movement tasks into component parts.

On a practical note, individuals with deficits in movement control present with both unique and variable patterns of functional limitations. Underlying impairments (presence of and significance of) must be linked to functional performance. Functional limitations may vary by the task, the environment, and the individual. A conceptual framework for intervention allows different postures, activities, and intervention techniques to be classified according to function. The terms *mobility, stability, controlled mobility,* and *skill,* originally used by the early neurophysiology theorist Margaret Rood, can be easily applied in a functional training intervention framework.

O'Sullivan and Schmitz (2001) have updated these original concepts into an approach that facilitates skill development through functional mobility training, using these commonly accepted motor control goals of mobility, stability, controlled mobility, and skill. It is now known that postural stability and mobility are not absolute and antagonistic functions. Functional movement requires that the *relative distribution* of stability and mobility be continuously adapted and changed. The most stable body part or segment needs some component of mobility for dynamic stability, and the most mobile body part needs some component of stability for the smooth grading of movement (Tscharnuter, 1993). Functional movement reflects this intricate relationship between mobility and stability. Intervention suggestions include progression through more difficult postures and activities, and intervention techniques are used to assist with movement as active voluntary control emerges. In a functional training approach and in functional mobility training, the therapist or assistant guides the patient/client in performing and practicing tasks that are relevant and important for optimal functional performance for that individual. This framework offers the clinician not only a practical starting point from which to start intervention but also a "user-friendly" framework within which to visualize and plan progression. The following sections, modified from material in O'Sullivan & Schmitz (2001), describe some clinical concepts and suggested techniques useful for functional mobility training as appropriate for individuals with neurological dysfunction.

■ *Strategies to Improve Mobility*

Initial **mobility** is characterized by the ability to move into a posture. Patients/clients with problems in initial mobility may demonstrate the following:

1. Poorly controlled movements that deteriorate as the demands for antigravity control and multiple body segments increase
2. May be too stiff to move as a result of abnormally high muscle tone (rigidity or spasticity)
3. May demonstrate impairments in flexibility such as contracture or limited active range
4. Decreased desire to move

The first step in clinical problem solving is for the therapist to discern the reason for the demonstrated lack of initial mobility. If the impaired mobility is due to limited ROM or muscle tone abnormalities, selected activities to ameliorate that impairment are indicated. If the difficulty is due to poor antigravity and multiple body segment control, postures and activities that minimize the demands for postural control should be attempted first, those ensuring the patient a wide base of support (BOS) and a low center of gravity (COG) (Fig. 6–17). Some patients may demonstrate decreased mobility due to weakness or decreased responsiveness. Activities to increase strength or to improve responsiveness and movement initiation would then be indicated (Fig. 6–18).

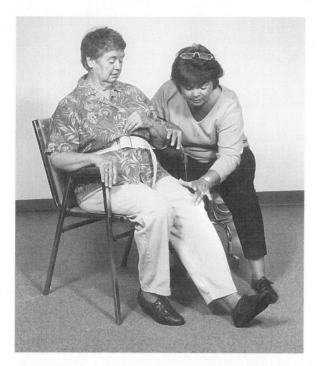

Figure 6–17. For the patient with poor antigravity control and multiple impairments, initial activities can be practiced in a position where the BOS is wider and the COG is lower. In this example, the patient can focus on understanding the concept of adequate knee extension as required for terminal stance as an intermediate step on working in upright.

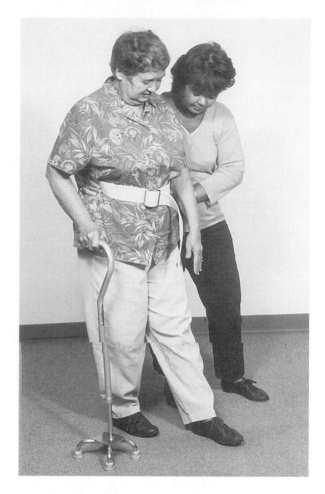

Figure 6–18. Practice achieving terminal knee extension can be practiced in upright, requiring increasing strength and movement initiation.

Facilitation techniques that activate and enhance initial muscle contraction, as described in Table 6–1, may be appropriate. These techniques should be viewed as a temporary bridge to voluntary control, withdrawn as soon as active control begins to emerge (O'Sullivan, 2001). The patient's initial movement attempts can be assisted and guided (Fig. 6–19). Equally important is that the therapist or assistant know when to offer guidance and when to withdraw it. Appropriate manual contacts can be used to enhance and support active movement attempts. PNF can be a very effective technique during this time, including the use of selective irradiation to activate muscular contraction (see Figs. 6–1 and 6–2). Continued practice of functional movements will serve to then strengthen the neuromuscular system, promoting integration, association, and enhanced motor learning.

▪ Strategies to Improve Stability

Stability or static postural control is characterized by the ability to maintain a stable posture, attained through muscular co-contraction to ensure the maintenance of upright posture. Stability is developed in weight-bearing postures. Patients who demonstrate problems

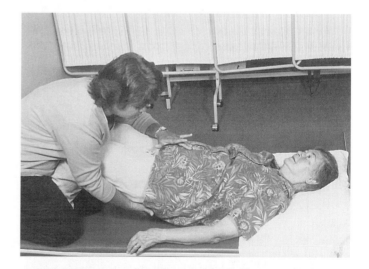

Figure 6–19. Patient's initial attempts at scooting in bed are facilitated by therapist who manually assists with pelvic control and lifting during bridging.

with stability control may demonstrate this functional impairment for a number of reasons:

1. Abnormal muscle tone or tonal imbalance around a joint or body segment
2. Decreased strength
3. Impaired voluntary control and too much random mobility
4. Hypersensitivity or heightened arousal

Effective strategies to enhance stability control include the facilitation techniques described as approximation and resistance (see Fig. 6–4A); activities to enhance proximal stability (Fig. 6–20); isometrics; rhythmic stabilization; weight-bearing activities (see Figs. 6–3, 6–16, and 6–20, including the use of developmental sequence positions [Table 4–2]); and aquatic therapy.

▪ Strategies to Improve Controlled Mobility

The ability to move while maintaining a stable upright posture is referred to as dynamic stability, or **controlled**

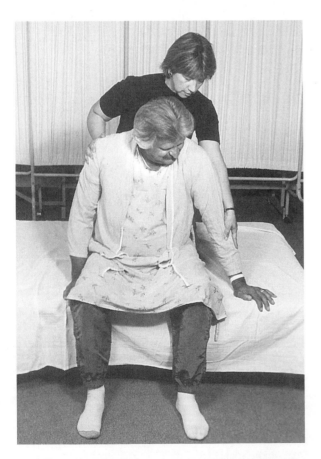

Figure 6–20. Therapist uses manual techniques to increase postural control and proximal shoulder stability: approximation through right shoulder to stabilize right upper extremity; approximation and weight bearing through left upper extremity; rhythmic stabilization and isometrics to activate postural stabilizers, all enhanced by visual and verbal feedback.

mobility. According to O'Sullivan (2001), controlled mobility represents the combined function of both mobilizing and stabilizing muscles, characterized by smooth coordinated movements with appropriate synergistic stabilization. Movement can be easily reversed, demonstrating effective interplay between antagonists. Examples of activities in which controlled mobility is utilized include weight-shifting activities and movement transitions (see Figs. 6–3 and 6–11). Individuals who demonstrate problems with controlled mobility are unable to maintain their posture while moving the body or limbs. A number of factors can produce deficits in controlled mobility, including the following:

1. Muscle tone imbalances
2. Limited ROM or hypermobility
3. Impaired proximal stabilization or poor muscular co-contraction strength

During controlled mobility activities, the therapist or assistant emphasizes movements with directional changes that encourage antagonist muscle actions. Movements are typically started small and then gradually progressed into larger increments of range. Assistance and guidance are given judiciously, with encouraged active movement and voluntary control from the patient/client. Varying transitional movements can be practiced. Focus is on eccentric control (moving out of a posture), as well as on concentric control (moving into a posture) (Fig. 6–21). Functional activities, such as bridging (see Fig. 6–19), and transitioning between sitting and standing (Fig. 6–21) are effective ways to integrate controlled mobility into an individual's movement repertoire. PNF is effective to establish and strengthen the agonist-antagonist relationship during movement. Any of the appropriate stimulation techniques used with PNF can be selected (see Table 6–2).

▪ Strategies to Improve Skill

Skill is a level of functional motor mastery that enables the individual to produce highly coordinated movement, characterized by precision in timing and direction. Skilled movement is consistent and efficient, allowing goal attainment with an economy of effort. Activities that are considered skills are novel exploratory or investigatory behaviors such as eye and head movements, manipulation skills, and oral-motor exploration. The demonstration of skilled movement allows for adaptive functions and interaction with the environment through body orientation, position, and movement, such as locomotion and exploration, advanced manipulation skills, and complex functional skills. Progression to skill level activities normally

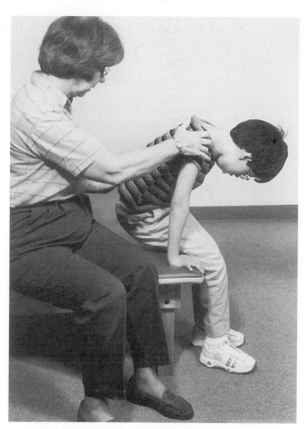

Figure 6–21. Sit to stand and stand to sit are effective choices for practicing concentric (sit to stand) and eccentric (stand to sit) control.

occurs after control in stability and controlled mobility activities have been achieved. Skills are classified as either open or closed, according to Gentile's classification as described in the previous chapter (Gentile, 1992, 2000). There are many reasons why individuals with neurological dysfunction encounter difficulty developing motor skills. Potential for performance may be limited by the following:

1. Significant cognitive impairment
2. Impaired motor planning
3. Impaired balance or coordination
4. Any of the limitations previously listed

When working on skilled activities, active practice of specific task-oriented activities is a prerequisite to the promotion of successful learning, problem solving, retention, and transfer (Duncan, 1997). A hands-on approach using facilitation techniques probably has a limited role during skill training. In the planning of intervention activities, the following may be useful: coordination tasks, multilimb tasks stressing the simultaneous control of multiple body segments (walking while turning the head, walking and holding a conversation), tasks that focus on postural control and balance, and tasks that emphasize agility and timing (Fig. 6–22).

PNF can still be applicable, emphasizing the use of resistance and timing for emphasis (see Figs. 6–1 and 6–2).

The Importance of Person-Centered Functional Goals

Without doubt, upon retrospective reflection on this path from the earliest intervention approaches to today's contemporary approaches to intervention with the person with a neurological impairment, one word comes to the forefront: *function.* Intervention has always and will continue to prioritize the individual person and how that individual functions optimally with a sense of self-worth and well-being in his or her world. *Function* is certainly the buzzword of today's practitioners. However, this is nothing new. Upon reading this chapter, as it traces intervention models from the beginning approaches through today, *function* has been threaded throughout every single approach. Wherever the clinician practices within the intervention setting, at the level of the therapist or the assistant, a commitment

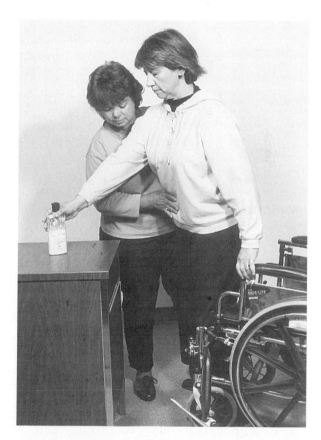

Figure 6–22. The ability to execute a sit to stand transfer in order to stand up, rotate, and reach for an item requires postural control and balance, multisegment strength and coordination, and timing.

to patient-centered functional performance is the cornerstone of clinical practice. Therapists develop the goals in concert with the patient, and all members of the intervention team participate in attempting to meet those goals successfully.

Functional goals are based on the needs and desires of the individual and on the functional impairments that have been identified by the therapist during evaluation (Ryerson, 2001). They should represent a desired significant change in the patient's level of independence, be practical, and reflect an improvement in a specific functional limitation. A functional limitation is a restriction of the ability to perform, at the level of the whole person, a physical action, activity, or task in an efficient, typically expected, or competent manner. Functional goals state the desired function and the expected level of performance (Randall & McEwen, 2000; Ryerson, 2001; Ryerson & Levit, 1997). According to the Guide to Physical Therapist Practice and the Guide to Occupational Therapy Practice, the use of functional goals promotes a patient-centered approach in which the therapists "actively facilitate the participation of the patient/client, family, significant others, and caregivers in the plan of care" (APTA, 1999, p. 3-1, 2001; AOTA, 1999). The reason for writing and following functional goals is because individuals are more likely to make the greatest gains when therapy focuses on activities that are meaningful to them and will make a difference in their lives (Lewthwaite, 1990; Randall & McEwen, 2000).

The process of identifying meaningful, achievable functional goals should be a collaborative one among the therapist, the therapy team (which includes the assistant), the patient/client, and the family, caregivers, or significant others. Randall & McEwen (2000) propose the following three-step process to be helpful:

1. Determine the individual's desired outcome of therapy.
2. Develop an understanding of the individual's self-care, work, and leisure activities and the environments within which these activities occur.
3. Establish and work toward goals with the patient/client as related to the desired outcomes.

The following Clinical Connection offers some suggestions for key interview questions that can be used in conversation with patients/clients to help identify functional goals for those individuals.

Clinical Connection:

In the clinic, home, or school setting, try using these questions to help the individual and his or her family to determine meaningful individual functional goals. It is also suggested that the treating therapist or assistant continue to have similar conversations with the patient during the course of therapy to ensure that the goal is still important and meaningful and that the relationship between therapy activities and the desired outcome is not forgotten.

Questions to Determine Desired Outcomes of Therapy

- If you were to focus your energies on one thing for yourself, what would it be?
- What activities do you need help to perform that you would rather do yourself?
- What are your concerns about returning to work, home, school, or leisure activities?
- How can I help you to be more independent?
- Imagine it's 6 months down the road. What would you like to be different about your current situation? What would you like to be the same (Randall & McEwen, 2000; Winton & Bailey, 1993)?

Functional goals should contain the following elements: Who will do what, under what conditions, how well, and by when (O'Neill & Harris, 1982).

An Integrated Approach to Intervention with Patients/Clients with Neurological Impairment at Any Age

Therapeutic intervention needs to include any combination of sensorimotor techniques, task-oriented analysis, functional training, and motor control/motor learning strategies to offer the individual the most appropriate and efficient route to functional independence or optimal quality of life. How each therapist and assistant combines the interventions with the individual's unique and specific needs will vary. Creativity in intervention is a hallmark of the effective, dynamic therapist. The intervention techniques presented in this chapter are universally applicable to the very young and the very old.

An integrated approach to management of the individual with neurological dysfunction subscribes to today's contemporary **top-down approach,** one that is so patient centered that it starts with an inquiry into how functional is the individual, whether there is adequate role competency for that individual in his or her own environment, and whether the role and ability to function are meaningful for that person. This approach is in contrast to a more traditional **bottom-up approach,** which focused on the deficits of components of function, such as strength, range of motion, and balance, believed to be prerequisites to successful occupational and functional performance (Trombley, 1993). Current views on intervention reflect a paradigm shift from the early sensorimotor and hierarchical theorists with a focus on *normality* of movement to a current focus on *functionality*. This functional approach to neurorehabilitation emphasizes the learning of motor abilities that are meaningful in the individual's environment to generate movement solutions for dilemmas that are perceived to be problematic for the individual, or in the case of a child, the child and family (Ketelaar, Vermeer, t'Hart, Beek, & Helders, 2001). The task of the therapist and assistant is to provide an environment that enables the individual to learn and practice self-initiated and goal-directed actions within naturally occurring contexts (Latash & Anson, 1996).

Contemporary motor control and motor learning theory, as well as present levels of knowledge in the areas of neuroscience, biomechanics, movement science, behavioral science, and ecological theory, all contribute to a perspective unique to today's treating clinician. In assessing and treating the patient with movement and motor control dysfunction, Hedman, Rogers, and Hanke (1996, with permission of Neurology Section, APTA) have proposed the asking of four pivotal questions when looking at the clinical picture presented by the individual:

1. *What is the problem?* Attempt is made to identify the problems that the individual is having with movement from among any or all of the following categories: mobility, force generation, muscle tone, sensory information, pain, speed, endurance, posture, balance, coordination, adaptive capacity, perceptual capabilities, and psychological/cognitive capacity. Any of these components could be altered, contributing to the movement problem. Solutions for solving some of these problems are offered in the chapters to follow.

2. *Where in the movement continuum does the problem interfere with function?* The movement continuum considers movement from its initial organization in the CNS to its outcome in the environment, further broken down into six interactive yet distinguishable stages: *initial conditions*—includes the state of the individual's systems and the environmental context; *preparation*—the period when the movement is being organized in the CNS, including identification of the stimulus, selection of a response, and programming of the movement response; *initiation of movement*—beginning of the actual movement, including timing, direction, and smoothness; *execution*—including the amplitude, direction, smoothness, and speed of the movement; *termination*—stopping the movement described by the parameters of stability, timing, and accuracy; and *outcome*—whether or not the goal was reached successfully.

3. *What are the underlying determinants of the problem?*

Any of the determinants of movement control may underlie the clinical manifestation of the movement from among the neural, musculoskeletal and biomechanical, and behavioral aspects of movement. The neural factors include the structures, pathways, and processes that participate in the control of movement. The musculoskeletal and biomechanical factors include the structure and function of the joints, muscles, and soft tissues involved in the execution of a movement. The behavioral factors include the cognitive, motivational, perceptual, and emotional processes, as well as the outcome of a movement framed within its goal and environmental context. Consistent with a dynamic systems approach, no one process is more vital than another, and it is the interaction of all these processes that must be appreciated.

4. *How do we treat the problem?* Intervention is then directed at helping to solve the movement dilemma by solving problems with the movement components (using an intervention technique to intervene) and assisting with strategy generation (such as modifying an environment) to produce effective, efficient functional movement.

These questions are displayed for easy clinical reference in Table 6–8. Students and clinicians are encouraged to use these questions not only clinically but also during the reading of the case studies at the end of this and subsequent chapters to help develop a problem-solving, integrated, and practical approach to intervention for individuals presenting a movement dilemma secondary to a neurological deficit. There are differences in practice scope between the therapist and the assistant; remember that all clinical decision making must fit within those practice constraints. *All members of the therapy team are involved at some level with practice-appropriate clinical decision making*, within the plan of care for the patient and the practice act of the profession.

The essence of functional training, functional mobility training, motor learning theory, and a dynamic systems approach has been integrated into the approach of this text, whereby human movement patterns are acknowledged as enjoying both similarities across the life span and differences between and among individuals. The authors in other cited works offer detailed descriptions of common functional movements and offer clear pictorial explanations to guide therapists and assistants in establishing or re-establishing functional movement (Carr & Shepherd, 1987, 2000; Davies, 1985; Dutton, 1995; O'Sullivan & Schmitz, 2001; Palmer & Toms, 1992; Ryerson & Levit, 1997). Functional movement is most necessary for retraining for individuals with movement problems secondary to a neurological insult. Chapters 7 through 10 will focus on specific

TABLE 6–8

Clinical Questions to Help Identify Movement Problem: A Pocket Guide

Question	Clinical Significance	Possible Clinical Action
1. What is the problem?	Attempt to identify the problems that the individual is having, such as: mobility, force generation, muscle tone, sensory information, pain, speed, endurance, posture, balance, coordination, adaptive capacity, perceptual capabilities, and psychological/cognitive capacity.	Assess or refer for assessment to discern contribution from any of these factors from any subsystem to the movement problem. Any of these components could be altered, contributing to the movement problem.
2. Where in the movement continuum does the problem interfere with function?	The movement continuum includes initial conditions, preparation, initiation of movement, execution, termination, and outcome.	Discern where in this continuum the individual is being confronted by the movement problem. Intervene, modify, or adapt at that point.
3. What are the underlying determinants of the problem?	Any determinant may underlie the clinical manifestation of the movement problem from among the neural, musculoskeletal, and biomechanical, and behavioral aspects of movement, as well as the goal itself or the environmental context.	Remember the equal and interactive contributions from all the systems contributing to movement: neural, biomechanical, and behavioral. None is more important than the other. They also must work together.
4. How do we treat the problem?	Intervention is directed at helping to solve the movement dilemma by solving problems with the movement components (using an intervention technique to intervene) and assisting with strategy generation (such as modifying an environment) to produce effective, efficient functional movement.	Choose from several main actions to help solve the problem: remediate effect of limitation or constraint; alter the context in which an individual performs; retrain with new components or strategies; modify the task or condition; adapt the environment; prevent maladaptive performance; or create circumstances that promote more adaptable performance in context (Dunn, Brown, & McGuigan, 1994).

Source: Adapted from Hedman, L. D., Rogers, M. W., & Hanke, T. A. (1996). Neurologic professional education: Linking the foundation science of motor control with physical therapy interventions for movement dysfunction. *Neurol Rep*, 20, 9–13. Reprinted from the Neurology Report with permission of the Neurology Section, APTA.

intervention solutions and suggestions for the following four commonly encountered clinical dilemmas pertaining to movement control for patients/clients with neurological disorders: problems with force production; deficits in postural control and balance difficulties; problems with upper extremity control, including manipulation; and problems with lower extremity control, including transfers and locomotion. This text will also attempt to emphasize the decision-making role of the individual patient/client, the meaningfulness of occupational choice, and respect for the importance of movement success in natural environments.

Prioritizing an individual's functionality and well-being is threaded throughout the practice guidelines and intervention approaches of both occupational and physical therapy, as reflected in both the "Guide to Occupational Therapy Practice" (Moyers, 1999) and the "Guide to Physical Therapist Practice" (APTA, 2001). The subsequent chapters on commonly encountered clinical dilemmas will adhere to the language promoted by these cornerstone documents. The Guide to Occupational Therapy Practice delineates four major intervention approaches to be used in an integrative fashion when treating a patient/client. These four intervention approaches are listed in Table 6–9. The Guide to Physical Therapist Practice delineates intervention as consisting of three major components as depicted in Table 6–9. From these lists, the interventions that will be the main focus of this text are those that are typically enlisted in the intervention with an individual with a neurological disorder. Procedural interventions such as therapeutic exercise, functional training, and the use of equipment and devices are often employed for remediation or compensation when working with an individual to solve a movement problem imposed by a neurological disorder. The language used in this text is complementary to both the guides, emphasizing the importance of person-centered functional goals, the remediation of impairments that interfere with function, the reduction or prevention of functional limitations, the importance of meaningful activity and occupation, and the minimization of disability. Intervention

TABLE 6–9

Intervention Approaches Typically Used in Neurorehabilitation

Occupational Therapy Intervention Approaches

Remediation/Restoration Changing the biological, physiological, psychological, or neurological process Teaching/training	Restoring or remediating impairments in performance components Establishing new skills, habits, or behaviors in performance components
Compensation/Adaptation Changing the task Changing the context	Adapting the task requirements, procedures, task objects Modifying or adapting the task environment
Disability Prevention	Safe occupational performances
Health Promotion	Lifestyle redesign

Physical Therapy Intervention Components

Coordination, Communication, and Documentation
Patient/client-related instruction
Procedural interventions, including: Therapeutic exercise   Functional training in work, community, and leisure and in self-care/home improvement   Manual therapy techniques   Prescription, application, fabrication of devices and equipment   Physical agents, mechanical modalities, and electrotherapeutic modalities

Sources: Adapted from American Physical Therapy Association (2001). Guide to physical therapist practice (2nd ed). *Physical Therapy*, 81, 9–744, with permission of the American Physical Therapy Association; and Moyers, P. (1999). Guide to occupational therapy practice. *American Journal of Occupational Therapy*, 53, 247–322. Copyright 1999 by the American Occupational Therapy Association, Inc. Reprinted with permission.

will be directed at remediating the impairments that can be affected by physical or occupational therapy or training the individual to develop new or adapted compensation strategies. The task or environment may also need to be modified. The focus is on enablement, not disablement.

Movement skills are derived, in part, from human ingenuity (Gentile, 2000). They represent a match among all the variables—the individual at a unique developmental phase with a unique set of capabilities and constraints, the task with all its idiosyncrasies, and varying environments. In trying to help the individual gain functional skills, rehabilitation therapists establish goals with the individual and arrange the environment in which the action takes place. It is really *only* the individual patient who must then organize the movement that matches the environmental and task demands, producing the desired outcome. The challenge for the therapist and assistant is to create a match between the individual patient/client and the plethora of intervention strategies that are available. What follows are two case studies, one from pediatric and one from adult practice, that illustrate the selection and application of key concepts from among all the currently available intervention options.

Case Studies

The following case studies describe an integrated approach to intervention with a child and an adult with neurological dysfunction. No one frame of reference or model is advocated, but rather clinicians are encouraged to be familiar with the many models and to choose the most appropriate insights and tools from among all of them in order to most effectively treat each unique patient. For each case study, guiding principles for that age phase are listed from the motor learning tools described in the previous chapter. When reading the case study approach and intervention suggestions, recognize the contributions from among all the theoretical background information available, and acknowledge the selection of the activities as reflective of intervention approaches as discussed in this chapter. The contributions from many approaches (sensorimotor approaches, motor learning theory, dynamic systems approach to motor control, functional training, and task analysis with goal-directed movement) and the integration of all available tools to serve these two individuals all work together to offer an effective intervention strategy for the specific movement problem presented. Both case studies are supplemented with figures demonstrating the intervention.

Case Study: Child

Elijah: Child with Hypotonia and Developmental Delay

History

Elijah is a 28-month-old boy, born at 38 weeks' gestation via a vaginal delivery at 7 pounds, 2 ounces. There were no indications of perinatal distress. Medical history has been uneventful except for an incidence of pneumonia requiring hospitalization at 4 months of age. History is negative for medications or seizures. Magnetic resonance imaging (MRI) is normal. Elijah is receiving Early Intervention services, including physical therapy and occupational therapy, for the presenting developmental delay and hypotonia, including delays in the attainment of all gross and fine motor milestones. Transdisciplinary assessments are periodically done, including physical therapy and occupational therapy evaluations. Services are delivered in both the home and day care center, within Elijah's natural environment, with his parents closely involved in all aspects of intervention.

Evaluation

Elijah is a delightful, pleasant boy who readily engages the examiner with smiles and eye contact. He is extremely social, appearing to enjoy interaction. His animation and interest in moving about to explore the world help him to be quite responsive to intervention. Elijah has a caring and supportive family who appear to be highly motivated to participate in therapy. Elijah is the third child in a family of two parents and two older siblings, ages 4 and 8. The mother is a full-time homemaker and the father works full time. The family's main concerns are expressed as worries about Elijah's lack of independent mobility and attainment of gross and fine motor milestones. There is a wealth of stimulating, interesting toys and books in this home. The day care center staff is capable and caring, willing to help Elijah to learn and function optimally within the center.

Elijah's preferred position is circle sitting on the floor or playing in supine. In supine, his head is in midline and he is able to play with toys with either hand, occasionally transferring from hand to hand. There is a full head lag on pull to sit, with assistance given at shoulders. Lower extremities are observed to kick randomly into some antigravity flexion, always widely abducted

and externally rotated. Elijah rolls to either side but prefers to roll to the right. Rolling is initiated by neck hyperextension and executed without evidence of segmental rotation. He does not usually pause for play in a side-lying position. In prone, Elijah props onto widely based forearms with fisted hands. Weight shift onto a single forearm is inconsistent with Elijah preferring to roll back into supine when visually engaged by a toy. He is not yet pushing up onto extended arms. In prone, he has just started to pull into a belly crawl to obtain objects placed out of reach. Lower extremities remain widely abducted and externally rotated; upper extremities remain abducted rather than underneath him for support. Movement appears to be a lot of work for Elijah. Elijah is not yet able to achieve sitting independently but will maintain sitting once placed. Sitting is characterized by a wide base of support, rounded trunk, neck flexion, capital extension and upper extremities retained adducted against the thorax, elbows flexed, and scapulae retracted. There is obvious instability. The pelvis is tilted posteriorly. Elijah tends to "stay safe," maintaining this quiet sitting posture for long periods. He is not able to transition independently out of a sitting position, but waits to be moved.

Muscle tone is low throughout neck, trunk, and all four extremities. Quality of tone is equally low throughout this distribution. Righting and protective responses are not yet evident in any position. If balance is disturbed while sitting, Elijah will either fall to the side or attempt to stabilize himself by pulling with his arms onto his lower extremities for support. There is no evidence of protective extension in sitting. From ventral suspension, Elijah will demonstrate a weak, delayed protective response onto partially extended upper extremities. The hips and shoulders are not extended to plane in the Landau position. There is no evidence of tonic reflex postures during movement.

Functionally, Elijah demonstrates incomplete antigravity control in all positions, including supine, prone, and sitting. Rolling is characterized by lack of emergence of segmental rotation. All transitions are executed with difficulty with apparent inability to combine flexion and extension movements. Spontaneous rotation is absent, and there is no dissociation between body segments. In prone, Elijah is able to prop onto forearms and inconsistently shift weight to reach for an object. Floor mobility is limited to rolling and belly crawling forward. Elijah will accept weight when passively placed in a standing position with full support. Hips are slightly flexed and knees extended to neutral. Foot alignment is appropriate for an early stance posture.

Range of motion is full without significant hypermobility or ligament laxity. Hips appear to be clinically stable with full and symmetrical range of motion. Spinal mobility is passively full, but there is limited active thoracic expansion in an upright position and limited thoracic extension in all positions. Respiration appears to be shallow, confirmed by a history of frequent upper respiratory infections. Vocalizations are limited to short strings of vowel sounds and low volume.

In summary, Elijah is a 28-month-old boy with hypotonia and developmental delay. Muscle tone is moderately low throughout all extremities, neck, and trunk. Antigravity strength is limited in all positions. Evidence of proximal instability and limited co-contraction is detected at the shoulder girdle, as well as the pelvis, with broadened base and limited weight-bearing capabilities. Segmental rotation and dissociation are not yet observed in his movements. Transitional movements are either absent or ineffective.

Present Movement Problem

Observation, evaluation, and family interview led to the discernment of several immediate problems of concern and meaning to both Elijah and his family. A movement problem identified as being of tantamount concern at this time is the limitation experienced by Elijah in independent mobility around his home and day care center, as he attempts to interact with siblings and peers. That movement problem is the focus of this case study, illustrating an integrated approach to intervention as the therapy team assists Elijah and his family in finding some movement solutions.

Intervention

The therapy team used the following concepts as guideposts in the therapeutic management of this child. The entire team of practitioners discussed these concepts with Elijah's family so that all are in agreement with these key guiding principles:

1. Throughout infancy and childhood, play is a child's work. Play activities assist the child in developing skills through engagement with objects and through interaction with caregivers and family members. Through play, the child practices and develops mastery of skills in motor planning and problem solving, developing form and space perception, equilibrium, and postural adaptability to the environment. Cognitive development during this time is fostered through repetition and combining of sensory and motor experiences. Movement and play that stimulate sensorimotor functioning and interaction are vital at this time.
2. Physical and occupational therapy intervention is a teaching and learning relationship. Familiarity with developmental theory (see Chapter 4) and learning theory (see Chapter 5) can help clinicians to assim-

ilate key developmental and teaching concepts into the intervention setting and interaction with children. To facilitate motivation for learning in children, emphasis should be placed on keeping the goals important and meaningful to the child, involving the child in the anticipatory and planning phases of the activity, offering opportunity for repetition and explorative learning, and giving reinforcement. Modeling is an extremely powerful teaching tool for use with children. Children tend to be more visually dependent than adults, who rely more on a combination of visual and proprioceptive input. Visual demonstration and nonverbal communication are important teaching tools to use when working with a young child.
3. Encouraging creative behaviors has been demonstrated to be a powerful way of enhancing motivation in children. Promoting some degree of flexibility in therapy could entail allowing and acknowledging a child's independent thinking and ability to generate a creative movement response. The therapist can support the child's attempts to express movements, allowing some originality in demonstration, so that movement exploration is an active process with a perceptual, cognitive, and motor aspect.
4. The use of functional activities that provide opportunities to explore and dynamically interact with the environment are of unquestionable value. If at all possible, involve the child in setting the goal, or indicate choice in an activity. Movements "preselected" by the child result in greater goal clarity and increased success, as well as superior performance as compared with movements or activities selected solely by the therapist.
5. Natural environments, within the interaction settings of home, school, and community, are the most functional contexts where practice and learning for transfer are most likely to occur.

All these principles served to guide both the therapists and family members in helping Elijah to develop a solution to his problem of being unable to move around his house. The physical therapy and occupational therapy teams alternated visits, each working closely with Elijah and his family to promote the acquisition of optimal sensorimotor development and independent functional movement. Discussion with caregivers and observation of Elijah resulted in the selection of preferred play activities that would motivate Elijah to move from place to place within the home and day care center. The therapists offered Elijah choices whenever possible.

The following summarize some of the intervention activities. The therapy goals and sample activities to meet these objectives are outlined here, to be integrated as play activities by all family members and day care staff as they encourage Elijah to move around the household and play environment. From these suggestions, as each individual task is used to assist Elijah in the development of mobility skills, the therapist analyzes each movement attempt at each task and the movement dilemma, as per Tables 6–6 and 6–8.

1. Elijah will actively participate in movement transitions and positioning choices utilized during activities of daily living. The therapists will work with the parents and caregivers to improve positioning, feeding, bathing care and dressing techniques, incorporating these techniques into Elijah's daily care activities. All caregivers will be included in therapy sessions so that movement strategies will be repeated by all facilitators, becoming a familiar and natural way to assist Elijah with active movement (Figure 6–23). This consistency will offer Elijah multiple opportunities to practice new movements as they emerge within various contexts, especially as integrated into activities of daily living and routine activities, with multiple facilitators. A stander and a gait trainer will be ordered so that a standing and ambulation program can be started, with standing encouraged at the kitchen counter, bathroom sink, and so on to promote the assimilation of upright abilities into functional activity (Figs. 6–24 and 6–25).

2. Elijah will demonstrate increased antigravity strength in multiple positions.
   a. Supine: development of antigravity movement out of supine and work on stability, as well as controlled mobility; for example, bridging incorporated into a game of forming a bridge over a push toy, initiation of transition out of

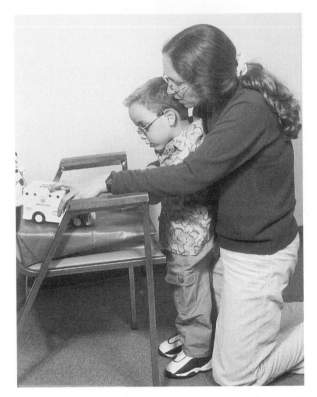

Figure 6–24. Practicing standing with support during play.

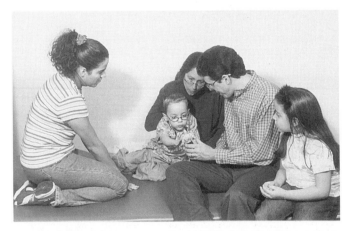

Figure 6–23. Inclusion of all caregivers in family teaching encourages practice of therapeutic play activities within natural environments, allowing for increased learning and carryover opportunities.

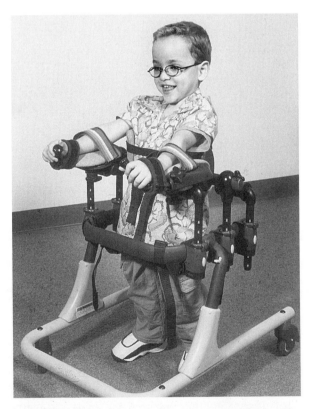

Figure 6–25. Use of a gait trainer will offer beginning experience with upright mobility.

supine with neck flexion and extremity movements (Fig. 6–26).

b. Prone: movement activities from the prone position to encourage weight bearing with arms in alignment beneath him when reading a book with family member or teacher; weight shift activities, such as reaching for toys while on his belly; narrow upper and lower extremity base in prone to encourage antigravity control and weight bearing; play activities to encourage weight bearing and pushing (Figs. 6–27 and 6–28).

c. Sitting: introduction of transitional sitting positions such as side sitting; reaching for toys at shoulder height in floor sitting to encourage trunk extension; sitting with upper extremities moving actively away from body while engaged in play (Fig. 6–29).

3. Elijah will incorporate rotation and dissociation into transitional movements (Figs. 6–30 and 6–31).

a. Transitions from supine or prone with dissociation to change positions or move toward a play activity.

b. Reaching away from midline for toys into a diagonal pattern in supine and sitting.

c. Pivoting in sitting, rotating sit to prone, prone to sit, quadruped to sit, and sit to quadruped.

4. Elijah will demonstrate effective postural responses during functional activity.

a. Introduce displacements and perturbations across positions, including sitting, and supported quadruped. Amplitude and speed of perturbations will be progressed as responses emerge. Play activities to encourage equilibrium responses can be done seated on a riding

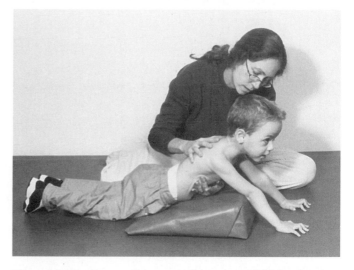

Figure 6–27. Play in the prone position will help develop shoulder stabilizers and upper extremity extensor muscles, as well as postural control of the head and upper trunk.

toy, a bolster, or the parent's lap. Introduce supported use of a rocking horse, "sit-and-spin," or riding toy. An excursion to a playground or on backyard play equipment is suggested.

5. Elijah will demonstrate increased varieties of independent floor mobility. All floor mobility activities are integrated into environmental exploration, moving to a desired target.

a. Belly crawling with increased ease and control.

b. Play in quadruped with proper support, alignment, and narrowed base of support of upper and lower extremities.

6. Elijah will explore increased varieties of upright alignment and postural control.

a. Institution of a supported standing program to promote acetabular development, bony miner-

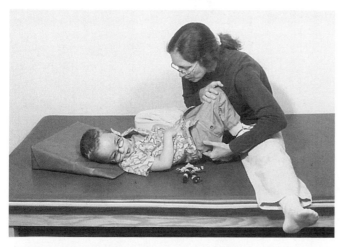

Figure 6–26. Bridging incorporated into play is a good activity for strengthening. Therapist is encouraging active antigravity hip extension with abdominal strengthening, which may contribute to improved pelvic control.

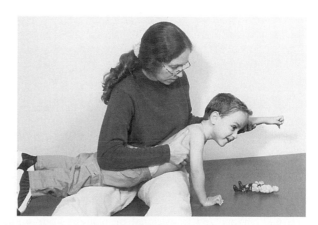

Figure 6–28. Weight-shifting activities in prone are easily incorporated into a reaching task.

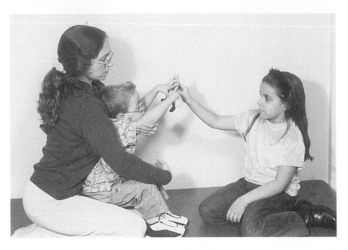

Figure 6–29. Reaching from supported sit offers practice with emerging trunk and UE control.

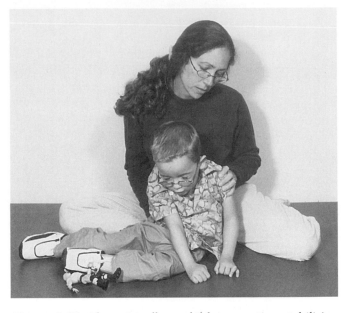

Figure 6–31. Therapist allows child to practice stabilizing with the upper extremity in weight bearing as she offers approximation and some manual assistance at the left shoulder and trunk.

alization, skeletal alignment, and visual regard of the environment in an upright position.

b. Available adapted equipment for supported standing to assess optimal position, alignment, and weight bearing. Stander used for play at the sink, kitchen counter, or table for fun activities. Gait trainer to introduce ambulation (see Fig. 6–25).

c. Begin pull to stand at furniture within the home and day care center (see Fig. 6–24).

d. Adapted seating as needed but not in replacement of Elijah's attempts to exercise emergent postural control (Fig. 6–32).

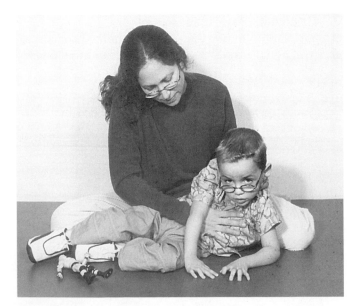

Figure 6–30. Practicing transitional movement from supine to sit requires practice of dissociation, rotation, and weight shifting.

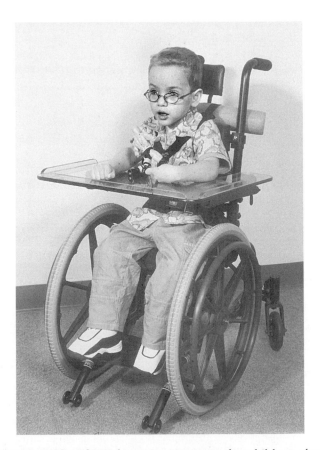

Figure 6–32. Adapted seating supports the child so that engagement in daily activity is encouraged.

Case Study: Adult

Kitty: Adult with Hemiplegia After CVA

History

Kitty is a 68-year-old woman who suffered a right CVA (middle cerebral artery infarct) 2 weeks ago. She was hospitalized for 5 days and has been participating in an inpatient rehabilitation setting for the past week. Kitty is medically stable, has regained some mobility skills, and has a supportive family, including a husband and two married daughters who live nearby. Discharge to home with outpatient therapy is being planned.

Evaluation

Kitty is a small, lively woman with a great deal of anxiety about being able to return to a premorbid level of independence, especially in the area of self-care. Kitty is rather petite, just barely 5 feet tall. She says that she is "fiercely independent" but somewhat private and modest about personal matters. Kitty has an attentive but somewhat shy husband, stating that he "keeps his nose out of women's business." He is eager to attend to any recommended environmental changes recommended for their two-story home but prefers to be a steadfast but retiring support in the background. Kitty has been the vocal leader in the family. Kitty's husband has already moved their bedroom into a first-floor recreation room, which has a bathroom within it. The bathroom can be adapted appropriately to accommodate Kitty's need for some increased space and open areas for improved maneuverability, since she is using an assistive device.

Kitty presents with a left hemiplegia. Muscle tone is high throughout both left extremities and the trunk on the left side. Spasticity in the left upper extremity is considered mild to moderate, distributed predominantly in the scapular retractors, elbow flexors, and finger flexors. She can demonstrate independent voluntary elbow extension and finger extension but still has difficulty fully protracting the scapula to bring the extremity forward, especially across midline. The trunk has some increased muscle tone, precipitating a frequent posture of shortening on the left side and delayed postural responses when balance is perturbed. In the left lower extremity, muscle tone is only mildly high, with signs of spasticity seen only during fast or unfamiliar movements or when Kitty is tired. Sensation is generally intact, with some decrease in proprioception discerned during intermittent episodes of mild positional edema in the distal parts of both left extremities. There are no range-of-motion limitations with the exception of slight limitations in full scapular protraction and active shoulder forward flexion on the left. Vision and hearing are within normal limits.

Kitty's postural control is limited by evidence of residual spasticity as described previously, with poor selective voluntary control of the following key muscle groups: trunk flexors and extensors, scapular protractors, shoulder flexors and adductors during skilled movements, and spontaneous elbow extension with smooth control of the wrist/hand for refined reach, grasp, and release. Sitting is stable with good balance as long as the chair is stable and Kitty's feet can be supported on the floor beneath her. Kitty demonstrates impaired balance when having to reach across midline and when not in a secure seat. She is quite the problem solver, actively engaged in "being able to do this myself," when she discusses her desire to independently perform routine self-care. Kitty is ambulating with a quad cane on level surfaces with contact guard for balance, safety, and reassurance; using stairs with minimal assistance of one; and has achieved independence in all transfers within the rehabilitation setting.

In summary, Kitty is a 68-year-old woman status post–right CVA with residual left hemiplegia. Muscle tone is hypertonic on the left side, with spasticity distributed predominantly throughout the left upper extremity and trunk. Postural control continues to re-emerge with increasing voluntary control of the involved extremities. There are residual deficits in postural control affecting automatic responses and dynamic balance on the left side. Functional mobility is improving with the ability to transfer and ambulate with an assistive device. Deficits in independent self-care are the dominant present issue.

Present Movement Problem

Observation, evaluation, and personal interview led to the discernment of several problems of immediate concern and meaning to both Kitty and her family. A movement problem identified as being of priority concern at this time was the limitation experienced by Kitty as the inability to dress herself. Heading home, Kitty is adamant that she needs to be able to dress herself each morning independently. That specific movement problem is the focus of this case study, illustrating an integrated approach to intervention as the therapy team assisted Kitty in finding a movement solution and solving several tasks associated with dressing.

Intervention

The therapists and assistants used the following concepts as guideposts in the therapeutic management of Kitty, an adult learner whose learning capabilities may be challenged by the recent CVA (see Chapter 5).

1. Adults tend to have a problem-solving orientation to learning and real-life situations, and problems are the main motivator for an adult learner. Most adult learners value the immediate application of learned information. Active participation in learning im-proves retention. Intrinsic motivation produces more pervasive and permanent learning. Kitty is highly motivated about the importance of being independent in dressing skills.

2. An adult's readiness to learn depends on his or her previous learning. Tasks that are more meaningful are more fully and easily learned. The fact that dressing is a familiar activity should promote learning for Kitty.

3. Learning is enhanced by repetition and needs to be presented in natural, environmentally correct contexts.

4. Adults exhibit unique learning styles that illustrate various learning theories, such as having personal strategies for coding information. It is important that the therapist engage in a discussion with Kitty regarding how she perceives herself as a learner and what teaching strategies may be preferred.

Available information about the challenges experienced by a learner after a CVA alerts the therapy team to the importance of active participation, the need for contextual interference (especially as a patient prepares to be discharged home), promotion of retention and transfer of the skill, and the value of both random and blocked practice. The value of added-purpose occupation, which promotes motivation and meaningfulness, is vital. All these principles serve to guide both the therapists and Kitty in helping Kitty to actively develop solutions to her problem of meeting her goal of independence in dressing.

The following summarize some of the intervention activities. The therapy goals and sample activities to meet these objectives are outlined next, accompanied by figures depicting the intervention. From the suggestions listed here, as each individual task is used to assist Kitty in the development of mobility skills required for activities of daily living, the therapist analyzed each movement attempt at each task and the movement dilemma, as per Tables 6–6 and 6–8. The therapists and assistants also adhere to the four steps suggested by the MRP approach to stroke rehabilitation: task analysis, including observation and comparison; practice of missing or problematic components; practice of the whole task; and then transference of the training to generalized situations.

1. Kitty will actively participate in selecting the environmental contexts and the regulatory conditions to be mastered during practice of initial dressing skills. Kitty and the therapist will agree on the position choice for the dressing activity and select the types of clothing to be donned and removed. Opportunity will be given for Kitty to practice in varying contexts. A home visit is planned immediately so that active problem solving can occur within that natural environment. In the meantime, mental rehearsal is used as Kitty anticipates the home environment and that environment is contrived within the rehabilitation setting. Conversations are held with her husband to offer suggestions about the dressing space in the converted recreation room, selection of a dressing area with a suitable chair and table, and equipping the area with adequate lighting and a mirror.

2. Kitty will demonstrate adequate upper extremity mobility to execute the dressing task.

   a. In sitting or in supine before arising in the morning: teach Kitty to self-mobilize her left scapula into protraction by using her right arm to grasp the left scapula and bring it forward around the rib cage. Kitty can then also clasp her hands, raise both arms to shoulder height extended in front of her, and self-mobilize the left upper extremity by performing forward reach and trunk rotation to the right (Fig. 6–33).

   b. Therapist to teach Kitty home exercise program consisting of activities (preferably functional and goal-directed) to increase active left shoulder protraction, flexion, internal and external rotation, abduction and adduction, elbow extension, wrist extension, and finger extension (Fig. 6–34).

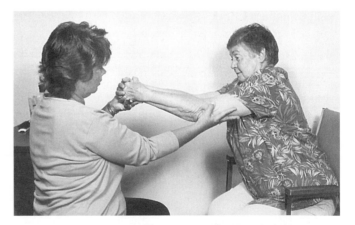

Figure 6–33. By raising her right upper extremity, clasping and grasping the left while reaching at shoulder height to the right, she effectively self-mobilizes her left scapula during daily tasks.

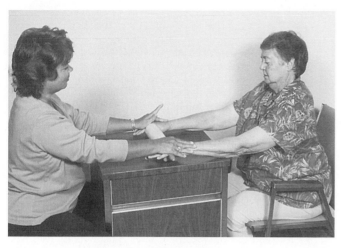

Figure 6–34. Practicing active scapular protraction, shoulder flexion, slight external rotation, and elbow extension while engaged in movement of a rolling pin.

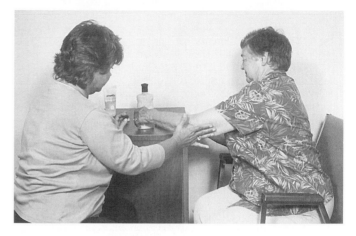

Figure 6–35. Practicing automatic postural responses and use of left upper extremity while reaching for objects across midline.

3. Kitty will demonstrate more accurate, automatic postural responses to challenged trunk balance while performing a functional activity.
   a. Sitting and reaching at and across midline to reach for objects and engage in the activities required for dressing (Fig. 6–35).
4. Kitty will demonstrate practice in varying dressing tasks, including selection of the type of clothing and closures, preparation for the execution of the task (clothing and body segment preparation), initiation, execution, and termination of the actual task.
   a. All the following teaching strategies are employed: mental rehearsal, active problem solving, practice, self-assessment, and solution regeneration.

Summary

This chapter has attempted to draw an intimate relationship between theoretical constructs and frameworks or models of intervention. As rehabilitation practitioners, our historical background arose from the early works of neurophysiologists and both occupational and physical therapists as they discovered and tried a clinical application using the neuroscience knowledge available at that time. The sensorimotor approaches, arising from the reflex and hierarchical theories, offered therapists valuable rudimentary tools for application to individuals with neurological dysfunction. As contemporary knowledge advances and refines a more dynamic systems approach to motor control, that perspective, in conjunction with simultaneous advances in motor learning theory and movement science, all contribute to a broader, more informed selection of intervention choices. Clinically, intervention should be patient centered and individualized, requiring that the therapist choose the most appropriate from among the many tools available from all the approaches (both time honored and new) as theoretical advances continue. An integrated approach to intervention is described, prioritizing optimal functional outcomes for the patient/client regardless of age or pathological condition. The next four chapters will focus on intervention, with four common clinical dilemmas affecting movement performance in the individual who is neurologically impaired. An integrated, eclectic intervention approach will be described, accompanied by patient/client photographs.

References

American Occupational Therapy Association (1994). Uniform terminology for occupational therapy—third edition. *American Journal of Occupational Therapy, 48,* 1047–1054.

American Occupational Therapy Association (1999). Glossary: Standards for an accredited educational program for the occupational therapist and the occupational therapy assistant. *American Journal of Occupational Therapy, 53,* 590–591.

American Physical Therapy Association (1999). *Guide to physical therapist practice* (Rev. ed., p. 3-1). Alexandria, VA: American Physical Therapy Association.

American Physical Therapy Association (2001). Guide to physical therapist practice (2nd ed.). *Physical Therapy, 81,* 744.

Arend, S., & Higgins, J. R. (1976). A strategy for the classification, subjective analysis, and observation of human movement. *Journal of Human Movement Studies, 2,* 36–52.

Ayres, A. J. (1973). *Sensory integration and learning disorders.* Los Angeles: Western Psychological Services.

Bennett, S. E., & Karnes, J. L. (1998). *Neurological disabilities: Assessment and treatment.* Philadelphia: Lippincott-Raven.

Bobath, B. (1965). *Abnormal postural reflex activity caused by brain lesions.* London: William Heinemann.

Bobath, B. (1969). The treatment of neuromuscular disorders by improving patterns of coordination. *Physiotherapy, 55,* 18–22.

Bobath, B. (1970). *Adult hemiplegia: Evaluation and treatment.* London: William Heinemann.

Bobath, K., & Bobath, B. (1984). The neuro-developmental treatment. In D. Scrutton (Ed.), *Management of the motor disorders of children with cerebral palsy.* Philadelphia: J. B. Lippincott.

Breslin, D. M. M. (1996). Motor-learning theory and the neurodevelopmental treatment approach: A comparative analysis. *Occupational Therapy in Health Care, 10*(1), 25–40.

Brunnstrom, S. (1970). *Movement therapy in hemiplegia: A neurophysiological approach.* New York: Harper & Row.

Bundy, A. C., Lane, S. J., & Murray, E. A. (2002). *Sensory integration: Theory and practice* (2nd ed.). Philadelphia: F. A. Davis.

Burke, D. G., Culligan, C. J., & Holt, L. E. (2000). The theoretical basis of proprioceptive neuromuscular facilitation. *Journal of Strength and Conditioning Research, 14,* 496–500.

Carr, J., & Shepherd, R. (1987). *A motor relearning programme for stroke.* Rockville, MD: Aspen Publishers.

Carr, J., & Shepherd, R. (1998). *Neurological rehabilitation: Optimizing motor performance.* Oxford: Butterworth Heinemann.

Carr, J., & Shepherd, R. (2000). *Movement science: Foundations for physical therapy in rehabilitation* (2nd ed.). Gaithersburg, MD: Aspen Publishers.

Craik, R. L., & Oatis, C. A. (1995). *Gait analysis: Theory and application.* Philadelphia: Mosby.

Davies, P. M. (1985). *Steps to follow: A guide to the treatment of adult hemiplegia.* New York: Springer-Verlag.

Davis, W. E., & Burton, A. W. (1991). Ecological task analysis: Translating movement behavior theory into practice. *Adapted Physical Activity Quarterly, 8,* 154–177.

DeGangi, G., & Royeen, C. B. (1994). Current practice among neurodevelopmental treatment association members. *American Journal of Occupational Therapy, 48,* 803–809.

Duncan, P. W. (1997). Synthesis of intervention trials to improve motor recovery following stroke. *Topics in Stroke Rehabilitation, 3,* 1–20.

Duncan, P. W., & Badke, M. B. (1987). *Stroke rehabilitation: The recovery of motor control.* Chicago: Year Book.

Dunn, W., Brown, C., & McGuigan, A. (1994). The ecology of human performance: A framework for considering the effect of context. *American Journal of Occupational Therapy, 48,* 595–618.

Dutton, R. (1995). *Clinical reasoning in physical disabilities.* Baltimore: Williams & Wilkins.

Farber, S. (1982). *Neurorehabilitation: A multisensory approach* (p. 122). Philadelphia: W. B. Saunders.

Fetters, L. (1991). Measurement and treatment in cerebral palsy: An argument for a new approach. *Physical Therapy, 71,* 244–247.

Fisher, A. G., Murray E. A., & Bundy, A. C. (1991). *Sensory integration: Theory and practice.* Philadelphia: F. A. Davis.

Flinn, N. (1995). A task-oriented approach to the treatment of a client with hemiplegia. *American Journal of Occupational Therapy, 49,* 560–569.

Gentile, A. M. (1992). The nature of skill acquisition: Therapeutic implications for children with movement disorders. In H. Forssberg & H. Hirschfeld (Eds.), *Movement disorders in children.* Basel: Karger.

Gentile, A. M. (2000). Skill acquisition: Action, movement, and neuromotor processes. In J. Carr & R. Shepherd (Eds.), *Movement science: Foundations for physical therapy in rehabilitation* (2nd ed.). Gaithersburg, MD: Aspen Publishers.

Gesell, A. (1954). The ontogenesis of human behavior. In L. Carmichael (Ed.), *Manual of child psychology.* New York: Wiley.

Gordon, J. (2000). Assumptions underlying physical therapy intervention: Theoretical and historical perspectives. In J. Carr & R. Shepherd (Eds.), *Movement science: Foundations for physical therapy in rehabilitation* (2nd ed.). Gaithersburg, MD: Aspen Publishers.

Guide to Physical Therapist Practice (2nd ed.) (2001). *Physical Therapy, 81,* 9–744.

Haugen, J. B., & Mathiowetz, V. (1995). Contemporary task-oriented approach. In Trombley, C. A. (Ed.), *Occupational therapy for physical dysfunction* (4th ed.). Baltimore: Williams & Wilkins.

Hedman, L. D., Rogers, M. W., & Hanke, T. A. (1996). Neurologic professional education: linking the foundation science of motor control with physical therapy interventions for movement dysfunction. *Neurology Report, 20,* 9–13.

Horak, F. (1991). Assumptions underlying motor control for neurologic rehabilitation. In M. Lister (Ed.), *Contemporary management of motor control problems. Proceedings of the II-Step Conference* (pp. 11–27). Alexandria, VA: Foundation for Physical Therapy.

Kabat, H., & Knott, M. (1953). Proprioceptive facilitation techniques for treatment of paralysis. *Physical Therapy Review, 33,* 53–64.

Kamm, K., Thelen, E., & Jensen, J. L. (1990). A dynamical systems approach to motor development. *Physical Therapy, 70,* 763–775.

Ketelaar, M., Vermeer, A., t'Hart, H., Beek, E. v. P., & Helders, P. J. M. (2001). Effects of a functional therapy program on motor abilities of children with cerebral palsy. *Physical Therapy, 81,* 1534–1545.

Kielhofner, G. (1997). *Conceptual foundations of occupational therapy* (2nd ed.). Philadelphia: F. A. Davis.

Knott, M., & Voss, D. E. (1968). *Proprioceptive neuromuscular techniques: Patterns and techniques* (2nd ed.). New York: Harper & Row.

Kohl, R., & Sheal, C. H. (1992). PEW (1966) revisited: Acquisition of hierarchical control as a function of observational practice. *Journal of Motor Behavior, 24,* 247–260.

Latash, M. L., & Anson, J. G. (1996). What are "normal" movements in atypical populations? *Behavioral and Brain Sciences, 19,* 55–106.

Lewthwaite, R. (1990). Motivational considerations in physical therapy involvement. *Physical Therapy, 70,* 808–819.

Long, T., & Toscano, K. (2002). *Handbook of pediatric physical therapy* (2nd ed.). Philadelphia: Lippincott Williams & Wilkins.

Majsak, M. J. (1996). Application of motor learning principles to the stroke population. *Topics in Stroke Rehabilitation, 3,* 27–59.

Martin, S., & Kessler, M. (2000). *Neurological intervention for physical therapist assistants.* Philadelphia: W. B. Saunders.

Mathiowetz, V., & Haugen, J. B. (1994). Motor behavior research: Implications for therapeutic approaches to central nervous system dysfunction. *American Journal of Occupational Therapy, 48,* 733–744.

McCormack, G. L., & Feuchter, F. (1996). Neurophysiology for the sensorimotor approaches to treatment. In L. W. Pedretti (Ed.), *Occupational therapy: Practice skills for physical dysfunction* (4th ed.). St. Louis: Mosby.

McCormacke, G. L. (1996). The Rood approach to treatment of neuromuscular dysfunction. In L. W. Pedretti (Ed.), *Occupational therapy: Practice skills for physical dysfunction* (4th ed.). St. Louis: Mosby.

Montgomery, P. C., & Connolly, B. H. (Eds.) (1991). *Motor control and physical therapy: Theoretical framework and practical applications.* Hixson, TN: Chattanooga Group.

Morris, S. L., & Sharpe, M. H. (1993). PNF revisited. *Physiotherapy Theory and Practice, 9,* 43–51.

Moyers, P. (1999). Guide to occupational therapy practice. *American Journal of Occupational Therapy, 53,* 247–322.

Newell, K. M., & Valvano, J. (1998). Therapeutic intervention as a constraint in learning and relearning movement skills. *Scandinavian Journal of Occupational Therapy, 5,* 51–57.

O'Neill, D. L., & Harris, S. R. (1982). Developing goals and objectives for handicapped children. *Physical Therapy, 62,* 295–298.

O'Sullivan, S. B. (2001). Strategies to improve motor control and motor learning. In S. B. O'Sullivan & T. J. Schmitz (Eds.), *Physical rehabilitation: Assessment and treatment* (4th ed.). Philadelphia: F. A. Davis.

O'Sullivan, S. B., & Schmitz, T. J. (Eds.). (2000). *Physical rehabilitation: Assessment and treatment* (4th ed.). Philadelphia: F. A. Davis.

O'Sullivan, S. B., & Schmitz, T. J. (2001). *Physical rehabilitation laboratory manual: Focus on functional training.* Philadelphia: F. A. Davis.

Padilla, R., & Peyton, C. G. (1999). Neuro-occupation: Historical review and examples. *Neuroscience and occupation: Links to practice* (Vol. 10). Rockville, MD: American Occupational Therapy Association.

Palmer, M. L., & Toms, J. E. (1992). *Manual for functional training* (3rd ed.). Philadelphia: F. A. Davis.

Poole, J. (1997). Movement related problems. In C. Christiansen & C. Baum (Eds.), *Enabling function and well-being* (2nd ed.). Thorofare, NJ: Slack.

Randall, K. E., & McEwen, I. R. (2000). Writing patient-centered functional goals. *Physical Therapy, 80,* 1197–1203.

Reed, E. (1982). An outline of a theory of action systems. *Journal of Motor Behavior, 14,* 98–134.

Reeves, G. D. (2001). Sensory stimulation, sensory integration and the adaptive response. *Sensory Integration, Special Interest Section Quarterly, 24,* 1–3.

Rood, M. (1962). The use of sensory receptors to activate, facilitate and inhibit motor response, automatic and somatic in developmental sequence. In C. Sattely (Ed.), *Approaches to the treatment of patients with neuromuscular dysfunction.* Dubuque, IA: Wm. C. Brown.

Rose, S. A. (1984). Preterm responses of passive, active and social touch. In C. C. Brown (Ed.), *The many facets of touch.* Skillman, NJ: Johnson & Johnson.

Ryerson, S., & Levit, K. (1997). *Functional movement reeducation.* Philadelphia: Churchill Livingstone.

Ryerson, S. D. (2001). Hemiplegia. In D. A. Umphred (Ed.). *Neurological rehabilitation.* St. Louis: Mosby.

Sawner, K., & LaVigne, J. (1992). *Brunnstrom's movement therapy in hemiplegia* (2nd ed.). New York: J. B. Lippincott.

Schoen, S., & Anderson, J. (1993). Neurodevelopmental treatment frame of reference. In P. Kramer & J. Hinojosa (Eds.), *Frames of reference for pediatric occupational therapy* (pp. 49–86). Baltimore: Williams & Wilkins.

Shah, S. K., Harasymiw, S. J., & Stahl, P. L. (1986). Stroke rehabilitation: Outcome based on Brunnstrom recovery stages. *Occupational Therapy Journal of Research, 6,* 365–376.

Shepard, K. (1991). Theory: Criteria, importance, and impact. In M. Lister (Ed.), *Contemporary management of motor control problems. Proceedings of the II-Step Conference* (pp. 5–10). Alexandria, VA: Foundation for Physical Therapy.

Sherrington, C. S. (1906). *The integrative action of the nervous system.* New Haven, CT: Yale University Press.

Shumway-Cook, A., & Woollacott, M. H. (2001). *Motor control: Theory and Practical Applications* (2nd ed.). Philadelphia: Lippincott Williams & Wilkins.

Smith, R. H., & Sharpe, M. (1994). Brunnstrom therapy: Is it still relevant to stroke rehabilitation? *Physiotherapy Theory and Practice, 10,* 87–94.

Stockmeyer, S. (1967). An interpretation of the approach of Rood to the treatment of neuromuscular dysfunction. *American Journal of Physical Medicine, 46,* 900–956.

Stockmeyer, S. (1972). A sensorimotor approach to treatment. In P. Pearson & C. Williams (Eds.), *Physical therapy services in the developmental disabilities.* Springfield, IL: Charles C. Thomas Publishers.

Styer-Acevedo, J. (1998). Physical therapy for the child with cerebral palsy. In J. S. Tecklin (Ed.), *Pediatric physical therapy* (3rd ed.). Philadelphia: Lippincott-Raven.

Taub, E. (1976). Movement in nonhuman primates deprived of somatosensory feedback. *Exercise and Sports Science Reviews, 4,* 335–374.

Trombly, C. (1993). Anticipating the future: assessment of occupational function. *American Journal of Occupational Therapy, 47,* 253–257.

Tscharnuter, I. (1993). A new therapy approach to movement organization. *Physical & Occupational Therapy in Pediatrics, 13,* 2, 19–40.

Uniform terminology for occupational therapy (1994). *American Journal of Occupational Therapy, 48,* 1047–1054.

Umphred, D., Byl, N., Lazaro, R. T., & Roller, M. (2001). Interventions for neurological disabilities. In *Neurological Rehabilitation* (4th ed.). St. Louis: Mosby.

Valvano, J., & Long, T. (1991). Neurodevelopmental treatment: A review of the writings of the Bobaths. *Pediatric Physical Therapy, 3,* 125–129.

VanSant, A. (1990). Brunnstrom's treatment approach in the light of contemporary motor-control concepts. In J. Schleichkorn, *Brunnstrom: Physical therapy pioneer, master clinician and humanitarian.* Thorofare, NJ: Slack.

Walsche, F. M. P. (1961). Contributions of John Hughlings Jackson to neurology. *Archives of Neurology, 5,* 99–133.

Weiss, S. (1986). Psycho physiological effects of caregiver touch on incidence of cardiac dysrhythmia. *Heart and Lung, 15,* 495–505.

Whiteside A. (1997). Clinical goals and application of NDT facilitation. *NDTA Network, Sept/Oct,* 2–14.

Winton, P. J., & Bailey, D. B. (1993). Communicating with families: Examining practices and facilitating change. In J. P. Simeonsson & R. J. Simeonsson (Eds.), *Children with special needs: Family, culture, and society.* Orlando, FL: Harcourt Brace Jovanovich.

7

Clinical Management of the Primary Neuromuscular Impairments That Interfere with Functional Movement

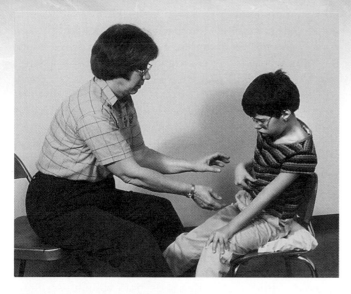

Cornerstone Concepts

- Differentiation between positive and negative features of brain damage and primary and secondary impairments

- Abnormal force production: definition, description, and clinical management

- Weakness

- Muscle tone abnormalities: abnormally low or abnormally high muscle tone

- Coordination problems: definition, description, and clinical management

- Muscle activation and sequencing problems

- Timing problems

- Involuntary movements

- The nature of functional movement problems in individuals with neurological impairment

Clinicians are cautioned to respect the fact that when an individual with a brain injury attempts a purposeful action, the movement pattern that emerges reflects the best that can be done under the circumstances, given the state of all of both the neural and musculoskeletal systems and the dynamic possibilities inherent in the linkages between all the subsystems involved in movement production and control (Carr & Shepherd, 1998). It is the clinician's task, responsibility, and opportunity to assist the patient/client in developing creative but individual solutions to movement problems given the strengths and challenges of that unique person.

221

Introduction

When faced with what appears to be a large problem, one of the strategies employed in attempts to problem solve is to try to step back from the problem, gain some perspective, and attempt to see the large (seemingly insurmountable) problem as a set of mini-problems or series of interrelated parts. An analysis of the smaller mini-problems, as well as an understanding of how these parts contribute to the whole issue, helps the problem solver to develop and enact a workable solution.

Clinical Connection:

For example, imagine that you are faced with the task of cleaning your apartment, house, or dormitory room. On initial inspection, the entire problem appears to be large and perhaps overwhelming. There are apparent (hard to miss) signs of disarray and disorganization all around you! Some of the "symptoms" of your disarray may be very obvious, others more apparent only in the limitations they contribute to (e.g., "I can't find my keys!"). Some of these signs of disarray may be the presence of trash and dirt, piles of papers, books, compact discs, and personal belongings, and perhaps even the presence of a persistently obnoxious odor that probably accompanies last week's late night snack. These signs of your lack of domesticity are very apparent to the naked eye (and nose!). Other symptoms or signs of your domestic disorder may include your inability to find things, an apparent lack of organization for proper storage of needed items, and the frustration you feel when trying to locate your class syllabus, checkbook, or car keys. These signs of your lack of domesticity are not necessarily easy to see, but they unmistakably contribute to your limited ability to function best within your dormitory world.

To solve your functional dilemma, the first thing that you have to do is develop a plan. The plan probably will include several steps, one of which is the identification of two major tasks. First, the removal of the visually apparent features of your untidiness: take out the trash, pile up the dirty clothes, locate and remove the evidence of last week's snack, locate the floor and then wash or vacuum it. Only then can you begin the second task of organizing your belongings and generating some kind of new intervention plan for keeping things in order, spurred onward by your resolution to maintain better order so that you can function better in the future. Breaking the task down into separate components helps to prioritize a management plan and organize the approach to the problem.   ▪

At first glance, intervention with the patient/client with neurological dysfunction may appear to be overwhelming, because this individual often presents with myriad clinical signs and symptoms. Students in the neurorehabilitation professions often feel overwhelmed with the complexity of the patient's clinical presentation and wonder, "Where do I start in trying to understand this patient's movement disorder so that I can then effectively help this patient?" Students and clinicians need to have a method for assessing and understanding the patient's clinical presentation so that these signs and features can be categorized into describable and manageable components. Clinicians and students need to have a method for recognizing the features of the patient's problem, knowing which of those features are due to the neurological damage, and understanding the impact of all the signs on the patient's ability to demonstrate safe functional movement. The contributing components can then be listed and prioritized, including discerning which features seem to have a recognizable impact on that patient's function, as well as recognizing which features can be changed or not changed.

These next four chapters do not intend to replace the primary texts on evaluations, tests, and measurements in physical therapy or occupational therapy education. Rather, for therapists, this text intends to be complementary to those texts, focusing on the main clinical dilemmas experienced by patients with neurological dysfunction and offering strategies for management. For therapist assistants, this text can serve as a practical guide to intervention and understanding of the patient/client with a neurological disorder. In fact, because evaluation is the responsibility of the therapist and beyond the scope of the assistant, this text will give descriptions of clinical presentations and offer a methodology for understanding how to clinically tackle the movement problem. Evaluation, per se, will not be covered. Although assistants do not evaluate, an effective assistant needs to have an understanding of the patient's movement dilemma to best treat that patient. Intervention with the patient/client, without a concurrent understanding of the signs, symptoms, and functional limitations facing the person, would be ineffective at best and most assuredly frustrating, not only for the therapist/assistant team but also for the patient or client.

In concert with the dynamic systems model, it is understood that individuals with a neurological disorder present with a complex set of impairments within the motor, sensory, cognitive, and perceptual domains of function. Because this is a text on clinical management of the impaired movement system in patients with neurological impairment the focus here is on the motor system, although the importance of the other domains, such as cognitive and social-emotional, cannot be minimized. A more comprehensive discussion of the vital contributions of those factors to movement success is beyond the scope and the intent of this text. The next four chapters will focus on the impairments, functional limitations, and intervention strategies most appropriate for solving the most common functional clinical problems associated with central nervous system (CNS) pathology:

1. Problems caused by primary neuromuscular impairments, including weakness, muscle tone abnormalities, coordination problems, and involuntary movements
2. Problems with postural control and balance
3. Problems with upper extremity control, including manipulation
4. Problems with lower extremity function, including locomotion

This chapter will describe the primary neuromuscular impairments that impose a major constraint on functional movement in the patient/client with neurological dysfunction. Clinical management of these common impairments will emphasize decreasing the effect of the functional limitation and optimizing or *enabling* the individual to function best within the limits imposed by these primary impairments.

Separating the Large Problem into "Mini-Problems"

Brain pathology produces a unique pattern of signs and symptoms associated with the nature and area of the neurological damage (Shumway-Cook & Woollacott, 2001). In the neurosciences, it has been typical since the time of Hughlings Jackson (Walshe, 1961) to consider the dyscontrol characteristics associated with upper motor neuron (UMN) pathology as either **positive features** or **negative features** (Table 7–1). Positive features are defined as abnormal behavior due directly to the lesion, including the presence of abnormal movement patterns such as pathological reflex responses (e.g., Babinski reflex) or hyperactive reflex responses such as a hyperreactive stretch reflex. Positive signs also include muscle tone abnormalities and the presence of involuntary movements (Stein, Pomerantz, & Schechtman, 1997). These positive features or signs are all really exaggerations of normal phenomena, considered to be due to the pathological involvement in the parapyramidal (around the pyramids) fibers in the brain (Burke, 1988; Shahani & Young, 1980). In contrast, negative features or signs are due to a loss in or deficit of motor behavior. Examples of negative features of brain damage are weakness, slowness of movement, loss of dexterity or coordination, and fatigability. There is mounting evidence that these negative features of damage may be more disabling to the patient than the changes in muscle tone or the hyperreflexia (Burke, 1988; Carr & Shepherd, 1998; Landau, 1988). Patients/clients are also more preoccupied with losses in strength and dexterity, stiffness associated with muscle changes, and with consequent loss in functional abilities. The negative factors experienced by the patient, such as difficulty activating muscle, generating appropriate force, and coordinating those muscle forces, need to be the primary targets of therapeutic intervention (Carr & Shepherd, 1998).

In addition to differentiating academically between positive and negative features of CNS damage, there is a similar delineation of impairments, including separation of impairments into primary and secondary impairments. CNS lesions can result in a variety of primary impairments affecting motor, sensory, perceptual, and cognitive systems. In addition to primary impairments, secondary impairments also contribute

TABLE 7–1		
Positive and Negative Signs Associated with Upper Motor Neuron Disorders		
Feature	Definition	Examples
Positive sign	Abnormal behavior due directly to the lesion; actually exaggerations of normal phenomena due to the pathological involvement in the brain	Presence of abnormal movement patterns such as reflex responses, including: • Babinski reflex • Hyperactive reflex responses such as a hyperreactive stretch reflex Presence of muscle tone abnormalities and involuntary movement
Negative sign	Due to a loss in or deficit of motor behavior	Negative features of brain damage include: • Muscle weakness • Slowness of movement • Loss of dexterity or coordination • Fatigability

Sources: Data from Burke, D. (1988). Spasticity as an adaptation to pyramidal tract injury. In S. G. Waxman (Ed.), *Advances in Neurology 47: Functional recovery in neurological disease.* New York: Raven Press; Carr, J., & Shepherd, R. (1998). *Neurological rehabilitation: Optimizing motor performance.* Oxford, U. K.: Butterworth Heinemann; Landau, W. M. (1988). Parables of palsy, pills, and PT pedagogy: A spastic dialectic. *Neurology, 38,* 1496–1499; and Walsche, F. M. P. (1961). Contributions of John Hughlings Jackson to Neurology. *Archives of Neurology, 5,* 99–133.

to the movement problems demonstrated by patients. Secondary impairments do not result from the CNS pathology directly, but rather develop as a result of the consequences of the pathology or primary impairment.

Clinical Connection:

A child with cerebral palsy (CP) may have a lesion (presence of the pathology) in the descending motor pathways, causing a primary impairment of muscular weakness and abnormal muscle tone. The child presenting for therapy may have secondary impairments of a hip flexion contracture and a dislocating hip because of the abnormal muscle pull caused by these primary impairments. It is important to realize that function can be limited by the abnormal muscle tone and weakness, as well as by the unstable hip and the hip flexion contracture. Intervention will be directed at many levels:

1. At the primary impairment level to reduce the effects of abnormal muscle tone by increasing voluntary control and muscle strength

2. At the secondary impairment level to increase hip range of motion, reduce the contracture, and promote hip stability

3. At the strategy level to assist with the development of more effective and efficient movement strategies or compensatory strategies

Neuromuscular impairments encompass a diverse group of problems that constitute a major constraint on functional movement in the individual with neurological dysfunction. The remainder of this chapter will describe the primary neuromuscular impairments associated with functional movement disorders in patients/clients with neurological dysfunction.

Abnormal Force Production: Definition and Description

The primary neuromuscular impairments associated with neurological dysfunction mainly center on abnormal muscle force production. The ability to produce and coordinate an appropriate movement response requires production of muscular force, activation and sustenance of muscle activity, and the coordination and timing of muscle activation patterns. The primary motor system impairments that interfere with functional movement are muscle weakness, abnormalities of muscle tone, coordination problems, and interference from involuntary movements. This author acknowledges and commends Anne Shumway-Cook and Marjorie Woollacott for organizing the impairments into such a "user friendly" fashion (Shumway-Cook & Woollacott, 2001).

Weakness

Weakness is defined as an inability to generate normal levels of muscular force and is a major impairment of motor function in patients with nervous system damage. Lesions within the CNS, peripheral nervous system (PNS), or muscular system can produce weakness. This text is focusing on weakness as an impairment following CNS damage. For a discussion of weakness associated with PNS pathology or primary muscle disorders, refer to other sources.

By definition, **upper motor neuron** lesions affect the CNS, anywhere from the spinal cord superiorly, producing signs of UMN syndrome, typically associated with hypertonicity, or hypotonicity, depending on the site of the lesion and the time of onset (acute versus chronic). Depending on the extent of the lesion, weakness in the patient with a CNS or upper motor neuron lesion can vary in severity from total loss of muscle activity, called paralysis or plegia, to a mild or partial loss of muscle activity, called paresis (Shumway-Cook & Woollacott, 2001). Paresis and plegia are described by their distribution, as described in Chapter 2. Paresis results from damage to the descending motor pathways, which interferes with the central (from the brain) excitatory drive to the motor units (Ghez, 1991). The end result is an inability to recruit and modulate the motor neurons, leading to a loss of movement.

Muscle force produced is dependent on the number and type of motor units recruited and the characteristics of both motor unit discharge and of the muscle itself. Firing of a single motor unit results in a twitch contraction of the innervated muscle fibers. With an increase in firing rate, these twitches summate to increase and sustain force output. An individual increases his or her muscle force by increasing the number of active motor units and increasing the firing rates of those active motor units. Motor units are normally recruited in an orderly pattern, with those that produce low force recruited first, followed by higher force-producing units as force requirements increase (Carr & Shepherd, 1998).

Damage to the CNS is accompanied by abnormal muscle tone and altered motor control, secondary to UMN lesions (Fredericks & Saladin, 1996; Shumway-Cook & Woollacott, 2001). The range of muscle tone abnormalities found within patients who have UMN lesions is broad, ranging from flaccidity or complete loss of tone to hypertonicity or spasticity (Shumway-Cook & Woollacott, 2001). Depending on the insult to the CNS, clinical manifestations of altered muscle tone will vary. However, *weakness and lack of normal voluntary control prevail*. Neural lesions affecting the ability to generate forces, both voluntarily and within the context of a functional task, are a major limitation in many patients who are neurologically impaired (Bertoti,

Stanger, Betz, Mulcahey, & Akers, 1997; Fredericks & Saladin, 1996; Shumway-Cook & Woollacott, 2001). The patient with spastic hemiplegia secondary to a cerebrovascular accident (CVA) or a child with spastic cerebral palsy both present with clinical weakness. Sensory feedback may also be altered or diminished.

After an upper motor neuron lesion, weakness is reflected in deficiencies in generating force and in sustaining force output (Bourbonnais & Vanden Noven, 1989). This occurs because of loss of motor unit recruitment, changes in recruitment patterns, and changes in firing rates. Additionally, changes occur in the properties of the motor units and in the morphological and mechanical properties of the muscle itself. These changes happen as adaptations to loss of innervation, immobility, and disuse.

In upper motor neuron lesions, reduced numbers of motor units and reduced firing rates of motor units have been reported (McComas, Sica, Upton, & Aguilera, 1973; Rosenfalck & Andreassen, 1980). Within 2 months of the insult, patients with hemiparesis resulting from a stroke show up to a 50-percent reduction in motor units on the affected side. Individuals with stroke display atrophy in motor units on the hemiparetic side. The remaining motor units require more time to contract, and they fatigue more rapidly. Craik (1991) suggests that altered recruitment and decreased motor unit firing account for this apparent weakness.

The degree of weakness may differ for different muscle groups. Given that the pyramidal tract is the primary pathway for voluntary goal-directed movement, it has been suggested that interruption of this pathway produces a greater impairment in prime mover muscles (Burke, 1988). In addition, because pyramidal innervation is denser for the distal muscles of the hand (including the extrinsic muscles that cross the wrist), there may be considerable deficits in hand functions, such as manipulation and prehension, with the greatest weakness observed in the intrinsic hand muscles.

Clinical Connection:

Patients/clients with neurological damage demonstrate deficits in strength. Clinicians have always been aware of the weakness observed in the limbs directly affected by the neurological insult, such as in the limbs on the affected side, contralateral to the CVA in the patient presenting with hemiplegia following a stroke. Experienced clinicians recently have contended that patients *also* present with weakness and signs of disturbed motor control in the unaffected limbs, perhaps due to the new or changed demands now placed on those limbs. A recent study by Andrews and

Bohannon (2000) demonstrates that strength deficits in the unaffected limb can be significant, less than 90 percent of normal. In concert with that study and clinical practice, clinicians should move away from designating limbs as "affected" and "unaffected" in deference to a more appropriate designation of referring to a weaker versus a stronger side or a stronger versus a weaker limb. This manner of referencing would also serve as a clinical reminder that *all* limbs, regardless of the underlying pathology, can benefit from individual assessment and strengthening if needed. ▪

Prolonged paresis, a primary neuromuscular impairment, also produces peripheral changes in the muscle, known as secondary musculoskeletal impairments. Changes in muscle tissue resulting from an upper motor neuron lesion suggest that muscle may not be as "strong" due to changes in the properties of the muscle and the presence of denervated muscle fibers (Craik, 1991). Specific changes at the motor neuron or muscle level, secondary to the UMN syndrome, can decrease a patient's ability to produce force. For example, the following changes, as summarized below, have been demonstrated in stroke patients:

- Motor neuron changes
  - Loss of motor units
  - Changes in recruitment order of motor units
  - Changes in firing rates of motor units
- Nerve changes
  - Changes in peripheral nerve conduction
- Muscle changes
  - Changes in morphological and contractile properties of the motor units
  - Changes in mechanical properties of muscles (Bourbonnais & Vanden Noven, 1989)

Without a doubt, individuals with CNS damage are weak.

▪ Clinical Management of Weakness in UMN Lesions

Traditionally, clinicians had believed that assessing strength and prescribing strength training was not valid or appropriate for patients with UMN pathology. Early sensorimotor theorists believed that spasticity was the primary impairment affecting functional performance and that strengthening a "spastic" muscle would increase the spasticity and have a deleterious effect on the recovery of functional performance. These assumptions have now been reexamined, and there is a new awareness that paresis, which is a negative feature of UMN damage, is as important a factor in impaired functional performance, as is the spasticity, a positive sign (Andrews & Bohannon, 2000; Bohannon & Walsh, 1992;

Bourbonnais et al., 1997). Given the demonstrated relationship between cortical and pyramidal tract activity and muscle force production, muscle weakness should be an expected result of *any* lesion involving corticomotorneuon cells, their projections, and their targets (Bohannon, 1989). Research has clearly demonstrated that improvements in strength do not only contribute to an improvement in functional performance, but that there is no indication of an associated increase in spasticity (Bertoti et al., 1997; Damiano, Kelly, & Vaughan, 1995; Damiano, Vaughan, & Abel, 1995; Darrah, Fan, Nunweiler, & Watkins, 1997; Fowler, Ho, Nwigwe, & Dorey, 2001; Haney, 1998; Teixeira-Salmela, Olney, Nadeau, & Brouwer, 1999).

■ Strength Training

In assessing strength, it is sometimes difficult to directly test the force-generating ability of individual muscles in the presence of spasticity, abnormal extensibility, and poor selective control. Functionally, strength can be assessed by identifying the individual's ability to move against gravity (concentric control), stabilize a body part (isometric strength), or lower a body part resisting gravity's influence (eccentric control) (Fig. 7–1). If the individual is able to isolate a voluntary contraction, manual muscle testing or measurement of isometric strength can be done.

Research has demonstrated the benefits of strength training in individuals with neurological impairment. Strength training is thought to not only improve voluntary motor control, but also appears to be a means for preventing or slowing down some of the mechanical changes and denervation changes seen in muscle tissue following UMN damage (Light, 1996; McCartney, Moroz, Garner, & McComas, 1988). The shift in emphasis to the functional significance of weakness in patients with CNS lesions has led to increased attention on strengthening programs for these patients/clients.

Techniques to improve strength can focus on either generating force to stabilize a body segment, move a body segment, or generating force to resist a movement. Strengthening programs can be designed to emphasize isometric, eccentric, or concentric contractions or the use of isokinetic equipment. Therapeutic exercise programs are developed based on the assessment findings and the patient's/client's functional abilities. Progression is directed at increasing strength, endurance, and coordination. The therapist and assistant have two broad options for progressing therapeutic exercise:

1. To progress the movement from gravity-eliminated positions to a movement that requires that the individual work against gravity
2. To alter the amount of assistance, facilitation, or resistance given by the therapist so that the individual has to develop more force or control

If the therapist or assistant observes that the individual is having difficulty executing the task or performing the strengthening activity, modifications can be made, the influence of gravity can be eliminated, assistance can be given, or the environment can be adapted. In most clinical practice settings, the therapist is the professional responsible for the design of intervention and establishment of goals, with the assistant actively engaged in intervention modification within the established plan of care, trained to be an astute observer and communicator with the therapist and the patient/client.

Clinical Connection:

As an intervention, a strength training program can be designed to start at the level of voluntary control demonstrated by the patient and then customized to focus on the individual's needs to build strength for the effective performance of functional tasks. For example, strengthening can be targeted to help the patient gain isometric, concentric, and eccentric control within the context of a functional activity. The following example is offered to illustrate task analysis and progression within this intervention approach:

Task: Getting a glass out of the overhead cabinet in order to get a drink of water.

To *target concentric control*: This is a good starting point, because concentric control is easier for patients than isometric or eccentric muscular control. Have the patient reach, concentrically contracting the shoulder flexors, to varying cabinet height levels. The amount of shoulder flexion required can be progressed as the patient gains antigravity strength and control, allowing the therapist to then progressively increase the demand by increasing the cabinet height. Assistance may or may not be given as indicated.

To *target isometric strengthening*: This is also a good starting point, depending on the angle of shoulder flexion selected for strengthening. Have the patient practice isometrically controlling the shoulder flexors with the upper extremity in the appropriate overhead position needed to retrieve the glass from the cabinet. Progression and strengthening can then focus on increasing the amount of time maintaining the position or altering the cabinet height (and therefore the angle of shoulder flexion).

To *target eccentric strengthening*: This is often the most difficult type of voluntary control to be achieved by the patient. Have the patient practice lowering the glass onto the counter, progressing from lower heights to higher cabinet heights, requiring progressively more eccentric control through increasingly greater ranges of motion. The weight and size of the glass can also be varied.

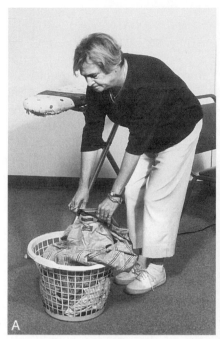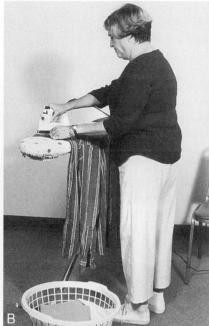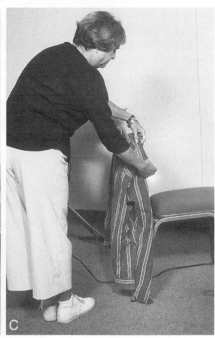

Figure 7–1. (A) Task requiring concentric hip extensor control—removing laundry from basket and then returning to a standing position. (B) Task requiring isometric hip extensor control. (C) Task requiring eccentric hip extensor control—maintaining stability while carefully placing ironed shirt onto a chair.

Strengthening programs can also include proprioceptive neuromuscular facilitation (PNF) and isokinetic training, both demonstrated to be effective for patients with neurological disorders. ▪

▪ Functional Task Training

Strengthening programs for patients with muscle weakness subsequent to neurological dysfunction often follow a progression of isometric contractions first and then practicing concentric and eccentric contractions, all practiced within the performance of a functional task. Isometric contractions are often first practiced in midrange, where the muscle can produce the greatest tension (see Fig. 7–1). Tasks that the individual has difficulty performing should become the major emphasis of the training program. These tasks should be practiced as whole-task activities whenever possible to allow the individual to learn or relearn and practice the task in its naturally occurring timing and sequence.

Clinical Connection:

The following example illustrates how a strengthening progression can be easily incorporated into a functional task. When transferring from a sitting position to standing, a patient/client could begin by practicing the task

standing from chairs with raised seats so that symmetrical movement patterns can be used, assisted partially through the initial range. The environmental modification of the raised seat helps to make the task more easily accomplished. As the movement becomes easier, lower seat heights and varying seat heights should be used to make the task more difficult, requiring that the muscles to be used in the task contract differently. This strategy also encourages the patient learner to generalize the skill to changed environmental contexts. Progression can also include asking the patient to stand without using the hands for support or having the individual hold an object while coming from sit to stand (Bennett & Karnes, 1998). ▪

▪ Physical Agents: Electrical Stimulation and Biofeedback

Electrical Stimulation

The efficacy of electrical stimulation for the purposes of strengthening has been extensively studied and is well established. Neuromuscular electrical stimulation (NMES) has been demonstrated to be effective in improving voluntary control and muscle strength in both children and adults with abnormal muscle tone, weakness, and difficulty with voluntary movement. Electrical stimulation has been clearly demonstrated to be a valuable facilitation tool for patients with primary movement disorders (Baker, 1979; Bertoti et al., 1997; Carmick, 1997a, 1997b; Comeaux, Patterson, Rubin, & Meiner, 1997; Hummelsheim, Maier-Loth, & Eickhof, 1997; Pease, 1998). In patients with spasticity, research and clinical practice are demonstrating that as strength increases and voluntary motor control emerges, the symptom of abnormal muscle tone clearly decreases. With the augmentation in muscular strength due to electrical stimulation, the symptom of spasticity or abnormally high tone decreases.

Basic science research has demonstrated that skeletal muscle, exposed to prolonged functional demands augmented by exercise and electrical stimulation, responds with changes in metabolic activity and then structural adaptation (Daly et al., 1996). Motor learning can then occur as the child or adult is supported, with the electrically induced contraction, into a functional use of the stimulated muscle contraction (Figs. 7–2 and 7–3). For the use of electrical stimulation to have any lasting effect on the patient's movement, stimulation, as any other augmentative intervention, must be done within a functional context. Parameters for application of therapeutic surface electrical stimulation are available elsewhere. Amplitude need be only adjusted high enough to achieve the desired motor response. Electrical stimulation has been successfully used to improve gait and hand function in children with CP and adults with hemiplegia (Baker, 1979; Bertoti et al., 1997; Carmick, 1997b; Hummelsheim et al., 1997). Carryover effects have been demonstrated, with translation of the training effects of the electrically facilitated movement into improved function when the stimulation ceases (Bertoti et al., 1997; Comeaux et al., 1997).

Neurorehabilitation focuses on using the electrical stimulation to elicit a contraction during an appropriate functional task requiring the activation of that muscle, such as in standing, stepping, or reaching. Success has been reported stimulating the following muscles during functional tasks: gluteus maximus, quadriceps, hamstrings, anterior tibialis, gastrocnemius, triceps, wrist extensors, and finger flexors. Clinically applied therapeutic functional electrical stimulation can be viewed as a motor learning assist, assisting the patient/client in increasing sensory awareness and relearning voluntary control.

Clinical Connection:

For facilitation of muscle strengthening and voluntary control, electrical stimulation can be used as follows, in the following functional positions:

1. Over the triceps muscle during upper extremity weight-bearing activities

2. Over the deltoid and supraspinatus muscles to aid in reduction of a subluxed shoulder

3. Over the hip extensors, quadriceps, or gastrocnemius muscles to assist with lower extremity stance stability

4. Over the anterior tibialis muscle to assist with foot clearance during the swing phase of gait

Therapists and assistants are reminded to adhere to published contraindications and precautions before using electrical stimulation (Nelson, Hayes, & Currier, 1999; Robinson & Snyder-Mackler, 1995). ▪

Biofeedback

Biofeedback is a process whereby the amount of motor unit activity is detected, amplified, and then converted into either an auditory or a visual signal. This augmented signal is used for the purpose of teaching an individual to increase or decrease the amount of that muscular activity. Biofeedback has been successfully used for individuals with neurological disorders to achieve either of two therapeutic training purposes:

- To increase the amount of voluntary muscle activity, biofeedback can be used with the sensors located over the weak muscle to assist the patient/client to direct his or her attention to recruiting more motor units or isolating the activation of that specific muscle. The threshold setting of the biofeedback unit is set so that the desired amount of motor unit recruitment results in the auditory or visual signal.
- To decrease undesirable motor unit activity in a muscle, biofeedback can be used with the sensors located over the hyperreactive muscle to assist the patient/client to direct his or her attention to relaxing

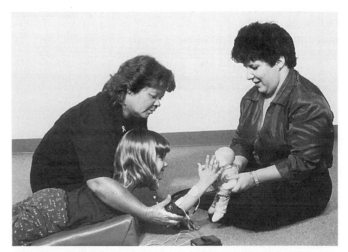

Figure 7–2. Electrical stimulation assisting active wrist extension during functional reach.

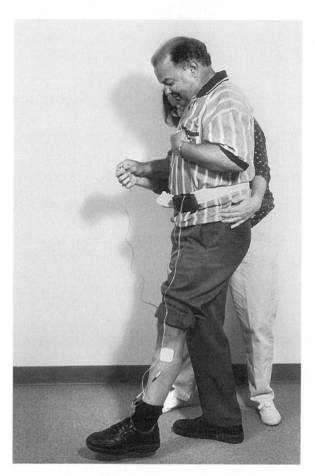

Figure 7–3. Electrical stimulation as a dorsiflexion assist to help foot clearance during swing phase of gait.

that muscle. Alternately, the sensors could be placed on the antagonist muscle so that as the individual voluntarily activates the antagonist, attention is directed to reciprocal inhibition (quieting of) the hyperreactive agonist.

As with any physical modality, the modality is only as effective as the creativity of the clinician using it as part of the intervention. Biofeedback can be a very effective teaching tool, useful in helping patients to regain kinesthetic awareness and then directing the individual to use that awareness to build voluntary motor control. It is of limited value with a patient with a severe cognitive disorder, because the relationship between the muscle activity and the resultant auditory or visual signal may be difficult for the patient with cognitive impairment to comprehend.

Muscle Tone Abnormalities

The concept of tone itself is vague, to say the least. Muscle "tone" at rest does not really depend on purely neural mechanisms; any resistance to passive move-

ment is due to mechanical factors or intrinsic properties of the muscle. There is no electrical activity in resting muscle or when muscle is passively stretched in a relaxed subject.

Muscle tone is defined as a state of readiness of skeletal muscle so that the muscular system is in a state of arousal prepared for the task demands to be placed on it. A certain level of muscle tone is typical of a normal muscle. It is determined by the level of excitability of the entire pool of motor neurons controlling a muscle, the intrinsic stiffness of the muscle itself, the absence of neuropathology, and the level of sensitivity of many different reflexes. Muscle tone can be viewed as a continuum, according to the following display (Shumway-Cook & Woollacott, 2001):

FLACCIDITY ↔ HYPOTONIA ↔
NORMAL ↔ SPASTICITY ↔ RIGIDITY

A hallmark of CNS pathology is the presence of abnormal muscle tone. Abnormally high (hypertonia) or abnormally low (hypotonia) muscle tone is a universally recognized clinical sign of nervous system pathology. It is considered to be a primary impairment of disorders of the motor system. It is not known, however, how much abnormal muscle tone contributes to the functional limitations experienced by patients. Flaccidity and hypotonia are states of muscle hypotonicity, and spasticity and rigidity are states of hypertonicity.

▪ Abnormally Low Muscle Tone

Abnormally low muscle tone is characterized by a clinical presentation whereby the muscles demonstrate no resistance to passive movement. The stretch reflexes are diminished (**hyporeflexia**) or absent (**areflexia**), the limbs are easily moved, and the limbs feel "floppy." Hyperextensibility and instability of joints are common. Abnormally low muscle tone is seen in both lower and upper motor neuron disorders. Although in either case the clinical presentation of the abnormally low tone will look the same, it is important to differentiate between these instances.

Lower motor neuron (LMN) lesions affect the anterior horn cell or the peripheral nerve, producing decreased or absent muscle tone along with associated symptoms of paralysis, signs of muscle denervation, and atrophy. In the case of an LMN lesion, weakness and paralysis are permanent, not replaced by any signs of hypertonicity.

Decreased muscle tone is also associated in UMN lesions affecting the entire cerebral cortex and the cerebellum or in the acute state of a CNS insult. When the nervous system is in a state of shock after a lesion of acute onset, there may be a profound depression of motor function in which all muscles of the affected body segments are involved (Denny Brown, 1950). This may be a temporary state, called spinal or cerebral shock, depending on the location of the lesion. In the patient with an acute CVA, the term **cerebral shock** is aptly used to describe the temporary flaccid state on the involved body side; in the person with a spinal cord injury, the term **spinal shock** is used. The neural explanation for hypotonia following an UMN lesion is that there may be insufficient descending fibers converging on the final motor neuron population to shape a complex movement or to even bring the motor neurons to the level of discharge frequency necessary for a tetanic muscle contraction (Landau, 1988). This results in profound weakness, slowness of movement, and loss of coordination.

▪ Flaccidity

Flaccidity is characterized as the complete loss of muscle tone. Flaccidity is often seen in the acute stage of injury, immediately following a CNS injury, but it can also be secondary to a lower motor neuron lesion. In patients with flaccidity, deep tendon reflexes (DTRs) are absent and there is no evidence of muscle contraction. In the CNS, flaccidity is often but not always a transient stage.

▪ Hypotonia

Hypotonia is defined as a reduction in muscle stiffness, often seen in spinocerebellar lesions and in developmental disorders such as a type of cerebral palsy or Down syndrome. Hypotonia is characterized by low muscle tone, weak neck and trunk control, poor muscular co-contraction, and limited stability. The patient with hypotonia demonstrates high fatigability, poor endurance, slowness or a paucity of movement, and often a listless affect. It is hard work to move with hypotonia!

▪ Clinical Management of Abnormally Low Tone

As a primary motor system impairment, abnormally low muscle tone presents with some recognizable clinical characteristics and common movement problems. Patients with hypotonia present with weakness, a decreased ability to sustain muscle activation, a decreased ability to co-activate muscle groups, abnormal joint mobility patterns, and a delayed or ineffective exhibition of normal postural responses. Clinically, it is vital that therapists and assistants offer additional physical support to flaccid extremities to prevent injury. Table 7–2 describes these common clinical problems

and the consequent functional limitations experienced by individuals with hypotonia, with some suggestions for therapeutic intervention. Figures 7–4 through 7–6 accompany the table to give a pictorial view of the problem, functional limitation, or intervention suggestion.

Sensorimotor Approaches

Sensorimotor techniques are often used to increase motor unit firing in flaccid muscles. For example, tapping on the muscle in a functional, gravity-eliminated position may elicit enough activation of the muscle to facilitate beginning regaining of voluntary control. Other sensorimotor techniques that may be employed include approximation, quick stretch, and visual input. To apply approximation, a weight-bearing position is used, with the clinician offering manual assistance as needed to stabilize the body segment. Examples include the use of weight bearing through the involved upper extremity onto a tabletop or leaning to the side as depicted in Figures 6–4*A*, 6–20, and 6–31. Recent evidence supports the effectiveness of upper extremity weight-bearing in activating corticospinal facilitation of motor units in the muscles of patients with hemiparesis (Brouwer & Ambury, 1994). In the lower extremity, approximation is accomplished easily in standing as the patient shifts weight from side to side. A splint or manual assistance may be needed to prevent knee buckling. Quick stretch is most effectively used to activate motor unit firing by giving a quick stretch to the muscle in the lengthened range, easily incorporated into use of a PNF diagonal in a passive or active assistive manner. Quick stretch or tapping, as discussed in Chapter 6, activates the monosynaptic stretch reflex arc, resulting in activation of the agonist muscle. This activation is a very phasic (brief) response, best used in conjunction with other techniques. It is extremely effective in helping patients to initiate or sustain a newly acquired voluntary muscle contraction, again best used in a functional context. Always, facilitation is only augmentative and should be incorporated during a functional activity (Fig. 7–7). Because the goal is to assist patients in relearning functional movement, these sensorimotor techniques need to be faded (decreased and then stopped) as soon as the patient/client begins to demonstrate independent control.

Clinical Connection:

The following example is offered to illustrate the effective use of sensorimotor techniques during the beginning stages of neurorehabilitation. When working with an individual with abnormally low muscle tone in the

TABLE 7–2

Common Clinical Problems, Functional Limitations, and Goals for the Patient/Client with Hypotonia as a Main Impairment

Clinical Problem	Functional Limitation	Goals
Weakness	Decreased strength Decreased antigravity control (Fig. 7–4A)	Increase voluntary strength: isometrically, eccentrically, and concentrically Increased antigravity control in functional positions (Fig. 7–4B)
Decreased ability to sustain muscle group activation	Inability to maintain postural alignment and control in static positions (Fig. 7–4A) Fatigability	Increased muscle activation through the use of sensorimotor techniques and strengthening procedures (Fig. 7–4C) Incorporation of endurance training into functional retraining, energy conservation
Decreased ability to co-activate muscle groups	Poor proximal stability, increased reliance on soft tissue support or biomechanical locking to stabilize a joint (Fig. 7–4B) Susceptibility to injury	Increased co-contraction and proximal stability with joint in open pack position, use of sensorimotor techniques such as approximation, weight bearing, and weight shifting in developmental positions (Fig. 7–5) Use of positioning, orthoses, and adaptive equipment (e.g., wheelchair lap tray)
Decreased postural control of head and trunk	Decreased ability to stabilize and move head and trunk in upright postures	Increased control of head and trunk in multiple positions when static, as well as during movement (Fig. 7–6)
Inefficient or ineffective demonstration of postural responses	Decreased ability to realign posture when displaced or while moving Poor balance, frequent falls	Increased response accuracy to postural changes Balance activities
Abnormal joint ROM	Incorrect joint excursion for required movement Hyperextensibility Abnormal "fixing," resulting in joint contracture	Joint excursion during functional movement Joint integrity and skeletal alignment Strategies to improve range of motion
Shallow breathing	Increased incidence respiratory infection Oral motor difficulties	Increased thoracic extension and trunk strength, breathing exercises Pulmonary hygiene

Sources: Adapted from Bertoti, D. B. (2000). Cerebral palsy: Lifespan management. In *Orthopaedic interventions for the pediatric patient, orthopaedic section home study course.* Alexandria, VA: American Physical Therapy Association.

upper extremity, a functional goal may be stable weight-bearing through that upper extremity to assist in a sit-to-stand transfer. In this case, the therapist or assistant manually assists the patient (either a child or an adult) to place the extremity on the arm of the chair. Visual and verbal cues are used as the patient's vision is directed to the desired task. Approximation is given with a downward pressure through the shoulder, asking the patient to assist by co-contracting the muscles around the shoulder girdle, elbow, and wrist. A series of taps to the triceps or a quick stretch accomplished using the patient's body weight activates the triceps to fire. As the patient is assisted in executing the transfer, manual guidance is offered, using the shoulder as a key point of control. This example illustrates that

the following techniques are "stacked" during this task, to augment the patient's motor learning of this important functional skill: tapping, quick stretch, approximation, manual contacts, key points of control, visual feedback, verbal instruction, and reinforcement. None of these sensorimotor techniques would be effective in isolation, but they can have an important, temporary role in the entire intervention approach used with the patient/client. ■

Training to Improve Motor Control and Functional Performance

The emphasis of intervention with individuals with abnormally low muscle tone should be on the establish-

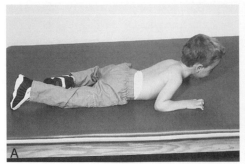
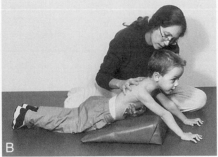
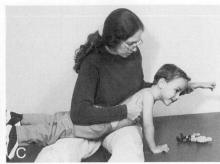

Figure 7–4. (A) Children with hypotonia often demonstrate limited antigravity strength and control. (B) Therapist assists child working on antigravity control in a functional position, as well as during a reaching task (C).

ment of stability in functional positions. Functional positions may include side lying, sitting, or standing. Intervention emphasis is on initiating stable postures and assisting the individual in functional movements that can then be repeated and practiced. For patients with very low muscle tone, such as flaccidity, rolling from side to side, basic bed mobility, and moving from supine to a sitting position may be difficult and require a great deal of initial guidance from the therapist or assistant. These important functional tasks, however, must be initiated early for pressure relief and basic hygiene. Repetitive practice of these tasks requires activation of intact muscles, facilitation of the involved body segments, weight bearing, and sensory stimulation through the involved body parts. Other functional tasks include transfers and engagement in mobility and self-care skill, depending on the ability of the patient/client.

As the individual begins to contract muscles in stable postures or moves without facilitation, the emphasis is on volitional muscle contraction and facilitation techniques are no longer used. Once stability in functional postures is achieved, controlled mobility activities are encouraged. Examples of controlled mobility activities include weight-shifting activities and movement transitions, which require synergistic activation of antagonistic muscle groups (see Chapter 6). Dynamic activities that combine mobility and stability are stressed. Voluntary control during independent or assisted transitional movements is practiced in functional contexts (see Figs. 6–3 and 7–7).

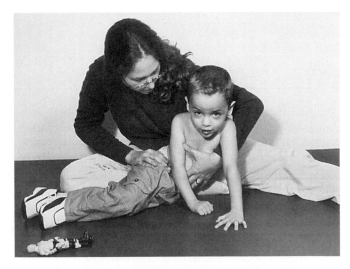

Figure 7–6. Child working on strengthening of upper extremity weight bearing and the development of postural head and trunk control during a transitional movement. Note how the therapist's judicious use of her hands supports and facilitates the child's movement attempts, using the child's pelvis and trunk as key control points.

Figure 7–5. Bridging can be a very effective activity for promoting strength increases and the development of proximal control and stability during a functional or playful activity.

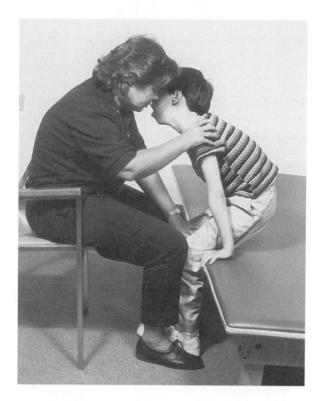

Figure 7–7. Therapist facilitates use of weight bearing and approximation through both the impaired upper and lower extremity in a child during performance of a functional activity. Note the therapist giving approximation through the child's shoulder and manual assistance at the knee.

▪ Abnormally High Muscle Tone or Hypertonia

▪ Spasticity

Spasticity is a state of hypertonicity of the muscle. The word *spasticity,* derived from the Greek word *spastikos,* means "to tug" or "to draw" (Albright, 1992; Preston & Hecht, 1999). It is defined as a motor disorder characterized by a velocity-dependent increase in the stretch reflex with exaggerated tendon jerks, resulting from hyperexcitability (Lance, 1980). Spasticity is typically seen as part of the upper motor neuron syndrome. The nature of the clinical presentation of "spasticity" remains a controversial issue. The term is typically used generically to encompass both negative and positive features: hyperreflexia, hypertonus, reflex changes, and weakness (Bourbonnais & Vanden Noven, 1989). The predominant hypothesis regarding the neural mechanism underlying spasticity is that it is due to changes in descending motor control activity, causing increased alpha motor neuron excitability, which results in increased tonic and phasic stretch reflex activity (Landau, 1980). It is more important to understand the clinical presentation of spasticity.

Clinically, the term *spasticity* is used to describe a wide range of abnormal motor behaviors, including the following (Horak, 1991):

1. Hyperactive stretch reflexes
2. Abnormal posturing of the limbs
3. Excessive co-activation of the antagonist muscles
4. Associated movements
5. Clonus
6. Stereotypical movement synergies

The key clinical sign of spasticity is the velocity-dependent increase in resistance of a muscle or a group of muscles to passive stretch. The neural basis for this increased stretch reflex activity (**hyperreflexia**) has been proposed to be because the alpha motor neuron pool at the spinal cord segmental level is hyperexcitable or because the amount of excitatory afferent input elicited by the stretch is increased or both. The hyperexcitability of the alpha motor neuron pool can be due to a loss of descending inhibitory input, postsynaptic denervation sensitivity, or collateral sprouting of the dorsal root afferents (Noth, 1991; Mayer, 1997).

Clinical Connection:

The most widely accepted tool for grading the degree of spasticity in a limb is the Modified Ashworth Scale for Grading Spasticity (Bohannon & Smith, 1987, Reprinted with permission of the American Physical Therapy Association):

Grade	Description
0	No increase in muscle tone
1	Slight increase in muscle tone, manifested by a catch and release or by minimal resistance at the end of the range of motion when the affected part is moved in flexion or extension
1+	Slight increase in muscle tone, manifested by a catch, followed by minimal resistance throughout the remainder (less than half) of the range of motion
2	More marked increase in muscle tone through most of the range of motion, but affected part is easily moved
3	Considerable increase in muscle tone; passive movement is difficult
4	Affected part is rigid in flexion or extension

The clinically observed increase in muscle tone results from both abnormal processing of the afferent (sensory) input and a defect in inhibitory modulation (change) from cortical centers and spinal interneuron pathways (Craik, 1991). Disorders in the stretch reflex mechanism will result in increased resistance to passive movement, especially when moving the limb quickly. A common clinical sign is **clonus,** spasmodic alternations of muscle contractions between antagonistic muscle groups, caused by hyperactive stretch reflexes. The DTRs of a muscle demonstrating spasticity are hyperactive. The **Babinski sign,** extension of the great toe with fanning of the other toes into abduction on stimulation of the lateral sole of the foot, is a classic diagnostic sign of spasticity. Dyssynergic movement patterns also occur, including co-activation of agonist and antagonistic muscle groups and abnormal timing. Prolonged agonist action and antagonist co-activation both contribute to a loss of smooth, voluntary muscle control in the patient/client with spasticity. There is increasing evidence, however, that the inappropriate recruitment of the agonist is more of a problem than undesired antagonistic muscle activity (Nwaobi, 1983; Sahrmann & Norton, 1977). Current research is showing that this inadequate recruitment and prolonged activation of agonist motor neurons, rather than increased activity in antagonist motor neurons, is the primary basis for the spasticity accompanying CNS lesions. It is to the agonist and voluntary muscle control that therapeutic intervention should direct its efforts.

Spasticity will also cause changes in the physical properties of the muscle. **Stiffness,** reflective of changes in the viscoelastic properties of the muscle tissue, and contracture are additional clinical signs. The muscles of patients with hypertonicity also may undergo an adaptation that involves formation of a higher proportion of binding cross-bridges (Carey & Burghardt, 1993). These physical changes in the muscular tissue contribute to the encountered increased resistance to passive stretch, perceived stiffness, and subsequent impaired movement.

Because the stretch reflex is velocity dependent and due to increased muscular stiffness, spasticity will limit a patient's ability to move quickly. Regardless of its complex neural basis, it is important to remember that spasticity is simply one of several symptoms of neurological damage and should therefore be treated as it interferes with function. Functional intervention approaches should focus primarily on improving active muscle control, in addition to reduction of the symptom of spasticity when it is severe enough to limit movement.

Clinically, transitional movements and balanced co-contraction of muscles appropriately at the joints in weight-bearing positions will be compromised when spasticity is present. The overall effect of spasticity on movement is the lack of novel movement patterns with the varying demands of the environment, with a subsequent reliance on stereotypical patterns of movement. Examples include the ambulation movement pattern of anterior pelvic tilt, lower extremity internal rotation, adduction, and knee flexion seen in a child with CP (Fig. 7–8) or the pelvic retraction, external rotation, adduction, and knee extended gait pattern seen in an adult with hemiplegia (Fig. 7–9). Other examples include the predominance of abnormal synergy patterns, as described in Chapter 6 (Fig. 6–7). In the presence of an UMN lesion, weakness is reflected in deficiencies in generating force and in sustaining force output.

▪ Clinical Management of Spasticity

Current research suggests that intervention practices directed primarily at reducing spasticity have limited usefulness in helping patients to regain functional independence. Spasticity is *not* the major obstacle to improved function. Abnormal muscle tone is *not* the primary culprit in motor control disturbances. Rather,

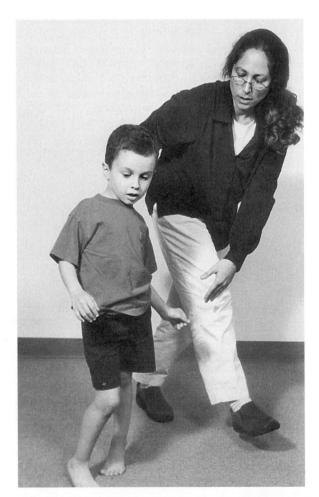

Figure 7–8. Child with spastic diplegic CP ambulating in characteristic posture of pelvic retraction, anterior pelvic tilt, internal rotation and adduction, knee flexion, and ineffective ankle control.

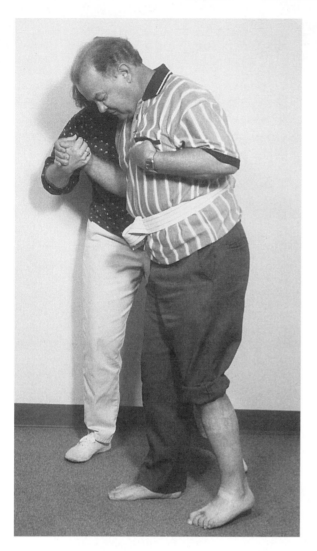

Figure 7–9. Patient with left hemiplegia ambulating in characteristic posture of pelvic retraction, external rotation and adduction, knee extension, and ineffective ankle control.

the primary factor limiting voluntary movement. Intervention for spasticity should be a component of an integrated approach to intervention for the patient, centered on the goal of maximizing functional performance and preventing undesirable secondary impairments. Table 7–3 summarizes the common clinical problems, functional limitations, and possible intervention solutions for the patient presenting with hypertonicity as a primary impairment. Figures 7–10 through 7–13 accompany Table 7–3. Intervention strategies are also expanded on in the following sections.

Positioning. An intact neuromuscular system allows automatic changes in muscle tone in response to the body movement or surface moving under the body, mediated by an intact sensory motor system. Changes in body position can significantly alter muscle tone or spasticity in individuals with an UMN lesion. In general, prolonged stretch can be used to induce relaxation in a spastic muscle. Patients with hip flexor spasticity benefit from positioning in prone to relax the spastic muscle and promote alignment. Modifying the influence of a reflex pattern on body position can be effective in promoting relaxation so that voluntary movement can be initiated or made more effective. In individuals with strong dominant influences of tonic reflexes on postural alignment, positioning will assist with decreasing that interfering influence of the reflex pattern on voluntary movement. Flexion of the head and lower extremities as depicted in Figure 6–5 will dampen the influence of the tonic labyrinthine reflex during supine positioning. Positioning in side lying is often used clinically to decrease the dominance of all the tonic neck reflexes, especially the tonic labyrinthine and the asymmetrical tonic neck reflex (ATNR). These interventions are most appropriate for the severely impaired individual where motor control is very compromised and the interfering influence of spasticity on movement is significant.

Sensorimotor Approaches

As discussed in Chapter 6, a sensorimotor approach using selected sensory stimulation techniques can either facilitate or inhibit muscle tone, depending on the use of the stimulus and how it is applied. For example, prolonged stretch, icing, or neutral warmth can be used to decrease the level of muscle activation. Techniques such as approximation can stimulate muscle activity, especially when the therapeutic goal is stability of a body part. These techniques are valuable tools to use as part of total patient management and as such are not really considered interventions in and of themselves, but rather they are helpful manual techniques to employ when guiding an individual in the attainment of a functional skill.

intervention needs to be directed at a multitude of factors that all contribute to the movement impairment, performance deficits, and functional limitations demonstrated by the patient/client. The presence of spasticity and its contribution to the individual's movement problem should be attended to as one of several variables requiring attention.

Clinical assessment of spasticity involves observations of resistance to passive movement, postural alignment, and volitional movements. It is important to differentiate between spasticity and other causes of stiffness. Little and Merritt (1988) list the following features that may contribute to a restraint of voluntary movement: contracture, hyperactive stretch reflexes, weakness, or central co-activation of antagonistic muscle groups. According to Bjornson (1999), the mere presence of spasticity does not mean it is

TABLE 7–3

Common Clinical Problems, Functional Limitations, and Goals for the Patient/Client with Hypertonicity as a Main Impairment

Clinical Problem	Functional Limitation	Goals
Weakness	Limited force production Limited strength in movements against gravity Poor voluntary control	Increased motor unit recruitment Increased concentric, isometric, and eccentric strength Improved voluntary motor control
Evidence of increased muscle tone, predominantly in the extremities	Stereotypical movement patterns (Fig. 7–10A) Inability to move fast	Improved voluntary, isolated muscle activation out of stereotypical patterns (Fig. 7–10B) Activation of functional muscle patterns
Decreased ability to activate isolated muscle groups in extremity (hip extensor, triceps) required for functional control	Decreased ability to accept or sustain effective weight bearing	Increased ability to accept loading onto upper or lower extremity as required for function through isometric work, use of developmental positions, sensorimotor techniques (Fig. 7–11)
Difficulty terminating certain muscle groups (hip flexors, adductors, internal rotators) as required for functional control; decreased ability to use eccentric control especially in hip and knee extensors	Decreased control of movement Difficulty with deceleration at end ranges Decreased ability to eccentrically stabilize a loaded joint	Increased ability to terminate muscle activation during movement Eccentric control during movement, as well as while holding postures (Fig. 7–12)
Decreased ability to balance flexors and extensors	Decreased ability to combine flexion and extension smoothly during posture and movement	Increased ability to balance flexors and extensors, especially trunk flexion in combination with extension, upper extremity extension as strong as flexion, and lower extremity flexion as strong as extension
Inaccurate muscle recruitment	High energy cost and slow, laborious movement	Increased variety of movement experiences within safe and familiar contexts
Decreased strength in the trunk	Poor static trunk control Inability to sustain antigravity postures	Improve active movement and trunk co-contraction (Fig. 7–13)
Decreased rotation and dissociation during movement	Poor movement transition Ineffective movement within postures	Practice combinations of movements and transitions involving trunk rotation (rolling, coming to sit, walking) Practice functional movement within static postures (reaching, dressing)
Inefficient or ineffective demonstration of postural responses	Decreased ability to realign posture when moving actively or make adjustments when being moved Fear of movement	Increased accuracy of responses to postural changes Balance activities
Decreased ROM	Limited excursion to complete functional movement, such as reaching, walking Risk for orthopedic deformities, pain	Restored or maintained functional ROM Preventative management, including ROM program, positioning, use of assistive devices, adaptive equipment, orthotic devices

Source: Adapted from Bertoti, D. B. (2000). Cerebral palsy: Lifespan management. In Orthopaedic interventions for the pediatric patient, orthopaedic section home study course. Alexandria, VA: American Physical Therapy Association.

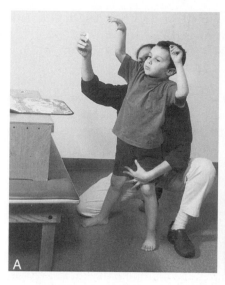
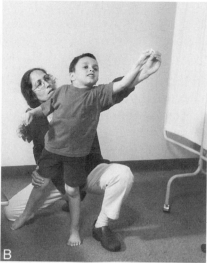

Figure 7–10. Child with hypertonicity reaching with an ineffective strategy, characterized by stereotypical posturing of the extremities and trunk (A). Child using isolated muscle activation patterns, as facilitated by therapist (B).

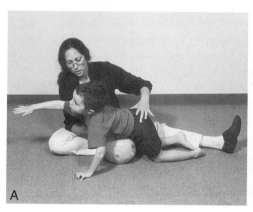
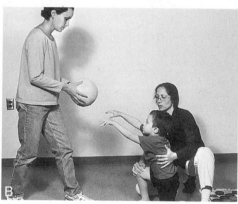

Figure 7–11. Use of developmental positions such as (A) quadruped or (B) half kneel to create opportunity for development of upper and lower extremity isometric strength and postural control of the trunk.

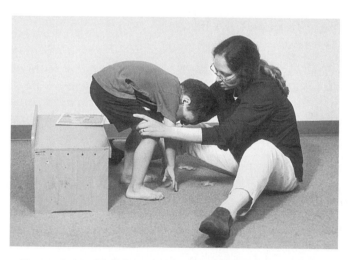

Figure 7–12. Work on eccentric control during movement.

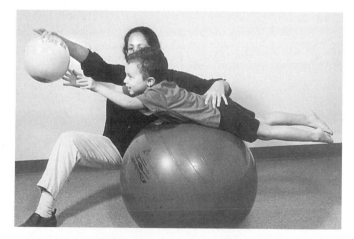

Figure 7–13. Playful activity used to encourage development of active movement, extensor strength, and trunk co-contraction.

Clinical Connection:

Consider the example of working with a patient with hypertonicity evidenced by scapular retraction, elbow flexion, and flexion of the wrist and fingers with the thumb flexed across the palm (sometimes called an "indwelling" or "cortical" thumb). If the clinical goal is to assist the patient in bed mobility, retraining the patient to use this upper extremity to push up to sitting from supine, the therapist or assistant may employ some sensory manual techniques as part of the intervention attempt. In this case, the clinician may use manual contact to gently guide the scapula into protraction, deep inhibitory pressure over the biceps tendon at the elbow to dampen the flexor spasticity, stroking and gently tapping to activate the triceps, slow stroking over the wrist and finger extensors to extend the wrist and open the hand, and a distal key point of control to bring the thumb out of the palm and into extension. All this physical "handling" is integrated into the clinician's physical guidance as the therapist or assistant teaches the patient to reorganize the skillful use of the upper extremity, within a functional task, repeated and practiced so that the limb becomes strengthened and motor control improves. These manual techniques are then "faded" as the patient gains more voluntary control and functional use of the extremity. ▪

Neurosurgical and Pharmacological Interventions. Neurosurgical interventions include selective posterior rhizotomy (SPR) or the use of an intrathecal baclofen pump. Although baclofen can also be considered as a pharmaceutical intervention, it will be discussed with SPR because of the similarities in mechanism between it and SPR. Basically, the mechanism of both these interventions is to suppress some of the overexcitation at the spinal cord area to decrease the negative effects of the symptom of spasticity. Both interventions uncover weakness that may then respond to therapeutic intervention.

SPR is a neurosurgical procedure performed to reduce spasticity in children with CP. The procedure involves the selective division of certain posterior rootlets of L2 through S2 spinal nerves, requiring a limited laminectomy. During the surgical procedure, the major muscle groups of the lower extremities are monitored via electrodes and the rootlets with abnormal responses are divided. By cutting these posterior (dorsal) roots, rhizotomy is thought to decrease presynaptic facilitory impulses to the interneuron pool, thereby decreasing some of the overexcitatory, afferent input onto alpha and gamma motoneurons (Peacock & Staudt, 1990). Selection criteria include the presence of severe spasticity that significantly interferes with function but is associated with no evidence of ataxia, dysto-

nia, hypotonia, or athetosis. The best candidates are children with spastic quadriplegia or diplegia when the spasticity is thought to be the *main* factor limiting the child's function or progress in therapy (Cioffi & Gaebler-Spira, 1989). SPR may uncover profound weakness and an altered sense of kinesthetic awareness. The main physical therapy and occupational therapy goals after rhizotomy are to improve alignment through range of motion (ROM), splinting, and positioning; facilitate active movement and motor re-education; strengthen and improve independent mobility; and ultimately improve gross motor function. Most studies demonstrate an improvement in function due to the ability to functionally strengthen key muscles without the undesirable effects of spasticity (Cioffi & Gaebler-Spira, 1989; Wright, Sheil, Drake, Wedge, & Naumann, 1998). SPR is becoming less commonly seen, in favor of a baclofen pump, which has a similar mechanism but is a reversible procedure.

Baclofen is delivered into the spinal fluid via a catheter inserted into the space at L1–2. (See the case study at the end of Chapter 10.) The catheter is connected to a pump, the size of a hockey puck, implanted under the skin of the abdomen (Albright, Barron, Fasick, Polinko, & Janosky, 1993). Baclofen affects spasticity in generally the same way as a rhizotomy. Baclofen, a gamma-aminobutyric acid (GABA), is an agonist of GABA and was initially developed as an anticonvulsant. Baclofen probably diminishes spasticity by binding to the GABA receptors in the spinal cord, impeding the release of excitatory neurotransmitters from afferent terminals (Albright, 1995). Baclofen can be delivered either orally or through the placement of a pump in the intrathecal space of the spinal cord for continual delivery. Oral doses are typically not as effective as an intrathecal pump, with drowsiness being a common adverse effect. As with SPR, the main indication for this intervention is severe spasticity when the spasticity is thought to be the *main* reason for interference with function. After placement of the pump, clinicians can expect to see a decrease in spasticity within 3 days. The pump needs to be refilled every 2 or 3 months. Adverse effects are minimal but may include infection, drowsiness, blurred vision, or dysarthria (Albright, 1995). The main physical therapy and occupational therapy goals are the same as for SPR: to facilitate active movement, motor re-education, and strengthening with the now weakened patient where the influence of spasticity has been pharmaceutically decreased.

Antispasticity medications are classified by their site of action in relation to the CNS as either centrally or peripherally acting. Centrally active drugs are active at numerous sites from the cerebral cortex to the spinal cord. Peripherally acting drugs influence spasticity at various sites from the anterior horn cell to the cellular structures of the muscle (Whyte & Robinson, 1990). Common pharmaceutical interventions for the management of spasticity include vigabatrin, tizanidine (a derivative of clonidine), dantrolene, and diazepam, all administered orally (Albright, 1995; Gormley, 1999). It is important for therapists and assistants to be familiar with the mode of action for a drug a patient is on and to be alerted to undesirable side effects. All centrally acting drugs will have a depressant effect on the CNS, perhaps causing sedation or interfering with concentration or attention to task. It is crucial that therapists and assistants be adept at observing the effects of medications that may be prescribed for their patient/client.

The pharmaceutical intervention in most widespread use today is the intramuscular administration of Botox. Botox, or botulinum-A toxin, is a neuromuscular blocking agent derived from the bacteria *Clostridium botulinum* (Koman, Mooney, & Smith, 1996). Botox, injected into the muscle at the anatomical locations of the myoneural junction, will produce a temporary chemical denervation. By blocking the release of acetylcholine at the neuromuscular junction, Botox can effectively cause a decrease in clinically observed muscle tone (Gormley, 1999). The target threshold is an amount sufficient to eliminate the presenting dynamic deformity (e.g., toe-walking or crouch gait) and therefore allow the antagonist muscle group to be activated and strengthened. Spasticity usually is observed to be decreased 12 to 72 hours after the injection, and the effects will last for 3 to 6 months. The main therapy goal is to stretch and strengthen both the injected muscle and the antagonist once the interfering, deleterious effects of spasticity are reduced, and to work on functional movement control (Albright, 1995).

Training to Improve Motor Control and Functional Performance. Current research clearly demonstrates that therapy directed at decreasing the functional limitations and promoting the attainment of meaningful function for the patient/client, in concert with a dynamic systems approach that integrates motor learning principles, is the most appropriate therapeutic orientation for approaching individuals with hypertonicity caused by neurological damage. Intervention is multifaceted, gathering the most appropriate tools from among the available resources. In combination with any medical management (such as medication or surgery), the therapist can chose from among a variety of tools, such as sensorimotor approaches, adaptive equipment, orthoses, positioning, and therapeutic exercise geared toward strengthening of voluntary motor control, to offer the patient an individualized management package built around meeting the individual's movement goals. The focus is not on the hypertonicity, because that is simply a symptom of disordered motor control, but rather on lessening the impact of the functional limita-

tions that result. Patients with spasticity should be trained to increase voluntary movement by improving motor neuron recruitment efforts rather than by reducing activity in the antagonistic muscle (Gowland, deBruin, Basmajian, Plews, & Burcea, 1992). Therapy directs its efforts to decrease the interfering effects of the abnormal muscle tone, build or re-establish strength, and assist in the development of strategies that will make movement effective and most efficient for that patient, given the constraints imposed by the pathophysiology.

Leaders in rehabilitation assert that the major objective in rehabilitation is to train the individual to improve voluntary control over motor output during the performance of essential actions (Carr & Shepherd, 1987, 1998, 2000; Duncan & Badke, 1987; O'Sullivan & Schmitz, 2001; Palmer & Toms, 1992; Ryerson & Levit, 1997). Although the training and the exercise may be aimed at improving motor unit recruitment in a weak muscle, training is directed overall at the behavioral consequences or the motor performance deficits of the central lesion. Such an approach makes one major assumption: that directing movement training toward improved performance of everyday actions (transfers, walking, reaching for an object, or manipulation) provides the system with the opportunities to readjust and to learn or relearn a pattern of neuromotor activity, using what is intact within the neuromotor system, so that the individual can attain a relevant movement goal. This contemporary approach assists the patient to learn motor control and develop strength and endurance during functional motor performance. As such, the patient practicing motor tasks under conditions similar to real life may best stimulate neural organization or reorganization.

▪ Rigidity

Rigidity is another form of hypertonicity, characterized by a heightened resistance to passive movement but independent of the velocity of that stretch or movement. Rigidity is associated with lesions of the basal ganglia and appears to be the result of excessive supraspinal drive acting on a normal spinal reflex mechanism (Jankovic, 1987). In addition, muscle stiffness is increased in individuals with rigidity due to changes in the peripheral mechanical properties of the muscle (Dietz, 1997). Contrary to spasticity, in rigidity resting muscle activity is higher than normal, suggesting that patients with rigidity have an inability to relax muscles voluntarily (Harburn & Miller, 1990; Marsden, 1982). There are two types of rigidity: lead pipe and cogwheel. A constant resistance to movement throughout the range characterizes lead pipe rigidity, whereas cogwheel rigidity is characterized by alternate episodes of resistance and relaxation. Cogwheel rigidity is recognizable clinically by a ratchetlike response to passive movement characterized by an alternate letting go and increased resistance to movement, very common in patients with Parkinson's disease. Rigidity tends to be predominant in the flexor muscles of the trunk and limbs and results in severe functional limitations. Patients demonstrate stiffness and inflexibility. Rigidity impairs the initiation, execution, and smooth termination of a motor activity. Numerous functional limitations result, including difficulty with bed mobility, transfers, postural control, gait, speech, and eating.

Significant corticospinal lesions can also result in clinical conditions known as decorticate or decerebrate rigidity. **Decorticate rigidity** (Fig. 7–14) refers to a state of sustained contraction and posturing of the trunk and lower limbs in extension, and the upper limbs in flexion. This type of rigidity is indicative of a corticospinal tract lesion at the level of the diencephalon, above the superior colliculus. **Decerebrate rigidity** (Fig. 7–15) refers to a state of sustained contraction of the trunk and all four limbs into extension, indicative of a brainstem lesion. **Opisthotonus** is a strong and sustained contraction of the extensor muscles so that the individual assumes a hyperextended posture. All these conditions are exaggerated, severe forms of hypertonicity and indicative of severe neurological damage (O'Sullivan, 2001).

Clinical Connection:

Intervention for individuals with severe, exaggerated forms of hypertonicity are typically directed at positioning and management for relief of discomfort, strategies to optimize ease of total care and prevent skin breakdown and other secondary problems. For these patients, positioning to decrease the overwhelming influence of the tonic neck reflexes and the predomi-

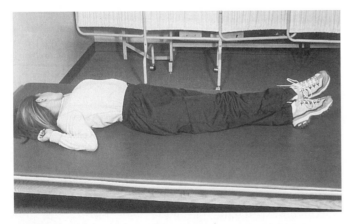

Figure 7–14. Posturing described as decorticate rigidity, where the trunk and lower extremities are rigidly extended and the upper extremities are flexed with scapular retraction.

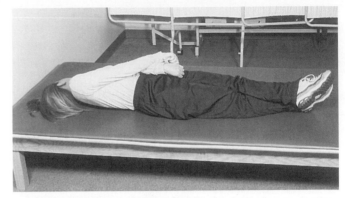

Figure 7–15. Posturing described as decerebrate rigidity, where all four limbs are rigidly extended.

nance of the described total body postures may improve ease of breathing, feeding, and swallowing and enhance quality of life. ■

Clinical Management of Rigidity

Clinical management of the functional limitations caused by rigidity are similar to those used to manage spasticity. In the cases of decerebrate or decorticate rigidity caused by severe brain damage, management very closely resembles that suggested for patients with severe spasticity (see Figs. 7–14 and 7–15). These types of rigidity often accompany the rare instances of significant brain damage, as seen in individuals in a comatose or "vegetative" state.

The most common cause of rigidity is the rigidity seen as a symptom of Parkinson's disease. There is a wealth of literature available for the management of Parkinsonian rigidity. Current research is demonstrating that therapeutic interventions directed at reducing the neural component of rigidity in these patients is of questionable meaningful benefit. Rather, intervention should be directed at enhancing functional movements and on cognitive retraining, not focusing on the rigidity as the main impairment responsible for difficulties with functional performance (Morris, 2000). Patients with Parkinsonian rigidity appear to have difficulty effectively using proprioceptive and exteroceptive feedback to initiate or monitor movement. Cognitive strategies that teach the patient to bring motor action under cognitive control may enable the individual to bypass the disordered neural circuitry that contributes to the faulty motor control in Parkinsonian rigidity (Harburn & Miller, 1990).

Pharmacological management of the rigidity associated with Parkinsonism is fairly successful; the most common medications used are levodopa and apomorphine. Clinical research data show that the effectiveness of medications can fluctuate throughout the course of the disease and that these medications appear to be most effective early in the disease (Morris, 2000; Morris, Iansek, & Churchyard, 1998; Selby, 1975). For this reason, clinicians need to ensure that they train people with Parkinson's rigidity to cope with movement disorders during the expected fluctuations in motor performance (Morris, 2000).

Coordination Problems

Coordinated movement involves multiple joints and muscles that are activated at the appropriate time and with the correct amount of force so that smooth, efficient, and accurate movement occurs (Shumway-Cook & Woollacott, 2001). The essence of coordinated movement therefore is the synergistic organization of multiple muscles, not just the capacity to fire an isolated muscle contraction. Coordination deficits occur when muscles fail to fire in sequence or when the CNS is unable to direct movement activities properly. Lack of coordination can impair the quality of movement or be so severe that it limits movement altogether. Incoordination can result from pathology in a variety of neural structures, including the motor cortex, basal ganglia, and cerebellum. In CNS lesions, several movement dysfunctions may occur, including movement decomposition and dysmetria. **Movement decomposition** is characterized by a breakdown of movements between multiple joints, resulting in movement of individual segments rather than movement as a fluid, coordinated unit. **Dysmetria** is characterized by overshooting or reaching beyond the target, sometimes referred to as past-pointing. **Incoordination** occurs when the firing rates of muscles are disrupted, resulting in loss of smooth reciprocal movement, or when the CNS loses its ability to direct movement activity that requires accuracy. Uncoordinated movement may be displayed through the manifestation of abnormal synergies, inappropriate co-activation patterns, and timing problems (O'Sullivan, 2001; Shumway-Cook & Woollacott, 2001).

Muscle Activation and Sequencing Problems

Pathology within the CNS can produce problems in activating and sequencing the appropriate muscles needed to execute functional tasks. This results in the production of unnecessary movements in joints and muscles not directly involved in a functional movement task. Lesions to corticospinal centers can also lead to the ability to recruit only a limited number of muscles controlling a movement. The result is the emergence of mass patterns of movement, referred to as abnormal synergies (see Chapter 6).

In traditional rehabilitation literature, the word *synergy* had most often been used in describing abnormal or disordered motor control (Bobath, 1978; Brunnstrom, 1970). Simply put, however, *synergy* means a group of muscles that often act together as if in a bound unit. In fact, in 1932 Nicolai Bernstein used the term *synergy* (as translated into English in 1967) to aptly describe the functional muscle groups that produce normal motor behavior. *Abnormal* synergies are stereotypical patterns of movement that don't change or adapt to environmental or task demands. Abnormal synergies reflect an inability to move a single joint without simultaneously generating movement in other joints. Movement out of the fixed pattern is often difficult if not impossible.

As described in the previous chapter in Table 6–4, there is a flexion and extension synergy of both the upper and the lower extremity. In the patient with hemiplegia secondary to a CVA, the flexor synergy in the upper extremity and the extensor synergy in the lower extremity often predominate the patient's movement. In the upper extremity, the flexion synergy is characterized by scapular retraction and elevation, shoulder abduction and external rotation, elbow flexion, forearm supination or pronation, and wrist and finger flexion. The scapular and elbow components are usually the first to emerge after the CVA and stay the strongest. In the lower extremity, the extensor synergy is characterized by pelvic retraction, hip extension, adduction, and internal rotation, knee extension, and ankle plantar flexion and inversion. The pelvic retraction and ankle plantar flexion components can be quite strong.

An example of a sequencing problem is *inappropriate* co-activation. Notice the emphasis in the clarifying adjective *inappropriate*. Co-activation, which means that the agonist and antagonist both fire, is normally present in the early stages of learning a skilled movement. Co-activation is commonplace in young children just learning to balance and during early walking patterns, as well as in adults attempting to learn a new task. In the neurologically intact adult, co-activation is atypical unless during the early stages of learning a new skill, requiring unnecessary energy expenditure and resulting in inefficient movement.

Inappropriate co-activation is commonly seen in CNS disorders in both children and adults. This inappropriate and ungraded co-activation of agonist and antagonist contributes to functional limitations in force generation. Sometimes termed "antagonistic restraint," this abnormal activation of the antagonist when the agonist is recruited to fire may be caused by misdirected descending motor signals, as well as by exaggerated phasic stretch reflexes activated during voluntary effort. Such co-activation has been demonstrated in patients after stroke and in children with cerebral palsy, during walking and the performance of common functional skills (Bertoti, 2000; Knutsson & Richards, 1979). Inappropriate co-activation is probably evidence of an unrefined form of coordination, indicative of a loss of skilled, refined movement patterns.

Timing Problems

Uncoordinated movement can also be manifested as an inability to appropriately time the action of muscles and thus the movement itself. There can be many facets to timing errors, including problems initiating the movement, slowed movement execution, and problems terminating a movement (Shumway-Cook & Woollacott, 2001). All these timing errors have been observed in patients with neurological damage.

Problems initiating movement, often referred to as **reaction time,** is the time between the patient's decision to move and the actual initiation of the movement. There are several factors that may affect reaction time (Shumway-Cook & Woollacott, 2001):

1. Inadequate force generation (inability to overcome gravity or recruit enough motor units)
2. Insufficient rate of force generation (not quickly enough)
3. Insufficient ROM to allow the movement
4. Reduced motivation to move or other cognitive factors
5. Abnormal postural control, specifically the inability to stabilize the body in advance of the movement

Slowed movement time may be another problem for individuals with neurological problems. **Movement time** is defined as the time taken to execute a task-specific movement once it has been initiated. Slowed movement time may be associated with a variety of neural pathologies, such as stroke, Parkinson's disease, and CP. Difficulty in terminating a movement manifests itself as an inability to stop a movement or an inability to change direction of a movement. This is thought to result from an inability to concentrically control the agonist and inadequate timing and eccentric control of the antagonist. The antagonist does not generate enough force or force at the proper time to smoothly brake a movement. Problems with terminating movements are common in individuals with cerebellar disorders, in CP, and in Parkinson's disease.

Clinical Connection:

Patients with cerebellar disorders often demonstrate difficulties in checking or halting a movement, resulting in what is clinically called a rebound phenomenon, whereby a limb moves involuntarily when isometric resistance to that limb is suddenly removed. Another example of movement termination problems is **dysdiadochokinesia**, the inability to perform rapid alternating movements. What a great word. How many points is it worth in a Scrabble game?   ▪

▪ Clinical Management of Coordination Problems

Coordination problems, characterized by problems in muscle activation, sequencing, and timing, can create a tremendous obstacle to efficient functional movement. Because coordination requires adequate strength and ROM, uncoordinated movement is often characterized by some degree of weakness or instability. All the suggestions described earlier for increasing strength and stability are very appropriate for patients/clients with coordination difficulties. Stability can be improved through isometric exercise, weight-bearing activities through the proximal joints, PNF, rhythmical stabilization, and functional tasks that emphasize control of proximal components versus distal manipulation (Bennett & Karnes, 1998). Several different training strategies have shown clinical evidence of success for application with individuals demonstrating coordination difficulties.

▪ Sensory Cues

External cues appear to help guide the uncoordinated individual effectively through the motor performance. These external cues can be visual, auditory, or proprioceptive in type. These external cues appear to remove the cognitive focus from the movement and allow automatic motor programs to be executed, usually with more success. Alternatively, external cues may allow the individual to focus attention on critical aspects of the movement that need to be regulated, such as weight transference to unload the leg or axial motion to assist in turning (Morris, 2000; Yekutiel, Pinhasov, Shahar, & Sroka, 1991). A very powerful sensory cue that can improve coordination is visual feedback. Visual feedback is provided early in training to facilitate acquisition of skill. Visual feedback should then be gradually withdrawn as patients are guided to depend on their own sensory processing for task performance. Rhythmical sensory cues, such as rocking the body from side to side, may sometimes be useful in assisting the initiation of movements such as walking or rolling over in bed (Schenkman et al., 1989). In patients with cognitive impairments, combinations of external cues, environmental restructuring, visual demonstration, and verbal instructions may be effective because these strategies are less reliant on complex information processing.

Clinical Connection:

When working with a patient or client with a coordination disorder, the task may initially need to be modified so that the ROM required is initially decreased, allowing the patient to practice moving through smaller ranges of motion. The speed of the movement may or may not be altered. Research and clinical practice have demonstrated that patients have more success if the speed of the motion closely resembles that of the naturally occurring movement. The addition of sensory cues that give the patient amplified feedback does help initially with movement execution but needs to be faded as soon as possible. The addition of light weights to the limb and manual guidance can increase the patient's kinesthetic sense. These sensory cues, similar to auditory and visual feedback, are best faded quickly so that the patient does not develop dependence on augmented feedback but rather uses the feedback to foster motor learning. ■

■ Functional Task-Specific Training

Task analysis and task-specific training, as described in the previous chapter, is a valid model for movement training. It is most appropriate that intervention and retraining take place in the environmental context that is most troublesome for the patient. Training in the person's home and community, including community ambulation skills such as road crossing and negotiation of obstacles, are often priorities. Environmental modifications should be considered.

Probably the most commonly used technique to improve coordinated movement is repetition and practice of a functional, task-specific movement. Therapists can select functional tasks with appropriate demands for accuracy, increasing the demands as improvement occurs or simplifying the task if progress is slow. The motor learning principles of practice and feedback are vitally important for learning to occur. If timing is the key problem (reaction time, movement time, or termination time), functional movements can be practiced under externally imposed time constraints. Having a patient/client perform a movement to music or in time to a specific beat or metronome is another successful approach used to influence timing.

Clinical Connection:

A common problem reported by individuals with movement disorders is difficulty turning over and getting out of bed. This complex sequential motor skill has many components. The following illustrates how a clinician could analyze this task for retraining (Morris, 2000):

1. Throwing back the bed covers
2. Shifting the pelvis toward the center of the bed so that, when the turn is completed, the body is not too close to the edge
3. Turning the head
4. Bringing the arm across the body in the direction of the roll or turn
5. Swinging the legs over the edge
6. Pushing up
7. Adjusting postural alignment to sit upright

You will have an opportunity to practice task analysis of common functional activities in an active learning experience in the companion workbook. ■

Functional movement activities emphasizing weight bearing and weight shifting can offer opportunities to improve proximal stability in functionally useful positions. Standing activities in parallel bars, or at a table or counter support, can be very effective. Functional locomotor activities typically include practice on key components of gait (see Chapter 10), braiding activities, walking sideways, walking within lines on the floor or on foot patterns drawn onto the floor, or stepping over and around obstacles (Figs. 7–16 and 7–17). Reaching for objects from standing can offer occupation-embedded opportunities to work on proximal control, distal accuracy, and weight shifting (see Figs. 7–1A,C and 6–22). Frenkel's exercises were designed to enable voluntary relearning of movement through the repetition of functional movement patterns. These exercises can be performed in supine, sitting, or standing and are described in other sources (Licht, 1965). Use of PNF diagonals is very effective in re-establishing smooth, reciprocal functional movement patterns. Timing for emphasis and rhythmical stabilization are very often used for individuals with incoordination.

Clinical Connection:

The tests used to assess coordination deficits (Schmitz, 2001) describe many functional tasks that can also be used as tasks to practice as part of intervention. Tasks to practice as intervention include drawing numbers or letters on the floor or in the air with upper or lower extremity, rapid alternating movements, tandem walking, tapping of hand or foot, finger opposition, finger to therapist's finger, standing eyes open or closed, unilateral stance, marching in place, stepping around obstacles, and stopping and starting abruptly while walking.

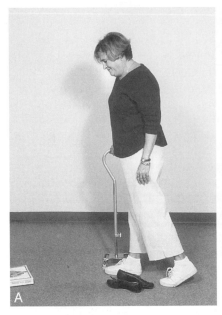

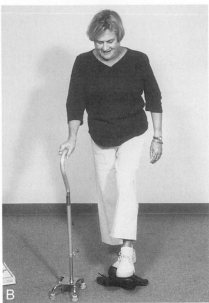

Figure 7–16. Functional locomotor activities may include offering opportunities for a patient to negotiate around obstacles commonly encountered on the floor within a living environment (A) or stepping over an obstacle (B).

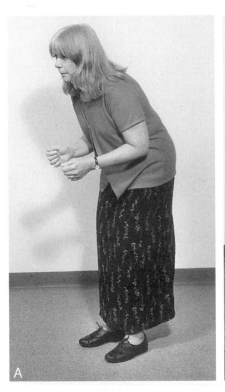

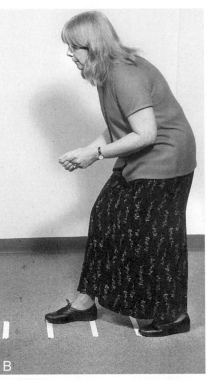

Figure 7–17. An example of a functional locomotor activity where a patient with a stooped posture and limited step length (A) practices stepping with an appropriate step length, aided by tape marks on the floor (B).

Other functional tasks that can be practiced as part of intervention include drawing on paper, practice writing, donning and doffing clothing, brushing teeth, combing hair, picking up small objects from a table (paperclips, pen, keys), negotiating different terrain or inclines, and repeatedly stepping up and down steps of varying heights. The therapist or assistant should try to emphasize practice of activities that are familiar and meaningful for the individual. For example, asking a child to reach into a crayon box to retrieve a crayon or

an adult to separate nuts from bolts or nails are better choices than the use of a pegboard or a rote exercise activity. Dialing a cell phone is vitally valuable to the teenager!

Involuntary Movements

Involuntary movements are a common sign of neurological damage and can take many forms, including dystonia, tremor, associated movements, and athetoid and choreiform movements (Shumway-Cook and Woollacott, 2001).

▪ Dystonia

Dystonia is defined as a syndrome dominated by sustained muscle contractions, often causing abnormal postures, twisting or writhing movements, and repetitive abnormal postures. The abnormal movements associated with dystonia are quite diverse, ranging from slow to quick patterns of movement and even co-contraction of the agonist and antagonist. Muscle tone is often disordered, accompanied by repetitive involuntary movements (Shumway-Cook & Woollacott, 2001). Intervention is largely related to the reduction of symptoms. Relaxation exercises and stress reduction education are commonly used, because dystonia appears to be exacerbated by stress and anxiety. Anticholinergic drugs and local injections of Botox have also been used successfully. Dystonic movements usually result from basal ganglia disturbances.

▪ Tremor

Tremor is defined as a rhythmical, involuntary, oscillatory movement of a body part (Deuschl, Bain, & Brin, 1998). Tremor results from damage to the CNS. Resting tremor is a tremor occurring in a body part that is not being voluntarily activated and is supported against gravity. Resting tremor is a symptom of Parkinson's disease, secondary to basal ganglia dysfunction. It is often the first symptom reported at the onset of Parkinson's disease. Presumably, it is due to an altered firing rate of the thalamic neurons, although the exact mechanism is unknown. Resting tremor disappears during movement and therefore does not interfere with the ability to perform everyday tasks. It also responds very well to levodopa. Less commonly, a **postural tremor** can be observed when the individual bears weight through the limb or encounters resistance to movement of the limbs, head, trunk, or neck (Selby, 1975). **Intention tremor,** sometimes called an "action tremor," is tremor evidenced upon purposeful movement of the body part, typically seen during reaching with the upper extremity or stepping with the lower extremity (Deuschl, Bain, & Brin, 1998; Shumway-Cook & Woollacott, 2001). Intention tremors often accompany cerebellar lesions.

▪ Associated Movements

We have all experienced mild demonstration of associated movements, when under stress or engaged in a novel or difficult activity. Associated movements are characterized by involuntary movement of one body part during the voluntary movement of another body part. Associated movements are often seen in the presence of abnormal muscle tone, especially spasticity. They are probably the result of lost supraspinal inhibitory mechanisms that normally suppress the coupling of movements between limbs (Lasarus, 1992). Associated movements are easily observable in patients with CNS damage, often evident during times of effort, stress, or fatigue. In Chapter 6, Figures 6–7 and 6–14 depict the demonstration of an associated movement characterized by increased expression of synergy patterns when an individual with a CVA is experiencing fatigue during an attempt at movement execution. Another example of an associated reaction is a response known as Raimiste's phenomenon, described in an active learning experience in the companion workbook.

Brunnstrom, credited with careful observations of patients with hemiplegia, drew the following currently relevant conclusions about associated movements as seen in individuals with a motor disorder (Sawner & LaVigne, 1992):

- An associated movement can be evoked in a limb that is essentially flaccid and may be the first sign of movement that can be elicited after an acute neurological insult. This elicited tension in the affected limb decreases rapidly after cessation of the stimulus (tapping or resistance) used to elicit it.
- Associated movements are commonplace in the presence of spasticity.
- Associated movements may be present years after the onset of the motor disturbance.

The presence of associated reactions is a symptom of disordered motor control. As such, their presence requires no direct intervention, but simply recognition of their presence as a symptom of a motor control disturbance.

▪ Athetoid and Choreiform Movements

The abnormal postures associated with these types of involuntary movements are diverse and can range from **athetoid** (slow involuntary writhing or twisting, usually involving the upper extremities more than the lower extremities) to quick choreiform movements (involuntary, jerky, rapid, and irregular movements). Pure **athetosis** is relatively uncommon and most often presents in combination with spasticity or hypotonia. The most common clinical presentation of athetosis is as a form of cerebral palsy. Choreiform movements are usually associated with a movement disorder known as Huntington's chorea. The movement disturbances characterized as choreiform or athetoid are often seen in combination, with the predominant features of abnormal movement control, repetitive involuntary movements, repetitive abnormal postures, and disordered, seemingly fluctuating muscle tone.

Muscle tone appears to fluctuate in an unpredictable manner from low to high. There is often a global increase in stiffness that is sometimes quite significant. The stiffness seems to fluctuate with a high-amplitude, low-frequency oscillation pattern. Individuals with athetosis tend to demonstrate involuntary movements, often moving between one extreme of range of motion to the other, in what has been described as a "writhing" pattern. Problems with co-activation and reciprocal inhibition result in these extreme ranges of movement. Muscles on both sides of the joint cannot be coordinated to stabilize that body segment, especially in midranges, resulting in the involuntary movement from one extreme to the other. This individual has great difficulty maintaining stability and is often observed to develop compensatory strategies whereby the person positions the hand or feet in an atypical or stabilizing posture in an effort to gain stability (Figs. 7–18 to 7–20). Individuals with athetosis and chorea demonstrate an inability to grade the initiation of muscle activity, effectively sustain muscle activity, and use eccentric control to efficiently terminate muscle activity (Styer-Acevedo, 1998). Motor control is disturbed with evidence of persistent immature patterns of movement, indicated by postures characteristically associated with the tonic reflexes (see Fig. 7–20A). Secondary impairments such as joint instability and contracture formation are common. Because the motor disturbance often includes the muscles of the face and mouth, problems with speech, drinking, and feeding are of tremendous concern. Breathing may then also be affected, with irregular breaths associated with the fluctuating muscle tone and poor chest expansion (Ratliffe, 1998).

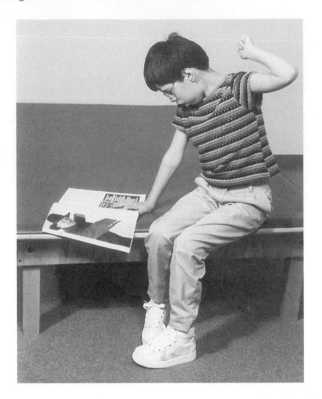

Figure 7–18. Child using a compensatory strategy whereby posturing the left upper extremity into a high on-guard position of scapular retraction may serve to increase trunk extensor tone in effort to increase postural stability needed to complete a task. This posture also resembles the posture of an ATNR reflex pattern.

▪ Clinical Management of Involuntary Movements

Rehabilitation strategies for treating involuntary movement focus primarily on compensating for the movement rather than on changing the movement itself. For example, because increased effort tends to magnify involuntary movements, patients can be taught to perform functional movements with reduced effort. Interestingly, patients do tend to develop compensatory strategies on their own, such as walking with their hands in their pockets to increase stability and decrease involuntary movements or grasping onto objects to decrease a tremor (see Fig. 7–20B) (Shumway-Cook & Woollacott, 2001).

Table 7–4 summarizes the common clinical prob-

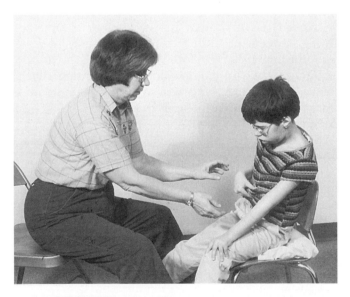

Figure 7–19. Child using a compensatory strategy of grasping her knee with an upper extremity while engaged in a dressing skill, in an effort to increase postural stability.

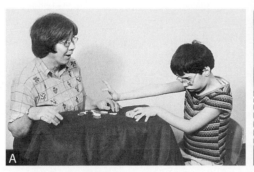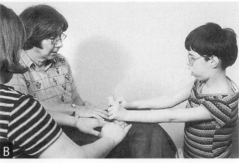

Figure 7–20. Reaching may be accomplished by using the ATNR as a preferred movement pattern (A). Use of an external handhold, such as a dowel block, may assist the child to increase her postural stability while practicing a fine motor task (B).

TABLE 7–4

Common Clinical Problems, Functional Limitations, and Goals for the Patient/Client with Dystonia as a Main Impairment

Clinical Problem	Functional Limitation	Goals
Weakness	Poor voluntary motor control (Figs. 7–18 and 7–20A)	Increased strength concentrically, eccentrically, and isometrically (Fig. 7–7)
Lack of midrange control and lack of co-contraction	Lack of postural stability (Figs. 7–18 and 7–21) Inability to hold body segment at various points within the range of motion (Fig. 7–20A)	Work within range in small increments Work on co-contraction, postural stability (Fig. 7–22)
Lack of muscle grading	Difficulty changing positions and combining functional movements	Work on trunk stabilization (Figs. 7–19 and 7–22) Facilitate proximal control for more accurate control (Fig. 7–7)
Lack of use of upper extremity (UE) or lower extremity (LE) in closed chain for support	Poor weight bearing Instability and unsafe movement (Fig. 7–23)	Weight bearing through UE and LE for stability and safe movement transitions (Fig. 7–24)
Fluctuations of abnormally high and abnormally low muscle tone	Postural instability Inefficient, ineffective movements	Increased ability to sustain postures Work on co-contraction and stability (Figs. 7–22 and 7–24)
Involuntary, uncoordinated movement	Poor movement transitions Involuntary movement Poor purposeful task execution	Increased ability to stabilize and transition with control (Fig. 7–25) Decreased involuntary movement by directing controlled movements
Asymmetry in posture and movement	Difficulty with midline control and symmetrical muscle action	Increased controlled symmetry and midline postural control through rhythmical stabilization (Fig. 7–22)
Inefficient or ineffective demonstration of postural responses	Decreased ability to realign posture when displaced or while moving Fear of movement	Increased response accuracy to postural changes Balance activities
Poor dissociation	Head movement usually affects posture of limbs or trunk Difficulty with functional movements such as rolling, coming to sit, and mobility	Practice functional movement

Source: Adapted from Bertoti, D. B. (2000). Cerebral palsy: Lifespan management. In *Orthopaedic interventions for the pediatric patient, orthopaedic section home study course.* Alexandria, VA: American Physical Therapy Association.

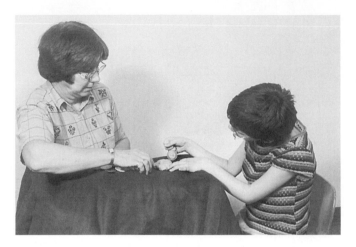

Figure 7–21. Children and adults with dystonia often demonstrate difficulty maintaining postural alignment and control, especially when challenged during the performance of a fine motor task. Performance in fine motor activities is compromised by fluctuating muscle tone, postural stability, and ineffective midline orientation.

lems, functional limitations, and possible intervention solutions for the patient/client presenting with dystonia as a primary impairment. Figures 7–18 through 7–25 accompany the table and a case study at the end of this chapter. Intervention strategies are similar to those described previously for management of the underlying weakness and functional limitations, with the following section highlighting any suggestions unique to the management of an individual with dystonia.

▪ Positioning and Adaptive Equipment

Because the symptom of dystonia results in impaired stability, poor muscular co-contraction, and involuntary movements, positioning to support functional achievement is more of a concern in this population. Midline stability of the head and trunk are vital so that the individual can optimize functional social, visual, and self-help skills, such as feeding. Because of the fluctuating muscle tone, adaptive positioning may help to promote alignment for more efficient functional control, as well as to prevent secondary impairments.

▪ Sensorimotor Approaches

Selected techniques from the sensorimotor approaches can be useful in facilitating maximal functional performance. The therapist's role with the individual with involuntary movements is often one of helping to achieve some level of organization and grading of the seemingly erratic movement behaviors. Usually, individuals with dystonia respond best to slow and steady movements from the therapist or assistant, giving the individual time to regulate his or her own motor responses. Because

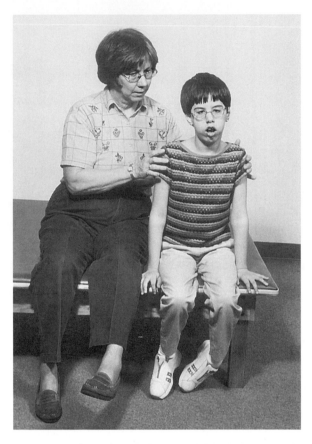

Figure 7–22. Therapist challenges child's balance and cues her to practice the development of postural control and upper extremity weight bearing as an adaptive strategy when balance is challenged from an outside force.

midline control and stability are intervention priorities, firm manual contacts, approximation, and weight-bearing and graded weight-shifting activities are good choices. Use of sustained joint compression through the spine, shoulders, and hips can aid in stimulating some muscular co-contraction around those joints. Children with dystonia, especially athetosis, have difficulty organizing and responding to sensory input. Firm, controlled pressure can help to provide a sense of stability and security. Firm, broad touch is usually more calming and supportive to movement efforts, as opposed to light or intermittent touch, which may accentuate a feeling of lack of control (Styer-Acevedo, 1998).

▪ Functional Training

As with all other types of motor disturbances, the development of functional skills is paramount. There was a time in physical therapy and occupational therapy history that "normalizing" tone was a goal and the postures associated with reflex patterns were thought to be undesirable. Recognizing now that reflex patterns of

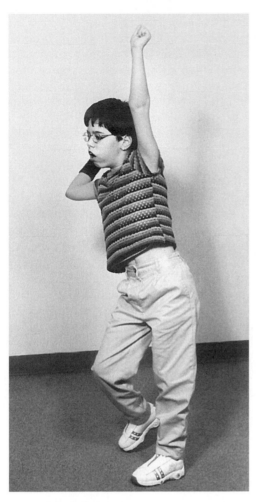

Figure 7–23. Gait characterized by asymmetry and instability with dystonic posturing predominant, precipitating frequent falls and difficulty negotiating new terrain.

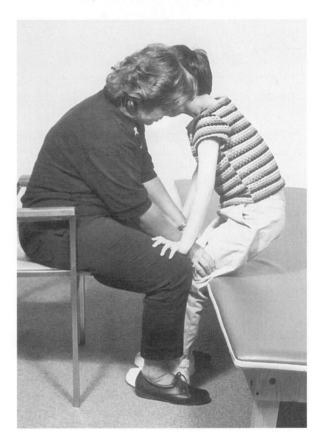

Figure 7–24. Practicing sit to stand and stand to sit offers the opportunity for practice of concentric, isometric, and eccentric muscle strength within a functional task. The therapist cues the child by emphasizing the weight borne through both the lower extremities (approximation through the knees to the child's feet) and the upper extremities (child bearing weight onto the therapist's legs).

movement may simply be the best movement pattern possible given the constraints imposed by the pathological condition, there is nothing inappropriate in allowing an individual to use a reflexive posture in the successful execution of a motor skill. For example, reaching may be accomplished through the posture recognizable as the ATNR reflexive posture (see Fig. 7–18 and 7–20A). Individuals with dystonia should be encouraged to use their ingenuity and to seek movement solutions. The therapist or assistant can be collaborative in this search, suggesting environmental modifications or preventative suggestions as appropriate.

Facilitation of slow, controlled movements can help the individual to develop postural control during movement transitions. Transitions between positions can help to develop stability and strength. Postural control may improve by special attention to the relationships between the head and trunk and associated movements of the limbs. Weight bearing and approximation have been found to be very helpful in increasing joint stabil-

ity and thereby decreasing the predominance of involuntary movements. Careful observation of movement may reveal a predictable pattern that can then be directly addressed in therapy.

Clinical Connection:

There are several creative solutions available for helping an individual with involuntary movements or dystonia to increase postural stability. Distal fixation can also be achieved by providing external handholds on wheelchairs, lap trays, or desks (see Fig. 7–20B). Wearing a weighted belt or simply placing a small amount of weight in the hip pockets may offer an increased sense of proprioception and give some degree of joint approximation through the lower extremities, increasing postural stability in upright positions. Similarly, the wearing of a weighted vest or shoulder pads may accomplish the same goal—to

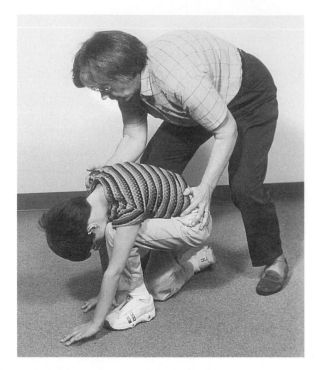

Figure 7–25. Rising to stand from the floor is an important functional task to practice, should the child fall. The therapist uses physical guidance, all key points of control and weight-shifting facilitation, along with coaching while practicing this skill.

increase upper extremity stability and control. Therapists and assistants need to experiment with some of these strategies and adjust the placement or amount of weight to accomplish the goal. ▪

The Nature of the Functional Movement Problem in Individuals with a Neurological Impairment

This chapter has described the most current explanation regarding the key aspects of the motor impairments affecting muscular force production seen in individuals who have damage to the nervous system. These patients/clients present with a complex of impairments and features, including muscle weakness; abnormal muscle tone; coordination problems as a result of difficulties with muscle activation, sequencing, and timing; and involuntary movements. Abnormal patterns of movement are no longer considered to be purely evidence of abnormal muscle tone or disinhibited lower centers. Rather, the observed abnormal patterns of movement may perhaps be explained, at least clinically, as a functional adaptation to motor performance that becomes apparent when an individual attempts to

move in the presence of muscle weakness and imbalance between stronger and weaker muscle groups. When an individual with a brain injury attempts a purposeful action, the movement pattern that emerges reflects the *best* that can be done *under the circumstances,* given the state of both the neural and musculoskeletal systems and the dynamic possibilities inherent in the linkages between all the subsystems involved in movement production and control (Carr & Shepherd, 1998). The movements that emerge may be distorted.

Problem-solving clinicians need to first identify what factor or factors seem to interfere the most with motor performance. The major impairments of weakness, uncoordinated movement, and the adaptive changes of muscle stiffness and abnormal posturing are typically among the factors that interfere the most with functional motor behavior. It appears likely that the development of disability will be less severe if soft tissue extensibility can be maintained and if intervention emphasizes training the individual to control muscle activity as required for specific actions, with task-related practice to improve muscle force generation and synergistic relationships between muscle groups. Encouraging the patient/client to be active seems to be a critical factor. Engaging the individual in meaningful, occupational-embedded tasks is crucial for success. Neurological rehabilitation should not only begin early but should also be active (Carr & Shepherd, 1987, 1998; Richards et al., 1991). Immobility, which leads to contractures and increased stiffness of soft tissue, is a major consequence of a brain lesion. If at all possible, immobility with its negative consequences should be minimized. Soft tissue length should always be maintained, if not actively, then by passive means, employing the use of splints, casts, orthoses, or positioning devices. Muscle stiffness, which limits active movement and appropriate tension development, can be effectively reduced by a brief stretch for a minute or two just before voluntary movement.

Following are some conclusions based on a thorough review of the current literature:

- The functional effects of abnormal muscle tone are unclear.
- A decrease in hyperreflexia, as a sign of hypertonicity, does not by itself enable a new action to be learned (Neilson & McCaughey, 1982).
- Strengthening exercise is associated with a decrease in hyperreflexia (Bertoti et al., 1997; Butefisch, Hummelsheim, Denzler, & Mauritz, 1995).

Based on the current knowledge available, Carr and Shepherd (1998) offer the following recommendations for rehabilitation intervention when working with patients with a neurological disorder who present with movement problems complicated by abnormal force generation:

- Intensive training and practice, including task-related exercise, directed at eliciting muscle activity, controlling force generation and synergistic muscle activity, and strengthening muscles
- Preserving length and flexibility of all tissues

Clinical Connection:

As a young therapist in the 1970s, I spent a great deal of time and energy on directing the efforts of my intervention at improving the "quality" of movements of a patient/client who had a neurological impairment. "Quality" was defined as movement devoid of obvious influence of reflex postures, associated or involuntary movements, or effects of abnormal muscle tone. Functional improvement was always the overall goal, but the way to achieve that functional improvement was with a focus on decreasing the abnormal features of the neurological disorder. Currently, the focus is on minimizing the interfering effects of neurological damage while maximizing voluntary control. Interestingly, with the current focus on functional improvement achieved through a retraining or a re-education approach that emphasizes empowering the patient with adequate strength, mobility, and stability skills, that long sought-after improved "quality" of movement appears to have become increasingly evident in our outcomes with patients/clients. ■

Case Studies

The following case studies illustrate an approach to intervention with a child or an adult presenting with a movement disorder characterized by upper motor neuron signs and abnormal muscle force generation, characterized by combinations of muscle weakness, abnormal muscle tone, coordination problems, or involuntary movements. This chapter has three case studies, so that all the pertinent neuromuscular impairments described in this chapter can be adequately illustrated.

Case Study: Child

Lori: 12-year-old Girl with Cerebral Palsy

History

Lori is a 12-year-old girl with cerebral palsy, athetoid type. She has normal intelligence and attends the seventh grade in her local elementary school. Lori lives at home with her parents and two brothers. The home is accessible to Lori, having only a few steps from the first to the second floor. Vision and hearing are within normal limits. Speech is intelligible but becomes labored and difficult to understand during periods of great excitement, stress, or fatigue.

Evaluation

Generally, muscle tone is low in her trunk and neck with predominantly hypertonic muscle tone throughout her extremities. Movement is characterized by fluctuations in tone and involuntary movements (see Figs. 7–18 and 7–20A). Functionally, Lori ambulates independently, although her gait pattern is characterized by instability and dystonic posturing, resulting in frequent falls (see Fig. 7–23). Although Lori is independent in all mobility at school, her parents and teacher are increasingly concerned about the precarious nature of Lori's movements. Safety and independence in open environments are a big concern as Lori prepares to enter high school.

Present Movement Problem

Lori and her family participated eagerly in the physical and occupational therapy evaluations, openly discussing the functional significance of the evaluation findings. The therapists carefully explained to Lori the underlying reasons for the neuromuscular impairments associated with athetoid cerebral palsy: abnormal muscle tone and stiffness, weakness, and lack of voluntary muscle control; muscular coordination difficulties, including problems with muscular activation, sequencing, and timing; and interference from involuntary movements.

The therapists used Table 6–8 from Chapter 6 to guide the clinical decision making to clarify Lori's main movement problem. It was decided that Lori's main movement problem was one of difficulty with appropriate and consistent force generation, instability, muscle pattern coordination deficits, and interference from disordered and involuntary movement.

Intervention was directed at the movement components needed for functional mobility, with an emphasis on strategies to improve stability and controlled mobility (see Chapter 6). Lori and her parents have agreed that improving functional postural control and functional use of all four extremities and her trunk is an important goal, to increase Lori's level of functional independence within her home and school.

Intervention

Intervention is directed at the impairments and functional limitations that are interfering with Lori's ability to move more safely within an increased variety of environments. Interventions include activities of daily living (ADL) training and functional training, with task adaptation as needed. The following short-term functional goals were agreed to at this phase:

- Lori will develop increased extremity strength, especially during movement transitions requiring weight bearing and weight shifting, so that movement patterns become more consistent across tasks and environments.
- Lori will demonstrate improved postural control during movement in many environmental contexts.

Therapy intervention occurred during scheduled home visits, school visits, and appointments in the outpatient pediatric rehabilitation center.

The following, accompanied by figures, describes some of the therapy activities. The focus of intervention was on an increase in functional skills within the limits of Lori's disability. The following activities all integrate within them techniques to accomplish the following:

1. Improve stability within positions and during functional movement
2. Improve postural control in varying positions
3. Improve voluntary control and decrease random or extraneous movements that interfere with movement control
4. Increase functional strength
5. Improve dynamic stability to allow for smooth synergistic stabilization to improve postural control
6. Improve the effectiveness and safety of selected movement choices within specific natural environments—the home and school setting, and across environmental contexts

Activities to Improve Stability

Stability is developed primarily in weight-bearing postures. Lori's problems with stability control may be due to a combination of factors, such as abnormal muscle tone or imbalance around all the joints, especially during weight-bearing activities, and decreased strength. Activities are done to increase proximal stability around the shoulder girdles and to increase effective muscular co-contraction during weight bearing. Effective strategies to enhance stability control would include using facilitation techniques described as approximation and resistance during functional activities, activities to enhance proximal stability (see Fig. 7–24), isometrics, rhythmical stabilization, and weight-bearing activities (see Fig. 7–22). Multiple positions, primarily sitting against support and pushing up to standing, would be practiced to emphasize strengthening of the upper extremity muscles during closed chain activities. Pushing through the upper and lower

extremities would be immediately practiced within functional tasks, so that Lori learns to use her new stability during functional movement (see Figs. 7–24 and 7–25).

Strategies to Improve Controlled Mobility

As discussed in the previous chapter, the ability to move while maintaining a stable posture is referred to as dynamic stability or controlled mobility. Controlled mobility represents the combined function of both mobilizing and stabilizing muscles, characterized by smooth coordinated movements with appropriate synergistic stabilization between antagonists. Examples of activities in which controlled mobility is utilized include weight-shifting activities and participation in movement transitions. Lori is asked to practice maintaining her trunk posture while moving into another position (see Figs. 7–24 and 7–25). Opportunity is given for practice of proximal stabilization or muscular co-contraction during the accomplishment of a functional task (see Fig. 7–19 and 7–20B).

During controlled mobility activities, the therapist or assistant emphasizes movements with directional changes that encourage antagonist muscle actions. Movements are typically started as small, and then gradually progress into larger increments of range. Assistance and guidance are given judiciously, with encouraged active movement and voluntary control from Lori. Varying transitional movements can be practiced (see Fig. 7–25). Focus is on eccentric control (moving out of a posture) (see Fig. 7–24), as well as concentric control (moving into a posture). Functional activities such as bridging, and transitioning between sitting and standing are practiced and used as functional strengthening activities.

This case study illustrates the clinical management of a child with dystonia, specifically athetoid cerebral palsy. The interventions described are directed at improving the main functional limitation of the individual, within the constraints of the pathophysiology. A specific, practical functional goal is defined and some strategies to meet that goal are described.

Case Study: Adult
Jake: 62-year-old Man Following CVA

For the purposes of illustrating the changing nature of some of the clinical features of a neurological disorder, this case study will present the clinical management of an individual who has suffered a stroke, focusing on two different phases of the recovery: acute and subacute.

Acute Phase

History

Jake is a 62-year-old man who has just sustained an infarct to the right middle cerebral artery, resulting in a left hemiplegia. Medical history includes a history of hypertension for which he has been pharmacologically managed since the onset of hypertension at age 56. Other than that, he has enjoyed good health until this hospitalization and worked as a plumber until retirement at age 61. Vision and hearing are within functional limits, with age-related changes including presbyopia, for which he wears reading glasses, and a slight hearing loss requiring no aid at this time. Before admission to this facility, Jake lived at home with his wife and son where he was independent in all ADLs. He enjoys cooking, reading, and woodworking. There is one step to enter the home and twelve steps to the upstairs bedroom. There is a small bathroom with a shower stall on the first floor.

Evaluation

Jake presents in a hospital bed on a medical-surgical floor, following 3 days in an intensive care unit (ICU) immediately after admission. He is medically stable. He presents with a flat affect and slurred speech. He is oriented to his surroundings and appears to understand that he has suffered a stroke. The nursing staff reports that Jake is cooperative and able to follow simple directions.

In the bed, the nursing staff positions Jake in supine, with his left upper extremity supported on a pillow. He appears to neglect his left body side, consistently looking to the right, but staff reports that he attends to his left side if cued. He can be transferred to a wheelchair, with a maximum assist of one. Posture in the chair is characterized by asymmetry with trunk leaning to the left, left arm dangling at the side unless placed into his lap, and head consistently oriented to the right. The following summarizes the evaluation findings.

Motor Control and Musculoskeletal Status. There is weakness throughout the left side of the body. Muscle tone is abnormally low, characterized by flaccidity. DTRs are absent and no muscular contraction can be elicited in any muscle group on the left side. On the right, muscle strength and voluntary control are functional. There is a painful subluxation of the left shoulder. All other range of motion is within functional limits.

Sensory Status. Sensation appears to be intact to light touch and pressure throughout. There is minimal edema evident in the left lower extremity, which appears to be positional.

Function. At this time, Jake is dependent for self-care.

He is just beginning to assist in bed mobility and transfers, using his right trunk and limbs while a nursing or therapy staff member supports the left side. When seated on the edge of the bed, trunk control is poor, requiring the physical support of one person. In the wheelchair, balance is fair, although Jake lists to the side when tired. He does not use his left upper extremity to help support himself but does attempt to compensate with his right upper extremity. During execution of the dependent transfer, standing balance is poor and Jake accepts limited weight through the left lower extremity.

Present Movement Problem

Jake was included in a discussion of the evaluation findings and the therapist carefully explained to Jake about the neuromuscular impairments that he was presenting with: weakness, flaccidity, and lack of muscle activation, complicated by a perceptual/ cognitive neglect of his left side. The therapist used Table 6–8 in Chapter 6 to guide the clinical decision making to clarify Jake's main movement problem. The therapy team decided that Jake's main movement problem was one of lack of mobility, an inability to generate muscular force in his flaccid left side, abnormally low muscle tone on the left, deficient perceptual capabilities secondary to the CVA, pain, and impaired balance and coordination. The reason for the pain in his left shoulder and an explanation about the left shoulder subluxation were also discussed with Jake. Along the movement continuum, Jake was experiencing most of his difficulties with the preparation, initial conditions, and initiation of movement phases of movement execution. Intervention was directed at the movement components needed for initial mobility and force generation as discussed under strategies to improve mobility and beginning work to improve stability (see Chapter 6). Jake appeared to understand the discussion and agreed that the functional short-term goal of regaining some independent mobility was paramount.

Intervention

Intervention is directed at the impairments and functional limitations that were interfering with Jake's ability to function optimally. Interventions included ADL training (bed mobility, transfer training, self-care activities) and functional training (task training or adaptation). During this acute phase, the following short-term functional goals were agreed on:

- Jake will assist with bed mobility, requiring less assistance from nursing staff.
- Sitting balance will improve as follows: from poor to

fair on the edge of the bed with the minimal assistance of one person and from fair to good in the wheelchair, with the assistance of a wheelchair lap tray.

- Jake will transfer from supine to sitting to standing with the minimal assistance of one person.
- Jake will transfer from sitting using a stand pivot transfer with the minimal assistance of one person.

Therapy intervention occurred both at bedside, in Jake's room, and in the physical therapy/occupational therapy gym.

The following discussion, accompanied by figures, describes some of the therapy activities. The focus of intervention was on the regaining of functional skills. To regain function, the therapist and assistant emphasized activities and techniques to increase voluntary muscle activation of the left upper and lower extremity, and the left side of the trunk. The following activities all integrate within them techniques to accomplish the following:

1. Increase kinesthetic awareness and perceptual integration of left body side into functional movement
2. Activate motor unit recruitment
3. Activate initial mobility
4. Increase strength
5. Increase muscular co-contraction
6. Improve stability

Positioning

Proper positioning at this flaccid phase is important for the following reasons: increasing sensory awareness, stimulation of motor function out of anticipated characteristic synergy patterns, improvement in respiratory function, skin care, and assistance in maintaining functional ROM throughout extremities and trunk, including stabilizing and protecting the subluxed left shoulder. In most cases, the pelvis and scapula on the affected side should be positioned in protraction to minimize the anticipated effects of spasticity that is characteristically distributed in the retractors and to promote a midline orientation of both body sides. Positioning should be varied between time on the affected side and unaffected side, including several different positioning choices. Examples are as follows.

Supine Positioning. In supine, the head and neck should be positioned in neutral flexion/extension and Jake should be encouraged to look toward his involved body side. Small towel rolls, placed under the scapula and pelvis on the affected side, will promote protraction. The involved upper extremity should be supported in external rotation and elbow extension with the forearm supinated, the wrist slightly extended, the fingers open, and the thumb abducted. A pillow under the extremity will assist with venous return and decrease dependent edema. The involved lower extremity is positioned in pelvic protraction, slight hip and knee flexion, and ankle dorsiflexion (Fig. 7–26).

Side lying. Side-lying positioning should be alternated between the involved and the uninvolved sides. Positioning on the involved side will increase proprioceptive awareness through weight bearing on that side. Positioning on the uninvolved side will encourage visual regard and beginning functional use of the involved side. On the involved side, it is important that the shoulder be protracted and positioned well forward, so that Jake doesn't lie directly on the involved shoulder, creating the opportunity for impingement. The elbow should be extended, forearm supinated, wrist slightly extended, fingers extended, and thumb abducted. The pelvis should be protracted, with the involved hip extended, knee slightly flexed. Both uninvolved limbs should be supported with pillows (Fig. 7–27). In side lying on the uninvolved side, the trunk and head should be aligned in midline, the involved upper extremity protracted on a small pillow, the elbow extended, the forearm in midposition, and the wrist and fingers open and relaxed. The lower extremity should be positioned with the pelvis protracted, the hip and knee slightly flexed, and the ankle dorsiflexed (Fig. 7–28).

Supported Sitting. Positioning in an upright, functional position should occur as soon as the patient is medically cleared and can tolerate sitting up. In supported sitting as in a wheelchair, the head and trunk should be aligned in midline and Jake should be encouraged to look toward his involved side. Both arms should be positioned in front of him, within the visual field. Clasping his hands together may increase sensory awareness of this involved hand and a lap tray on the wheelchair supports both arms in this forward, functional position. The lower extremities are positioned in flexion with towel rolls to prevent pelvic

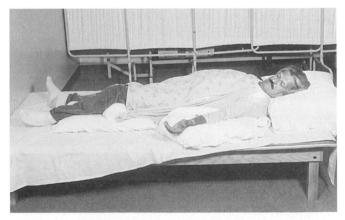

Figure 7–26. Supine positioning depicting support of left side.

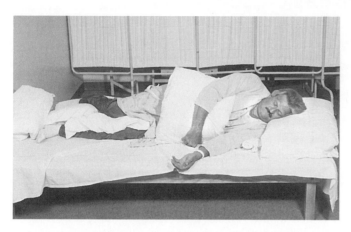

Figure 7–27. Side-lying positioning on involved (left) side.

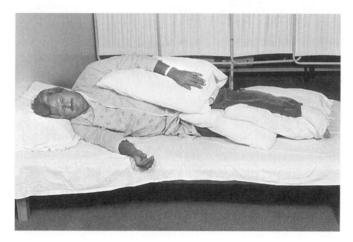

Figure 7–28. Side-lying positioning on uninvolved (right) side.

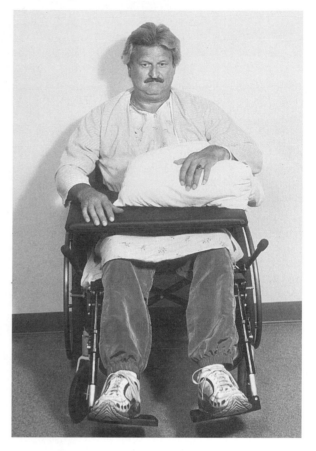

Figure 7–29. Positioning in wheelchair to encourage alignment.

retraction or hip external rotation on the left side. Footrests encourage weight bearing through the feet with the ankles in neutral (Fig. 7–29).

Early Mobility Activities

Early mobility activities include bed mobility, functional upper extremity activities, and functional movement transitions. Strengthening activities are incorporated into early mobility and functional training activities. Examples are as follows.

Early Functional Mobility Activities. An example of a functional mobility activity for the lower extremities that can be tried early in neurorehabilitation is bridging. Bridging (Fig. 7–30) is a functional task that activates weight bearing through the lower extremities in a symmetrical movement pattern, combining flexion and extension muscle groups. The clinician can use various sensorimotor techniques during bridging to activate motor units and increase the beginnings of voluntary control (see Fig. 7–30). Techniques such as approximation, tapping, and verbal cues are especially effective.

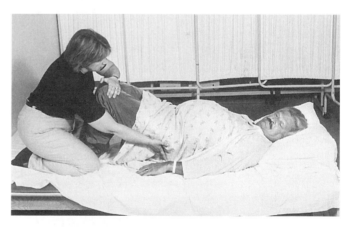

Figure 7–30. Bridging is a good functional task that can be combined with use of sensorimotor techniques such as weight bearing, resistance, and tapping to cue lower extremity muscle activation.

Very early in neurorehabilitation, Jake is instructed in performing self-directed scapular mobilization and upper extremity elevation. Jake clasps his hands together (thumb of involved hand on top of right thumb) and uses his uninvolved right upper extremity

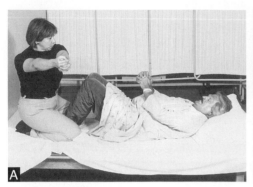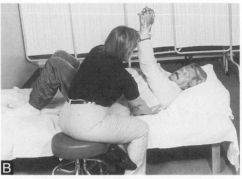

Figure 7–31. Jake is taught to clasp his hands together (A) while the therapist facilitates carryover of bridging into the functional task of scooting in bed (B).

to guide the left upper extremity forward, mobilizing the left scapula into the functionally important position of protraction.

Activities such as rolling and scooting in bed are important early mobility activities that are not only functionally important but also encourage activation of and use of both body sides in a coordinated effort (Figs. 7–31 and 7–32). Scooting in bed is a natural progression from work on bridging and upper extremity self-directed mobility activities. Jake is instructed to clasp his hands together and push off through the lower extremities to scoot to both sides and up and down in bed. The therapist or assistant assists with the bridge or from under the involved scapula to facilitate trunk movements. This activity is an example of integration of sensorimotor techniques, the use of key points of control and physical guidance, and functional strength training all incorporated into a functional task.

Rolling to both sides is another functional activity that could begin immediately during early mobility training. Rolling to the involved side is usually easier because Jake can initiate the roll by using his uninvolved arm and leg to cross over to his left side. To roll,

Jake is instructed to clasp his hands with the shoulders flexed forward, look to the left, and use momentum to roll to the involved side. Rolling to the uninvolved side is much more difficult. The assistant or therapist may need to first flex the hips and legs so that the weight is shifted over toward the right side. Jake is instructed to look to his right and with his hands clasped together and arms flexed forward, roll to the right side, assisted by the therapist or assistant to rotate the head and trunk. A compensatory strategy often used is depicted in Figure 7–32, whereby hooking the uninvolved lower extremity under the involved lower extremity allows the one limb to move the other.

Transfers

Transfer training is an extremely important functional activity that promotes strengthening, voluntary motor control, and a sense of well-being and returning independence. Early functional mobility tasks that are incorporated into transfer training include work on supine to sitting, transfers from sit to stand, and transfers out of bed to a chair.

Transitions from supine to sitting should be practiced from Jake's involved and uninvolved side. It is extremely important that practice be offered in both directions, and even on different mats and beds, so that the task can be generalized to different conditions. In coming to sit with the uninvolved side, Jake is instructed to roll to the uninvolved side and to use his uninvolved right lower extremity to assist in moving both lower extremities off the side of the bed, after which he uses his uninvolved upper extremity to push up to sit (Fig. 7–33). The therapist or clinician instructs Jake in properly positioning his left upper extremity onto his lap so that this subluxed extremity is safe from injury during the movement. Trunk support is offered as necessary. In coming to sit with the involved side, the same initial steps are taught, including rolling first to the side and moving his lower extremities off the side of the bed, but usually more assistance is required. The therapist or assistant uses manual cues to assist.

Once in sitting, bedside activities to improve align-

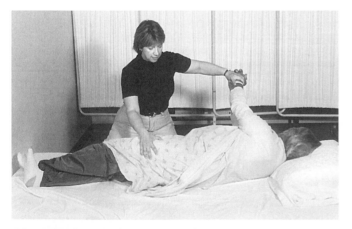

Figure 7–32. Therapist teaches rolling, allowing Jake to use two compensatory strategies to assist in movement: clasping the upper extremities and hooking the involved lower extremity over the stronger uninvolved opposite lower extremity.

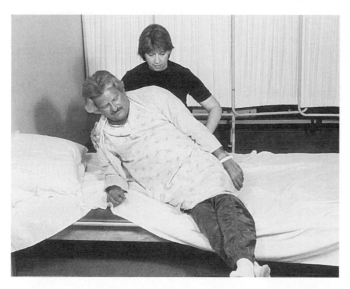

Figure 7–33. Jake moves hooked lower extremities off the bed while the therapist cues him in using uninvolved upper extremity to push to sit. Manual cues and trunk support are offered by therapist as needed.

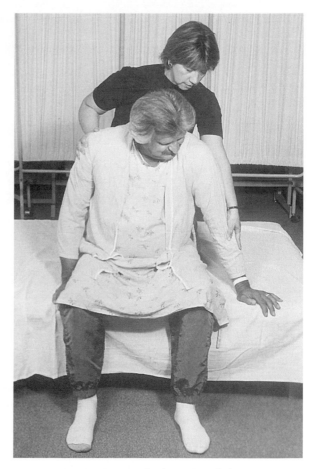

Figure 7–34. Once sitting, rhythmical stabilization, approximation, and weight bearing can be used to promote weight bearing through the involved left upper extremity.

ment and voluntary trunk control can be incorporated into the intervention session. Rhythmical stabilization can be used to increase trunk co-contraction and a mirror can offer important visual feedback. Approximation, tapping, and rhythmical stabilization can be used to promote weight bearing at the side through the involved left upper extremity (Fig. 7–34).

Transfer training from sitting to standing and sitting to and from a wheelchair are then practiced. The therapist or assistant may use many of the techniques advocated by neurodevelopmental intervention experts to promote use of both body sides, weight shifting during the movement, and optimal head and trunk control (Fig. 7–35). The stability of the involved lower extremity is closely monitored by the clinician to prevent knee buckling.

Subacute Phase

Evaluation

Jake has now been participating in inpatient neurorehabilitation for 2 weeks, having had the stroke 16 days ago. He is alert and oriented but appears to be depressed; he is tearful several times during this reassessment. Jake now presents in a standard wheelchair wearing an ankle-foot orthoses on the left foot. The following summarizes Jake's present clinical picture.

Motor Control and Musculoskeletal Status

There is continued evidence of weakness throughout the left side. Muscle tone is characterized by spasticity, distributed predominantly in the left scapular retractors, shoulder flexors, elbow flexors, and finger flexors and the hip retractors and adductors, knee extensors, and plantar flexors in the left lower extremity. DTRs are hyperreactive. The left extremities are typically postured in a flexor synergy pattern of the upper extremity and an extensor synergy pattern in the lower extremity. There is some voluntary control out of synergy beginning to be demonstrated. Motor control deteriorates during times of stress or fatigue. According to Brunnstrom's recovery stages, Jake is presenting at stage three (see Table 6–5 in Chapter 6). On the right side, muscle strength and voluntary control are functional. The left glenohumeral joint subluxation has decreased, and there is minimal pain reported. All other range of motion is within functional limits.

Function

At this time, Jake is able to propel his wheelchair for short distances, using his right extremities. He is able to perform all transfers with the minimal assistance of one person. Functionally, Jake's sitting balance is as

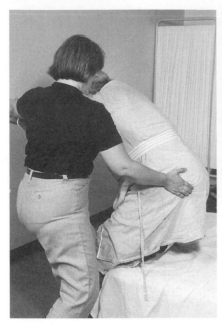 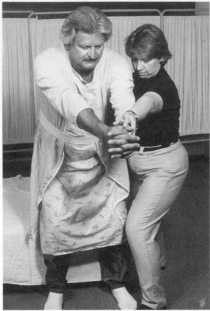

Figure 7–35. Therapist promotes use of both body sides and alignment during practice of transfer techniques.

follows: good in supported static sitting, poor in supported sitting during dynamic movement, and poor in unsupported sitting. While in stance with a wide-based quad cane, static balance is poor, and dynamic balance is very precarious. Jake is independent in all mat mobility, but movement transitions are accompanied by increased posturing in an upper extremity flexor synergy pattern. He uses his left side during movement inconsistently. Jake walks with the assistance of a wide-based quad cane and the moderate assistance of one. Several gait deviations are noticeable: lack of heel strike on the left, hyperextension at the left knee, and consistent hip retraction on the left contributing to a shortened step length and an ineffective swing phase of that left lower extremity.

Present Movement Problem

Jake has been consistently included in discussions of his progress during therapy. He is looking forward to eventual return home, after a stay in an intermediate care facility. To clarify Jake's main present movement problem, the therapist and assistant used Table 6–8 in Chapter 6 as a guideline, elucidating the following summary statements regarding Jake's functional abilities. Jake's present movement problem is centered around ineffective force generation and abnormally high muscle tone on the left body side and difficulties with posture and balance, interfering with his adaptive capacity. He appears to have difficulty in the initiation of movement and the execution of that movement, resulting in inconsistent and sometimes unsafe outcomes. Intervention is directed at key movement components and to assist Jake with effective strategy

generation, including compensatory strategies. Jake has agreed that the functional short-term goal of regaining safe and independent mobility is paramount.

Intervention

Intervention is directed at the impairments and functional limitations that are interfering with Jake's ability to be safe and independent in mobility skills. Interventions include activities to improve postural control and functional balance, transfer training, gait training, and functional training in simulated environments with appropriate task adaptation. Activities to improve stability and controlled mobility (see Chapter 6) are emphasized. The following short-term functional goals were agreed to at this subacute phase:

• Jake will perform all transfers with a contact guard of one person.
• Sitting balance will improve as follows: in unsupported sitting to good with integration of left extremity into postural support as needed; fair in stance and during ambulation. Improved sitting and standing balance will translate to improved safe independence in ADLs.
• Jake will demonstrate increased stance stability and weight acceptance onto the left lower extremity.
• Jake will walk a distance of 100 feet with a wide-based quad cane with minimal assistance.
• Gait quality will improve, as evidenced by decreased knee hyperextension and pelvic retraction on the left, resulting in a longer step length and a more effective swing phase.

Therapy intervention occurs throughout the facility,

in the hallways and sunroom near Jake's room, and in the physical therapy/occupational therapy gym.

The following describes some of the therapy activities. The focus of intervention was on the regaining of functional skills. To regain function, the therapist and assistant emphasized activities and techniques to increase voluntary motor control of the left upper and lower extremity and increase strength of the muscles on the left side. The following activities all integrate within them techniques to accomplish the following:

1. Increase automatic integration of the left body side into functional movement
2. Decrease interfering influence of synergistic muscle activation patterns
3. Improve postural control
4. Increase strength and voluntary motor control
5. Improve stability
6. Increase controlled mobility combined with stability as needed during functional movement
7. Increase functional independence

Activities to Improve Postural Control and Functional Balance

In *sitting*, activities to encourage active weight shifting in both anteroposterior and lateral directions are used to stimulate the activation of automatic postural responses. The therapist or assistant uses rhythmical stabilization to activate co-contraction of the trunk muscles, isometrically at small increments within midrange. Weight bearing through either upper extremity at the side is encouraged as needed, with efforts to increase proximal stability at the shoulder girdle and increase functional elbow extensor strength. Electrical stimulation can be effectively used around the left shoulder muscles or over the triceps belly to augment muscle strengthening. Manual resistance can also be used at the trunk as strength and control improve. Functional activities in sitting, such as reaching to both sides and overhead, are used to integrate the returning strength and control into a functionally meaningful activity (Fig. 7–36). Trunk control activities are practiced during dressing and self-care activities.

In *standing*, work continues on postural control and functional strength. During the sit-to-stand transition, the therapist or assistant guides Jake from his pelvis, cueing Jake to maintain symmetrical body alignment and to decrease the tendency for hip retraction on the left. Using the pelvis as a key point of control offers the assistant or the therapist an effective method of maintaining pelvic alignment, offering approximation as a feedback when an appropriate position is attained. Manual contacts over the gluteus maximus may be needed to cue appropriate activation of the hip extensors. Jake is wearing an orthotic device, which is

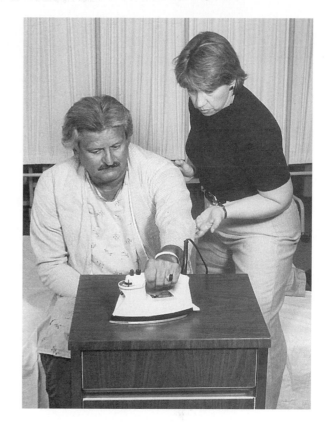

Figure 7–36. Jake happens to enjoy the task of ironing, so this was an effective choice for practicing a functional task using re-emerging trunk control and use of the left upper extremity while sitting.

assisting with heel contact and prevention of knee hyperextension. Manual contacts to the posterior aspect of the knee assist with prevention of hyperextension. In standing, activities to encourage effective weight bearing and weight shifting in all directions are encouraged. Small, controlled weight shifts are most effective at this stage. As Jake performs weight shifting activities in stance, the clinician observes for the activation of standing balance responses, such as activation of muscles around the ankle (ankle strategy) or hip (hip strategy) or the elicitation of a stepping strategy. These strategies will be described in Chapter 8. Functional activities can be done in standing to integrate the postural control responses into a functional task.

Functional Training and Strengthening Activities: Transfer and Gait Training

The sit-to-stand transition, standing activities, transfer, and gait training all progress along a continuum that is difficult to arbitrarily divide into completely separate tasks. Recognize that although these tasks are presented separately for academic purposes, in the clinic and within natural contexts, these activities

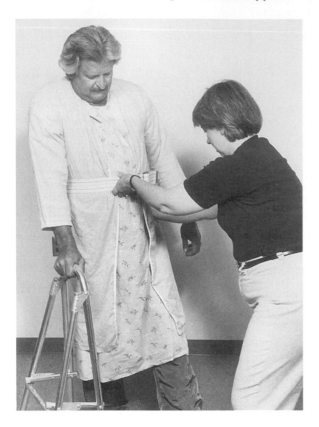

Figure 7–37. Use of quick stretch to left hip protractors activates the incorporation of active hip protraction into swing phase of gait.

should flow into each other as parts of a whole task, as functional movement activities.

Transfer training emphasizes safety and consistency at this phase. The therapist breaks the task down into component parts and encourages strengthening and postural control during all phases of transfer execution. Repetition of the transfer activity offers multiple opportunities for practice of concentric, isometric, and eccentric muscle control, as the therapist or assistant pauses Jake throughout the task execution for the purpose of gaining strength and control. When strength and control have improved, practice is done of the entire transfer, with feedback and knowledge of results discussed with Jake. Practice is done within a variety of contexts with varying environmental settings, so that Jake learns the rules for transferring, rather than an isolated technique. Opportunity is offered for practice in varying environments so that the skill can be generalized.

Gait training includes all the aspects of gait from effective stability in stance, to unloading and weight shift, to limb advancement and initial contact and limb loading. These activities will only be briefly described here, because lower extremity control and gait activities are to be covered in depth in Chapter 10. For Jake, func-

tional gait activities are primarily done within a functional context while he uses his assistive device. Use of the parallel bars is kept to a minimum and only used on occasion to emphasize a specific component skill. For Jake, gait-training activities are primarily directed at encouraging and strengthening effective pelvic protraction on the left, with consequent improvement to step and swing length. The therapist uses the pelvis as a key point of control and facilitates left hip protraction as Jake swings that leg forward. Quick stretch at the beginning of swing, followed by selective resistance, is an effective strengthening activity for the pelvic protractors (Fig. 7–37).

The purpose of this case study was to focus on the clinical management of the primary neuromuscular impairments of muscular weakness, abnormally low and high muscle tone, disturbed postural control, and the subsequent functional limitations in a patient who presents with a hemiplegia as a result of a CVA. Remember that the purpose of this particular text is to focus on the movement impairment. Although the perceptual and cognitive impairments following a stroke cannot be underemphasized, management of those impairments is not within the scope or purpose of this text.

Case Study: Adult

Betty: 58-year-old with Parkinson's Disease

History

Betty is a 58-year-old widow who was diagnosed with Parkinson's disease 8 years ago. Symptoms have been managed quite well pharmaceutically, but she is recently experiencing an exacerbation of symptoms. Betty is active and independent, having been widowed now for 14 years. She lives alone with her dog and is actively engaged in volunteer activities at her local church. She resides in a single-story dwelling and enjoys gardening in her beautifully manicured backyard.

Evaluation

Betty presents with muscle tone characterized by signs of Parkinsonian rigidity, cogwheel type. She has mild muscle stiffness. Sitting and standing posture is typically stooped, with trunk flexion, neck flexion, and capital extension, hips and knees slightly flexed (see Fig. 7–17A). She demonstrates difficulty initiating all voluntary movements and executes functional movement tasks in a jerky, stiff manner. Betty is independently ambulatory with gait characterized by a stooped posture, minimal reciprocal arm swing, and small, shuf-fling steps (see Fig. 7–17). She appears to have diffi-culty with appropriate acceleration and deceleration during a walking task, often overshooting her desired target. Betty has a tremor at rest, but this does not interfere with functional activity. Betty expresses frus-tration with her functional limitations affecting her movement efficiency, and her family is worried about her safety because she lives alone with her dog, Max.

Present Movement Problem

Betty participated eagerly in the physical and occupa-tional therapy evaluations, openly discussing the func-tional significance of the evaluation findings. The therapists carefully explained to Betty the underlying reasons for the neuromuscular impairments associated with Parkinson's disease: rigidity and stiffness; muscu-lar coordination difficulties, including problems with muscular activation, sequencing, and timing; and the presence of the resting tremor. The therapists used Table 6–8 in Chapter 6 to guide the clinical decision making to clarify Betty's main movement problem. It was decided that Betty's main movement problem was one of difficulty with appropriate force generation and coordination. On the movement continuum, Betty was experiencing difficulties with preparation for move-ment, initiation, execution, and termination of move-ment, all contributing to inconsistent and sometimes precarious outcomes. Betty was engaged in a dialogue with the evaluating team, centered on the following focus questions, as discussed in the previous chapter:

- If you were to focus your energies on one thing for yourself, what would it be?
- What activities do you need help to perform or do you feel unsafe performing?
- What are your concerns about functioning optimally at home, during leisure activities, and in your community?
- How can I help you to stay safe and independent?
- Imagine it's 6 months down the road. What would you like to be different about your current situation? What would you like to be the same?

Betty's main concerns centered around being able to remain safely independent in her own home.

Intervention was directed at the movement compo-nents needed for functional mobility and force genera-tion as discussed under strategies to improve mobility and controlled mobility in combination with stability (see Chapter 6). Strategies emphasized helping Betty with coordination activities to assist with timing and sequencing of movement so that movement could be executed more smoothly. Betty eagerly participated in the discussion and agreed that the functional short-term goal of functional retraining to learn some compensatory strategies to improve movement coordi-nation was paramount.

Intervention

Intervention is directed at the impairments and func-tional limitations that are interfering with Betty's ability to function optimally. Interventions include ADL train-ing (self-care activities) and functional training (task training or adaptation). The following short-term func-tional goals were agreed to:

- Betty will perform functional movement with improved coordination, demonstrated by smoother movement initiation, execution, and termination.
- Betty will demonstrate improved functional postural control and balance during dynamic movement activities.
- Betty will develop compensatory strategies that will enable her to execute functional movement activi-ties in a safe and consistent manner.

Therapy intervention occurred both during sched-uled home visits and during outpatient appointments in the physical therapy/occupational therapy gym.

The following, accompanied by figures, describes some of the therapy activities. The focus of interven-tion was on the retraining of functional skills and learn-ing some compensatory strategies. To maximize safe and independent function, the therapist and assistant emphasized activities and techniques to improve postural control and dynamic stability during the performance of functional movement activities. The following activities all integrate within them techniques to accomplish the following:

1. Improve the control of multiple body segments during functional movement
2. Improve the effectiveness of muscle activation and movement initiation
3. Improve voluntary control and decrease random or extraneous movements that interfere with move-ment control
4. Increase functional strength
5. Improve dynamic stability to allow for smooth synergistic stabilization to improve postural control
6. Improve the efficiency of movement initiation, execution, and termination within a variety of natu-ral environments

Activities to Improve Stability, Including Dynamic Stability

Activities to improve stability are performed in func-tional positions that require co-contraction and coordi-nation between antagonistic muscle groups. Because "freezing" is a common characteristic of patients with

Parkinson's disease, these activities are incorporated into stabilizing during the performance of functional activity. Practice in holding a variety of postures, such as sitting and standing, are combined with the performance of ADLs within these positions. The therapist or assistant uses techniques such as rhythmical stabilization and alternating isometric contractions within a small range of increments to assist Betty in gaining a sense of stability and control. Opportunity is given for pausing during execution of a movement task, requiring that Betty demonstrate isometric control (Fig. 7–38). Compensatory strategies, such as environmental adaptation ensuring secure seating or leaning against the bath or kitchen counter, are encouraged to become second nature. Betty is asked to concentrate on developing cognitive strategies to compensate for the movement difficulties caused by the Parkinson's disease. Energy conservation is stressed.

Dynamic stability, also known as controlled mobility, represents the combined function of both mobilizing and stabilizing muscles. Examples of activities that require this smooth interplay between antagonistic muscle groups include weight-shifting activities and

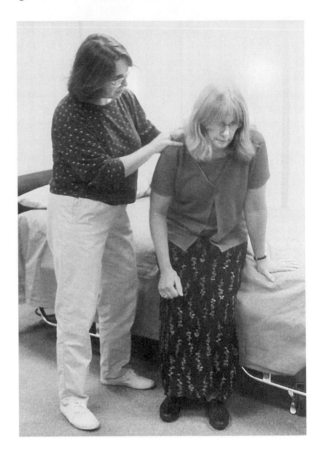

Figure 7–39. Practice is offered in movement tasks requiring weight shift and movement and transitions.

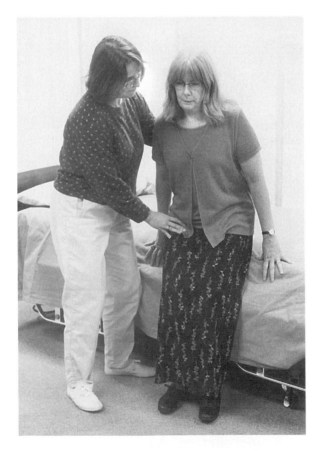

Figure 7–38. Therapist offers cues during instruction to pause while practicing transfer training, offering an opportunity to develop eccentric and isometric muscle control.

movement transitions (Fig. 7–39). During these activities, the therapist or assistant emphasizes directional changes that encourage antagonistic muscle activation. Movements are first started small and then incrementally increase, requiring more control and activation of more motor units. Focus is given to a variety of transitional movements, including those requiring eccentric control (lowering onto a bed) and those requiring concentric control (arising from sitting) (see Figs. 7–38 and 7–39). PNF can be effectively used as an exercise choice to strengthen muscles, retrain agonist/antagonist muscle patterns, and work on timing and sequencing. PNF patterns can be performed independently using pulleys or elastic tubing, so that Betty can perform the exercise at home.

Functional Retraining, Including Compensatory Strategies

Parkinson's disease produces symptoms of akinesia, as evidenced by difficulty with initiation (seen as hesitancy or "freezing"); absence or reduction in the amount of movement; difficulty stopping movement, especially once momentum has taken over; and difficulty monitoring posture and making postural adjustments. The presence of akinesia requires that therapists and assistants be creative in providing a means for Betty to relearn some functional movement strategies and to be educated about the symptoms associated with her disease.

Imitation, verbal and tactile cues, rhythm, and visualization or imagination have all been used successfully in retraining movement skills for individuals with akinesia secondary to Parkinson's disease. Observing and copying another person performing may serve to "unfreeze" the body part when Betty encounters initiation or hesitancy difficulties. Verbal and tactile cues can also assist in the release of akinesia. A light touch or a verbal cue may assist Betty in the initiation, initial weight shift, or weight transfer during a movement. Rhythm can be a very useful movement initiator and maintainer of movement, and because Betty enjoys singing, singing a rhythmical phrase may prove helpful when movement becomes disorganized. Visualizing a movement or an object doing the moving may help Betty overcome difficulties with hesitancy. All these cognitive strategies can be practiced in a variety of natural environments so that Betty becomes proficient at utilizing these adaptive strategies during her daily activities at home.

This case study was used to illustrate the neuromuscular impairments of rigidity and stiffness and uncoordinated movement, such as difficulties in muscle activation, sequencing, and timing, as commonly seen in patients with Parkinson's disease. The clinical management of these impairments and functional limitations requires a very dynamic, practical approach to offering solutions for the individual's movement dilemma. Strategies for intervention with patients/clients with Parkinson's disease often require cognitive retraining, as described in this case study. As part of clinical management of a patient with Parkinson's disease, communication with the physician and integration of medication dosage and administration are also extremely important because it is known that a person's movement difficulties may fluctuate around the medication schedule.

Summary

This chapter, as the first of four clinical management chapters, described the primary neuromuscular impairments that accompany neurological dysfunction. The positive and negative features of damage to the CNS were described and explained. Clinical management of the following impairments was detailed and described, in both text and figures: weakness; abnormal muscle tone, including abnormally low and abnormally high muscle tone; coordination problems, including problems with muscle activation, sequencing, or timing; and interference from involuntary movements, including dystonia, tremor, associated movements, and athetoid or choreiform movements. Three case studies were presented at the end of the chapter in an attempt to illustrate the clinical management of each of these common neuromuscular impairments. A focus of functional training and enablement was the cornerstone of the interventions described.

References

Albright, A. L. (1992). Neurosurgical treatment of spasticity: Selective posterior rhizotomy and intrathecal baclofen. *Stereotactic and Functional Neurosurgery, 58,* 3–13.

Albright, A. L. (1995). Spastic cerebral palsy: Approaches to drug treatment. *CNS Drugs, 4,* 17–27.

Albright, L. A., Barron, W. B., Fasick, M. P., Polinko, P., & Janosky, J. (1993). Continuous intrathecal baclofen infusion for spasticity of cerebral origin. *Journal of the American Medical Association, 270,* 2475–2477.

Andrews, A.W. & Bohannon, R.W. (2000). Distribution of muscle strength impairments following stroke. *Clinical Rehabilitation, 14,* 79–87.

Baker L. L., Yeh C., Wilson D., & Waters R. L. (1979). Electrical stimulation of wrist and fingers for hemiplegic patients. *Physical Therapy, 63,* 1967–1974.

Bennett, S. E., & Karnes, J. L. (1998). *Neurological disabilities: Assessment and treatment.* Philadelphia: Lippincott-Raven.

Bertoti, D. B. (2000). Cerebral palsy: Lifespan management. In *Orthopaedic interventions for the pediatric patient, orthopaedic section home study course* 10:2:4. Alexandria, VA: American Physical Therapy Association.

Bertoti D. B., Stanger M., Betz R. R., Akers J., Moynihan M., & Mulcahey M. J. (1997). Percutaneous intramuscular functional electrical stimulation as an intervention choice for children with cerebral palsy. *Pediatric Physical Therapy, 9,* 123–127.

Bjornson, K. F. (1999). Management of spasticity. In *Topics in pediatrics: In touch home study course* (2nd ed., Lesson One). Alexandria, VA: American Physical Therapy Association.

Bobath, B. (1978). *Adult hemiplegia: Evaluation and treatment.* London: William Heinemann Medical Books.

Bohannon, R. W. (1989). Is the measurement of muscle strength appropriate in patients with brain lesions? A special communication. *Physical Therapy, 69,* 225–236.

Bohannon, R., & Smith, M. (1987). Interrater reliability of a modified Ashworth scale of muscle spasticity. *Physical Therapy, 67,* 206–207.

Bohannon, R. W., & Walsh, S. (1992). Nature, reliability, and predictive value of muscle performance measures in patients with hemiparesis following stroke. *Archives of Physical Medical Rehabilitation, 73,* 721–725.

Bourbonnais, D., Bilodeau, S., Cross, P., Lemay, J-F., Caron, S., & Goyette, M. (1997). A motor reeducation program aimed to improve strength and coordination of the upper limb of a hemiparetic subject. *NeuroRehabilitation, 9,* 3–15.

Bourbonnais, D., & Vanden Noven, S. (1989). Weakness in patients with hemiparesis. *American Journal of Occupational Therapy, 43,* 313–319.

Brouwer, B. J., & Ambury, P. (1994). Upper extremity weight-bearing effect on corticospinal excitability following stroke. *Archives of Physical and Medical Rehabilitation, 75,* 861–866.

Brunnstrom, S. (1970). Movement therapy in hemiplegia: A neurophysiological approach. New York: Harper and Row.

Burke, D. (1988). Spasticity as an adaptation to pyramidal tract injury. In S. G. Waxman (Ed.), *Advances in neurology 47: Functional recovery in neurological disease.* New York: Raven Press.

Butefisch, C., Hummelsheim, H., Denzler, P., & Mauritz, K-H. (1995). Repetitive training of isolated movements improves the outcome of motor rehabilitation of the centrally paretic hand. *Journal of the Neurological Sciences, 130,* 59–68.

Carey, J. R., & Burghardt, T. P. (1993). Movement dysfunction following central nervous system lesions: A problem of neurologic or muscular impairment? *Physical Therapy, 73,* 538–547.

Carmick, J. (1997a). Guidelines for the clinical application of neuro-muscular electrical stimulation (NMES) for children with cerebral palsy. *Pediatric Physical Therapy, 9,* 128–136.

Carmick J. (1997b). Use of neuromuscular electrical stimulation and a dorsal wrist splint to improve the hand function of a child with spastic hemiparesis. *Physical Therapy, 77,* 661–671.

Carr, J., & Shepherd, R. (1987). *A motor relearning programme for stroke.* Rockville, MD: Aspen Publishers.

Carr, J., & Shepherd, R. (1998). *Neurological rehabilitation: Optimizing motor performance.* Oxford, U.K.: Butterworth Heinemann.

Carr, J., & Shepherd, R. (2000). *Movement science: Foundations for physical therapy in rehabilitation* (2nd ed.). Gaithersburg, MD: Aspen Publishers.

Cioffi, M., & Gaebler-Spira, D. J. (1989). Selective posterior rhizotomy and the child with cerebral palsy. In *Topics in pediatrics: Lesson 10.* Alexandria, VA: American Physical Therapy Association.

Comeaux, P., Patterson, N., Rubin, M., & Meiner, R. (1997). Effect of neuromuscular electrical stimulation during gait in children with cerebral palsy. *Pediatric Physical Therapy, 9,* 103–109.

Craik, R. L. (1991). Abnormalities of motor behavior. In M. J. Lister (Ed.), *Contemporary management of motor control problems: Proceedings of the II-Step conference.* Alexandria, VA: Foundation for Physical Therapy.

Daly, J. J., Marsolais, E. B., Mendell, L. M., Rymer, W. Z., Stefanovska, A., Wolpaw, J. R., & Kantor, C. (1996). Therapeutic neural effects of electrical stimulation. *IEEE Transactions on Rehabilitation Engineering, 4,* 218–229.

Damiano, D. L., Kelly, L. E., & Vaughn, C. L. (1995). Effects of quadriceps femoris muscle strengthening on crouch gait in children with spastic diplegia. *Physical Therapy, 75,* 658–667.

Damiano, D. L., Vaughan, C. L., & Abel, M. F. (1995). Muscle response to heavy resistance exercise in children with spastic cerebral palsy. *Developmental Medicine and Child Neurology, 37,* 731–739.

Darrah, J., Fan. J. S., Chen, L. C., Nunweiler, J, & Watkins, B. (1997). Review of the effects of progressive resisted muscle strengthening in children with cerebral palsy: A clinical consensus exercise. *Pediatric Physical Therapy, 9,* 12–17.

Denny Brown, D. (1950). Disintegration of motor function resulting from cerebral lesions. *Journal of Nerves and Mental Disorders, 112,* 1–45.

Deuschl, G., Bain, P., & Brin, M. (1998). Consensus statement of the Movement Disorder Society on tremor. *Movement Disorder, 13,* 2–23.

Dietz, V. (1997). Neurophysiology of gait disorders: Present and future applications. *Electroencephalography and Clinical Neurology, 103,* 333–355.

Duncan, P. W., & Badke, M. B. (1987). *Stroke rehabilitation: The recovery of motor control.* Chicago: Year Book.

Fowler, E. G., Ho, T. W., Nwigwe, A. I., & Dorey, F. J. (2001). The effect of quadriceps femoris strengthening exercises on spasticity in children with cerebral palsy. *Physical Therapy, 81,* 6, 1215–1223.

Fredericks, C. M., & Saladin, L. K., (1996). *Pathophysiology of the motor systems: Principles and clinical presentations.* Philadelphia: F. A. Davis.

Ghez, C. (1991). Voluntary movement. In E. Kandel, J. H. Schwartz, & T. M. Jessell (Eds.), *Principles of neuroscience* (3rd ed., pp. 609–625). New York: Elsevier.

Gormley, M. E. (1999). Management of spasticity in children. Part I: Chemical denervation. *Update on Pharmacology, 14,* 2, 207–209.

Gormley, M. E. (1999). Management of spasticity in children. Part 2: Oral medications and intrathecal baclofen. *Update on Pharmacology, 14,* 97–99.

Gowland, C., deBruin, H., Basmajian, J., Plews N., & Burcea, I. (1992). Agonist and antagonist activity during voluntary upper-limb movement in patients with stroke. *Physical Therapy, 72,* 624–633.

Haney, N. B. (1998). Muscle strengthening in children with cerebral palsy. *Physical & Occupational Therapy in Pediatrics, 18,* 149–157.

Harburn, K. L., & Miller, J. A. (1990). Parkinsonian mechanisms of rigidity and occupational therapy approaches. *Occupational Therapy Practice, 1, 4,* 34–43.

Horak, F. (1991). Assumptions underlying motor control for neurologic rehabilitation. In M. Lister (Ed.), *Contemporary management of motor control problems. Proceedings of the II-Step Conference* (pp. 11–27). Alexandria, VA: Foundation for Physical Therapy.

Hummelsheim, H., Maier-Loth, M. L., & Eickhof, C. (1997). The functional value of electrical muscle stimulation for the rehabilitation of the hand in stroke patients. *Scandinavian Journal of Rehabilitation Medicine, 29,* 3–10.

Jankovic, J. (1987). Pathophysiology and clinical assessment of motor symptoms in Parkinson's disease. In W. Koller (Ed.), *Handbook of Parkinson's disease.* New York: Marcel Dekker.

Koman, L. A., Mooney, J. F., & Smith, B. P. (1996). Neuromuscular blockade in the management of cerebral palsy. *Journal of Child Neurology, 11,* S23–S28.

Knutsson, E., & Richards, C. (1979). Different types of disturbed motor control in gait of hemiparetic patients. *Brain, 102,* 405–430.

Lance, J. W. (1980). Symposium synopsis. In R. G. Feldman, R. R. Young, & W. P. Koella (Eds.), *Spasticity: Disordered motor control.* Chicago: Year Book.

Landau, W. M. (1980). Spasticity: What is it? What is it not? In R. G. Feldman, R. R. Young, & W. P. Koella (Eds.), *Spasticity: Disordered Motor Control.* Chicago: Year Book.

Landau, W. M. (1988). Parables of palsy, pills, and PT pedagogy: A spastic dialectic. *Neurology, 38,* 1496–1499.

Lasarus, J. C. (1992). Associated movement in hemiplegia: The effects of force exerted, limb usage, and inhibitory training. *Archives of Physical and Medical Rehabilitation, 73,* 1044–1052.

Licht, S. (1965). *Therapeutic exercise.* New Haven, CT: Elizabeth Licht Publisher.

Light, K. E. (1996). Clients with spasticity: To strengthen or not to strengthen. *Neurology Report, 15,* 19–20.

Little, J. W., & Merritt, J. L. (1988). Spasticity and associated abnormalities of muscle tone. In J. Delisa, D. Currie, B. M. Gans, P. Gatanes, & M. McPhee (Eds.), *Principles and practice of rehabilitation medicine.* Philadelphia: J. B. Lippincott.

Marsden, C. D. (1982). The mysterious motor function of the basal ganglia: The Robert Wartenberg Lecture. *Neurology, 32,* 514–539.

Mayer, N. H. (1997). Clinicophysiologic concepts of spasticity and motor dysfunction in adults with upper motoneuron lesion. *Muscle and Nerve Supplement, 6,* S1–S13.

McCartney, N., Moroz, D., Garner, S. H., & McComas, A. J. (1988). The effects of strength training with selected neuromuscular disorders. *Medicine and Science in Sports and Exercise, 20,* 362–368.

McComas, A. J., Sica, R. E. P., Upton, A. R. M., & Aguilera, N. (1973). Functional changes in motoneurons of hemiparetic patients. *Journal of Neurology, Neurosurgery, and Psychiatry, 30,* 183–193.

Morris, M. E. (2000). Movement disorders in people with Parkinson disease: A model for physical therapy. *Physical Therapy, 80,* 578–597.

Morris, M. E., Iansek, R., & Churchyard, A. (1998). The role of physiotherapy in quantifying movement fluctuations in Parkinson's disease. *Australian Journal of Physiotherapy, 44,* 105–114.

Neilson, P. D., & McCaughey, J. (1982). Self-regulation of spasm and spasticity in cerebral palsy. *Journal of Neurology, Neurosurgery, and Psychiatry, 45,* 320–330.

Nelson, R. M., Hayes, K. W., & Currier, D. P. (1999). *Clinical electrotherapy* (3rd ed.). Norwalk, CT: Appleton and Lange.

Noth, J. (1991). Trends in the pathophysiology and pharmacotherapy of spasticity. *Journal of Neurology, 238,* 131–139.

Nwaobi, O. M. (1983). Voluntary movement impairment in upper motor neuron lesions: Is spasticity the main cause? *The Occupational Journal of Research, 3,* 132–140.

O'Sullivan, S. B. (2001). Assessment of Motor function. In S. B. O'Sullivan & T. J. Schmitz, *Physical rehabilitation: Assessment and treatment* (4th ed.). Philadelphia: F. A. Davis.

O'Sullivan, S. B., & Schmitz, T. J. (2001). *Physical rehabilitation laboratory manual: Focus on functional training.* Philadelphia: F. A. Davis.

Palmer, M. L., & Toms, J. E. (1992). *Manual for functional training* (3rd ed.). Philadelphia: F. A. Davis.

Peacock, W. J., & Staudt, L. A. (1990). Spasticity in cerebral palsy and the selective posterior rhizotomy procedure. *Journal of Child Neurology, 5,* 179–185.

Pease, W. S. (1998). Therapeutic electrical stimulation for spasticity: Quantitative gait analysis. *American Journal of Physical Medicine and Rehabilitation, 77,* 351–355.

Preston, L. A., & Hecht, J. S. (1999). *Spasticity management rehabilitation strategies.* Bethesda, MD: American Occupational Therapy Association.

Ratliffe, K. A. (1998). *Clinical pediatric physical therapy: A guide for the physical therapy team.* St. Louis: Mosby.

Richards, C. L., Malouin, F., Dumas, F., & Wood-Dauphine, S. (1991). New rehabilitation strategies for the treatment of spastic gait disorders. In A. E. Patla (Ed.), *Adaptability of human gait: Implications for the control of locomotion.* New York: Elsevier.

Robinson, A. J., & Snyder-Mackler, L. (Eds.). (1995). *Clinical electrophysiology: Electrotherapy and electrophysiologic testing* (2nd ed.). Baltimore: Williams and Wilkins.

Rosenfalck, A., & Andreassen, S. (1980). Impaired regulation of force and firing pattern of single motor units in patients with spasticity. *Journal of Neurology, Neurosurgery, and Psychiatry, 43,* 907–916.

Ryerson, S., & Levit, K. (1997). *Functional movement reeducation.* Philadelphia: Churchill Livingstone.

Sahrmann, S. A., & Norton, B. J. (1977). The relationship of voluntary movement to spasticity in the upper motor neuron syndrome. *Annals of Neurology, 2,* 460-465.

Sawner, K. & LaVigne, J. (1992). *Brunnstrom's movement therapy in hemiplegia* (2nd ed.). New York: Lippincott.

Schenkman, M., Donovan, J., Tsubota, J., Kluss, M., Stebbins, P., & Butler, R. B. (1989). Management of individuals with Parkinson's disease: Rationale and case studies. *Physical Therapy, 69,* 944–955.

Schmitz, T. J. (2001). Coordination assessment. In S. B. O'Sullivan & T. J. Schmitz, *Physical rehabilitation laboratory manual: Focus on functional training.* Philadelphia: F. A. Davis.

Selby, G. (1975). Parkinson's disease. In P. J. Vinken & G. W. Bruyn (Eds.), *Handbook of clinical neurology* (2nd ed.). Amsterdam: Elsevier.

Shahani, B. T., & Young, R. R. (1980). The flexor reflex in spasticity. In R. G. Feldman, R. R. Young, & W. P. Koella (Eds.), *Spasticity: Disordered motor control.* Chicago: Year Book.

Shumway-Cook, A., & Woollacott, M. H. (2001). *Motor control: Theory and practical applications* (2nd ed.). Philadelphia: Lippincott Williams & Wilkins.

Stein, A. B., Pomerantz, F., & Schechtman, J. (1997). Evaluation and management of spasticity in spinal cord injury. *Topics in Spinal Cord Injury Rehabilitation, 2,* 70–83.

Styer-Acevedo, J. (1998). Physical therapy for the child with cerebral palsy. In J. S. Tecklin (Ed.), *Pediatric physical therapy* (3rd ed.). Philadelphia: Lippincott-Raven.

Teixeira-Salmela, L. F., Olney, S. J., Nadeau, S., & Brouwer, B. (1999). Muscle strengthening and physical conditioning to reduce impairment and disability in chronic stroke survivors. *Archives of Physical and Medical Rehabilitation, 80,* 1211–1218.

Walsche, F. M. P. (1961). Contributions of John Hughlings Jackson to neurology. *Archives of Neurology, 5,* 99–133.

Whyte, J., & Robinson, K. M. (1990). Pharmacologic management. In M. B. Glenn & J. Whyte (Eds.), *The practical management of spasticity in children and adults* (pp. 201–226). Philadelphia: Lea & Febiger.

Wright, F. V., Sheil, E. M., Drake, J. M., Wedge, J. H., & Naumann, S. (1998). Evaluation of selective dorsal rhizotomy for the reduction of spasticity in cerebral palsy: A randomized controlled trial. *Developmental Medicine and Child Neurology, 40,* 239–247.

Yekutiel, M. P., Pinhasov, A., Shahar, G., & Sroka, H. A. (1991). A clinical trial of re-education of movement in patients with Parkinson's disease. *Clinical Rehabilitation, 5,* 207–214.

Management of Disorders of Postural Control and Balance

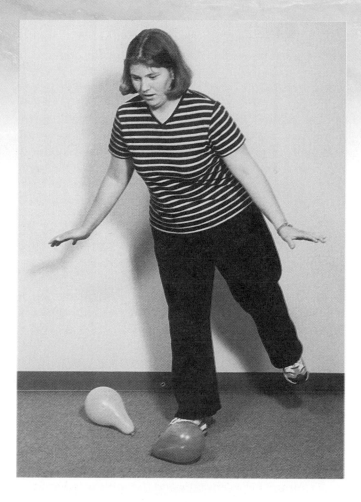

Catherine Emery,
MS, OTR/L, BCN

It is good to have an end to journey toward; but it is the journey that matters in the end.

Ursula Le Guin

Cornerstone Concepts

- Balance: differentiation between postural control and balance
- Theoretical models of postural control and balance:
  - Reflex-hierarchical
  - Systems approach
- Components of postural control and balance:
  - Musculoskeletal mechanisms
  - Neuromuscular mechanisms
  - Sensory mechanisms
  - Perceptual mechanisms
  - Cognitive mechanisms
- Strategies for recovery: sensory and motor
- Age-related differences to postural control and balance
- Assessment of postural control and balance
- Intervention for postural control and balance problems

Introduction

The ability to keep the body steady while engaged in activities that use the limbs is critical to functional independence. Control of posture provides the stable base from which balance is achieved in a variety of body positions, whether the body is still, preparing to move, or preparing to stop (Wade & Jones, 1997).

Clinical Connection:

Imagine getting onto a bus while jostling packages, a magazine, and a wallet. The search for exact change occurs simultaneously to walking onto the bus steps. This results in a misjudgment of the height of the step and causes a trip. Recovery of balance is achieved by steadying pressure against the bus followed by mounting the steps to deposit the coins. A search for a seat ensues while the bus lurches forward, requiring a rapid movement in the opposite direction of the bus's movement to avoid falling down or spilling the packages. The task is completed upon sinking into an open seat, arranging the packages on the floor, and reading the magazine as the bus moves toward the destination. ▪

The many tasks involved in this example illustrate the complexity of the postural control and balance systems. These systems involve recovery from instability, *as well as* the ability to anticipate and move to avoid instability (Shumway-Cook & Woollacott, 2001). These mechanisms are the focus in this chapter. It will describe the systems that keep a person in balance, as well as the abnormalities that can occur to those systems, and approaches to use in intervention to help patients/clients to re-establish stability and balance for optimal function.

Postural Control

Postural control is the most basic of voluntary movements; it provides stability to the body so that interaction with the environment using the upper and lower extremities is possible (Gallahue & Ozmun, 2002). Because postural problems often result in injury and because stability is essential to leading an independent lifestyle, it is of great concern (Wade & Jones, 1997).

Definition and Description

Postural control is defined as the ability to maintain a steady position in a weight-bearing, antigravity posture. As mentioned in Chapter 4, it represents a functional relationship between stability (holding an antigravity position steadily) and mobility (movement). To achieve stability, the **center of mass** (**COM**; the

center of all the body parts) is maintained within the limits of a stable base—whether sitting, standing, or moving (O'Sullivan & Schmitz, 1999). Postural control requires stability and orientation (Shumway-Cook & Woollacott, 2001). As previously mentioned, stability is achieved by keeping the body within the boundaries of space defined by the **base of support** (the plane defined by the surface of the body in physical contact with the environment). When a device is used for mobility, the base of support extends to include that device (see Fig. 6–12). Stability develops from postural adjustments made through our postural control systems (Wade & Jones, 1997). These adjustments serve to reduce or eliminate a displacement of the center of gravity to allow safe movement (Frank & Earl, 1990).

To maintain this stability, coordinated muscle contractions must occur around the joints. This coordination must be flexible enough to allow for adjustment to changes in the environment. Co-contraction needs to occur continuously and be somewhat removed from voluntary suppression (Littell, 1990). In other words, it is important to have the muscles that stabilize the joints working at all times to keep the body upright. It is equally important to limit the ability of the conscious brain to reduce this action. Many small corrective muscle actions are made to prevent falling whether the body position is standing quietly; doing the simplest of movements, such as waving to a friend; or engaging in complex motions such as those required when trying to regain balance after a slip on an icy surface (Cohen, 1999).

The second element of postural control is **orientation**—defined as keeping the body segments in an appropriate relationship with each other and the environment to complete functional tasks. An important goal of postural control is to provide stability to both sensory and motor systems. This stability optimizes the influx of sensory information while moving (Wade & Jones, 1997).

Balance

From the perspective of the clinician, balance is seen as a continuum between static and dynamic balance. Static balance contains the elements of postural control already discussed, whereas dynamic balance indicates movement of muscles while simultaneously keeping the body upright against the resistance of gravity.

Clinical Connection:

In the clinic, therapists evaluate static balance while a patient/client is sitting or standing. Usually this is a measure of a patient's ability to sit or stand upright without support and when presented with a challenge in the form of an anterior/posterior and lateral push.

Postural control is what is really being assessed here. Dynamic ability is also measured while a patient is sitting or standing without support and with challenges to stability as described earlier. Here the intent is to see to what extremes of the base of support a patient can reach before using a postural adjustment strategy (these will be presented later in this chapter). Balance ratings (e.g., good, fair, or poor) are based on how far within or beyond the security of the base of support a person can reach without losing balance. ▪

Definition and Description

Balance is a concept similar to postural control with the added dimension of adjusting to voluntary limb movements and external disturbances (Light, Rose, & Purser, 1996). **Static balance** is the stability component of postural control and is used interchangeably with stability in most texts. **Dynamic balance** is considered to be the ability to move without falling even to the extremes of the base of support. This differentiation seems artificial at best; current systems theories propose that postural control and balance exist on a continuum of movement from the stereotypic reflexive activity of the infant to the vast realm of movement available in the mature system (Wade & Jones, 1997). Movement, as has been stated, is determined by the context in which it occurs. In the same way, sitting and standing activities require different mechanisms to achieve and maintain stability because the characteristics of the support bases are different. When sitting, the support base is the area defined by the thighs and buttocks and the COM is lower, which both contribute to increased stability. When walking, the support base is much smaller as the area between the feet defines it and the COM is higher, contributing to decreased stability. To accommodate for these differences in the support base, different mechanisms are required of the postural control systems.

Clinical Connection:

When children are practicing getting on and off a chair, they will use several approaches. They can access the seat from the front or the side or even over the arms by leveraging their lower extremities onto the seat with their upper extremities. The child learns what approach works on various surfaces (e.g., a rocking chair versus an armchair) through trial and error. As the body matures, a person analyzes the surface and evaluates the conditions of the task before selecting the method of approach. By noticing the stability of the transfer surface (e.g., deep, soft sofa cushions versus rolling desk chair), unsteady approaches are dismissed in the preplanning stage and the risk of injury due to falling is reduced. ▪

Stability develops from postural adjustments made through the postural control systems (Wade & Jones, 1997). These adjustments serve to reduce or eliminate a displacement of the center of gravity to allow safe movement (Frank & Earl, 1990). The type of adjustment attempted depends on the perceived need for safe maintenance of the COM (i.e., how dangerous a fall would be in the particular environmental circumstance) and on the goal of the movement (Frank & Earl, 1990; Hines & Mercer, 1997). Anticipatory adjustments, or **postural preparations,** occur before execution of a planned movement and appear to be related to the stability requirement of a task (Hines & Mercer, 1997). The goal is to increase postural stability by increasing the base of support (e.g., reaching for a handrail when beginning to climb a flight of stairs) or stiffening the joints (e.g., keeping the knees stiffly straight when skating around the ice rink).

Associated adjustments, or **postural accompaniments,** occur simultaneously with the movement. Adjustment made to posture during movement is a very efficient motor strategy for postural stability, but it relies on knowing the task conditions. If unanticipated changes occur during execution, accompaniments can be as destabilizing as the original movement (e.g., reaching for that hand rail as the step is missed but the hand rail detaches from the wall when it is grabbed) (Frank & Earl, 1990).

Adjustments can also be made after a balance challenge has occurred; these are known as **postural reactions.** These adjustments are the best defense against unanticipated, external changes and rely on sensory receptors to alert automatic postural mechanisms for recovery. Upright posture develops from the position of the head relative to the trunk relative to the base of support (Gibson, 1966), as well as being subject to the force of gravity (Wade & Jones, 1997). In other words, postural adjustment starts with the righting reactions that align the parts of the body to each other and to vertical, adds equilibrium that positions the body over its center of mass, and includes orienting reactions to position the body in optimal relationship to objects in the environment. The interaction of these processes seeks stability in reference to gravity and to a person's three-dimensional position in space.

Theoretical Models of Postural Control and Balance

The two models used to explain the neural control of balance are the reflex-hierarchical model and the systems model (refer to Chapters 3, 4, and 6). Briefly, the reflex-hierarchical model proposes that postural control develops over time through reflex integration and increasing central nervous system (CNS) control of movement. The highest levels of the nervous system (selection, planning, and initiating) control the middle levels (specific firing instructions for the effecter muscles) that in turn control the lowest levels (the movement that is observed). The systems model claims that it is the interaction of several systems (not just the CNS), as well as the characteristics of the task itself and constraints of the environment that influence postural control and balance (Mathiowetz & Haugen, 1994; Merla & Spaulding, 1997). In occupational therapy's uniform terminology (Mathiowetz & Haugen, 1994), the systems model attends to the interaction between the person (sensorimotor, cognitive, and psychosocial) and the performance context (physical, socioeconomic, and cultural) as these result in occupational performance (activities of daily living, productive activity, and leisure). In physical therapy practice, the systems model—or dynamic systems theory—proposes that task performance results from the interaction and cooperation of the body's segments and the environmental context, or systems of the environment. The exact wording used by each discipline may differ but the importance of action in context is acknowledged in both practice areas.

The two models are *not* mutually exclusive. The motor skills required for postural control and balance develop in an **ontogenetic sequence** (one skill builds on attainment of another in order), supportive of the reflex-hierarchical model. Each new situation may demand a different approach in order that balance is maintained. The development of strategies in the mature system represents the contribution of the systems model of postural control (Gallahue & Ozmun, 2002). As the infant develops, reflexive movements are replaced with voluntary actions. The component skills are refined through experience in different environments and situations. This exposure to alternate approaches allows for effective integration of the systems that influence postural control and balance.

Reflex-Hierarchical Model

Reflexes are the first form of human movement. The information-gathering role of these movements is strongly linked to motor development and, later, to voluntary movement (Gallahue & Ozmun, 2002). Although the sequence of motor development is predictable, the rate is not; milestones are less accurately linked to an age than they are to each other in sequence and to experience in the environment (Gallahue & Ozmun, 2002). Remember from Chapter 4 that simple reflexes provide a framework to the movements seen in the newborn. The reflexes support motor development by providing consistent, predictable responses. The

postural reflexes automatically allow for maintenance of an upright body posture in relation to the environment. Every movement begins with a weight shift, which in turn stimulates vestibular receptors and proprioceptors to adjust posture. These adjustments are present throughout adulthood as righting and equilibrium reactions. These reactions for early postural adjustment and the lessons of gravity build the skills necessary for the development of strategies to counter challenges to postural control and balance presented by task or the environment (Mathiowetz & Haugen, 1994).

▪ Righting Reactions

The **righting reactions** represent attempts to realign the head or body parts to each other or to the environment. The righting reactions appear within the first few months of infancy. **Labyrinthine righting** (impulses arise from the otolith of the vestibular apparatus of the inner ear) initially dominates the infant's responses but gets replaced by **optical righting** (movement that is initiated by the eyes) by about 6 months, when vision becomes more important. **Neck and body righting** (named for the body part that leads the change in body alignment) also emerge at about 6 months. These reactions contribute to the infant's forward movement around the end of the first year (Gallahue & Ozmun, 2002).

▪ Equilibrium

To re-emphasize a point presented in Chapter 4, **equilibrium** is the act of re-establishing balance after it is lost. The equilibrium reactions allow the body to adjust to a change in the body's orientation in space. **Equilibrium reactions** cause body movement over the base of support or cause enlargement of that base and are sometimes referred to as "tilting reactions" (Shumway-Cook & McCollum, 1991). For example, if the trunk is pushed sideways (laterally), a person will reach out or take a step to stay upright. Equilibrium reactions seem to emerge at each stage of development (i.e., in prone, supine, sitting, quadruped, and standing) before a child's achievement of the next developmental milestone (Shumway-Cook & McCollum, 1991). These basic skills of systems cooperation are necessary for the child to gain independence in sitting and eventually stance.

▪ Orienting Reactions

The **orienting reactions** work to move the head or body in order to bring an object in the environment into clearer vision or into reach. To want to use an object in the environment, one must be aware that it is there. This awareness requires the development of thalamocortical connections—that is, sensory impulses from the periphery being transferred along the neurons to the cortex where conscious attention occurs (Littell, 1990). For that pathway to be established, an infant must have varied sensory stimuli in the environment and experience the success of bringing an object of interest into closer range. This is an example of one of the critical or sensitive periods of development discussed in Chapter 4. Primitive reflexes such as suckle, palmer grasp, and asymmetrical tonic neck reflex (ATNR) allow the newborn to interact with the environment without having to plan the movements to do so. These predictable reflexes develop into voluntary reach and movement as motor development progresses so the infant can explore everything in the environment. With maturity comes selection of what to attend to from the environment; the orienting reactions allow objects to be moved into the best position for the sensory receptors to gain the most information from them (Gallahue & Ozmun, 2002).

Clinical Connection:

When a person walks down the street and notices a familiar figure in his or her peripheral vision, a turn of the head allows examination of the face directly in order to decide if it really is that person's best friend or just another long-haired brunette. Another example is when a therapist climbs the stairs while reading the case history of the next patient on the caseload. As the toes encounter the upright of the step, an automatic lift of the foot results in successful achievement of that higher step. These types of reactions are possible due to the orienting reactions. ■

Meaningful contact with objects is absolutely necessary to develop manipulation or fine motor skills, including reach, grasp, and release, and follows locomotion skills (Gallahue & Ozmun, 2002). Arnold Gesell saw locomotion in the child as the series of sequential postural adjustments; that is, the child is adapting to a new set of conditions with each step (Gesell, 1946; Shumway-Cook & Woollacott, 2001). These skills are the subject of Chapters 9 and 10 in this text.

Systems Model

Currently, the development of movement is viewed as much more than the integration of the reflexes. Contributions of the developing musculoskeletal, neuromuscular, sensory, perceptual, and cognitive systems influence the output strategies available to an individual for postural control (Shumway-Cook & Woollacott,

2001). Each person develops a unique blend of these contributing factors to achieve postural control and balance. In addition, each task presents a new set of conditions that must be met; even tasks that are seen as similar may require different strategies for success. Furthermore, every task is different when the conditions surrounding it change. It is the interaction of these factors that contributes to successful performance at rest or when answering challenges to postural control and balance.

■ Head Control

The first goal of systems interaction is **head control.** This is the ability to maintain an upright position of the head despite changing body positions. It starts as a desire to explore the new, nonuterine environment as infants. The vestibular and proprioceptive systems work together in providing information on the location of the head in space, in relationship to the body, and on its movement (Horak, Shupert, Dietz, & Horstmann, 1994). An important result of head control is that movement becomes isolated. Once the head can be oriented in relationship to the body, eye movement can be separated from head movement and body movement can occur without head movement.

Clinical Connection:

When a baby is held upright and then tilted away from the body, the infant's head will move in a way that keeps it upright. This requires the proprioceptors to indicate a change in body position relative to the head and the vestibular receptors to indicate that movement in the correcting direction has occurred. It also relies on muscle strength and coordination to achieve the desired position change. Once this is done without external support, the infant can be held with less body contact, resulting in greater liberties in moving through space. In turn, this movement contributes to the development of the vestibular system and spirals into greater independence of movement initiated by the child. ■

■ Independent Maintenance of Sitting and Standing

Later, reactions develop to keep the head and trunk in a functional relationship to each other and to the world. If a child is lying in his or her crib and the legs are turned to the side, the upper trunk will rotate to align the vertebral column (Littell, 1990). This is the beginning of the process to gain trunk control, which requires a more sophisticated level of integration of postural adjustments of the head and the trunk and any challenges to stability or balance. The control that was learned for head control must be expanded to the muscles of the trunk and then integrated with those used for the head. One challenge to this integration is postural **sway,** which is the movement that results from these muscular adjustments that keep the trunk upright. The developing infant must learn to incorporate this sway into the movement plan that will result in alignment of the head and trunk. This is a challenge because it asks for the correction of movement even while seeking movement. When it is accomplished, the infant can sit independently.

■ *Movement*

Muscle control is practiced in each developmental position (i.e., supine, side lying, sitting) before integration of movement is attempted in each position. Eventually, control will be integrated in all the developmental positions culminating in independent stance.

The goal of this control in all the postures is skilled movement (Shumway-Cook & Woollacott, 2001). In the remaining chapters of this text, the concepts of limb movement will be explained. The postural control component of these movements is in providing a stable base or framework to support movement. The action or skilled movement becomes the primary objective, and the stability provided by our postural control systems takes a secondary role at that time.

Components of Postural Control and Balance

In the previous section, components of the postural control system were defined in terms of interacting systems built onto the reflex movements. In this section, the components that make up those systems will be clarified.

Musculoskeletal Mechanisms

As was previously mentioned, postural control and balance rely on the integrity of the muscles to make effective adjustments. To recover from a change to the COM, full range of motion (ROM) and strength are required. Limitations caused by pain, restricted ROM, muscle weakness, or limited endurance can affect the availability of movement strategies and the maintenance of equilibrium (Horak, 1987). Musculoskeletal disorders can occur secondary to a neurological lesion or injury. For example, patients with Parkinson's disease experience a loss of spinal flexibility that contributes to the immobility seen (Shumway-Cook & Woollacott, 2001).

Clinical Connection:

Children with cerebral palsy often show limited ROM at many joints due to pressure of abnormal muscle tone in the muscles that normally allow smooth movement. Contractures develop as the systems work to gain stability despite the disorganized system; because muscles do not respond in the normal way to a request to contract, the soft tissue remains immobile. This firming of the "soft" tissues actually provides stability when the child with cerebral palsy is trying to move. The longer the same position is held, the greater the reliance on the stability provided by that position. This prolonged reliance on contracted positions will lead to shortened muscle. Without intervention to elongate the muscle and prevent the soft tissue contracture, this may become a permanent change to the normal alignment of muscles and severely limit mobility and recovery from balance challenges. ■

If movements appear uncoordinated, an assessment of the basic musculoskeletal components can differentiate a CNS disorder from a biomechanical structure dysfunction. Because a limitation of ROM, strength, or endurance can restrict the postural preparations, accompaniments, and reactions available to a person, the musculoskeletal system has an important part in postural control and balance. However, a detailed discussion of these concepts is beyond the scope of this text, and the reader is referred to the excellent texts that are available on this subject (Basmajian & Wolf, 1990; Kisner & Colby, 2002).

Neuromuscular Mechanisms

The nervous system organizes the production, coordination, and grading of muscle forces fundamental to the control of posture. Three factors contribute to successful organization and achievement of postural control (Shumway-Cook & Woollacott, 2001):

- Postural alignment
- Muscle tone
- Postural tone

Postural alignment is keeping the body centered about the vertical midline (Fig. 8–1). Proper alignment reduces the effects of gravity by limiting the use of internal energy required to move against gravity. Muscle tone represents the readiness of the muscle to shorten or contract. The amount of muscle tone varies from person to person in the normal, relaxed state of being. Because postural control relies on muscle activation to achieve stability, muscle tone sets a level of readiness when adjustments are needed. **Postural tone** is the activation

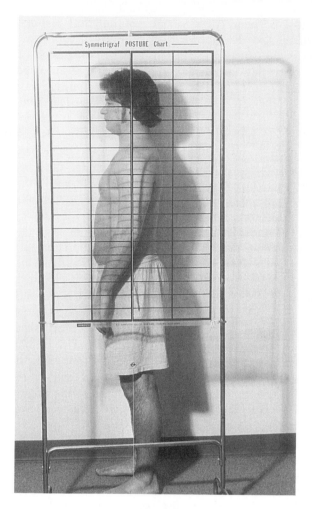

Figure 8–1. Side view of an adult with postural alignment line superimposed.

of specific antigravity muscles. These muscles stabilize the weight-bearing joints and the trunk and are tonically active.

Neuromuscular impairment has a widespread effect; it can influence musculoskeletal problems, create conditions of abnormal muscle tone, or affect coordination via muscle synergies. This can appear as timing difficulty (i.e., use of a strategy is initiated too late to be effective) or incoordination (i.e., shifting weight onto the weaker side without reaching out to increase the support available). Cerebellar involvement causes tremors or ataxia, which interferes with maintenance of postural control.

Sensory Mechanisms

To adjust the body within the base of support, there must be an internal concept of where the body parts are in space and whether they are moving. This involves intact sensory and perceptual systems. Researchers agree on three primary sensory systems (i.e., visual, vestibular, and somatosensory) whose input directly affect postural control and balance. The information received from each of the systems is redundant; that is, it repeats and confirms each of the others'. This allows for a large safety margin for stability to be regained (Merla & Spaulding, 1997), also permitting a person to remain stable in a variety of environments where one or more of the senses is unavailable (Montgomery & Connolly, 1991). Each one also has particular contributions to postural stability and balance.

▪ Vision

A detailed description of the visual system anatomy is beyond the scope of this text and is available in other sources (Cohen, 1999). Briefly, the structures of the eye itself all function to focus light rays on the retina, where light energy is converted into neural impulses. From the retina, these impulses are carried by nerve fibers bundled together to form the optic nerve until they are joined by fibers from the opposite retina at the chiasm and become the optic tract (Lundy-Ekman, 2002) (see Fig. 3–4). It is important to note that the optic tract carries impulses from both eyes and corresponding visual fields (see Fig. 3–4). The optic tract projects to three known areas, the largest of which is the **lateral geniculate nucleus of the thalamus,** where retinal impulses are represented cortically: Shading and colors become identifiable objects. From this nucleus, projections carry the visual image to the occipital lobe or primary visual cortex. It is in this lobe that images take on meaning as specific objects or people. The second projection of fibers from the optic tract goes to the **superior colliculus,** where the information is coded for movements within the field of vision, even those movements that result from body motion. Somatosensory information from the spinal cord and the medulla also project to the superior colliculus contributing information for the control of eye movements (Cohen, 1999). The last set of projections from the optic tract form the **accessory optic tract,** which seems to provide a feedback loop for eye movement control via the inferior olivary nucleus of the pons and cerebellar flocculus (Cohen, 1999).

Vision is really the integration of many processes rather than a singular one. The visual system is critical to interest in the environment and in motivating body movement. Vision skills, and the subsequent interest in the environment, start the infant's attempts to extend the neck, rotate the trunk, and eventually to roll over. After neck control is achieved through neck righting reactions, the eyes are able to move independently of the head and body. In the absence of stability, the body becomes an extension of the movement rather than the base from which it develops, and visual exploration is not supported (De Benabib & Nelson, 1991). Eye skill development, as presented in Chapter 3 (e.g., fixation, saccades, pursuits, and accommodation), relies on this stability (De Benabib & Nelson, 1991). In turn, these skills allow activation of the feed-forward system to initiate movement: "We perceive in order to move, but we must also move in order to perceive" (Epstein & Rogers, 1995).

The visual system predominates other sensory input in humans. Humans have come to rely on the rapid intake of immense amounts of stimulation afforded us by the visual apparatus, so much so that it is accepted as the most accurate even in the presence of profound impairment (Warren, 1999).

Clinical Connection:

By observing patients and their family members, it is noticeable that some people sway more than others, while quietly standing. The eyes and ankle proprioceptors provide feedback to stop this sway when both are functioning normally. People who are nearsighted cannot visually detect this movement during quiet stance even with normal vestibular and somatosensory input. Despite the input from their proprioceptors, patients' visual input carries the most weight, and conscious awareness of swaying does not occur as soon as is noted with people who have normal acuity (Lee, 1989). ▪

Vision serves two main purposes (Wade & Jones, 1997):

- To recognize and identify objects in the environment, a function also known as using **focal vision**
- To generate field-of-view information for motion, the "Where is it?" or big picture function also called **ambient vision**

Visual input seems to be the dominant information source for low-frequency stimulation such as postural sway and gait (Wade & Jones, 1997); if visual input indicates misalignment with the environment, sway is initiated to bring us into upright orientation as compared with this external, stable reference (Merla & Spaulding, 1997). However, nonvisual information also contributes to spatial orientation; this coordination of input allows us to gain far more information when we move than when we do not (Wade & Jones, 1997).

▪ Vestibular

The vestibular system is named for its location posterior to the vestibule of the inner ear. Sensory receptors are contained in the semicircular canals and the labyrinth (see Fig. 3–8). The three semicircular canals are arranged almost perpendicular to one another and respond to changes (acceleration or deceleration) of rotary movements (i.e., turning the head). This response is based on Newton's law of inertia, which states that an object in motion will stay in motion and an object at rest stays at rest unless acted on by an outside force. Head movement causes the fluid of the canals (**endolymph**) to move, which stimulates the embedded hair cells to send a neural impulse along the vestibulocochlear nerve (cranial nerve [CN] VIII). The labyrinth, meanwhile, responds to linear movement (e.g., the forward lurch of the bus in the earlier example) and gravity in much the same fashion; however, within the endolymph are otoconia crystals sitting atop the hair cells whose pressure against those hair cells provides the stimulus we call gravity (Cohen, 1999). Any changes in head movement, including weight shifting to regain posture and balance, stimulate the vestibular end organs, or hair cells. The semicircular canals and the otoliths work in pairs so that stimulation of paired receptors sends a directional signal about the movement. The vestibular system is divided further into central and peripheral areas; this becomes important in diagnosing disorders of the system. **Central vestibular disorders** are those that involve the projection fibers/tracts, whereas **peripheral vestibular disorders** affect the structures of the inner ear themselves (Adams, 2000).

The vestibular fibers of the vestibulocochlear nerve (CN VIII) project to the vestibular nuclei in the brainstem, maintaining their spatial distribution in part (Cohen, 1999). Once in the vestibular nuclear complex, information is modified by complex input from many pathways. It is here that the fibers of the accessory optic tract discussed earlier interact with vestibular input to influence eye movement (Cohen, 1999). Some fibers of CN VIII project directly to the vestibulocerebellum or floccular lobe of the cerebellum, where the information is combined and compared with other sensorimotor input to produce smooth voluntary movements (Cohen, 1999). Two descending vestibulospinal tracts, the medial and the lateral, project to the spinal cord for postural control. The lateral vestibulospinal tract influences the physiological extensors of the neck, trunk, and knees, whereas the medial vestibulospinal tract forms the basis of the labyrinthine righting reactions seen in infants (refer to p. 270) (Cohen, 1999). The three main contributions of the vestibular system are (Cooke, 1996):

1. Regulation of eye position in the orbit to ensure that a steady image is held on the retina during movement, called the **vestibular ocular reflex (VOR)**.
2. Influence of muscle tone for postural support.
3. Provision of conscious awareness of spatial orientation.

The vestibular system (see Figs. 3–7 and 3–8) alerts the CNS to the position and motion of the head and the direction of gravity; it can only provide input on head movement, not any other body segment (Horak & Shupert, 1994). The vestibular apparatus serves a sensory and motor purpose, but its role is difficult to isolate from somatosensory input due to the convergence of input from these structures within the brainstem nuclei (Horak et al., 1994). Vestibular receptors judge the position and motion of the head and then orient the head to vertical (Horak & Shupert, 1994). The body moves to align itself with the head and attains vertical positioning. The information may be ambiguous; fast, high-frequency stimulation may override other input. Examples of high-frequency stimuli are striking the heel as a step is taken during walking and sudden tripping (Horak & Shupert, 1994). Studies have demonstrated the direct role of the vestibular apparatus on postural corrections after a push to the head or shoulders and more recently have isolated corrections affecting the trunk and legs (Horak et al., 1994). This seems to indicate that vestibular input has an influence beyond adjusting head position, but the primary role of the vestibular system seems to be to stabilize the head in space to ensure a steady gaze during movement, whether that movement is voluntary or not (Horak et al., 1994). The importance of vestibular input to postural control seems to increase where somatosensory cues aren't good (Horak et al., 1994). In general, when head stabilization is crucial to performance or when somatosensory input is lacking, the vestibular system assumes a very important role in postural control (Horak & Shupert, 1994). The role of this system during movement seems more straightforward.

▪ Somatosensory

The somatosensory system includes tactile receptors and proprioceptors in muscles, tendons, and joints to provide subconscious input on body position and movement. The receptors of primary importance to postural control include joint receptors of the ankle, knee, and hip; muscle spindles of the legs, back, and neck; and tactile receptors of the feet. Input from the proprioceptors is used in conjunction with visual and vestibular information as a feed forward, or alerting, response during postural change. Often these receptors trigger corrections to posture before awareness of any disturbance; the postural preparations were discussed earlier (Merla & Spaulding, 1997).

Clinical Connection:

Walking across the lawn presents a perfect example of adjustments made before an awareness of their need. The lawn appears to be a flat surface evenly covered by lush, cushioning grass. The lawn is really a series of small hills and valleys. Yet walking across it does not result in a feeling of unsteadiness; the sensory input to the feet results in ongoing changes to the muscles of the legs to accommodate the unevenness of the surface. This all happens without conscious awareness of those adjustments. ▪

Perceptual Mechanisms

Even when the sensory receptors are functioning properly, the ability to make sense of their signals can be disrupted. Adding meaning to the impulses sent by the sensory receptors is the definition of **perception.** Perception is the incorporation of multiple receptor impulses (e.g., tactile stimulation across the fingertips) and multiple sensory modalities (e.g., tactile, visual, and kinesthetic) by the cortex. Because the receptors can only respond to features of the stimulus object, object identification (or naming) requires combining all the feature signals available.

Although all sensory modalities are perceived, it is vision that dominates the development of spatial perception and cognition. Vision is one sense that extends beyond the basic process of stimulus response. The occipital lobe encodes visual stimuli in addition to skeletal, visceral, and subcortical input before sharing visual information with other structures in the brain. Therefore, the visual image is understood according to its shape, distance, color, and size even before any other sensory information is integrated with it (Siev, Frieshtat, & Zoltan, 1986).

One of the foundation skills to perceptual awareness is the formation of body image and body scheme. Often used interchangeably, the terms are actually quite different (Siev et al., 1986). **Body image** is similar to self-image, the mental representation and thoughts associated with your body. **Body scheme** is a postural model, an understanding of the position of your body and the relationship of your body parts to each other and to the whole. These perceptions develop from awareness and movement as an infant.

Initially, movements are bilateral, and it is only through continued exploration that an internal awareness of the two sides of the body—**laterality**—develops. **Directionality,** or the sense of position relative to oneself, is learned as the child continues environmental explorations and develops postural control. Successful exploration and control establishes orientation of the body to the environment. With the interaction of the body and the environment, the child's self-image provides a reliable point of origin for encoding external features. This postural model becomes the basis for other movement because it is only through awareness of the parts of the body and their relationship to each other that a person knows how to move.

Cognitive Mechanisms

Perhaps least understood are the cognitive contributions not only to performance of strategies but also to compliance with intervention (Shumway-Cook & McCollum, 1991). Cognitive processes include the following:

- **Arousal** (being alert to the environment)
- **Attention** (directing cognitive processes to a significant feature of the environment)
- **Memory** (learning and recalling information)
- **Judgment** (discerning the appropriateness of a particular action)
- **Decision making** (selecting from an array of possible actions)

Identifying each of these separately during clinical examination is difficult and often arbitrary (Siev et al., 1986). Cognitive skills are not easily isolated from one another, as each builds on the others during functional activity, which creates the difficulty in establishing their individual roles in postural control and balance.

Although it is beyond the scope of this chapter to thoroughly examine cognitive functioning, it is critical for the therapist and assistant to recognize the importance of cognitive skills to performance of any activity. An apparent deficit in postural control or balance may be caused by inattention or judgment problems related to the cause of injury. Appropriate testing of these skills is needed when performance indicates a possible deficit.

Clinical Connection:

A patient who has sustained a traumatic brain injury may appear unable to execute movements in order to sit without support or to walk. Careful observation of this behavior often leads to the discovery of attention deficits rather than weakness or instability. The patient/client is unable to focus his or her mental energies on the therapy session because the clinic environment provides too many distractions. Intervention in a quieter area would be the effective intervention strategy rather than initiating a strengthening program. ■

Strategies for Recovery

Sensory Strategies

Sensory strategies are ways of organizing sensory input to alert the motor systems to make changes to the plan or execution of movement. Reducing the amount of conflicting sensory input and coordinating sensory information with motor aspects of postural control are the methods of organization that seem to be used. Effective postural control requires the ability to generate forces to control the body's position in space and to know where the body is in space and whether it is moving (Shumway-Cook & Woollacott, 2001). All the sensory systems discussed previously contribute to maintaining the postural control in the absence of challenges.

In the presence of challenges, each sensory system appears to take on a different role in correcting balance. This is due in part to the limitation of each system: The visual system cannot distinguish between body movement and environmental movement without vestibular input. Likewise, the vestibular system can't distinguish head movement, such as a head nod, from combined head and body movement, such as a forward bow, without contributions from the proprioceptors (Umphred, 2001). When the brain becomes aware of abnormal signals, the normal sensory input gains importance for position in space to be perceived accurately (Umphred, 2001). When the brain is unable to determine which system is providing erroneous input, an attempt is made to decrease input in order to evaluate each system. For example, **vertigo** (a sense of movement when there is no actual movement) is sometimes experienced after rising to a standing position. Closing the eyes can reduce the discomfort it creates, effectively reducing the sensory input being gathered by an overwhelmed system.

Clinical Connection:

Remember the strategies used when visiting the amusement park over summer vacation? As the merry-go-round rotates, the riders focus on one spot in order to reduce the risk of vomiting as they disembark. Another instance where input is reduced is during ice skating or skiing activities. Muscles are tensed to give an increased experience of control, as well as to reduce the extraneous movement felt. ■

The sensory strategies seem to be selected in a hierarchy to better ensure that the appropriate sense is selected for the task (Shumway-Cook & Woollacott, 2001). The selection process also varies based on age, the task at hand, and the context in which the task is occurring.

Motor Strategies

Researchers (Horak & Nashner, 1986) have identified automatic movements used to keep the COM over the base of support. The responses are stereotypical; they match the direction and degree of the challenge given (Umphred, 2001). For example, if a person is pushed to the right side, the automatic response is a shift to the left to re-establish midline. The harder the destabilizing challenge, the greater the movement to realign the body as body segments are activated to oppose the reaction forces (Frank & Earl, 1990). Environmental features, true to the systems model, do have an influence on the production of strategies; in a new environment, a person may take a step earlier than might have happened in a more familiar, less anxiety-provoking situation.

Increasingly, the contribution of trunk and hip input is being studied as more important to shaping the balance strategy than lower leg input, as was originally thought (Allum, Bloem, Carpenter, Hullinger, & Hadders-Algra, 1998). These postural adjustments serve to minimize the displacement of the center of gravity to allow safe and efficient voluntary movement (Frank & Earl, 1990). Interestingly, this selection of muscles is presumed to be shaped by vestibular input developed in early infancy to prevent falls (Allum et. al., 1998).

▪ Ankle Strategy

Postural control that is initiated from the ankles and feet is called an **ankle strategy**. This is the most common automatic adjustment to anterior-posterior sway

(Horak, 1987). As depicted in Figure 8–2, use of this strategy results in the head and body moving as a unit over the feet with minimal hip and knee movement. Typically, this is the preference when the challenge is small, slow, and near midline (Umphred, 2001). Success requires that the support surface is large and firm in order that the forces generated by the ankle rotation are resisted. For example, for a standing bus passenger, the "floor" moves in an anterior-posterior motion when the bus pulls away from the stop and the rider compensates by swaying at the ankles until midline is re-established.

Originally, it was believed that ankle input triggered responses in lower leg muscles, causing the distal-to-proximal balance correction seen with the ankle strategy. Research has shown that triggers in the trunk and neck are occurring simultaneously with the ankle triggers, suggesting that other proprioceptive input contributes to postural responses (Allum et al., 1998).

▪ Hip Strategy

Control of posture that comes from the pelvis and trunk is called a **hip strategy.** Figure 8–3 depicts that use of this strategy results in the head and hips moving in opposite directions. Larger postural challenges result in hip flexion/extension to shift the body's COM; the body segments counterbalance each other as equilibrium is

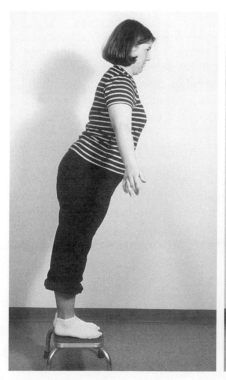
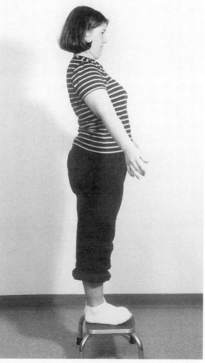

Figure 8–2. An individual using the ankle strategy.

regained. Hip strategy is preferred when the challenge is large or fast or if the support surface is too small to accommodate the ankle forces mentioned previously (Horak, 1987). For example, as a person attempts to walk along the raised rail border of a flower garden and begins to lose balance, compensation can occur using hip movements to realign the body segments on the narrow support base.

▪ Stepping Strategy

Lastly, the stepping strategy is depicted in Figure 8–4. Reaching with the arms to steady oneself is also in this category (Fig. 8–5). This strategy is used for very large or very fast changes and results in realignment of the COM with the base of support using steps or hops in the direction of the change (Horak, 1987). For example, when descending the stairs and missing a step, a person will rapidly reach for a rail or the wall to avoid a fall.

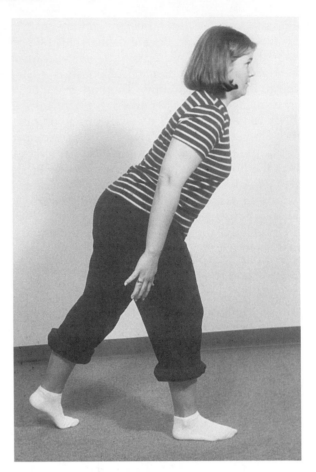

Figure 8–4. An individual using the stepping strategy.

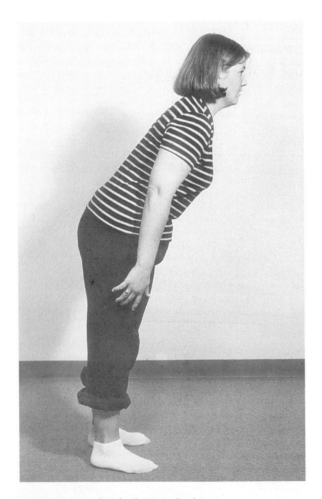

Figure 8–3. An individual using the hip strategy.

Clinical Connection:

The use of these strategies occurs regularly in everyday situations. Imagine standing in line, patiently waiting to get a lunch tray. Suddenly, someone steps into the line and grabs a tray. The automatic response is to shift weight from the balls of the feet to the heels to avoid contact. A slight lean back might be needed; this is the ankle strategy at work to keep the body balanced and avoid a fall. Another situation is when climbing back to a seat on the bleachers for the second half of an exciting basketball playoff. Trying not to spill soda into the people already seated, a weight shift at the hips is used. The upper body moves forward and back because there is limited space for foot movement. The hip strategy has just saved another person from tumbling down those bleachers. Over- or underestimating the height of a stair results in a flailing of arms and legs to regain postural control and balance. This is a demonstration of the stepping strategy at work protecting us from a fall.

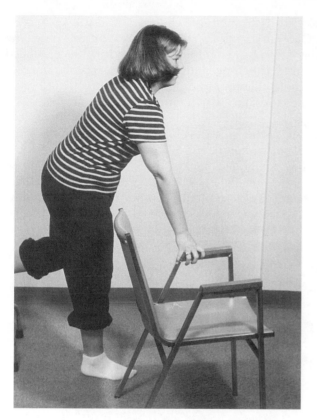

Figure 8–5. An individual using the reaching strategy.

Age-related Differences to Postural Control and Balance

Chapter 4 offers a thorough description of the development of motor skills through the lifespan. This chapter will highlight some of these skills needed for postural control as they develop and change as the body ages.

Early Development

Control of the head and neck is one of the first tasks the newborn faces. It is the first battle a newborn wages with gravity. Success means that the infant can lift the head up from a prone or supine position. With this movement comes dawning awareness of the environment and attempts to interact with its contents. Once mastery of the head and neck muscles is demonstrated, the infant needs to extend that control to the muscles of the trunk and lumbar region. Lifting the chest off of the surface when in prone and turning over from supine to prone are two indications of increasing trunk control. Motor control is practiced in each of the developmental

positions (e.g., prone-on-elbows, sitting, all-fours) in order for it to become steady. Once steadiness is gained in each of the positions, movement can be added within the base of support offered (controlled movement) and eventually to the extremes of that support (skilled movement). Generally, proximal body segments learn to stabilize the body so that distal segments are free to function (O'Sullivan & Schmitz, 1999).

Motor learning of stability postures seems to develop from weight-bearing postures. Head, upper trunk, and shoulder control are promoted by the prone-on-elbows position, which provides the conditions of a large base of support and low COM. Lower trunk, hip, and elbow control are added during practice in quadruped, which serves to decrease the base of support and raise the COM (Gallahue & Ozmun, 2002).

Upper trunk control often occurs before lower trunk control and is heralded by independent sitting. As the ability to sit alone develops, the infant is gaining coordination of the upper extremities and increasingly seeking environmental interaction. An upright posture provides the greatest freedom of movement for our upper extremities. Sitting develops first due to having a moderately sized base of support providing greater stability. To maintain a sitting posture, the head and trunk are held in vertical midline with the extensors of the pelvis and lumbar spine providing antigravity control. **Reactive control** (movement made in response to ongoing feedback) is needed for changes in the support surface or COM. For example, as weight is shifted forward when the infant reaches for a toy, increased muscle contraction results from the increased muscle stretch. **Anticipatory control** (preparations for movement that relate to the task and the environment as it currently exists) is needed to prepare for voluntary movements. Using the same example as earlier, this is what resulted in the initial weight shift (O'Sullivan & Schmitz, 1999).

Standing is more challenging due to the reduction in the size of the support base and higher COM relative to that base. Stability in standing is dependent on the distance between the feet, their length, and the height and weight of the person. Although a small amount of spontaneous sway is normal, all body joints are vertically aligned. Muscle activity is primarily seen in antigravity muscles throughout the trunk and lower extremities. The prolonged postural control required of standing relies on the sensory input of the vestibular system, which indicates the effect of gravity on the head; the somatosensory input (tactile and proprioceptive) from the support surface, which indicates movement and body position; and the visual cues about the environment and the body's relationship to objects within the environment (O'Sullivan & Schmitz, 1999).

Clinical Connection:

Think of that infant in the first few months of life. As head control is mastered, the baby pushes up onto the arms to get a better look. Fatigue causes this action to last only a few moments at first. With enough pushes, the shoulder muscles are strengthened and the prone-on-elbows position can be supported for longer periods. Rocking is noticed as the child tries to get the legs underneath for support also. None of these actions happens without days or weeks of practicing the motor components and coordination required of each task. The effects of gravity and the strategies required to fight it are incorporated into the child's movement paradigm. Baby's first steps are often missed because the patient waiting for that moment is filled with false starts and near successes. ▪

Childhood

The postural control and balance goals of the child are to develop and refine abilities in a wide range of stability movements (Shumway-Cook & Woollacott, 1985). Children explore the movement and stability potentials of their bodies; they have conquered the force of gravity in limiting movement but now seek control in active opposition to gravity's restrictions (Gallahue & Ozmun, 2002). Old lessons are relearned as the body itself grows and dimensions change. As mentioned in Chapter 4, different levels of developmental skill exist among the body segments, perhaps resulting in the appearance of clumsiness as new tasks are attempted.

Childhood is a time to develop skilled movements that serve as the stabilizing framework of future movement. Rolling is a fundamental stability movement as it creates a disturbance within the semicircular canals to which the body must adjust. Movement through space develops as tasks are attempted during which the body has no contact with a support base. **Dodging,** the rapid deceleration and redirection of movement, requires new adjustments by the postural control systems. Balance is challenged through one-legged support and walking in **tandem,** toe-to-heel foot placement while walking in a straight line (Gallahue & Ozmun, 2002). By late childhood (10 to 12 years), the postural control goal is increased efficiency of movement while maintaining balance. Postural control and balance strategies are at the adult level by age 7 to 10.

An important factor to re-emphasize is the critical need for experiences that require development of mature patterns of movement. Encouragement, practice, and instruction are crucial for skill attainment at this stage of development. Inadequate opportunities for physical activity in the child can lead to weakness and ROM limitations affecting postural control strategy use. Care must be taken to engage in normal levels of activity rather than overemphasizing a particular area (e.g., strength training) in order to avoid damage to growth plates (Gallahue & Ozmun, 2002). Inactivity can limit experience with body motion and moving visual stimuli, impacting the development of systems integration vital for postural control during disturbances. Lack of exposure to movement in space limits the development of perceptual skills such as body image and body scheme, already mentioned as vital to maintaining postural control and balance.

Clinical Connection:

Remember those favored games of childhood: walking along a curb without falling, twisting the ropes holding the swing seat and then spinning in a circle until the ropes were straight again, or tumble sets done from the bedroom all the way into the kitchen on the way to breakfast? All these activities are opportunities to practice the skills needed to provide postural control and balance. ▪

Adolescence

During adolescence, mature stability and movement patterns are applied to particular sports or activities of daily living (ADL). Teenagers have often selected a particular sport they prefer and work to be better at it. Activity becomes a means of self-expression, and skills are refined to meet personal preferences. The desire for greater independence results in taking more responsibility for environmental maintenance. Activities of daily living are expanded as routines are established. The postural control systems that have been learned are adjusted for dimensional differences, advancing perceptual motor skills (refer to Chapter 9), and specialized movements (Gallahue & Ozmun, 2002). Teenagers are learning to adjust to physical changes in their bodies and emotional changes caused by the onset of puberty. It is during adolescence that the ideal adult posture develops (refer to Chapter 4) as children take on adult body proportions (see Fig. 8–1).

Adulthood

As was stated in Chapter 4, the healthy adult chooses the most appropriate postural pattern for the task-in-context interaction. Righting and equilibrium reactions are coordinated and smoothly performed. Generally, the adult experiences less formal participation in sport or physical activity. It is an oversimplification to state that decline is inevitable in middle age. Task performance becomes even more dependent on systems interaction. Task elements such as degree of difficulty, duration of activity, and need for speed or accuracy all influence successful participation by adults. The aging of different physiological systems occurs at a rate unique to each person. Disease and lifestyle combined with age can result in performance differences. An analysis of each postural control component is examined in the next section as many of these changes are in progress during adulthood (Gallahue & Ozmun, 2002).

Aging

Age-related changes are observed in our postural control system (Hageman, Leibowitz, & Blanke, 1995), although the information on the exact nature of these changes is controversial (Shumway-Cook & Woollacott, 2001). Beginning with the various definitions of "elderly," these studies seem to draw contradictory conclusions about the very nature of aging. Defining these changes has been the focus of recent research efforts because falls account for 32 percent of the deaths to adults age 85 years and older (McClenaghan, Williams, Dickerson, Dowda, Thombs, & Eleazer, 1996), and the risk of falling causes some older adults to become more sedentary, therefore limiting their sensory experiences and leading to decay of skilled responses to challenges (Poole, 1991). There seems to be no single cause for the increased falls experienced by the elderly, and current studies indicate several contributing factors are at work, including internal changes and environmental characteristics that result in the increased risk (Shumway-Cook & Woollacott, 2001). In this section, the focus will be on the internal changes to each of the postural control system components.

Several changes occur to the musculoskeletal system as we age. Muscle strength decreases 40 percent by the age of 80. Diminished ROM and loss of spinal flexibility, often occurring as a result of arthritis, further hinder recovery efforts. There is also a posterior shift in vertical alignment bringing the COM back over the heels (Shumway-Cook & Woollacott, 2001). Evidence supports a reduced control of muscles of the toes associated with postural instability (Tanaka, Hashimoto, Noriyasu, Ino, Ifukube, & Mizumoto, 1995). Additional studies demonstrate that aging affects lateral stability, causing decreased function in standing, walking, and climbing stairs (McClenaghan et al., 1996). Response time for motor performance increases despite no special increase in accuracy (Hageman et al., 1995). Finally, older adults seem to have lost to some degree the ability to combine movements needed for balance with those required for completion of an ongoing task (Shumway-Cook & Woollacott, 2001).

Study of the control and coordination of the muscles, a neuromuscular function, has been conducted during periods of quiet stance and during changes to the support surface. Muscle activation and use of recovery strategies are monitored. During quiet stance, postural sway is noted to increase as we age (Marsh & Geel, 2000). Sway seems most prevalent among those older adults with a history of falls and does not show significant increase in those with neurological impairment such as Parkinson's disease. When support surface changes are made, greater use of the hip strategy occurs in elderly persons, as well as co-activation of the agonist and antagonist around a joint to compensate for the noted change. It has been suggested that the greater use of the hip strategy results in more falls due to the sheer forces of the feet not getting resistance from the support surface, such as when walking on ice (Shumway-Cook & Woollacott, 2001).

With aging, sensitivity to tactile stimulation seems to diminish and there is a loss of vibration sensitivity (Poole, 1991). The loss of vibratory sense seems related to sway more than falls, whereas the loss of proprioception is more likely to contribute to falls. Vision undergoes many changes as we age. The loss of peripheral vision is of particular interest to the examination of balance because it is most sensitive to movement for postural adjustments (Poole, 1991). A loss of hair cells in the vestibular system reduces the input available. Dizziness or vertigo often accompanies vestibular dysfunction and compounds the problem of postural control and balance, especially in an environment of reduced visual or proprioceptive information (Shumway-Cook & Woollacott, 2001). The integration of these sources of sensory input may decline the most as we age. When descending stairs, a person uses tactile and kinesthetic information to get the "feel of the tread" and looks in order to accurately place the foot on the stair (Poole, 1991). As each system has diminished ability to give input when needed, the performance disintegrates and falls are more likely to occur.

As people age, their postural control ability may diminish in novel situations where attention to the environment or new demands take their attention from the task at hand but can function quite well in familiar settings in which the focus can be on the task (Shumway-Cook & Woollacott, 2001). Marsh and Geel (2000) studied the demands of postural control tasks paired with concurrent attention tasks in a dual-task paradigm. The data suggest the older adult may be at greater risk for falls when engaged in a concurrent task, even when that task is considered automatic (Marsh & Geel, 2000). Comparisons have been made between fallers and nonfallers, but few if any have explored the question not only of the impact of the fear of falling on balance assessments but also on actual performance (Shumway-Cook & Woollacott, 2001). At this point, little research evidence is available on the impact of cognitive functioning on postural control and balance, but it is an area that would benefit from further scientific inquiry.

Assessment of Postural Control and Balance

So far, this chapter has focused on describing normal development of skills permitting postural control and balance and their changes over the life span. However, those people seen by occupational and physical therapists are having difficulty in maintaining stability and/or safe mobility due to an abnormality (i.e., poor skill development, injury, or disease process) acting on one of the components of postural control and balance. The reasons for these disturbances are many, and they are further complicated by the use of compensatory behaviors. Because these movement and postural strategies work to keep an abnormal system upright, they can mask the true nature of the problem (Shumway-Cook & Woollacott, 2001) and lead to ineffective intervention.

Assessments that examine postural control and balance are grouped by type of approach. Currently, no single test covers the many aspects of postural control and balance. Most clinical assessments of postural control and balance rely on initial observations to arrive at some decision regarding the possible causal factor for imbalance. "Nudge or push tests" (Umphred, 2001) are used to evaluate a person's postural responses. This entails attempts to displace the person's COM by pushing in anterior-posterior and both lateral directions while that person is sitting or standing. This test provides a rough grading (e.g., good, fair, poor) of the person's balance ability. The limitations to this technique are that the ratings are subjective and the findings lack reliability (Umphred, 2001). The reader is cautioned to use more reliable measures to add validity to intervention plan development. Possible alternatives are presented in this section.

A thorough examination of postural control and balance would not be complete without gaining information on the patient's current symptoms and concerns, in addition to completing a medical and social history. Knowing what activities lead to the appearance of symptoms is important to the intervention planning process. Medical conditions and medications contribute to the risk of falls as much as environmental factors (e.g., poor lighting) and problems with balance or mobility (Whitney, Poole, & Cass, 1998). Use of more than one test is recommended because each category provides different but important information for intervention. Safety is of utmost concern regardless of the method chosen for testing. Although instability must be experienced for assessment to be constructive to intervention planning, the patient should be guarded against falling at all times. Refer to Table 8–1 for a comparison of the balance assessments mentioned here.

Functional Assessment

The purpose of functional tests is to provide clinically useful evaluations of balance during common activities (Light et al., 1996). Because most falls seem to occur when an individual is engaged in an everyday task (e.g., reaching into a high cupboard), there is a high correlation between balance and functional activity assessments (Merla & Spaulding, 1997). The limitations to functional assessment use are that they do not assess balance under changing conditions or contexts; they do not rate the quality of the movement used; and the underlying problem cannot be specifically assigned to a postural control mechanism because they measure disability, not impairment (Umphred, 2001).

Two common screening measures to assess functional balance are presented first. Using the Timed Get Up and Go Test, a patient is asked to stand up from a chair, walk 3 meters, turn around, and return to the chair while being timed (Podsiadlo & Richardson, 1991; Whitney et al., 1998). As practical as it is simple, the Timed Get Up and Go Test provides the examiner with a rudimentary picture of any functional balance problems experienced by the patient. Another screening measure, the **Functional Reach Test,** was developed to determine the risk of falls among elderly people (Umphred, 2001) (Fig. 8–6). It is believed that a more limited boundary of stability seen in elderly persons is a reflection of compensation for impaired postural control mechanisms (Duncan, Weiner, Chandler, & Studenski, 1990); this test intends to measure a proportional decline in limited reach. For this test, a patient is asked to stand near a wall, raise his or her arm to 90 degrees of shoulder flexion, and reach the fisted hand forward as far as possible along a measuring stick attached to the wall.

Functional reach is defined as the distance a person can reach forward beyond arm's length while keeping a fixed base of support in the standing position. It expands on the ideas behind one of the dynamic balance tests, called the center of pressure excursion (COPE), without requiring the expensive equipment required for that measure (Duncan et al., 1990). Whereas the COPE uses a force platform to measure the center of pressure as a subject leans forward, backward, and side to side, the Functional Reach screening test attempts to measure the margin of stability provided by a person's base of support as a more functional reflection of postural control.

TABLE 8–1

Comparison of Balance Assessment Tools

Test	Sample test items	Tools	Time required (approx.)
Timed Get Up and Go	Patient stands up from a chair, walks 3 meters, turns, walks back to the chair and sits down.	Chair Stopwatch 3-meter walkway	1–2 min
Functional Reach	Patient reaches forward (arm extended at 90 degrees shoulder flexion) along a yardstick placed at shoulder height.	Yardstick Wall space Method to attach yardstick to wall	1–2 min
Clinical Test of Sensory Interaction and Balance (CTSIB)	Patient stands on both feet with eyes open and closed. Conditions are changed by adding a dome to occlude vision and by having patient stand on foam with eyes open and closed.	Foam Dome–adapted	5–7 min
Tinetti Balance Test of the Performance-Oriented Assessment of Mobility Problems	Patient moves from sit to stand and from stand to sit, turns 360 degrees, turns the head, leans backward, stands on one foot, picks an item up from floor.	Chair Stopwatch 5-pound object 15-foot walkway	10 min
Berg Balance Scale	Patient moves from sit to stand and stand to sit, transfers from bed to chair, stands with eyes closed, stands with feet together, looks over shoulder, alternates placing each foot on a stool.	Chairs (2) or bed Stopwatch Ruler Stool	15 min

The limitation of screening measures is that they only provide information that the systems are not working normally and that a person is at greater risk for falling. More comprehensive tests include the examination of postural control and balance during movement and transitions between support surfaces. In this way, the falls risk is examined more closely and mobility skills are assessed; two such assessments are presented here. Tinetti's Balance and Mobility Scale provides a rating scale for 16 items related to balance (sitting, rising, and standing) and gait (Tinetti, 1986). Berg's Functional Balance Scale rates 14 items related to balance (sitting and standing supported and unsupported), transitions (standing to sitting, transfer to another surface), reach (forward and to pick an item off the floor), and gait (turning the head, turning the whole

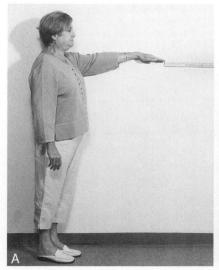
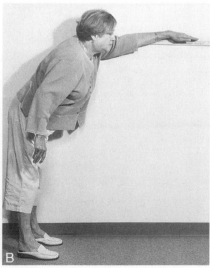

Figure 8–6. A person completing the Functional Reach Test. The figure depicts the start position (A) and a functional reach (B).

body) on a four-point scale (Shumway-Cook & Woollacott, 2001). Both provide a more functional picture of postural control and balance.

Systems Assessment

The purpose of systems assessment is to locate the mechanism or problem at the root of postural instability and imbalance and to identify the recovery strategy that is being used effectively by the patient. Dizziness is a common complaint of patients experiencing dysfunction (Horn, 1997). Dizziness, however, is a vague description requiring detective work to locate the cause. Because the intervention approach will differ based on the impaired mechanism, it is important to differentiate the cause. Once the mechanism is known, working with the patient to develop the use of a strategy might be an effective intervention technique leading to a decreased risk of falls to the patient. It is important to note that there does not need to be a disorder directly to one of the three main components of our postural control and balance system; musculoskeletal, neurological, cardiovascular, and even psychological illness may negatively impact a person's balance system (Merla & Spaulding, 1997).

The Romberg Test is a classic example of a systems assessment. It was originally designed to measure dorsal column (i.e., somatosensory) disorders (Umphred, 2001). The patient is asked to stand with feet parallel under eyes open and eyes closed conditions. The examiner judges the amount of sway; an excessive amount is considered to be a sign of abnormal somatosensory input. Immediate sway upon eye closure

would indicate visual dependency for balance. Because vestibular loss may result in difficulty using hip strategy required here, the precision of this test in isolating somatosensory dysfunction is in question (Umphred, 2001).

The Postural Stress Test is a quantifiable, reliable push test (Umphred, 2001). Weights in proportion to body weight pull the patient backward via a pulley attachment to a waist belt worn by the patient. The expected response is a forward adjustment to compensate for the backward displacement of the COM (Umphred, 2001). Following vestibular dysfunction, the body position in space is lost or impaired, and a patient may reach the posterior limit of stability before adjusting forward.

The modified Clinical Test for Sensory Interaction in Balance (CTSIB) is based on Nashner's concepts to assess sensory conditions of postural control (Fuller & Huber, 1995). The CTSIB establishes a base-line of performance in standing (Fig. 8–7A), then systematically eliminates vision (Fig. 8–7B), changes the support surface characteristics using medium density foam (Fig. 8–7C), and, finally, changes the accuracy of visual input (Fig. 8–7D) (Shumway-Cook & Horak, 1986; Herdman, 2000). Scoring gives an indication of whether a patient is dependent on visual, vestibular, or proprioceptive input or whether there is difficulty adapting sensory information for postural control (Cohen, Blatchly, & Gombash, 1993). Lacking research evidence on the dynamics of standing on foam, the accuracy of the interpretation based on these con-ditions is limited because the foam changes the dynamics of force production related to postural adjustments (Shumway-Cook & Woollacott, 2001).

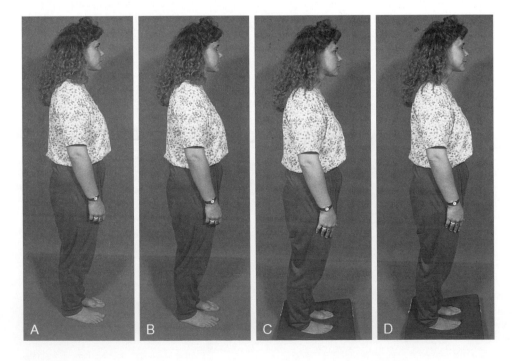

Figure 8–7. The four parameters of the modified Clinical Test of Sensory Integration of Balance. See text for explanation. (From Herdman, S. [2000]. *Vestibular rehabilitation* [2nd ed., p. 349]. Philadelphia: F. A. Davis.)

The Sensory Organization Test (SOT) uses a computerized force plate and the same conditions as the CTSIB. Body sway is measured when vision, vestibular, and somatosensory input are available and used as a reference to compare when each sensory system is absent or inaccurate. The advantage of the SOT is valid and reliable information; the disadvantages are the need for specialized equipment and that the scores have not been correlated to functional abilities (Fuller & Huber, 1995).

The visual system is assessed using oculomotor tests of **motility** (eye movement), **saccades** (precise eye movements from target to target within the visual field), and **pursuits** (smooth eye movements following a target as it moves throughout the visual field). Normal execution of these tests indicates the ability of the eyes to orient the head during movement (Umphred, 2001). Visual-vestibular interaction is examined using the **vestibular-ocular-reflex (VOR)** test. The patient is asked to focus on a target while moving the head in a horizontal (e.g., left to right), vertical (e.g., up and down), and diagonal (e.g., upper left to lower right) plane (Umphred, 2001). The interaction is normal if the patient is able to keep the gaze steady while moving. Eye movement control can help differentiate central and peripheral vestibular dysfunction as well, because the pathways are together in the medial longitudinal fasciculus (Horn, 1997). **Nystagmus,** an involuntary, rhythmic oscillation of the eye generally more to one side than the other, is an eye movement that assists in this differentiation. Complaints of vertigo usually accompany nystagmus. Nystagmus caused by peripheral vestibular disorder can be inhibited with visual fixation, whereas the type caused by central vestibular disorder cannot.

Stimulating the semicircular canals can make further differentiation of a vestibular lesion. One technique used to do this is the Hallpike-Dix maneuvers (Fig. 8–8). Although also used as an intervention technique for benign paroxysmal positional vertigo (Horak & Shupert, 1994), this maneuver puts the patient in a vertigo-stimulating position. For example, moving rapidly from sitting to supine with the head tilted so the affected ear is 35 to 40 degrees below the horizontal will stimulate the posterior canal. The response of vertigo should be brief but if it persists can be an indication of central vestibular disorder.

Intervention for Postural Control and Balance Problems

Resolving or preventing impairments, developing effective strategies and adapting them to be performed in different contexts, and retraining function are the goals of a task-oriented intervention approach. These goals are developed more specifically in this section.

Impairment Level

Intervention can begin to correct those impairments that can be changed and to prevent the development of secondary ones (Shumway-Cook & Woollacott, 2001). Musculoskeletal problems such as limited ROM, weakness, and limited flexibility can be addressed using traditional intervention techniques of exercise, strengthening regimen, or modalities (O'Sullivan & Schmitz, 1999). Studies have indicated the importance of not only addressing motor performance but also facilitating sensory input—that is, joint position sense or tactile sensitivity—for improving balance deficits (Tanaka et al., 1995).

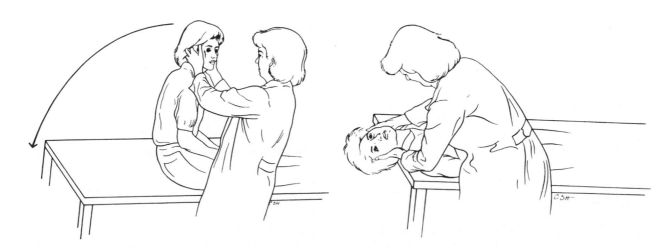

Figure 8–8. A person being positioned in all Hallpike-Dix maneuvers. See text for explanation. (Reprinted from Herdman, S. J. [1990]. Treatment of benign positional vertigo. *Physical Therapy*, 70, 381–388.)

Neuromuscular disorders often affect motor control, which in turn disrupts normal muscle recruitment in preparing or adjusting to postural challenge (O'Sullivan & Schmitz, 1999). **Neuromuscular facilitation techniques** are traditional approaches used to reduce the effects of impairments and improve function through motor recovery. Involved segments of the body are targeted to prevent learned disuse and overcompensation by intact segments. Sensory stimulation is a component of neurofacilitation techniques used to elicit movements before the presence of a stretch reflex. Exercise techniques are then added to decrease muscle tone, promote ROM, and facilitate active movement (O'Sullivan & Schmitz, 1999).

Sensory impairments can be addressed through sensory re-education techniques. The goal of these programs is to improve detection and processing of sensory information (Trombly, 1995). Habituation exercises, familiar to sensory integration (SI) therapists, are intended to promote physiologic fatigue and reduce motion-induced symptoms primarily aimed at the vestibular and tactile-kinesthetic systems (Herdman, 1994). Sensory integration uses vestibular stimulation to influence balance, postural adjustment, and movements against gravity. Gaze stabilization exercises are practiced to retrain oculomotor control during head movements (Cooke, 1996). Adaptation of the VOR to specific stimuli is the rationale for these exercises; vestibular adaptation is context specific, and learning within one sensory context may not work within another (Fuller & Huber, 1996).

Vestibular rehabilitation is an approach to the intervention of vestibular perception, specifically to dizziness or vertigo. The strategies are planned to be specific to the underlying cause of the dizziness due to the context specific nature of learned strategies (Herdman, 1994; Cronin, in press).

In the presence of cognitive impairments, adaptations can be made to the intervention program to reduce confusion, improve attention, and encourage participation through reinforcement consistency. It is important to note that focusing attention on the task has been shown to improve the motor performance of patients with Parkinson's disease. The mechanism at work seems to be that the increased cortical control of otherwise automatic movements overrides the basal ganglia circuitry affected by Parkinson's disease (Smithson, Morris, & Iansek, 1998).

Strategy Level

The purpose of intervention at the strategy level is to provide a means for patients/clients to recover or develop effective sensory and motor strategies to meet the demands of a functional activity (Shumway-Cook &

Woollacott, 2001). Development of appropriate sensory strategies requires that the person learn to select information for postural control during situations of sensory conflict (O'Sullivan & Schmitz, 1999). This requires analyzing the task at hand thoroughly and practicing in real-life situations. If a person is relying on visual information, use of diminished lighting or adaptations to reduce peripheral vision or visual acuity during rehabilitation activities teaches the use of other systems to determine postural control. Reliance on somatosensory input can be reduced through the use of tilt boards, thick carpet, and foam, which change the input received from the proprioceptors whether sitting or standing. The use of vestibular input is encouraged when both vision and somatosensory changes are made while asking for successful task completion (Shumway-Cook & Woollacott, 2001).

Scanning and gaze stabilization can be enhanced by activity also. Scanning the walls for posters while being pushed in a wheelchair is one technique. Having a patient read a letter or word target on the wall during an activity builds gaze stabilization. Use of obstacle courses when retraining balanced mobility increases scanning skills in a practical way.

Motor strategies are retaught through repetition and grading of environmental demands. When a COM that is shifted posteriorly causes imbalance or falls, alignment exercises might be in order. A common exercise is to have the patient match a tapeline on the shirt to a vertical line drawn on a mirror (Shumway-Cook & Woollacott, 2001). Incorporating neurodevelopmental handling techniques during the functional performance enhances the relearning of normal postural adjustment strategies better than with artificially imposed balance challenges (Merla & Spaulding, 1997). Alignment exercises also teach the patient to maximize stability by centering the COM over the base of support in a position of efficiency for the task at hand (see Chapter 6).

Once postural stability is achieved, strategies for balance during movement are added. Specific activities can address the ankle, hip, and stepping strategy; for example, having a patient balance with the toes on the edge of a telephone book while reaching develops the ankle strategy. Hip strategy can be developed by asking the patient to reach beyond his or her range for items while keeping the feet planted in the same spot. Basically, the strategies taught focus on keeping the COM within the base of support when that base is stationary and changing the base of support when the COM must move beyond it (Shumway-Cook & Woollacott, 2001). This requires coordinated, multijointed motion to be successful with the task within the range of stability.

During balance training activities, the therapist must alternate relatively easy tasks with more difficult activities to vary the balance challenge. Activities intended to address strategy level naturally incorporate components of the impairment. The focus is not on correcting the impairment; rather the focus is on giving the patient/client the feeling of successful postural stability and reducing falls. Patients are asked to become consciously aware of their actions and use movements or sensory strategies that limit the experience of postural insecurity or imbalance felt. A critical component is the application of learning theory and meta-cognitive processing to problem solve the task at hand (Abreu, 1992). Successful carryover of strategy use depends on successful experiences and enough practice and active attention to remember the method used and repeat it quickly and accurately (see Chapter 5).

Functional Task Level

Using real-life activities and environments, an ideal opportunity exists to immediately address the problem performance in the situation in which it is likely to occur (Merla & Spaulding, 1997). Because postural adjustments appear to be task specific, use of real-life activities ensures transfer of training to the natural situation where they will be needed (Poole, 1991). The goal is to expose the patient to successful performance of a variety of functional tasks in a variety of contexts (Shumway-Cook & Woollacott, 2001). To experience success, the intervention begins with simple instructions and activities with minimal processing demands. A multisensory approach is taken with each task. As improvement is seen, predictability of the conditions must be changed. Task performance is requested when the patient expects a challenge and when the patient does not. The patient must assume the task of self-monitoring to know when a response (strategy use) has been successful without relying on outside feedback. Combining changes to the environment, the postural support, and the position of the body during task completion increases the performance level required from the patient. The desired outcome is that the patient/client selects the appropriate strategy and performs it without cues in a variety of natural environments (Abreu, 1992).

Case Studies

The following case studies are presented to examine intervention with a neurologically impaired child and adult. Each disorder is characterized by neuromuscular, sensory, perceptual, and cognitive impairments and is used to illustrate the postural control and balance problems discussed in this chapter. Intervention ideas will focus on approaches to use for management of postural control and balance training.

Case Study: Child

Katarina: 13-year-old Girl Struck by a Car

History

Katarina is a 13-year-old girl who was struck by a car while riding her bicycle. She and her family (mother, father, and 8-year-old sister) were vacationing in Maine at the time of the accident. Originally from Ecuador, the family now lives in New England, where Katarina's father is a researcher at a university hospital. Katarina was in coma for 2 weeks and remained hospitalized for 1 month following the accident. She has now been transferred to an inpatient rehabilitation facility for therapy.

Evaluation

Katarina is medically stable. She opens her eyes when her name is called and seems to recognize her family, as demonstrated by increased movement of all extremities, and attempts to speak when she looks at them. Orientation to place or time cannot be tested at this time due to her limited verbal skills. Katarina is beginning to localize her responses and can follow simple commands such as "Lift your arm" and "Hold your head up." These efforts are brief due to fatigue. Katarina also demonstrates impaired motor control due to the imbalance of muscle tone (more flexor tone is noted on her right side) and muscle weakness (noted on the nondominant left side of her body). Upper extremity movements lack coordination, and asymmetrical body alignment is noted. When moved into a sitting position, Katarina's trunk is positioned in kyphosis with a loss of lordosis due to spastic abdominal, spinal, and paraspinal muscles; her lower extremities assume an extended position with a posterior pelvic tilt. She is having difficulty with head and trunk control and gets nauseous when sitting upright for more than 5 minutes. This nausea is considered to be post-traumatic benign paroxysmal positional vertigo (BPPV). Deep tendon reflexes are normal in all extremities. Thorough sensory, perceptual, and cognitive skills evaluations await recovery beyond the generalized response stage.

Intervention

The long-term intervention goals established at Katarina's current stage of recovery were to increase responsiveness to specific stimuli; to develop more normal movements of the head, trunk, and extremities; to improve postural control for tolerance of upright

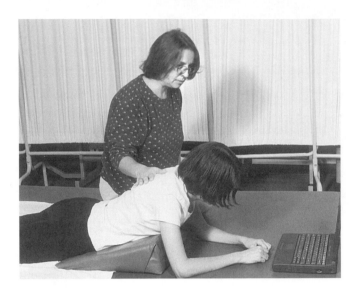

Figure 8–9. Katarina (model) positioned prone on elbows with upper body support while watching a video.

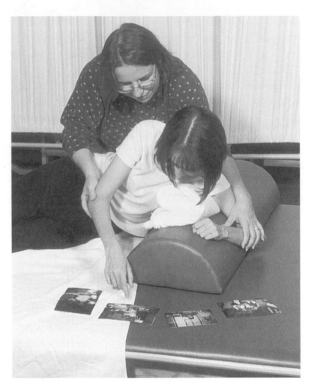

Figure 8–10. Katarina side lying with wedge cushion under upper body and knees flexed, reaching toward family pictures.

positions; and to initiate training in basic ADLs (Reed, 2001).

Short-term goals include the following:

1. Through increased upper extremity and trunk strength, Katarina will sit symmetrically using upper extremity support as needed for completion of grooming activities.
2. Through decreased positional vertigo, Katarina will sit out of bed for 20 minutes.
3. Through increased balance, Katarina will complete upper body bathing and dressing with moderate assistance.

Activities to address each goal include the following:

1. a. Position Katarina in prone on elbows on a mat. Provide bolster support of her upper body, being sure that she is putting weight through her upper extremities. This will increase strength and proximal stability. Katarina could watch a video to help her tolerate the position (Fig. 8–9).
   b. Position Katarina in side lying on her left. Provide upper body support using a wedge bolster, and use knee flexion to facilitate extensor tone reduction. Place pictures of her family in an array in front of Katarina and ask her to touch the correct picture when you say something about that person, such as "Who is your sister?" (Fig. 8–10).
   c. To address lower extremity strength, work with Katarina to move from supine or side lying to sit. Neuromuscular techniques are used to enhance the learning of normal postural adjustments during transitional movements. Using

key points to guide her movements, begin with upper trunk on lower trunk rotation to move into side lying from supine (Fig. 8–11A). Hip and knee flexion follow as the lower extremities are lowered off the side of the bed or mat (Fig. 8–11B & C). When Katarina is able to tolerate vertical positions, further strengthening could be accomplished with sit-to-stand transitions.

   d. While seated on a bolster, Katarina will be supported posteriorly by the therapist. She will be asked to reach out and push a switch to activate a radio playing her favorite music tape (Fig. 8–12). The switch device should be alternated to her left and right sides and handling techniques applied to ensure weight shift from side to side.
   e. Using a flashlight attached to her waist, Katarina can work on trunk alignment in supported standing. Using cutouts in a box frame, Katarina is asked to shine the light through the hole in the box to make shadow pictures on the wall (Fig. 8–13). The box is positioned such that Katarina needs to align her trunk to produce the pictures.
2. As Katarina is able to tolerate, five sets of Hallpike-Dix exercises will be performed twice daily to habituate Katarina's vestibular system to her new experience of upright positioning (see Fig. 8–8).

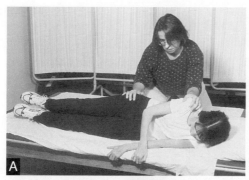

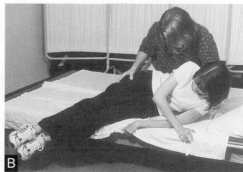

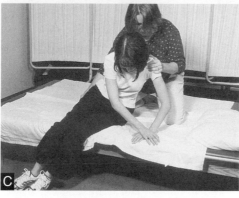

Figure 8–11. Katarina moving from supine (A) to side lying (B), showing upper on lower trunk rotation. Therapist uses key points of control to assist completion of transition to sitting (C).

3. a. Have Katarina long sit on a mat. She will be asked to shift her weight from side to side but keep her trunk upright (Fig. 8–14). The therapist can provide encouragement for greater excursions using key points.

   b. While sitting on a therapy ball, Katarina's balance will be disturbed by a gentle roll side to side and front to back. She will be cued to move in the opposite direction to correct her upright posture (Fig. 8–15). She will also be verbally guided to recognize the disturbance to her posture until automatic adjustments are noted in her reactions.

   c. In standing, Katarina will be asked to play balloon volleyball requiring moderate excursions from her base of support while retaining her balance (Fig. 8–16). Use of the various motor strategies should be noted and encouraged.

This case illustrates the clinical approach to postural control and balance impairments. The interventions

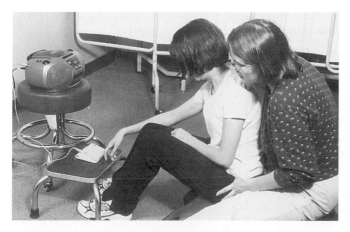

Figure 8–12. Katarina sitting on oblong bolster with therapist sitting behind using the hips as the key point to shift her weight, allowing reach for the modified control switch on the radio.

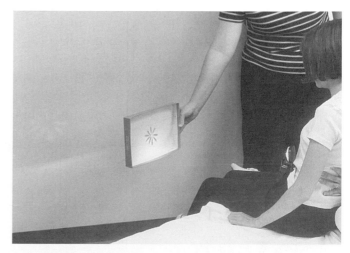

Figure 8–13. Katarina in supported sitting uses a cutout box to make shadow pictures on the wall.

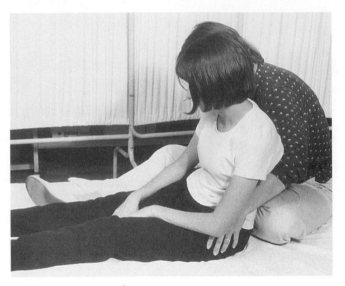

Figure 8–14. A therapist works with Katarina, who is positioned in long sit, leaning her from side to side to elicit righting reactions.

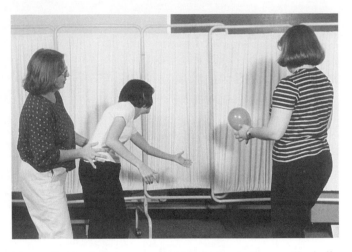

Figure 8–16. Katarina engaged in playing balloon volleyball.

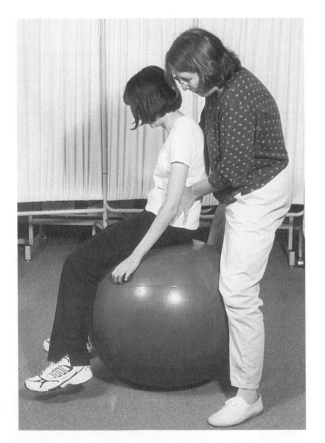

Figure 8–15. Katarina on a therapy ball being rolled from side to side by the therapist to correct posture.

described are directed at improving head, trunk, and extremity movement control to build functional skills. The impact of the components of the postural control system (i.e., musculoskeletal, neuromuscular, sensory, perceptual, and cognitive) on recovery was provided. Some attention has been given to illustrating the techniques used for management of benign paroxysmal positional vertigo; the reader is cautioned to seek proper training before administration of these specialized techniques.

Case Study: Adult

Robert: 55-year-old Man with Parkinson's Disease

History

Robert is a 55-year-old man diagnosed with Parkinson's disease 4 years ago. Medical history is significant for hypertension (controlled with medication) and cataracts (for which he received surgery several years ago). Bob and his wife, Dorothea, moved into an adult condominium community after his retirement from the postal service 2 years ago; neither of his adult children lives in the area. After his diagnosis, modifications were made to the home to allow first-floor living and included a wheelchair-accessible bathroom. Bob used the equipment provided during the renovation (e.g., a pole in the shower area and grab bars around the toilet) for self-care, requiring only minimal assistance for lower extremity dressing despite a significantly increased completion time. No exterior maintenance is required in the community; Bob assists his wife with meal preparation, grocery shopping, and cleaning. Bob's hobbies include growing tomatoes and bird watching. Due to a recent exacerbation of his Parkinson's symptoms, Bob has lost some mobility skills and is concerned about his wife's ability to provide care for him as his condition deteriorates. Discharge to home is planned after rehabilitation.

Evaluation

Robert is alert; oriented to person, place, and time; and displays a dry sense of humor despite the lack of facial expression familiar to Parkinson's disease. He appears realistic about the progressive nature of Parkinson's disease and expresses concern about his physical management over time, as his wife is not in good health.

Robert presents with limited AROM and flexibility, especially in trunk rotation and shoulder flexion greater than 90 degrees. Anterior pelvic tilt is limited, also resulting in kyphotic posture. The limited ROM also causes him to use very short steps when walking and to move without apparent upper or lower trunk rotation. His body alignment is pitched forward when standing, increasing his risk of falling forward.

Sensory testing indicates generally intact performance in all extremities. Corrected vision and hearing appear within normal limits. The presence of rigid tone affects Bob's postural control, and his reduced reaction time limits effectiveness of control strategies. Sitting is stable although moving from sitting to standing is complicated by the diminished pelvic tilt mentioned previously. As Robert rises to stand, his COM is held posterior to his support base. With limitations in hip flexion, the movement requires moderate assistance. Once standing, Robert uses a roller walker with standby assistance, especially when managing doorways, crossing thresholds, and on carpeted floors. Robert no longer uses stairs because he has moved his bedroom to the first floor.

Bradykinesia and tremor limit Bob's ability to make movements necessary for balance. Impaired initiation of movement results in slowed onset of automatic reactions and accompaniments in response to instability.

Robert is in good spirits but occasionally appears depressed when faced with struggles in therapy. He is in the hospital as the doctor re-evaluates his medication levels and requested therapy to address transfers on and off various seat surfaces and to improve balance recovery.

Intervention

The long-term intervention goals established with Bob are to increase initiation and quality of movement, increase mobility and prevent deformities; and increase or maintain independent performance of basic and instrumental ADLs.

Short-term goals include:

1. Through increased ROM and flexibility of the trunk, pelvis, and upper extremities, Robert will retrieve toiletries placed laterally and slightly posterior during shower activity.
2. Through increased upper on lower trunk rotation, Robert will complete rolling side to side independently and sit to stand with standby assistance and equipment as needed.
3. Robert will transfer from sitting to standing with minimal assistance through increased initiation and speed of movements.
4. Robert will have no loss of balance during standing and walking through increased body alignment and timely use of motor strategies for postural stability.

Activities to address each goal include the following:

1. Use therapeutic exercise used for increased ROM and flexibility utilizing proprioceptive neuromuscular facilitation (PNF) diagonals (see Figs. 6–1 and 6–2). Incorporate functional activities while Robert is in standing or sitting requiring rotational movements at all involved joints (Fig. 8–17A and B). Placing a firm wedge behind Bob's back while sitting will reorganize the COM; the hip proprioceptors alert the muscles to flex forward (Fig. 8–18). Eventually, the wedge can be removed as the internal representation of the COM has shifted.
2. While Bob is in side-lying position on the therapy mat, engage him in a game of checkers. Position the board closer to the floor, which will cause Bob to turn his upper trunk to reach the game pieces (Fig. 8–19).
3. Practice vertical alignment using a mirror and a beanbag toss game. Mark Bob's shirt with a vertical tape strip and place one on the mirror also. Bob will need to lean forward and to the side to pick up a beanbag and then realign his posture using the tape guides before he can toss the bag at the target. Using a metronome timer to gauge his toss will address the slowed reaction time (Fig. 8–20).

This case study was used to illustrate the neuromuscular impairments of rigidity, muscular activation, and timing characteristic of Parkinson's disease. The key goals focusing on initiation and quality of movement coupled with exercises to increase or maintain ROM are incorporated into intervention activities. The focus was on techniques to improve postural control and balance applied to everyday activities.

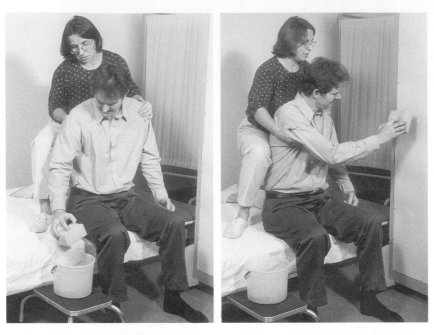

Figure 8–17. Robert (model) using PNF movement patterns during functional activities.

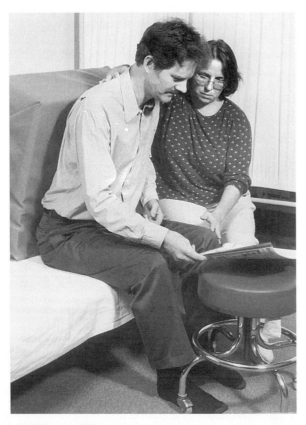

Figure 8–18. Robert profiled while in a sitting position showing a wedge cushion used to shift COM forward.

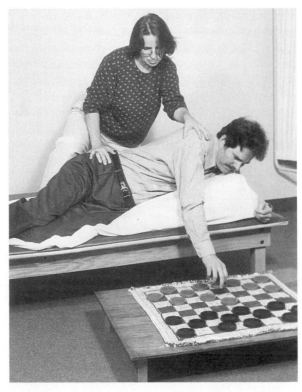

Figure 8–19. Robert positioned in side-lying position and playing checkers.

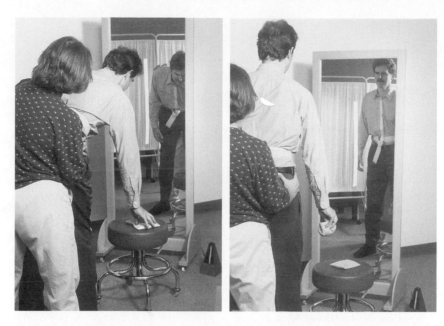

Figure 8–20. Robert with tape in a midsagittal plane on trunk facing a mirror, engaged in a beanbag toss activity with metronome for timing of movements.

Summary

This chapter has explained the management of postural control impairments and imbalance by identifying the components required for these skills and addressing the intervention approaches that are successful. The development of postural control skills was described in terms of the reflex-hierarchical and systems models. The importance of righting and orienting reactions was noted. The development of postural control was described in terms of developmental stages or milestones that represented integration of the many components into a functioning system. Detailed descriptions of those components were provided and their contributions to the task of balance during stable and mobile positions explained. Age-related differences in the availability of postural control mechanisms and components were also outlined. The changes experienced as the body ages were detailed, and implications to the prevention of falls by the elderly were discussed as this is the focus of many studies of balance. Strategies and intervention techniques were provided and applied through case study presentations. The following chapters add dimension to postural control and balance as they explain the development, control, and integration of upper and lower extremity mobility.

References

Abreu, B. (1992). The quadraphonic approach: Management of cognitive-perceptual and postural control dysfunction. *Occupational Therapy Practice, 3,* 12–29.

Adams. (2000). Neurology in primary care. Philadelphia: F. A. Davis.

Allum, J., Bloem, B., Carpenter, M., Hulliger, M., & Hadders-Algra, M. (1998). Proprioceptive control of posture: A review of new concepts. *Gait and Posture, 8,* 214–242.

Basmajian, J., & Wolf, S. (Eds.). (1990). *Therapeutic exercise* (5th ed.). Baltimore: Williams & Wilkins.

Cohen, H. (1999). *Neuroscience for rehabilitation* (2nd ed.). Philadelphia: Lippincott Williams & Wilkins.

Cohen, H., Blatchly, C., & Gombash, L. (1993). A study of the clinical test of sensory interaction and balance. *Physical Therapy, 73,* 346–354.

Cooke, D. (1996). Central vestibular disorders. *Neurology Report, 20,* 22–29.

Cronin. (in press). *Vestibular rehabilitation for the treatment of vertigo and imbalance: A rehabilitation handbook.* Aspen Publishers.

De Benabib, R., & Nelson, C. (1991). Efficiency in visual skills and postural control: A dynamic interaction. *Occupational Therapy Practice, 3,* 57–68.

Duncan, P., Weiner, D., Chandler, J., & Studenski, S. (1990). Functional reach: A new clinical measure of balance. *Journal of Gerontology: Medical Sciences, 45,* 192–197.

Epstein, W., & Rogers, S. (Eds.). (1995). *Perception of space and motion.* San Diego, CA: Academic Press.

Frank, J., & Earl, M. (1990). Coordination of posture and movement. *Physical Therapy, 70,* 109–117.

Fuller, K., & Huber, L. (1996). Improving postural control through integration of sensory inputs and visual biofeedback. *Topics in Stroke Rehabilitation, 1,* 32–47.

Gallahue, D., & Ozmun, J. (2002). *Understanding motor development: Infants, children, adolescents, adults.* Boston: McGraw-Hill.

Gesell, A. (1946). The ontogenesis of infant behavior. In L. Carmichael (Ed.), *Manual of child psychology.* New York: Wiley.

Gibson, J. (1966). *The senses considered as perceptual systems.* Boston: Houghton Mifflin.

Hageman, P., Leibowitz, M., & Blanke, D. (1995). Age and gender effects on postural control measures. *Archives of Physical Medicine Rehabilitation, 75,* 961–965.

Herdman, S. (1994). *Vestibular rehabilitation.* Philadelphia: F. A. Davis.

Herdman, S. (2000). *Vestibular rehabilitation* (2nd ed.). Philadelphia: F. A. Davis.

Hines, C., & Mercer, V. (1997). Anticipatory postural adjustments: An update. *Neurology Report 21,* 17–22.

Horak, F. (1987). Clinical measurement of postural control in adults. *Physical Therapy, 67,* 1881–1885.

Horak, F., & Nashner, M. (1986). Central programming of postural movements: Adaptation to altered support-surface configurations. *Journal of Neurophysiology, 55,* 1369–1381.

Horak, F., & Shupert, C. (1994). Role of the vestibular system in postural control. In F. Horak, C. Shupert, V. Dietz, & G. Horstmann (1994). Vestibular and somatosensory contributions to responses to head and body displacements in stance. *Experimental Brain Research, 100,* 93–106.

Horn, L. (1997). Differentiating between vestibular and nonvestibular balance disorders. *Neurology Report, 21,* 23–27.

Kisner, C., & Colby, L. (2002). *Therapeutic exercise: Foundations and techniques* (4th ed.). Philadelphia: F. A. Davis.

Lee, W. (1989). A control systems framework for understanding normal and abnormal posture. *American Journal of Occupational Therapy, 43,* 291–301.

Light, K., Rose, D., & Purser, J. (1996). The functional reach test for balance: Strategies of elderly subjects with and without disequilibrium. *Physical & Occupational Therapy in Geriatrics, 14,* 39–52.

Littell, E. (1990). *Basic neuroscience for the health professions.* Thorofare, NJ: Slack.

Lundy-Ekman, L. (2002). *Neuroscience: Fundamentals for rehabilitation* (2nd ed.). Philadelphia: W. B. Saunders.

Marsh, A., & Geel, S. (2000). The effect of age on the attentional demands of postural control. *Gait and Posture, 12,* 105–113.

Mathiowetz, V., & Haugen, J. (1994). Motor behavior research: Implications for therapeutic approaches to central nervous system dysfunction. *American Journal of Occupational Therapy, 48,* 733–745.

McClenaghan, B., Williams, H., Dickerson, J., Dowda, M., Thombs, L., & Eleazer, P. (1996). Spectral characteristics of aging postural control. *Gait and Posture, 4,* 112–121.

Merla, J., & Spaulding, S. (1997). The balance system: Implications for occupational therapy intervention. *Physical & Occupational Therapy in Geriatrics, 15,* 21–36.

Montgomery, P., & Connolly, B. (1991). *Motor control and physical therapy: Theoretical framework and practical applications.* Hixson, TX: Chattanooga Group.

O'Sullivan, S., & Schmitz, T. (1999). *Physical rehabilitation laboratory manual: Focus on functional training.* Philadelphia: F. A. Davis.

Podsiadlo, D., & Richardson, S. (1991). The Timed "Up & Go": A test of basic functional mobility for frail elderly persons. *American Geriatric Society, 39,* 142–148.

Poole, J. (1991). Age related changes in sensory system dynamics related to balance. *Physical & Occupational Therapy in Geriatrics, 10,* 55–66.

Reed, K. (2001). *Quick reference to occupational therapy* (2nd ed.). Gaithersburg, MD: Aspen Publishers.

Shumway-Cook, A., & McCollum, G. (1991). In P. Montgomery & B. Connelly (Eds.), *Motor control and physical therapy: Theoretical framework and practical applications.* Hixson, TN: Chattanooga Group.

Shumway-Cook, A., & Woollacott, M. (1985). The growth of stability: Postural control from a developmental perspective. *Journal of Motor Behavior, 17,* 131–147.

Shumway-Cook, A., & Woollacott, M. (2001). *Motor control: Theory and practical application* (2nd ed.). Baltimore: Lippincott Williams & Wilkins.

Siev, E., Freishtat, B., & Zoltan, B. (1986). *Perceptual and cognitive dysfunction in the adult stroke patient: A manual for evaluation and treatment.* Thorofare, NJ: Slack.

Smithson, F., Morris, M., & Iansek, R. (1998). Performance on clinical tests of balance in Parkinson's disease. *Physical Therapy, 78,* 577–592.

Tanaka, T., Hashimoto, N., Noriyasu, S., Ino, S., Ifukube, T., & Mizumoto, Z. (1995). *Physical & Occupational Therapy in Geriatrics, 13,* 1–17.

Tinetti, M. (1986). Performance oriented assessment of mobility problems in elderly patients. *Journal of the American Geriatric Society, 34,* 119–126.

Trombly, C. (Ed.). (1995). *Occupational therapy for physical dysfunction* (4th ed.). Baltimore: Williams & Wilkins.

Umphred, D. (2001). *Neurological rehabilitation* (4th ed.). St. Louis, MO: Mosby.

Wade, M., & Jones, G. (1997). The role of vision and spatial orientation in the maintenance of posture. *Physical Therapy, 77,* 619–627.

Warren, M. (1999). *Occupational therapy practice guidelines: Adults with low vision.* Bethesda, MD: American Occupational Therapy Association.

Whitney, S., Poole, J., & Cass, S. (1998). A review of balance instruments for older adults. *American Journal of Occupational Therapy, 52,* 666–671.

Management of the Impaired Upper Extremity

9

Doré Blanchet, MS, OTR/L

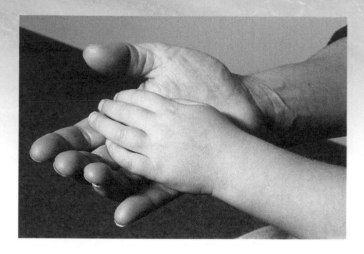

Man by the use of his hands, as they are energized by mind and will, can influence the state of his own health (Riley, 1962).

Introduction

Having read about the basic structure and theory behind movement and function, the reader's clinical eye can now turn to a study of the upper extremity. It is difficult to list many functional activities that do not require upper extremity use. From self-care to vocation to play and leisure, the upper extremity plays an integral role in an individual's successful ability to interact within the environment. Development of skillful use of the upper extremity relies on the coordinated efforts of a multitude of different systems and the ability of these systems to adapt to changes within the environment.

This chapter will examine the functional components of upper extremity (UE) use and the systems that support them. This description of components will be followed by an exploration of the developmental tasks of the upper extremity as they change throughout the life span. Common neurological problems and their effect on UE function will be explored. A discussion of useful intervention strategies enhancing upper extremity function and control will follow. The chapter will conclude with pediatric and adult case studies, illustrating some of the key management concepts discussed in this chapter.

Cornerstone Concepts

- Functional tasks of the upper extremity
  - Regard
  - Reach
  - Grasp and manipulation
  - Release

- Upper extremity function across the life span

- Neuromuscular impairments resulting in impaired upper extremity function
  - Weakness
  - Abnormal muscle tone
  - Incoordination

- Upper extremity problems associated with common neurological disorders: clinical management

Functional Components of Upper Extremity Function

The complex task of upper extremity control is accomplished through the coordination of postural control, vision and visual perception, somatosensory function, cognition/volition, and fine motor skills. Each of these components will be discussed separately, but remember that successful use of the upper extremity is made possible through the coordinated efforts of these many systems.

In Chapter 8, the functional implications of postural control were discussed. During fine motor activities, postural control through the trunk and shoulder girdle allow for distal mobility. This proximal stability afforded from the trunk provides a stable base from which distal movements can occur. Refer to Chapter 8 for more detail on postural control and stability, which serve as prerequisite skills for many upper extremity movements.

Clinical Connection:

Imagine sitting on a high stool with your feet unable to touch the floor and your desktop at chest height. Now you have to take notes for your anatomy class. Fortunately, no one in college is grading your penmanship. In grade school, however, poor handwriting is of concern to many teachers and may lead to a referral for therapy. Proper seating for children during writing activities is extremely important to provide stability and allow optimal distal mobility to accomplish writing activities. For optimal functional performance, children should sit with their feet flat on the floor, hips and knees flexed to 90 degrees, trunk supported, and the desk height 2 inches above a flexed elbow (Benbow, 1990). In this position, the feet and trunk provide the stability needed for good penmanship. The forearm resting on the writing surface at the proper angle also provides stability through the shoulder girdle, elbow, and wrist. Proper positioning during writing activities is often the first area to be addressed by the therapist. ▪

The central nervous system's control of upper extremity movement is a combination of motor function, sensory feedback, integration of this sensory information, and the ability to sequence and plan movement (Pehoski, 1995). Different areas of cortical control are used for these important functions. The control of the arm and the hand are represented separately in the central nervous system with the "primary purpose of the arm to place the hand in a position of function…and

the purpose of the hand to act on the environment" (Pehoski, 1995, p. 13).

The somatosensory system, along with the vestibular system, provides the foundation for postural control, as well as for reach and grasp. Proprioceptive input, received through joint receptors, Golgi tendon organs, and muscle spindles, transmits the information that tells the movement system how to position the extremity in space by activating certain muscles (Fig. 2–10). "The major sense working alongside vision is proprioception, providing information about movements and position of the body and its parts" (Sugden, 1990, p. 133). An example of proprioceptive input and vision working together can be observed in catching a ball, whereby vision provides the information concerning the object, speed, and trajectory while the proprioceptive system provides the information needed to position the upper extremity to catch the ball (Sugden, 1990).

The tactile system, another important component of the somatosensory system, provides additional input about the environment. Somatosensory information through the tactile and proprioceptive systems is vital for developing skilled movements of the hand (Pehoski, 1995). Initially this is a survival system in the infant, in whom tactile stimuli stimulate motor responses. An example of this is seen in the rooting reflex, in which tactile input to the cheek causes head turning and mouth opening for feeding. Early in development, however, the tactile and proprioceptive information gained through exploration by the hand and mouth help to provide the basis for skilled movement of the hand and refined **in-hand manipulation skills.** Tactile information is important for discrete finger movements and varying grip force, whereas proprioceptive feedback relays information important for handling objects of varying weight (Eliasson, 1995).

Vision, as stated in Chapter 8, is a powerful sensory system influencing the control of movement. When input from the environment is unclear, the information from the visual system will override other systems. Vision gives information about the environment in which an individual is attempting to place his or her hand to reach, grasp, and manipulate. **Visual perception** is the ability to make meaning of what one is seeing. Visual perception contributes to the ability to anticipate movement, also known as **feed-forward input,** by giving the individual information based on past experiences, on which he or she can anticipate movement. As has been described throughout this text, the context of the environment and the individual's ability to adapt are important for successful interactions. The ability to perceive how much pressure is needed to lift a Styrofoam versus a ceramic coffee cup is an example of the functional value of visual perception.

This skill incorporates the ability to recognize, discriminate, and recall previous experiences (Levine, 1991). Tactile and proprioceptive feedback also play a role in this example, as they provide information based on past experience related to shape and weight and texture of the cups that help with planning movement.

Cognition, of course, plays a part in how perceptions are interpreted. These interpretations are highly unique, based on each individual's past experiences within an ever-changing environment (Leonard, 1998). Cognition and volition enable the individual to make sense of the sensory input that has been registered. How this information is processed and perceived is through the coordinated efforts of all the systems. **Volition,** or the drive and desire to interact with the environment, often engages the individual in purposeful movement.

Fine motor skills are the end product of the interactions of the above systems. These skills include smooth coordinated movements of the upper extremity that are involved in functional skills such as writing, opening a door, throwing a ball, and waving goodbye. In studying the functional tasks of the upper extremity, the basic mechanisms can be broken down into the following main component functions: regard, reach, grasp, manipulation, and release (Duff, 1995).

Regard

The versatile and adaptive nature of the upper extremity does not begin with the motor responses observed in the shoulder, arm, and hand. Retinal receptors in the eyes are the first to detect what it is that will be approached with the upper extremity. Visual regard and perception, along with volition, begin the process of reaching for an object. The upper extremity has more neuroanatomical connections to the visual system than any other appendage (Leonard, 1998). It is this close relationship with the visual system that allows for quick and adaptive responses of the upper extremity.

Eye-hand coordination begins with coordination between eye and head movements (Leonard, 1998). Head and neck control facilitate smooth and quick visual tracking and location of objects outside the central visual field. To locate an object for visual regard, the person may need to use eye movements; eye and head movements; or eye, head, and trunk movements (Shumway-Cook & Woollacott, 2001). It is vitally important that clinicians assess the individuals' ability to visually regard the objects that they are being asked to reach for and manipulate. The treating therapist will need to determine if visual regard problems are due to eye movements; the coordination of eye and head movements; or coordination of eye, head, and trunk movements (Shumway-Cook & Woollacott, 2001).

Many **oculomotor components** facilitate successful visual regard. For the purpose of this chapter, the following are reviewed: visual fixation, vestibuloocular reflexes, saccades, accommodation, and vergence.

- **Visual fixation** is used to sustain gaze on an object when looking at a stationary target. This is then a building block for the ability to shift our gaze and then scan an object (Schneck, 2001).
- Vestibulo-ocular reflexes (VORs) allow the person to maintain visual fixation during fast movement of the head (Leonard, 1998).
- During the location and scanning of an object, certain rapid eye movements called saccades occur (Leonard, 1998). Researchers have found that eye saccades and arm and neck movements arise from neurons in the premotor cortex of the CNS (Shumway-Cook & Woollacott, 2001). Both intact saccadic movements and VORs allow for smooth tracking of an object during visual regard.
- **Accommodation** and **vergence** are two important visual receptive components that allow for accurate and clear regard of an object. Accommodation is the ability to focus on a near object and then a far object, which is important mainly for up-close activities such as buttoning a shirt (Chaikin, 2001). Vergence is the ability to move both eyes outward (divergence) or inward (convergence) toward midline so that a single image is viewed (Chaikin, 2001). This allows the person to regard a single object clearly whether it is near or far in his or her visual field (Chaikin, 2001).

Following visual regard of an object, the person begins the process of visual perception, or the ability to take in visual stimuli from the environment, and using cognition, make sense of the input. This process includes **visual discrimination**, **visual memory**, **visual recall,** and **visual cognition** (Cech & Martin, 1995; Schneck, 2001).

Head and neck control, along with these important contributions from the visual components, prepares the individual for placing the arm in space to allow the hand to interact within the environment.

Reach

Once a person has regarded an object using both the stability of the head, neck, and trunk and the function of the visual system, coupled with the desire to obtain the object, the process of reach begins. The goal of **reach** is to attain a target within the constraints of time and space (Exner, 2001). The overall desire is to bring the hand to an object with the correct timing and precision and prepare the hand for the task of grasping. The factors of the individual's abilities, along with the limitations of the environment and the actual task or object being obtained, must also be considered (Shumway-Cook & Woollacott, 2001).

Clinical Connection:

When determining an activity to be used during therapy, the therapist must look at the following:

- The strengths and limitations of the patient/client
- The environment in which the activity is being performed and whether the environment supports or hinders performance
- The components of the task and the properties of any objects being manipulated (e.g., the size or weight of an object may be important)
- The context and individual's motivation surrounding that activity

The speed and movements that encompass the ability to reach depend largely on the goal of the reaching task (Shumway-Cook & Woollacott, 2001). The velocity of arm movements when reaching toward an object changes based on the nature of the task, the properties of the object, and the environmental context. For example, when reaching to grasp a small glass ornament, the velocity of the reach will be much slower than when picking up keys off a table. Reaching movements could also change based on the environmental context, such as performing these tasks while rushing out the door late for a kinesiology class.

The goal of bringing the hand to the object for manipulation can only be accomplished with adequate mobility of the shoulder girdle. The glenohumeral joint is the most mobile joint in the body (Erhardt, 1992), allowing the hand to be positioned in a variety of ways for functional activities that range from eating to catching a baseball to typing on a computer. The shoulder girdle can accomplish this task effectively with adequate stability of the scapula on the rib cage and the humeral head, allowing the humerus to maintain or hold its position in space (Boehme, 1988; Shumway-Cook and Woollacott, 2001). As mentioned in Chapter 8, trunk stability provides the base for free movement of the humerus through space. Movements of the elbow, forearm, and wrist can help orient the hand to perform a task, as well as to provide stability for active hand grasp and manipulation.

The visual and proprioceptive systems are two more important components that allow for smooth and precise reaching patterns. Muscle spindles and joint receptors that provide proprioceptive feedback are important during movement of the arm (Leonard, 1998; Schumway-Cook & Woollacott, 2001). Studies have shown that input from the Golgi tendon organs and joint receptors have a faster response time than visual feedback (Shumway-Cook & Woollacott, 2001). In other words, the information received from the proprioceptive system is able to deliver the message to the CNS with a shorter latency than the information received via the visual tract. Therefore, proprioceptive feedback is important during quick movements of the upper extremity (Leonard, 1998).

Vision plays a large role in the ability of a person to successfully reach for a target. **Visual-motor control** is the process by which a person uses visual information to perform smooth and precise movements (Duff, 1995). In the motor learning literature, vision is described as an important component in the aiming movement of a limb toward an object. Vision first assists in the movement preparation and decides the certain movements that are to be used. The second phase, in which the UE starts to move, uses less vision and is called the initial flight phase. The third phase, when the target is reached, relies heavily on visual feedback for error correction and is called the termination phase (Mcgill, 2001). Authors also describe the function of visual feedback during reaching as the fine-tuning of the approach that helps to improve accuracy (Shumway-Cook & Woollacott, 2001).

Clinical Connection:

When working with the neurological involvement patient during a reaching task, the therapist is often very aware of the postural and musculoskeletal components needed for the task. The visual components needed are often overlooked. To improve a patient's ability to perform a reaching task, be aware of any visual limitations that the patient may have, such as a field-cut or an acuity problem. Also, simply make sure that patients are wearing their glasses if they have them. Check to see if the patient is able to visually regard the object he or she is reaching for and encourage the patient to look at his or her arm during a reaching activity, as this will help improve accuracy. You may also want to break down the activity into reaching for an object and then actually grasping it.

Grasp and Manipulation

Once the humerus has positioned the hand so that it can obtain an object, the process of grasping begins. The modeling of the hand in anticipation of the object that it will soon grasp and manipulate begins during the reaching phase. Research has demonstrated that the components used for reaching versus grasp appear to be carried on different descending neural pathways. The reaching phase of the upper extremity appears to be controlled by the midbrain and brainstem and the grasping phase by the pyramidal pathway (Shumway-Cook & Woollacott, 2001). The ability to grasp requires integration of input from the visual, tactile, and proprioceptive systems along with past experiences to help form internal representation or memories of an object's properties (Eliasson, 1995). **Internal representation** allows the person to anticipate how to mold the hand and is called **anticipatory control** (Shumway-Cook & Woollacott, 2001; Eliasson, 1995). This perception also gives information regarding size, shape, and perceived weight and texture based on past visual and somatosensory input and experiences. Anticipatory control uses sensory perceptions and experiences to give us the ability to form sensory motor memories that allow us to adapt our reach and grasp.

Grasp and manipulation patterns have been classified by a variety of professionals and continue to be studied and reviewed. Although initially devised in 1956, Napier's classification of grasp patterns continues to be used today (Duff, 1995). Napier divided grasp into two categories: power grasp and precision grasp. **Power grasp** is grasping in which the whole hand is used with the thumb held close to the other digits such as in the grasp used to pick up a large object. **Precision grasp** is one in which the thumb is held in opposition and is often used to grasp small or medium objects (Napier, 1956). These grasps were further refined in 1971 by Weiss and Flatt (Exner, 2001). Power grasps were elaborated on as hook, power grasp, and lateral pinch (Figs. 9–1 and 9–2). Precision grasps include cylindrical grasp, spherical grasp, pad-to-pad pinch, two-point pinch, and three-point pinch or three-jaw chuck (Exner, 2001) (Figs. 9–3 to 9–5).

During power grasps, the stability of the proximal musculature is again essential for successfully grasping and transporting large objects. With precision grasps, the opposition of the thumb is paramount. "Rotation of the thumb into an opposing position is a requirement of almost any hand function, whether it be strong grasp or delicate pinch" (Strickland, 1995, p. 36). Through movement of the carpometacarpal (CMC) joint, the thumb can be placed with its pad in opposition to the index finger pad, as well as the other digits. Because of the wide range of movement permitted at the CMC joint, stability of this joint through intact ligamentous structures is necessary for most prehensile activities (Strickland, 1995). It is this varied movement of the thumb that distinguishes the human species and allows human hands the versatility of a variety of in-hand manipulation experiences (Duff, 1995).

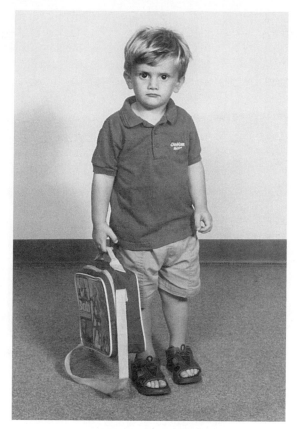

Figure 9–1. Hook grasp.

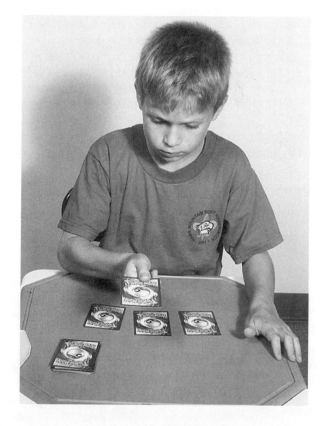

Figure 9–2. Lateral pinch.

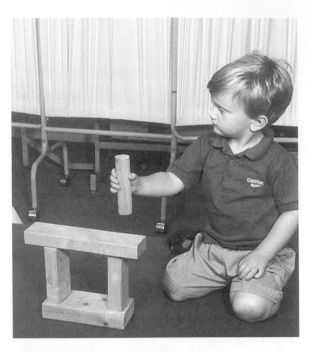

Figure 9–3. Cylindrical grasp.

Clinical Connection:

Grasping and picking up objects are only a fraction of what we do with our hands. Take the task of putting the top back on a gallon of milk. First you regard the top and determine the speed and distance that it will take for you to move your hand to the cap. Then during this approach your hand is molding to the shape it must take to grasp the cap with your thumb in opposition; your fingers slightly flexed; and your wrist, elbow, and shoulder stabilizing your movement along with your

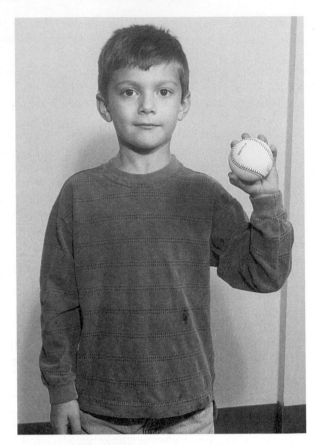

Figure 9–4. Spherical grasp.

trunk. You then grasp the cap and placed it on the milk carton. Now the intricate in-hand manipulation skills required to twist the cap are put into action while stabilization of the container is accomplished with your other hand.

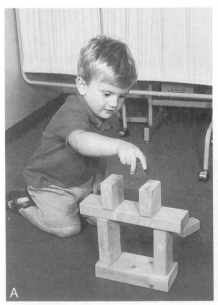

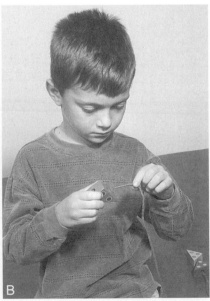

Figure 9–5. (A) Three-point pinch. (B) Two-point pinch.

Once an object has been obtained through grasping, the hand's perceptual functions and manipulative abilities can occur. The hand can be viewed as having powerful and precise motor functions, such as those needed to grasp and carry items or manipulate small objects. As Gibson (1966, pp. 123–124) states, "The perceptual capacity of the hand goes unrecognized because we usually attend to its motor capacity, and also because the visual input dominates the haptic in awareness." **Haptic perception** is active touch in which the hand integrates tactile and proprioceptive information concerning particular properties of an object, such as shape, weight, texture, and size, during manual manipulation (Stilwell & Cermak, 1995). The word *haptic* comes from the Greek origin and means "to lay hold of"(Gibson, 1966, p. 97). An example of the use of haptic perception is seen when an individual is able to identify an object placed in his or her hand, such as a coin or paperclip. Haptic perception, along with visual perception, begins to develop in infancy and continues to mature into early adolescence (Stilwell & Cermak, 1995).

In-hand manipulation is the ability to move an object within the hand after grasp (Exner, 2001). An example of this is writing with a pencil and then rotating it to erase a mistake. The use of intrinsic and extrinsic musculature within the hand is needed, as well as appropriate sensory feedback. Exner divides in-hand manipulation into three categories: **translation**, **shift,** and **rotation.** Definitions and examples are discussed in Table 9–1. In-hand manipulation skills are used by all of us each day as we carry out our functional activities. Activities such as using keys to open a door, opening containers, retrieving change from pockets, writing a letter to a friend, and the intricate tool use of a surgeon or computer technician are all examples of the multifaceted skills we possess at our fingertips.

Release

The release of an object following grasp can be done in a very precise manner or in a fairly crude manner. A 2-year old child dropping a toy versus an adult throwing a dart at a target is an example of the versatility with which an object can be released. The ability for accuracy during release, as required to release a small object into a container, is a developmental process and will be discussed in the next section.

Upper Extremity Function Across the Life Span

In this next section the different facets of regard, approach, grasp, manipulation, and release will be explored as they change over the life span. Due to maturation in the adult and older adult, many of the individual tasks of reach are accomplished and therefore will not be discussed individually. Please refer to Chapter 4 for a detailed discussion of fine motor development.

Infant

When analyzing upper extremity movements, attention is often focused on how the arm works in an open-chain, dynamic fashion, allowing the ability to grasp and manipulate things within the environment. In the early stages of development, as the patterns of reach and grasp are developing, the upper extremity also spends a lot of time in weight-bearing positions. The developmental positions as seen in the infant of prone,

TABLE 9–1		
In-Hand Manipulation Skills		
Classification	**Description**	**Example**
Finger-to-palm and palm-to-finger translation	Moving an object from the fingertips to the palm or palm to fingertips	Moving a coin from your fingertips to your palm or your palm to your fingertips
Shift	Moving an object or adjusting an object on the fingertips	Moving your fingers on your pencil to get an appropriate grip
Simple rotation	Rolling an object along the fingertips, which act as a unit to the opposed thumb	Screwing a cap onto a container of milk or spinning a top
Complex rotation	Turning an object 180 or 360 degrees in the hand with the fingers stabilizing and the thumb rotating, or the converse	Turning a marker over to remove the cap

Source: From Exner, C. E. (1992). In-hand manipulation skills. In Case-Smith J., & Pehoski C., (Eds.), *Development of hand skills in the child* (pp. 35–46). Bethesda, MD: American Occupational Therapy Association. Copyright 1992 by the American Occupational Therapy Association, Inc. Reprinted with permission.

with the base of support (BOS) over the head and shoulders progresses to prone on elbows and then four-point quadruped. The upper extremity is engaged in closed-chain activities during this developmental stage that help to facilitate proximal stability throughout the shoulder girdle and weight bearing through the small muscles of the hand. These activities also help provide tactile and proprioceptive input to the upper extremities that is important for later development. Jane Ayres, the founder of sensory integration assessment and intervention, reported that the tactile, proprioceptive, and vestibular systems are the precursors for many adaptive responses to the environment and that the tactile system in particular is foundational in the development of reach, grasp, and hand use (Ayres, 1987).

A myriad of functional skills encompass upper extremity use during this stage of development. The newborn uses the tactile and proprioceptive input from the upper extremities to begin to explore its surroundings as he or she gains input through this system. The tactile system is fully developed at birth and is integral in parent-infant bonding (Duff, 1995). As visually guided reach and purposeful grasp develop, the infant is constantly exploring objects, as well as his or her own body to gain more insight into the environment. Haptic perception begins at 6 months of age and helps the infant to further develop perceptions of different objects through tactile and proprioceptive input gained through the hand and mouth. These experiences will help to later facilitate more advanced grasping and manipulation skills. During this stage, the infant is also engaging in hand use for feeding, first with the bottle and then finger feeding, and later with utensil use. The functional use of the upper extremity for exploration and play are constant during this stage of development.

▪ Regard

During the newborn stage, the infant is able to briefly visually fix and follow, although eye movements are dependent on head movements (Alexander, Boehme, & Cupps, 1993). Newborns appear to have the ability to initiate a reaching pattern, which is triggered by vision (Shumway-Cook & Woollacott, 2001), but lack the motor coordination to contact the target. Through the emergence of the asymmetrical tonic neck reflex (ATNR) at approximately 2 months, the hand is brought into the visual field. Between the fourth and fifth month, when greater head and trunk control are present, visually guided reach emerges (Erhardt, 1992; Shumway-Cook & Woollacott, 2001). At 6 months, the infant is able to track objects in all planes and has intent when reaching for a target (Alexander et al., 1993). The ability to regard and track an object continues to improve during the first year of life, with visual monitoring of the upper extremity during reaching need-

ed for improved accuracy (Erhardt, 1992). As discussed in the previous section on regard, vision initiates the baby's movements and objects that are perceived in the visual field engage the infant who has the internal drive, or volition, to want to interact with what he or she sees. This interaction is initially seen as generalized motor activity because the infant lacks smooth and directed movements.

▪ Reach

Reach as it begins in the newborn is initiated by vision, as well as by tactile and proprioceptive input. Primitive reflexes, which were thought to control early reaching, are now thought to emerge concurrently with eye-hand coordination (Erhardt, 1992; Shumway-Cook & Woollacott, 2001). The stimulation that is present in the environment provides the context for the infant who has something to regard and reach for.

As described in Chapter 4, the infant begins reaching behaviors through visually guided movements in which the object is randomly contacted. Visually guided reach, in which corrections to the movement trajectory are made based on visual information, is replaced by a **ballistic style of reach,** in which corrections of the arm's movement are made at the end of the trajectory (Schumway-Cook & Woollacott, 2001). As stability develops within the head, neck, and trunk along with righting reactions, reach improves. Through the use of vision along with sensory input and stability of the trunk and shoulder girdle, the infant is successfully able to reach a target, if in a stable position, at 4 to 5 months (Duff, 1995). At this time, symmetry and the ability to bring hands together and to the mouth for further exploration also provide important sensory input. The infant continues to develop upright postures and righting and equilibrium reactions during the first year of life (see Chapters 4 and 8). Weight-bearing positions of the upper extremity help to facilitate increased shoulder girdle stability to allow for greater freedom during reaching activities. Upright positions also allow the infant to be able to reach in different planes in space. This allows a greater ability to interact and adapt to the environment. By 9 months of age an infant is able to produce a smooth and coordinated reach to attain an object. As the infant continues to refine his or her upright postural control and locomotion skills, eye-hand coordination continues to refine, improving upper extremity reach through practice and feedback.

▪ Grasp and Manipulation

Grasp is initiated in the infant by tactile and proprioceptive input in which contact to the **volar** (palmar) surface of the hand produces the reflexive response of the fingers tightly grasping around the object. With reflexes providing a foundation for movement in the early months of life, the infant is also using the hand as a weight-bearing surface while in prone positions. As described previously, this helps to provide the needed input to the intrinsic and extrinsic muscles of the hand, which will later be used for in-hand manipulation activities. **Voluntary grasp,** which emerges between 3 to 5 months of age, is accomplished by the ability of the infant to move the forearm and wrist in the right place to allow the hand to grasp an object (Boehme, 1988). At this age the infant is also bringing his or her hand to midline and to the mouth. The early stages of exploration of the haptic properties of objects begin but are limited by the amount of voluntary movement available in the arm and hand (Case-Smith, 1995). Forearm rotation is initially facilitated in prone by the 4 to 5 month old during lateral weight shifts while in a propping position. Forearm supination/pronation is further refined through practice by the infant, first against a stable surface such as the floor or the trunk and then, by 10 to 12 months, without environmental stability (Boehme, 1988).

The movement of the thumb, which is paramount to grasp, starts in an adducted position in early infancy and moves to a more opposed position at 7 to 9 months. By 12 months the thumb has developed opposition to the tip of the index finger and the infant is able to pick up small items such as Cheerios during self-feeding. This ability to produce refined pinch on objects along with the ability to transfer objects from hand to hand and produce a controlled release are all accomplished by the first 12 months and allow the infant to begin to actively explore objects and further develop in-hand manipulation skills (Case-Smith, 1995). The infant's ability to begin to orient his or her hands to the shape of an object also begins as early as 4 to 5 months but becomes more precise with increased age (Case-Smith, 1995; Shumway-Cook & Woollacott, 2001). This is accomplished using anticipatory control gained through somatosensory and visual experiences.

Clinical Connection:

In their research on the development of grasp in infants, Case-Smith, Bigsby, and Clutter (1998) found that haptic perception (the ability to discriminate different attributes of an object, such as size or texture) is paired with the development of grasp patterns. Haptic attributes of an object tend to produce different grasping patterns. Therapeutic implications of this finding include the importance of varying the objects being grasped during assessment to appreciate the full range of grasp patterns available to the infant. Additionally, toys with many different attributes, such as texture and moving parts, tend to enhance development of haptic

perception and manipulative skills in the infant. Toys that are textured tend to encourage more in-hand movement, whereas toys that are different in shape tend to increase transferring and rotation of the object (Case-Smith, 1995). ▪

When discussing grasp and in-hand manipulation skills, many different systems are needed to perform the complex tasks of planning the grasp pattern, molding the hand to fit the object with the appropriate pressure and speed, and manipulating the object within the hand. This coordination of multiple systems tends to be supported more effectively by a dynamic systems approach versus a hierarchical model. During the early stages of development, the infant is laying the groundwork for later refinement of in-hand manipulation skills, which begin to emerge in the preschool years (Exner, 2001). Exner (2001, p. 300) lists the following prerequisites for in-hand manipulation, developed during the first years of life:

- Forearm supination and the ability to hold this position in varying degrees
- Wrist stability
- Controlled and isolated movement of the thumb and index
- Control of the transverse metacarpal arch
- Disassociation of the two sides of the hand

Many of these prerequisites are established during upper extremity weight-bearing activities, which the infant engages in before the development of upright locomotion and through object manipulation and exploration.

▪ Release

Release in the infant is initially controlled by primitive reflex behaviors and tactile and proprioceptive input. Initially, objects drop randomly from the infant's hand or have to be removed by the parent. This is due to the strong grasp reflex, which begins to become integrated by 4 to 5 months. Once the grasp reflex is no longer prevalent, the infant releases an object through stabilization of the object on another surface. This often begins at approximately 5 months, when the infant is bringing hand to mouth. For example, the infant will bring a toy to his or her mouth and will stabilize it there and then release his grasp. Soon hand-to-hand transfer of toys begins, followed by purposeful release of objects. The infant no longer needs external stability by 9 months of age, and dump-and-fill activities begin. As in-hand manipulation skills and haptic perception begin to develop, the ability to grasp objects that vary in size and texture increases and the infant begins to refine release skills. By 12 months of age, the baby can release small objects using the stability through the shoulder girdle, elbow, and wrist, which allows for finger extension. Due to immaturity of the in-hand manipulative skills, finger extension during release is excessive in 1 to 2 year olds (Exner, 2001). Refined release continues to be practiced through play activities and feeding. At 2 years of age a child is usually able to release a small object into a small container. Examples of some activities in which refined release is practiced at this age include simple puzzles, shape sorters, and building with blocks.

Preschool/School Age

■ Regard

Visual regard and the ability to bring an object into the visual field, fix, and follow are mature by the preschool age. Visual perception continues to become more refined through the child's varied experiences and exposure to different daily tasks. By age 9, most of the visual perceptual abilities needed to carry out everyday tasks are developed (Schneck, 2001).

■ Reach

Most of the major motor components and stability/mobility foundations are achieved during the first 2 years of life, with the young child now able to put his or her hand in most positions. The speed and accuracy of reaching continue to develop, along with the ongoing maturation of the visual system. Intrinsic feedback from the visual system and the proprioceptive and vestibular systems assist to refine reaching behaviors of the preschool and school-aged child. Hay (1990) found that children between the ages of 4 and 6 were able to make fairly accurate reaching movements without visual feedback. At age 7, however, this behavior decreases, with the children relying more on visual feedback. It is interesting that this decrease in the use of somatosensory information and the increase in the use of visual input for reaching also coincide with a time in school when visual skills through reading are at a peak. By age 11, accuracy with reaching has matched adult levels (Shumway-Cook & Woollacott, 2001).

■ Grasp, Manipulation, and Release

Grasping patterns in the preschool-aged child improve with respect to strength and efficiency. The 3-year-old child has a difficult time grading force with grasp and will often apply too much pressure when holding and grasping things. This begins to improve at 4 years of age, as anticipatory control becomes more refined. Children at this age also have more difficulty with in-hand manipulation skills. Similarly, immature patterns

are used for releasing objects when manipulating them. The child will often need to stabilize an object on an outside surface to rotate or change the object's position within the hand (Pehoski, 1995). During this developmental stage, when the child is learning to grade movements within the hand, activities such as blocks, large Legos, Play-Doh, finger paint, and other **manipulatives** provide variation in texture, size, and weight, which helps provide rich sensory input to further develop hand dexterity. At age 4, the child begins to perform in-hand manipulation activities without using an external surface as an assist (Pehoski, 1995). It is also at this time that functional tasks such as dressing become more prevalent, as the child gains independence. Fasteners such as large buttons, zippers, snaps, and Velcro closures all help to facilitate improved intrinsic hand use, as well as providing rich tactile experiences.

During the preschool years, children have opportunity for an increase in tool use, such as utensils, crayons, and scissors. In-hand manipulation skills are developed in conjunction with grasping patterns and are necessary for skilled use of different tools (Exner, 1992). The practice and mastery of using different tools will later translate into tool use important for the occupational tasks of the student and adult.

The 4, 5, and 6 year old continues to improve in regulating grip force, as well as sequencing finger movements. The sensory systems of vision and tactile input continue to provide the needed input for appropriate output. Reaching and grasping are accomplished with the help of vision, and in-hand manipulation is guided by the tactile and proprioceptive systems (Pehoski, 1995).

The use of writing tools begins in the preschool years and gets refined as the child attends elementary school. The developmental progression of pencil grip is illustrated in Figure 9–6. An efficient grasp on the pencil is achieved with the shoulder and forearm stable, and the wrist in slight extension. The preschool child initially uses a full palmer grasp on the crayon and moves the arm as a unit to produce marks. This can be due to a lack of stabilization of the forearm and wrist, as well as a lack of development of the small muscles in the hand and immature in-hand manipulation skills. Proper wrist position occurs when the child is able to stabilize the wrist in extension through the balance of antagonistic muscles within the wrist and hand. Wrist position in turn influences the finger's position, which in turn influences the ability to hold a writing implement (Benbow, 1995). Wrist extension during writing allows for the most efficient and precise finger movements.

To encourage development of wrist stability in the young child, coloring and drawing on vertical surfaces such as easels and chalkboards, which place the child's wrist in extension, are advocated by many therapists (Myers, 1992).

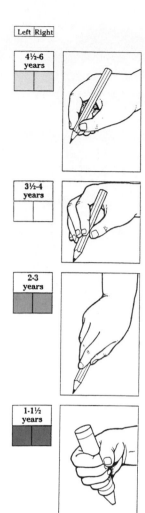

Figure 9–6. Developmental progression of pencil grasp. (Illustrations from *The Erhardt Developmental Prehension Assessment*, from *Developmental Hand Dysfunction*, 2nd Edition, copyright © 1994 by Rhoda P. Erhardt. Published by Erhardt Developmental Products, 2379 Snowshoe Court, Maplewood, MN 55119, USA, (651) 730-9004. Reprinted by permission.)

Clinical Connection:

Vertical surfaces can easily be introduced in preschools and elementary schools by the therapist to encourage efficient pencil grip. An empty three-ring binder placed horizontally on a child's desk with a clip at the top can serve as a makeshift raised clipboard. Taping paper to the blackboard or using easels during painting and coloring is another example (Fig. 9–7). ■

In addition to wrist stability, Benbow (1995) states that an open web space, stable hand arches, differentiation of the two sides of the hand, and good translation and rotation skills are needed for a successful handwriting outcome. An open web space allows full rotation of the CMC joint to permit complete thumb abduction and rotation in opposition to the finger pads. This position during writing allows the fingers to move the pencil efficiently, with little movement of the arm needed. Stability throughout the three arches in the hand—the distal and proximal transverse arches and the longitudinal arch—allows for shaping of the hand during grasp and in-hand manipulation. Differentiation is also important between the ulnar or power side of the hand and the radial or precision side of the hand. This can be demonstrated in scissor use, in which the ulnar digits stabilize the scissors to assist with thumb manipulation of the scissors (Benbow, 1995). In this example, the two sides of the hand must work together to accomplish the task of cutting across the paper. Translation and rotational skills (see Table 9–1) assist with precise handling of the writing implement.

Other sensorimotor components that influence handwriting include the following (Amundson, 2001):

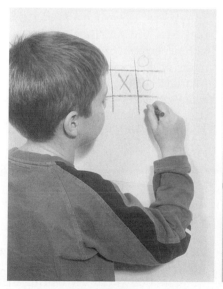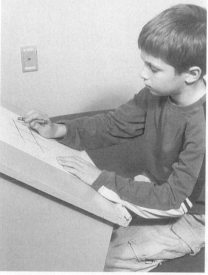

Figure 9–7. Vertical surfaces used with a child to encourage wrist extension and efficient pencil grip.

- Tactile and proprioceptive input to give feedback regarding grasp of the writing tool and smooth movement on the writing surface and pressure on the tool
- Kinesthesia for input regarding movement of the hand, weight of the pencil/pen, and appropriate pressure
- Visual-motor integration to allow the ability to form letters, trace, and color within boundaries
- Crossing midline to cross the midline of the body during writing tasks
- Bilateral integration to use both hands, one for writing and the other for stabilizing the paper
- Laterality for consistent use of a dominant hand
- Praxis for planning, sequencing, spacing, and forming letters and words

For the school-aged child a large portion of the day is spent on fine motor tasks. McCale and Cermack (1992) observed six classrooms to determine the percentage of time spent on fine motor tasks. They found that 30 to 56 percent of time was spent doing fine motor tasks, with 85 percent of these tasks being paper and pencil. Schneck and Henderson (1990) found that there was a distinct developmental progression of pencil and crayon grip and developed a more complete scale, including 10 grip postures. In their study of 320 nondysfunctional children, the **dynamic tripod grasp** was found to be the most common. The **lateral tripod grasp** was also observed in one-fourth of the children and is an acceptable form of a mature grasp for writing (Fig. 9–8). Burton and Dancisak (2000) observed 60 children performing a variety of precision writing tasks using different implements. They found that all the grips observed could be identified using Schneck and Henderson's 10-point scale (see Fig. 9–9 for a reprint of this scale). These researchers recommend that clinicians use this scale for documentation.

"As a child matures into adolescence, interest and experience further guide the refinement of prehensile skills" (Duff, 2002, p. 451). Practice of tasks that require complex abilities of grasp, manipulation, and release include such activities as schoolwork, playing a musical instrument, sports, and prevocational skills. Grip and pinch strengths increase in males and females in the late teens and may assist in increased abilities to perform certain skills (Duff, 1995). By the time an individual reaches adolescence, prehensile abilities are similar to those of an adult.

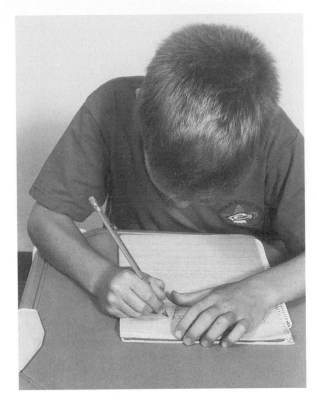

Figure 9–8. Child displaying a lateral tripod grasp during writing, in which thumb contacts the lateral surface of the index finger.

movements, such as needed by a carpenter. Individuals in this age range are usually cognizant of their abilities and may steer toward activities and tasks that they know they will be successful in. Adults, like children, can also improve their prehensile skills through practice and perseverance.

Adulthood grip strength continues to increase through age 20 (Duff, 1995). After this time, strength and abilities can be maintained if practiced. Adults who are experts in certain fields, such as sports or surgery, may have greater "innate abilities" than the typical individual. In converse, learning the task-specific components of a certain activity may determine their success (Starkes, 1990). In these expert vocations, as well as many other jobs that require repetitive upper extremity use, the problem of cumulative trauma disorders, such as carpal tunnel syndrome, tendonitis, and bursitis, are common (Duff 1995). These disorders can be avoided through education, rest, proper alignment, and possible adaptation of workstation or tool design (Duff, 1995).

Adulthood

During adolescence and adulthood, upper extremity movements are refined and often relate to personal occupational goals. Vocational choice may relate to the individual's ability to perform certain arm or hand

Older Adult

Older adults have many challenges when performing **prehensile** activities based on the changes in their different body systems. During reaching and regarding, the older adult often has to compensate for a decrease in

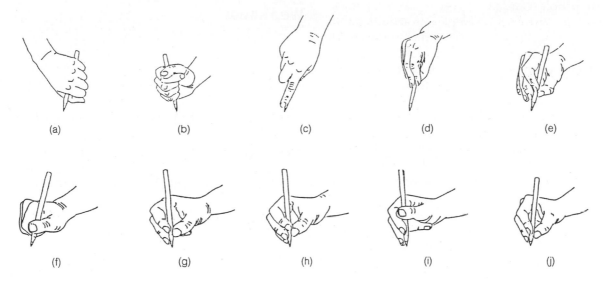

Figure 9–9. Schneck and Herderson's 10-point grip scale. (From Schneck, C. M., & Henderson, A. [1990]. Descriptive analysis of the developmental progression of grip position for pencil and crayon control in nondysfunctional children. *American Journal of Occupational Therapy* 44, 893–900. Copyright 1990 by the American Occupational Therapy Association, Inc. Reprinted with permission.)

acuity and visual processing (Duff, 1995). Cataracts are often common during this age, as is presbyopia, a thickening of the lens, which causes an inability to see things at reading distance (Cech & Martin, 1995). Reaching is hampered by the many normal changes in the musculoskeletal system that occur with aging. Muscle mass and velocity of synaptic firing decrease. These changes can cause a decrease in strength and speed during reaching. Bony changes, such as decrease in bone mass (as seen in osteoporosis) and damage to articular cartilage from years of use, can hinder the individual's capacity to reach freely overhead. The somatosensory system also undergoes changes, including decreased proprioception, tactile discrimination, and increased threshold for vibration (Cech & Martin, 1995; Kauffman, 1994). The changes that occur with aging cause the older adult to reach for objects with decreased speed to ensure accuracy. Velocity toward a target therefore decreases with more time spent in the approach phase of the reach (Shumway-Cook & Woollacott, 2001). It has been determined that older adults can improve reaching skills with practice and can retain these skills as well as young adults (Shumway-Cook & Woollacott, 2001).

Grasping and in-hand manipulation skills also decline with age. This can be due to decreases in joint mobility, diminished tactile and proprioceptive feedback, and decreases in grip and pinch strength. Often an older adult will grip something without grading the force of his or her effort due to decreased feedback from the somatosensory system. These limitations in sensory feedback and joint mobility impede the older adult from performing many daily activities, such as

opening containers, manipulating keys, and fastening buttons and snaps. In a study by Shiffman (1992), older adults' grip patterns were compared with younger adults' during selected functional activities. The older adults demonstrated the same prehension patterns during the activities as their younger counterparts, but with increased frequency. This increased frequency was often due to repositioning of the hand, which Shiffman surmises may be due to decreases in strength, inaccurate placement on the target, or decreased sensory information.

Clinical Connection:

When working with elderly individuals who have upper extremity impairments, therapists must remember the normal decline in sensory systems when assessing their patient. For example, an elderly individual who has a neurological impairment may be unable to grade the force with which he or she grasps objects in the involved hand. This may be due to the normal aging process as well as purely due to the neurological insult. If one side is unaffected, remember to check the grasp ability in that hand to get an appreciation of what is typical for that particular individual. ▪

Although older adults will have age-related changes that affect reach and grasp, the higher centers of cognition are least affected, enabling older persons to learn new skills. Ferguson and Trombly (2001) found that by adding meaning to tasks, performance improves with elderly people. Gardening, cooking, board games, and self-care are just some examples of activities that the older adult could engage in during therapy sessions. Ma and Trombly (2001) also found that functional tasks taught to the elderly person as a whole task, versus breaking down the task into parts, resulted in a better outcome. In their study, Ma and Trombly (2001) looked at the task of signing one's name in elderly subjects without motor problems. The researchers found that there was increased quality of movement for the whole task condition, in which the participant was asked to sign his or her name, versus the part task condition, in which the task was broken into three steps with a two- to three-second pause between steps. This study stresses the importance of using functional and meaningful tasks and having clients attempt to do the whole task versus practicing parts of the task.

Neuromuscular Impairments Resulting in Impaired Upper Extremity Function

Now that a picture of upper extremity function throughout the life span has been presented, attention will be directed to areas of dysfunction and the functional limitations that occur. "Loss of arm function is one of the most common long-term effects of neurologic pathology and one of the biggest contributors to disability" (Ryerson & Levit, 1997, p. 131). This is not surprising if one just looks back on the past few hours of a typical day and tries to calculate how many activities involve engagement in reaching, grasping, or manipulation skills to complete a given task. Most day-to-day activities are accomplished through use of the upper extremities.

Consistent with Chapter 7, this chapter will first look at neurological dysfunction of the upper extremity with respect to three functional impairment categories:

1. Abnormal force production or weakness
2. Abnormal muscle tone
3. Coordination problems

Patients who have central nervous system (CNS) damage often have upper extremity dysfunction affecting aspects of reach, grasp, and manipulation (Shumway-Cook & Woollacott, 2001). Although these components will be presented separately, it is important to remember that upper extremity function is a compilation of the functions of many different systems such that dysfunction in one area often affects another area. The final section of this chapter will describe characteristic problems of the upper extremity seen in common neurological disorders and intervention strategies targeted at improving function.

Weakness

Muscle weakness is one of the primary causes of decreased arm function in the patient/client with neurological impairment. Weakness is due to reduced or absent firing of the muscle motor units, which causes an inability to generate muscle force (Bennett & Karnes, 1998). When thinking about the upper extremity and weakness, a useful strategy employs looking again at the main functional components of arm movements: regard, reach, grasp, manipulation, and release.

▪ Regard

Vision is paramount to the development of reach, grasp, and release. When a patient displays muscle weakness, which affects neck and trunk stability, the ability to visually regard a target may be impaired. The patient may not be able to position the head appropriately to locate the target. The individual may also be unable to maintain head position in order to locate and track a target due to poor head and neck control. Oculomotor musculature, which controls eye movement and the ability to visually track objects, is commonly affected in many neurological impairments. Eye movements should be assessed before intervention in relation to its affect on regard and visual skills.

▪ Reach

Weakness in the upper extremity will also affect the person's ability to reach for objects. Weakness in the shoulder girdle often causes instability that can lead to subluxation in extreme cases and decreased range of motion (ROM) in moderate and mild cases. Decreased strength can also lead to increased fatigue. During reaching, this may be seen when the demand requires that the individual attempt to position the arm for grasp and hold that position. A person with decreased strength in the upper extremity often will compensate for this weakness with atypical movement patterns. A common pattern seen with weakness in the arm includes scapular elevation with humeral abduction and elbow flexion during forward reach (Ryerson & Levit, 1997) (Fig. 9–10). Patients will also compensate for arm weakness with their trunk, by laterally flexing their torso during reach or possibly assisting the weak extremity with the noninvolved arm. Stability and alignment within the trunk are also important during reaching tasks. When patients have poor proximal control due to weakness, their ability to use the distal function of their arm can be compromised. As with normal development of reach, trunk stability is needed to enhance distal arm movements during reach.

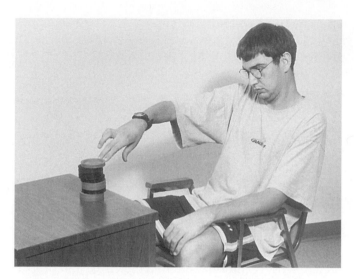

Figure 9–10. Individual displaying internal rotation of the humerus, shoulder girdle elevation, and elbow flexion during reach.

Weakness in the trunk is often present when there is weakness within the arm. See Chapter 8 for more detail concerning weakness related to postural stability.

▪ Grasp and Manipulation

Grasp and manipulation skills can be affected by limited strength due to lack of proximal stability in the trunk and shoulder girdle, which hampers distal mobility. Correct placement of the hand in space for grasp can also be limited due to weakness. Strength needed for sustained grasp and pinch on objects, as well as the intricate task of shaping the hand, relies on the intrinsic (muscles that have their origin within the hand) and extrinsic muscles (muscles' bellies of the forearm) within the hand. If weak, the patient may have a hard time with sustained pinch and grasp and full-digit ROM. Difficulty may also be seen with in-hand manipulation skills due to fatigue. Grasp and manipulation deficits limit a variety of daily skills, such as fastening clothing during dressing, writing, opening containers, and working appliances, to name a few.

▪ Release

Controlled release of an object is difficult in the patient with upper arm weakness. The individual may have difficulty with precision during release, such as poor placement or timing, or may release objects unintentionally due to inability to maintain a grasp.

Abnormal Muscle Tone

Abnormal muscle force production seen in flaccidity and spasticity of muscle tone presents a challenge to the clinician working with a patient/client with a neurological impairment (see Chapter 7). Decreased muscle tone as seen in hypotonicity or flaccidity results in decreased stability and increased joint range or laxity. Increased muscle tone or hypertonicity (spasticity) often results in decreased range of motion and limited movement patterns. Patients with fluctuating tone often have full ROM available to them but can stabilize joints only in the extreme end ranges of flexion or extension (Exner, 2001). Difficulty with reach, grasp, and manipulation, due to abnormal muscle tone, can hinder all areas of activities of daily living, leisure, and work.

▪ Regard

Beginning with visual regard, some of the problems discussed in the section on weakness can also occur in a patient with abnormal tone. Muscle tone, whether it is abnormally high or low, may prevent proper head positioning for visual regard. Patients with hypertonia may also have a lack of inhibitory control of primitive reflexes such as the ATNR or Moro (refer to Chapter 4 for reflex descriptions). Either of these reflexes could hinder visual regard by changing the position of the patient's head due to a stereotypic reflexive response.

Visual field deficits, often seen in stroke patients, limit the visual field and can limit the ability to reach and grasp accurately for a target (Shumway-Cook & Woollacott, 2001). **Visual neglect**, in which the patient has decreased awareness of visual stimuli on the contralateral side, will also decrease his or her ability to locate a target or an obstacle (see Fig. 3–5) (Shumway-Cook & Woollacott, 2001). Compensatory techniques, such as specific placement of objects, or cognitive cues to scan the environment are sometimes helpful. For example, for a child with a left-side visual neglect, a red line down the left side of the paper can be used as a strategy to teach the child to visually scan all the way to the left of the paper until he or she sees the red line. Once the child finds the red line, he or she can then begin to practice writing or reading from left to right.

▪ Reach

When examining the reaching component in clients with abnormal muscle tone, low, high, and fluctuating tone are considered. One would surmise that many of the same problems that occur with upper extremity weakness could be observed in the flaccid extremity. Joint laxity and difficulty stabilizing the glenohumeral joint during reach can make accuracy and speed in positioning the hand very difficult.

In the hypertonic upper extremity, the range and trajectory of the arm during reach may be limited due to muscle spasticity. Increased muscle tone, causing a decrease in active range of motion (AROM), may hinder the person's ability to extend the arm to contact a target. The timing and control observed during reaching are also longer, as seen in the patient/client with hypertonia due to cerebral palsy or stroke (Shumway-Cook & Woollacott, 2001).

Compensatory patterns during reach may arise due to underlying weakness of the shoulder musculature. Spasticity in the biceps and difficulty with reach may be primarily due to weakness in the antagonist muscles and an inability to recruit these muscles (Shumway-Cook & Woollacott, 2001). Therapists who follow a systems approach will often work on strengthening both the spastic and weak antagonist muscles as long as proper alignment can be achieved. This helps to promote stability around a joint (Bennett & Karnes, 1998).

▪ Grasp and Manipulation

Abnormal muscle tone within the intrinsic and extrinsic muscles of the hand can make in-hand manipulation skills a daily challenge. A lack of balance between the muscles of the hand can lead to limited movements, as seen in the hypertonic patient, or decreased stability around the joints of the fingers, most commonly the metacarpal phalangeal (MP) and CMC joints in the hypotonic patient. Individuals with an increase or decrease in muscle tone have many obstacles to overcome. Hygiene of a hand hard to open, even passively, is often a significant clinical issue. Cleaning the area and preventing skin breakdown becomes an important factor in daily living skills. Abnormally high or low muscle tone often leads to poor anticipatory hand formation during grasp as an object is approached. The grading of grip forces on objects is also decreased in patients with abnormal tone causing them to hold too tightly onto an object or drop the object due to a loose grasp.

Often, in the person with hemiplegia, the noninvolved hand will perform many of the in-hand manipulation skills, with the involved hand as an assist. Shumway-Cook and Woollacott (2001) note that in studies of children with cerebral palsy, as well as poststroke patients, the nonhemiparetic hand had mild impairments in grasp and object manipulation. This is felt to be due to the small percentage of fibers in the lateral corticospinal tract that are uncrossed.

▪ Release

Grading grip force is difficult in the individual with abnormal tone, as described earlier. The ability to release an object is equally affected. The individual may have too tight a grasp and be unable to actively release the object. The converse may be that the object drops

from the hand. In addition, an inability to grade forces may hinder slow or precise releases, such as releasing a glass when setting the table for dinner.

Incoordination

Smooth and precise movements, used to reach and interact with the environment, utilize the coordination of multiple systems within the CNS. "Incoordination occurs when the firing rates of muscles are disrupted, resulting in loss of smooth reciprocal movement, or when the CNS loses its ability to direct movement activity that requires accuracy" (Bennett & Karnes, 1998, p.158). Coordinated movements of the upper extremity require sensory information from the visual and proprioceptive system to assist with body position, movement, speed, and anticipatory control (Bennett & Karnes, 1998). The cerebellum is the primary center for coordinated movements, with contributions from the basal ganglia and sensory and motor cortexes (Bennett & Karnes, 1998) (see Chapter 7 for more details). Cerebellar or basal ganglia lesions lead to an impairment of smooth and coordinated movements. In the following section, the effects of incoordination on regard, reach, grasp, and manipulation and release will be explored.

▪ Regard

In patients with incoordination due to cerebellar lesions, oculomotor movements can also be affected. This can cause difficulty with smooth visual pursuits of a target. Limited ability to locate and maintain gaze on a target is also caused by "an inability to adapt the VOR to changes in task demands due to cerebellar lesions" (Shumway-Cook & Woollacott, 2001 p. 498). Incoordinated movements, which hinder eye-head coordination, may also limit smooth visual tracking of objects.

▪ Reach

The accuracy and timing required for smooth reach is impaired in patients with incoordination problems. Their ability to perform fast or reciprocal movements is challenging. A common problem occurs when more than one joint is involved in the reaching behavior. Impaired multijoint coordination causes reach to be a combination of movement segments rather than one smooth, fluid movement (Shumway-Cook & Woollacott, 2001; Bennett & Karnes, 1998). Reaching deficits also include difficulty with accuracy in reaching a target. Overshooting, missing the target, and extraneous movement to compensate for poor accuracy may be seen during reaching behaviors in the patient with incoordination problems. A common compensation is to slow down when reaching and use synergistic muscles rather than activation of agonist muscles and inhibition of antagonist muscles (Bennett & Karnes, 1998).

▪ Grasp, Manipulation, and Release

Inability to regulate and adjust force affects the ability to grasp, manipulate, and release objects. Inappropriate force may cause the patient to hold something too tightly and not be able to manipulate or release it. The converse problem, in which the object is held too loosely, can result in dropping the object. The inability to initiate grasping patterns and in-hand manipulation skills can be observed in patients with basal ganglia lesions. This can hinder activities of daily living (ADL) skills such as dressing, hygiene, and feeding.

Upper Extremity Control Problems Associated with Common Neurological Disorders

Cerebral Palsy

The primary functional limitations encountered in children with cerebral palsy (CP) are often in the areas of posture, movement, and atypical muscle tone. Abnormal muscle tone can present as hypotonic, hypertonic, or mixed. Children who present with increased muscle tone are more prevalent than those with decreased or mixed tone (Fetters & Kluzik, 1996). Secondary impairments that can occur due to muscle imbalance include joint contractures and orthopedic deformities. Because CP occurs during the prenatal period or within the first year of life, lack of varied sensory experiences, which are paramount in the early development of movement and visual perception, may lead to some of the motor disturbances seen by occupational and physical therapists.

▪ Regard

Visual limitations are present in 40 to 50 percent of children with cerebral palsy (Pellegrino, 1997). It has been found that children with CP who are perceptually impaired have a higher incidence of motor impairment (Schneck, 2001). As discussed at length throughout this chapter, the role of the visual system is vital in most aspects of upper extremity movement. Common visual deficits include the following (Rogers, 2001; Schneck, 2001):

- Problems with acuity
- Poor coordination
- Weakness of eye musculature
- Strabismus
- Nystagmus
- Convergence difficulties
- Poor visual perception

These deficits can lead to decreased ability to visually regard, track, or maintain visual fixation on an object. Difficulty with visual perception has also been found to lead to decreased bilateral manipulative skills (Schneck, 2001).

Many children with CP have poor postural control. Deficits in postural control can lead to poor head-neck control. As discussed previously in this chapter, in order to have adequate visual regard, head-neck control is needed to allow visual appreciation of a target. Without a stable base, development of eye movements to orient to the environment is hampered. "With inadequate alignment of the head in relation to the base of support, the visual system accumulates distortions and inconsistent input, which leads to formation of an inadequate perceptual base for later learning" (Nelson, 2001, p. 269).

Children with delayed development of motor control may continue to present with stereotypical movement patterns associated with primitive reflex patterns. The functional consequence in the case of a strong or obligatory ATNR, for example, may contribute to loss of regard of an object. For example, in the child who has not moved out of the primitive movement pattern seen in an ATNR response, tracking an object with head turning may cause the child to assume this strong reflexive pattern.

▪ Reach

The importance of postural stability for movement of the upper extremity cannot be stressed enough when thinking about the child with CP. Often clinicians will observe a child who presents with hypertonia in the extremities and poor trunk and postural control. This deficit in postural stability decreases the availability of varied distal strategies for reach and grasp. The position of the trunk and pelvis influences the mechanics of the shoulder girdle. The balance between flexors and extensors throughout the extremities is often severely limited, causing movement synergies and stereotypical movements of the upper extremity during reach. Movement patterns observed when extensor tone is increased include extension of the head, neck, and spine; adduction of the hips and scapulae; extension of the humerus; and flexion of the elbows, wrist, and hands (Danella & Vogtle, 1992).

Another common pattern seen in CP is hypotonia in the trunk, as characterized by a posterior pelvic tilt, lumbar flexion, head-neck extension, and hypertonic extremities. In both of these patterns a limitation is present throughout the shoulder complex, which decreases the child's ability to reach. These patterns, maintained over time, can lead to secondary shortening and contractures of the involved joints and muscles. Tight adduction of the scapula limits the synchrony of movement between the scapula and humerus. This can lead to limited range of motion of the humerus for overhead reach (Boehme, 1988). Common compensatory movements for reaching include internal rotation of the humerus, shoulder girdle elevation, and lateral flexion away from the reaching arm (Danella & Vogtle, 1992) (see Fig. 9–10).

▪ Grasp and Manipulation

Grasp and manipulation skills in the child with CP often hinder the child's ability to perform many activities required for basic activities of daily living and school-related tasks such as writing. Lack of good shoulder girdle stability contributes to poor grasp and manipulative skills (Scherzer & Tscharnuter, 1982). In a study by Cope and Trombly (1998), the grasping patterns of children with and without cerebral palsy were analyzed. The authors found that children with CP, like their noninvolved counterparts, did have use of anticipatory control when reaching for an object. The children with CP were able to shape their hand before contact, in anticipation of what they were grasping. This indicated that the children were able to use sensory information, specifically visual input, and past experiences to preshape their hand. The subjects with CP tended to have more exaggerated hand openings than the typical children. The researchers concluded that children with CP are sensitive to task constraints and that a task-oriented approach may be beneficial when working on reach and grasp.

Clinical Connection:

The study just discussed emphasizes the importance of therapists analyzing the tasks they are using during their intervention of children with CP. When working on grasping, remember the importance of visual regard, as this assists with the children's ability to preform their hand to the object they are attempting to grasp. Children with CP will also need more time to reach a target when attempting to grasp. Therapists also need to closely look at the properties of the object. The size and shape of the object should be appropriate for the grasp or pinch pattern they are working on with the child. ▪

Tactile and proprioceptive information is needed to determine how much grip force is needed to hold an object and perform in-hand manipulations. This registration of sensory information can be impaired in children with CP (Shumway-Cook & Woollacott, 2001), who have poor grasp and manipulation skills. Posturing of fingers in flexion during early development of upper extremity weight bearing limits the amount of tactile and proprioceptive input into the hand, which may lead to limited sensory processing in the hand. Some grasp and manipulation problems observed in children with CP include the following (Shumway-Cook & Woollacott, 2001):

- Exaggerated opening and closing of the hand
- Decreased ability to grade grip forces
- Poor differentiation between the ulnar and radial side of the hand
- Lack of precision and accuracy within small hand movements

▪ Release

To release an object, the child needs control of wrist and finger extensors, as well as cognitive and perceptual skills. Many children with CP have perceptual and cognitive deficits along with their motor and postural impairments (Pellegrino, 1997). The distal mobility required for controlled and graded release, as well as accurate proprioceptive feedback, is often lacking. Children with moderate to severe hypertonicity have difficulty with controlled release, and some cannot initiate release at all (Danella & Vogtle, 1992). The common atypical pattern seen during release is wrist flexion, which offers a mechanical advantage for the fingers to extend. When the wrist is flexed, this position causes the finger extensor tendons to passively elongate, favoring finger extension (Fig. 9–11). This pattern is often inefficient; therefore, accuracy and timing when releasing an object is lost. Other children with CP with mild hypertonicity or hypotonia may have difficulty sustaining grasp on an object, and therefore their release of an object may be uncontrolled and unwanted.

▪ Clinical Management of Cerebral Palsy

Upper extremity management is a clinical intervention goal for both physical and occupational therapists and assistants who work with children with CP. Even in the child with a diagnosis of spastic diplegia, in which the lower extremities are the most motorically affected, the upper extremities are often impaired. In an attempt to

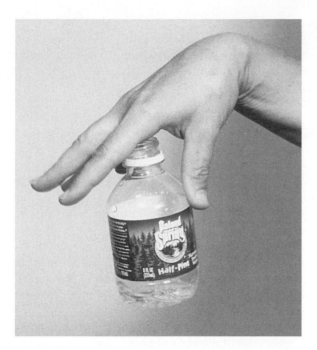

Figure 9–11. Individual using wrist flexion to facilitate finger extension.

provide continuity in the discussion of clinical management of the child with cerebral palsy, the areas of regard, reach, grasp and manipulation, and release will be used to organize and present clinical suggestions.

■ Regard

Visual limitations are very common in the children with CP. Clinicians must remember this during intervention activities and attempt to obtain any information regarding the child's visual status before intervention, if possible. An inability to visually fix and follow a target may be a starting point for intervention planning and therapeutic intervention. For example, if poor head control does not allow a child to visually regard objects, this may be a place to start intervention or an area where the clinician can provide the child with some outside stability through seating and positioning.

Specific visual training activities are beyond the scope of this text, and readers are referred to other sources (Downing-Baum, 1995; Menken, Cermak, & Fisher, 1987; Scheiman, 1997). An ophthalmologist or optometrist specializing in pediatrics may be able to address and evaluate very specific visual deficits and provide intervention recommendations.

■ Reach

Stability is a main component of reach that is often lacking in the child with CP. Gaining proximal stabil-

ity throughout the shoulder girdle is foundational for controlled reach in all planes. Weight bearing in different developmental positions can begin to build strength and stability around the shoulder girdle. Putting the young child in prone or quadruped positions and introducing subtle weight shifts begin the process of shoulder disassociation (Fig. 9–12). Graded reach activities in these positions can then be introduced (Fig. 9–13). The therapist must also determine if full scapular and humeral ROM is available both actively and passively. If passive ROM (PROM) is limited in the shoulder girdle, it should be determined whether this is due to tissue shortening or an abnormal muscle pull, resulting in contracture. Inhibitory sensorimotor techniques such as gentle sustained traction and vibration may help to decrease muscle spasticity during intervention (Danella & Vogtle, 1992). (See Chapters 6 and 7 for more information on management of abnormal muscle tone.)

Reaching activities in gravity-eliminated planes, such as side lying, may be beneficial to the children with hypotonia or underlying weakness. This position also provides some proximal stability and facilitates head and hands to midline and hands within the visual field (see Fig. 9–27). Another way to assist the child with managing the demands of gravity is to have the child use the support of a table in sitting to support the arm during reach.

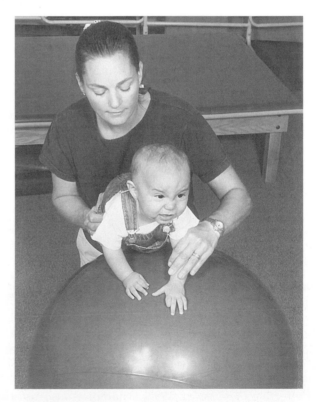

Figure 9–12. Therapist facilitating weight shifts and open-hand weight bearing in the quadruped position.

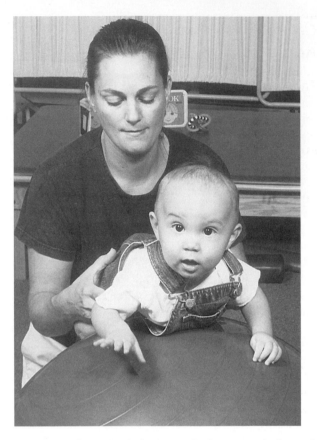

Figure 9–13. Therapist helping to facilitate graded reach while in prone.

Clinical Connection:

When working with children with cerebral palsy, therapists are reminded to be cognizant of the activities that they choose. They should be age appropriate and motivating to the child. An activity or toy that is visually interesting or tactilely stimulating may interest some children and overstimulate others. Knowing the child's strengths and challenges, along with the typical developmental sequence, will help therapists to choose the appropriate activity.   ■

■ Grasp and Manipulation

For the child with hypertonicity and a fisted hand, activities to decrease muscle tone and increase voluntary control may be beneficial. Boehme (1988) uses firm pressure and oscillating massage within the hand to increase expansion. Weight bearing on an open hand may also help to decrease a fisting posture (Fig. 9–14). If contractures are present, serial casting and splinting can be effective (Yasukawa, 1992). Therapists also use soft and hard splints to provide stability in the hand for those children with decreased muscle tone, who often

present with poor stability around the CMC joint. This instability can cause limited ability to maintain an open web space and inefficient thumb opposition. Stabilizing the thumb CMC joint through the use of splints can be helpful for activities such as coloring or building with blocks.

Once stability is gained proximally, grasping is most effective with the wrist in neutral or slight extension. Again, the choice of the object being grasped is important. The clinician must take into account the child's interest and volition, the sensory properties of the object, and the shape and weight of the object. Different objects elicit different grasp responses based on their haptic properties (Case-Smith, Bigsby, & Clutter, 1998). The grasp pattern that the treating therapist is striving to achieve must also be considered. Activities that use practice and verbal feedback can be helpful with children who are working on the intricate aspects of grasp.

When working on in-hand manipulation skills, the properties of the objects being manipulated are very important. Remember that in-hand manipulation relies more heavily on the tactile and proprioceptive senses. For children with CP, in whom these senses are

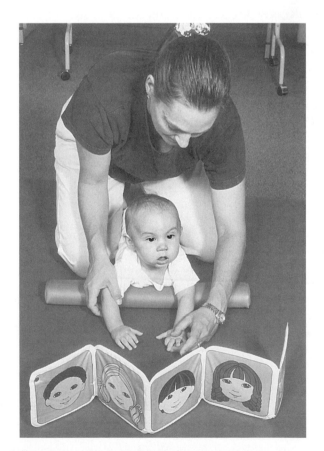

Figure 9–14. Open handed weight bearing while in prone, over a roll.

often limited, textured objects such as a small kush ball may encourage more exploration and build haptic abilities. For children with a higher level of cognition, smaller objects can be used with demonstration and verbal cues can be given as to how the objects are to be moved within the hand. Again, engaging the child and performing activities that can translate into functional skills needed for daily activities are important.

Children with CP who demonstrate limited grasp may also benefit from adapted toys, utensils, and writing implements to assist them with their daily activities. Lightweight and built-up handles on toys and pencils may assist a weak grasp by requiring less grip strength and hand ROM. Large or visually striking targets may help to visually guide reach. Adaptive keyboards and switch access to different electronic devices may provide children with the independence they desire and need. The decision regarding the type of adaptive equipment needed should be determined collaboratively with input from the team members and, most importantly, the family and child.

Clinical Connection:

A hand splint may be an appropriate device to increase function in the child with cerebral palsy. A wrist cock-up splint can help to position the wrist in extension for function. Splints that help provide an open thumb web space or a stable carpometacarpal joint, for example a short opponens splint, position the thumb functionally in opposition. Splints, such as a resting hand splint, also are used to prevent deformity or reduce loss of motion. Soft splint material such as Neoprene or low temperature thermoplastics can be used to fabricate splints. The needs of the child and goal of the splint help to determine the appropriate material to be used by the therapist. ■

■ Release

Release of objects using wrist flexion is common in children with spastic cerebral palsy. Intervention strategies should focus on establishing adequate ROM to begin training of release with wrist in neutral. As in the normal developmental sequence, practice of release can begin with external stabilization by using the other hand (Boehme, 1988; Duff, 2001). Intervention can then progress to release without external stabilization and then release into containers (Duff, 2001). In children in whom contractures prevent active release and hinder hygiene, serial casting, splinting, and botulinum toxin (Botox) injections may be helpful (see Chapter 7).

Cerebrovascular Accident and Adult Hemiplegia

There are 600,000 new cases of cerebrovascular accident (CVA) each year in the United States (Roth, Olson, & McGuire, 2001). "Loss of arm function is one of the most common long-term effects of neurologic pathology and one of the biggest contributors to disability" (Ryerson & Levit, 1997, p. 131). In the acute stages of recovery, patients who have had a stroke typically present with flaccidity or weakness in the extremities on the side contralateral to the CVA. In approximately two-thirds of patients, spasticity will develop (Roth et al., 2001), usually within the first few weeks following the stroke. In most of these patients, ambulation will be possible. Recovery of the upper extremity is, however, not as promising. Many of the functional limitations caused by upper extremity impairment hinder independence in daily activities and return to a premorbid lifestyle.

As in the section on cerebral palsy, the areas of regard, reach, grasp and manipulation, and release will be discussed as they relate to the individual who has suffered a stroke. This will be followed by discussion of the general clinical management of these functional component areas.

■ Regard

Visual problems are prevalent in the patient/client who has had a stroke. The most common types of visual deficits are discussed next. Approximately 26 percent of patients after CVA display a homonymous hemianopsia in which vision is impaired on the contralateral side of each eye (O'Sullivan, 2001b) (see Figs. 3–4 and 3–5). Unilateral neglect, or neglect of one side of the body due to visual and sensory losses on that side, is commonly observed in the patient with hemianopsia. The ability to visually regard an object, when neglect is present, is obviously limited. Difficulties with oculomotor control and acuity are also common following stroke (Unsworth & Warburg, 2001).

Other contributing problems, such as impaired head-neck control and postural instability, may limit the patient's ability to visually attend to an object that the therapist is encouraging him or her to reach for. Patients in the acute stage of a stroke who present with flaccidity and poor postural control may not be able to orient their head, and therefore their eyes, to regard, track, or visually fix on an object. Agitation, disorientation, and cognitive difficulties may also be complicating factors. Therapists and assistants must always remember to be aware of the context in which they are asking the person to perform a certain activity. Familiar activities such as basic ADLs (e.g., bed mobility, dressing, eating), done in the appropriate context, may provide the therapist with a starting point for engagement with the client.

▪ Reach

Reach relies heavily first on sensory input (feedback) and then movement is initiated from the shoulder girdle to start the reaching process. In the patient/client who has suffered a CVA, the complications of concurrent impairment at the shoulder girdle are numerous. Often, patients initially present with mild to severe flaccidity in the involved upper extremity. As the patient begins to progress, incomplete return of muscle function, hypertonicity, loss of joint alignment, secondary joint and muscle complications, and pain and **edema** can result. Improper positioning, inappropriate physical handling of the flaccid arm during transfers, and poor ROM techniques can cause or increase pain.

With the development of abnormally high muscle tone, a muscle imbalance may exist, contributing to certain recognizable recovery patterns. Typically, strength in scapular elevators, shoulder abductors, internal rotators, and wrist and finger flexors develops first, before the development of the opposing muscles (Ryerson & Levit, 1997). This recovery pattern causes a common pattern of shoulder elevation and abduction; internal rotation; and elbow, wrist, and finger flexion.

Scapular alignment and support of the glenohumeral joint are often compromised in the patient with hemiplegia, leading to shoulder subluxation. In the flaccid extremity, there is insufficient muscle tone to hold the glenohumeral joint in proper alignment due to the forces of gravity and the weight of the arm. The scapula is placed in a downwardly rotated, abducted position

(Ryerson & Levit, 1997). In the extremity with spasticity, unbalanced muscle activation can contribute to downward depression and retraction of the scapula (O'Sullivan, 2001b). Ryerson and Levit (1997) have described three major patterns of shoulder subluxation and compensatory reaching strategies associated with these patterns (Table 9–2).

Pain in the hemiplegic shoulder is a common factor encountered by many therapists and assistants treating patients with CVA. Shoulder pain occurs in 70 to 80 percent of stroke survivors and typically occurs during active movement (O'Sullivan, 2001b). Pain and its relationship to subluxation are controversial. Whereas some authors feel that subluxation causes pain, other researchers have found evidence that does not support the relationship between pain and subluxation (Zorowitz, 2001). Regardless of the primary cause, shoulder pain and edema are complications that many clinicians face when working with patients who have had a CVA. Limb positioning, decreased movement, and poor drainage by the venus and lymphatic systems can cause edema, a secondary complication (Duff, 2001; Ryerson, 2001). Both edema and pain interfere with the patient's ability to reach and the retraining of functional tasks. Edema in the hand can be associated with **shoulder-hand syndrome,** which often starts with swelling in the hand (Ryerson, 2001). Although edema in the hand does not always lead to shoulder-hand syndrome, the common characteristics are listed in Table 9–3.

▪ Grasp and Manipulation

Difficulty with grasp and manipulation occurs often in the patient/client with neurological impairment. In the

TABLE 9–2			
Shoulder Subluxation			
	Inferior Subluxation	**Anterior Subluxation**	**Superior Subluxation**
Muscle tone	Most common Muscle weakness and hypotonia	Hypertonicity and unbalanced muscle return	Hypertonicity and unbalanced muscle firing in middle deltoid, pectorals, and deltoid
Position	Downward position of scapula Humerus falls below glenoid fossa	Scapula pulled from downwardly rotated position into elevated forward position Humeral head migration anterior to glenoid fossa	Scapula moves at all times with humerus Humeral head lodged under coracoid process, elevated and internally rotated
Movement patterns with reach	Internal rotation of humerus Elbow extension and forearm pronation	Trunk backward rotation and anterior pelvic tilt Elbow flexion and forearm supination	Internal rotation of humerus Elbow flexion Wrist radial deviation Thumb extension

Sources: Data from Byrne, D., & Ridgeway, M. (1998). Considering the whole body in treatment of the hemiplegic upper extremity. *Topics in Stroke Rehabilitation, 4,* 14–34; Gillen, G. (1998). Upper extremity function and management. In G. Gillen & A. Burkhardt, *Stroke rehabilitation: A function based approach* (pp. 109–151). St. Louis, MO: Mosby; and Ryerson, S., & Levit, K. (1997). *Functional movement reeducation: A contemporary model for stroke rehabilitation.* New York: Churchill Livingstone.

TABLE 9–3

Shoulder-Hand Syndrome Stages

Stage 1	Edema primarily in the hand dorsum, complaints of severe pain and stiffness in shoulder, pain spreading to wrist and hand, decreased shoulder ROM in abduction, flexion and external rotation; vasomotor changes include mild skin discoloration; may have hypersensitivity to touch, pressure, or temperature.
Stage 2	Decreased pain, muscle and skin atrophy, vasospasm, hyperhidrosis, course hair and nails, early osteoporosis.
Stage 3	Progressive atrophy of skin, muscles, and hair, minimal pain and vasomotor changes, articular changes; hand becomes contracted in a clawed position and flattened, with thenar and hypothenar atrophy.

Source: Adapted from O'Sullivan, 2001, p. 538, with permission.

person who has suffered a CVA, there are many factors that may cause changes in distal functioning. These are not limited to but often include the following (Gillen, 1998):

- Unbalanced muscle pull
- Weakness or paralysis
- Changes in distal alignment due to shoulder girdle position
- Decreases in sensation
- Secondary joint changes
- Pain and edema

Due to any combination of these factors, abnormal movement patterns emerge during grasp and manipulation. In the flaccid hand, the components of internal shoulder rotation, elbow extension, forearm pronation, wrist flexion, and flattened palmer arches are often seen (Ryerson & Levit, 1997). In the hand in which muscle tone has increased, unbalanced muscle pull into flexion is more prevalent. The pattern that develops includes internal rotation and elevation at the shoulder, elbow flexion, forearm supination or pronation, and wrist and finger flexion. If this position of finger and wrist flexion continues for long periods, wrist and finger flexor tendons shorten. This causes increased difficulty in active or passive opening of the hand. Therapists may use splinting or serial casting to address these issues. Low load and prolonged stretch of the tight tendons are provided by the serial application of splints or casting and can increase ROM.

▪ Release

Similar to children with CP, adults with neurological impairments have common difficulties. In the hypotonic hand, grasp may be so limited that release is not controlled. Objects may fall out of the involved hand involuntarily. In the patient with hypertonicity, abnormal movement patterns may be used to facilitate release. These patterns include wrist flexion to mechanically extend the fingers and abduction of the humerus along with elbow extension in a synergistic pattern

(Boehme, 1988). The patient may also use the noninvolved hand to pry the object free or fling his or her hand in an attempt to release it (Boehme, 1988). All these patterns may produce the desired end product, release of the object, but accuracy and control are compromised. Varying muscle tone, along with sensory losses in the hand, hinders timing and graded release in patients with neurological impairments.

▪ Clinical Management of Adult Cerebrovascular Accident and Hemiplegia

Most therapists and assistants will work with a patient with upper extremity hemiplegia at some point in their clinical practice. Management of the upper extremity can be very challenging, especially in the patient/client who has had a CVA, who may have sensory deficits, visual and cognitive limitations, and pain and edema as confounding factors. Many of the patients seen are older adults who, regardless of their neurological impairment, have decreases in muscle strength and endurance and decline of sensory and visual systems as part of the normal aging process (see earlier sections on adult and older adult development). Clinicians may choose a variety of **frames of reference (FOR)** when working with the patient who has had a CVA. Some of the more common FOR used with this population include motor learning and control, neurodevelopmental treatment (NDT), proprioceptive neuromuscular facilitation (PNF), and task-oriented approaches (see Chapter 6). As in the previous sections, clinical management will be outlined specific to regard, reach, grasp and manipulation, and release.

▪ Regard

Visual deficits that often accompany a cerebrovascular accident are numerous, as explained previously. For the treating clinician, this area has an enormous impact on the ability of the individual to engage in reaching behaviors. Some common techniques for working with the patient with visual neglect and hemianopsia include teaching the patient to scan his or her visual field (Niemeier, Cifu, & Kishore, 2001) and using visual imagery to address the problem of **visual inattention** or neglect. In using the imagery of a lighthouse's beacon sweeping across the horizon, Niemeier and colleagues (2001) found increases in patient's ability to scan the environment and perform better on functional tasks.

Specific visual interventions are outside the scope of this text. The reader is encouraged to read Barbara Zoltan's (1996) manual, which discusses evaluation and intervention techniques used for visual and cognitive deficits in the adult with a neurological impairment.

▪ Reach

Reaching behaviors occur with a stable base and an aligned shoulder girdle. Both of these factors are often impaired in the person who has had a CVA. Pain and edema are also confounding factors, and their management will be discussed later. The posture of the trunk can influence the position of the scapula and humerus for reach. Ryerson and Levit (1997) describe four common patterns of decreased trunk control seen in the patient with neurological impairment:

- Excessive trunk flexion causes increased scapular abduction with the humerus positioned in front of the body.
- Excessive trunk extension causes scapular adduction with the humerus positioned in adduction and internal rotation or shoulder hyperextension.
- Lateral trunk flexion on the hemiplegic side causes scapular rotation downward. If flexion is on the noninvolved side, the scapula will be elevated.
- Trunk flexion on the hemiplegic side with lateral flexion as well causes the scapula to be abducted and downwardly rotated.

To begin to provide proper alignment of the scapula and shoulder girdle complex, trunk alignment should be addressed. Facilitating good trunk alignment during functional activities is often a good place to start. Rolling in bed and getting to sitting is a good way to start to reintegrate the hemiplegic side and encourage symmetry (see Figs. 7–32 and 7–33). Sitting with good alignment of the trunk, with feet flat and upper extremities as support, can be incorporated into activities in which subtle weight shifts are introduced. A more detailed account of intervention strategies for postural control can be found in Chapter 8.

Once trunk alignment is attained or achieved through an outside support (such as seating or positioning), upper extremity control for reaching can be a focus of the therapy session. Upper extremity weight

bearing in different positions, such as sitting, standing, and quadruped, is an early activity that can begin to stimulate shoulder stabilizers, as well as elbow, wrist, and finger extensors (O'Sullivan, 2001b). Weight shifting in these positions can also provide gentle scapular mobilization. ROM of the involved extremity is also important, as joint changes and edema may result without proper movement. ROM activities should be done carefully, so as not to cause increased pain or trauma to the affected limb. Some guidelines for correct PROM that O'Sullivan (2001) has recommended include careful attention to external rotation and extraction of the humerus, especially in overhead ranges greater than 90 degrees, and mobilization of the scapula in upward rotation to prevent tissue impingement. Always consider the premorbid ROM that was available to the patient as the individual's appropriate goal. The normal aging process does affect ROM such that full ROM may not be the baseline for the elderly patient. AROM is always more beneficial than PROM, and many therapists and assistants teach self-ROM activities that patients do independently.

If edema is present, it should be treated aggressively while it is soft and pitting to the touch, as its presence hinders mobility of the joints and tissues and is associated with pain (Ryerson & Levit, 1997). Edema that is not reduced can begin to adhere to underlying tissue and become hard and lumpy (Ryerson, 2001). In the early stages, edema should be decreased through gentle active motion, retrograde massage, and elevation. Some therapists also use elastic gloves and garments and distal-to-proximal bandage wrapping to reduce edema in this early stage.

Pain in the hemiplegic shoulder has many causes, both primary and secondary. Regardless of the underlying cause, pain decreases return of functional mobility and therefore must be assessed and treated. Ryerson and Levit (1997) list the following causes of pain in the hemiplegic shoulder:

- Poor joint mechanics at the shoulder causing misalignment
- Muscle and soft tissue pain due to spasticity or active shortening
- Impairment of sensory systems
- Chronic pain syndromes (shoulder-hand syndrome)

Intervention strategies for poor alignment include proper positioning and alignment of the humerus and mobilization of the scapula. Slings should be used with caution. They cannot reverse a subluxation but rather help maintain proper positioning of the glenohumeral joint, which has been achieved during therapy (Ryerson, 2001). There are many types of slings; therapists are referred to Ryerson and Levit's text (2001) for specific slings and their characteristics. Alternate positioning strategies include therapeutic taping of the shoulder and functional electrical stimulation (Woodson, 1995). An intervention strategy for decreasing muscle and soft tissue pain can include slow, pain-free stretching of the spastic muscles. Clinicians must pay careful attention to subjective reports of pain and decrease stretch if pain increases. Often, painful shoulders originate from painful therapy (Ryerson & Levit, 1997). When treating patients with sensory impairments and chronic pain syndromes, consistency is needed. Ryerson and Levit (1997, pp. 160–161) have listed the following stages in intervention of chronic arm pain:

1. Eliminate pain from intervention and patient's routine.
2. Desensitize the arm and hand to touch.
3. Eliminate hand edema.
4. Introduce pain-free arm movements.
5. Gradually increase movement demands.

▪ Grasp and Manipulation

Proximal control throughout the shoulder girdle assists with functional reach and places the hand in a position to begin the formation of grasp through anticipatory control. In patients/clients with neurological problems, in whom distal control may be hindered due to high or low muscle tone or secondary joint impairments, intervention strategies mirror that of the proximal joints. Providing joint alignment, increasing ROM, improving voluntary movement control and strength, and decreasing spasticity are some common goals. Practice of movements of the hand using functional and task-related activities tends to engage the patient and translate into increased carryover compared with rote exercises (Trombly & Wu, 1999). Intervention often begins with the establishment of a power grasp through activities using different objects. This is then followed by progression toward more precise pinch patterns, such as lateral pinch, three-point pinch, and two-point pinch (see Figs. 9–1 to 9–5) (Duff, 1995; Shumway-Cook & Woollacott, 2001). The objects being grasped need to be considered because their attributes influence anticipatory hand formation and grasping patterns based on experiential perceptions. In-hand manipulation activities using different sized and textured objects can be incorporated into intervention using the principles of motor learning, in which practice and verbal or visual cueing are provided. Everyday functional activities such as writing, money handling, and securing buttons and snaps can be incorporated into intervention for in-hand manipulation tasks. For extremely contracted and tight hands, in which hygiene is of major concern, serial casting, splinting, and botulinum toxin (Botox) injections may be helpful (see Chapter 7).

▪ Release

For individuals who have difficulty with active release due to spasticity, techniques to reduce muscle tone, such as vibration, tapping, or slow, sustained stretch, may help to begin the process of release. As in the section on CP, the typical sequence of developing mature release starts with external support, such as a table or opposite hand, and may be a place to start with the individual with decreased control. Attempting to work on release with wrist in the neutral position or slight extension, compared with flexion, also decreases the abnormal pattern and begins to work on active strengthening of the antagonist muscles.

Parkinson's Disease

Parkinson's disease is a chronic, progressive disease that affects approximately 1 million adults in the United States (Morris, 2000). As described in Chapter 7, individuals with Parkinson's disease (PD) have motor disturbances that include bradykinesia (slowness of movement), akinesia (absence of movement), tremor (at rest), rigidity (resistance to passive movement), and postural abnormalities (Montgomery, 1995). If present, any of these movement disorders can have an effect on the person's ability to reach, grasp, and manipulate objects. In the following section, impairment of upper extremity function due to Parkinson's disease and clinical management techniques will be discussed.

▪ *Regard*

Individuals with PD can have specific visual impairments that can limit their ability to regard objects. Visual disturbances include blurry vision, decreased acuity, and lack of smooth visual pursuits due to impaired saccadic eye movements and disconjugate gaze (O'Sullivan, 2001a). Many people with PD use their visual system to help override some of the motor disturbances. It is therefore important to determine if underlying visual impairments exist, especially if the therapist is using vision as a compensatory strategy to assist with functional movement.

The hallmark movement disturbances of rigidity, bradykinesia, and akinesia can affect the individual's ability to visually regard objects by decreasing the opportunity for the person to turn his or her head or body to visually track an object. The common posture in patients with PD is that of a forwardly flexed trunk with flexion of the neck, hip, and knees (O'Sullivan, 2001a) (Fig. 9–15). This posture may also decrease the ability to visually attend to objects in the environment due to head position.

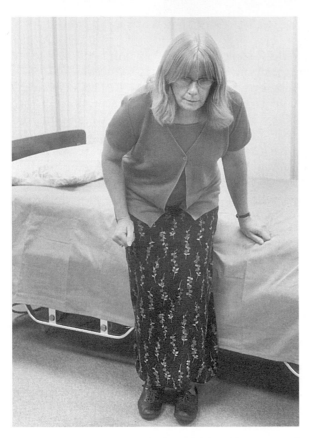

Figure 9–15. Model displaying forward flexed posture when getting out of bed.

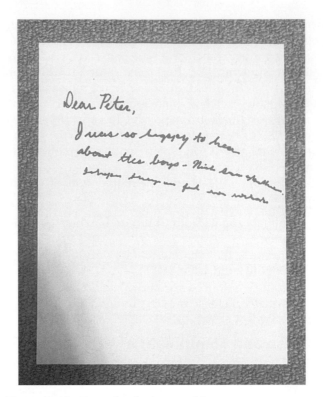

Figure 9–16. Example of micrographia.

▪ Reach

The impairment of reach can be varied in the individual with PD. Motor disturbances described earlier (bradykinesia, akinesia and rigidity) often hinder the person's ability to initiate reach. If the person can reach for something very slowly and does not need to use multiple joints and movements to attain the object, the reach may be successful (Shumway-Cook & Woollacott, 2001). If the movement amplitude is increased and the person is attempting to reach for something with increased speed and accuracy, reach capability may be decreased. Success in reach for the person with PD also depends on the task itself and the context. More difficulty in reach and grasp is noted in tasks that have multiple steps or use complex action sequences (Morris, 2000). Because many daily tasks, such as bathing, grooming, eating, and toileting, require multiple steps, individuals with PD are unable to complete these tasks or can only accomplish them extremely slowly.

▪ Grasp and Manipulation

Because grasp and manipulation require movement coordination across multiple joints, patients with PD have difficulty with many fine motor skills. Their ability to complete fine motor tasks that have multiple steps is hindered by the inability to string movements together and to initiate multiple movement sequences. Regulating grip forces, both generating enough force to lift something and sustaining grasp on an object, are impaired (Shumway-Cook & Woollacott, 2001). Time to generate grip force is often increased, which can cause excessive grip force to be generated. An example of a fine motor task that is extremely difficult for individuals with PD is handwriting. Handwriting uses coordination of multiple joints and multiple movements. Therefore, a person with PD has increased time and effort when writing. Typically, the person with PD starts off writing at a normal speed and strokes are within normal limits. As the task continues, speed decreases, as does size and legibility of the strokes, leading to **micrographia** (abnormally small handwriting) (Morris, 2000) (Fig. 9–16).

▪ Release

Difficulty with release or delayed release is present in the individual with Parkinson's disease. When grasp and release are completed at the patient's preferred speed, release may be without impairment. When the patient is asked to increase his or her speed, release time is decreased (Shumway-Cook & Woollacott, 2001). Initiating release, if it is part of a multitask activity, may be difficult for persons with PD due to their limited ability to string tasks together and use internal cues.

▪ Clinical Management of Parkinson's Disease

It is difficult to separate intervention techniques for the individual with PD into regard, reach, manipulation and grasp, and release due to the generalizability of techniques for all the components. Therefore, this section will give an overview of intervention approaches for upper extremity impairment in the individual with Parkinson's disease.

Therapists and their assistants working with individuals with PD can decrease functional impairments by using cortical input to help bypass basal ganglia pathology (Morris, 2000). What this translates into as therapists is that external cues (verbal, visual, tactile, and proprioceptive) can assist the patient with PD in performing motor sequences. Examples of this are providing visual cues, such as lines on the floor to help with step length or lined paper to assist with handwriting strokes (Morris, 2000). However, the clinician must be aware of any visual limitations the patient has, if using vision as an external cue. Proprioceptive cues, such as rocking, can help to initiate movements like rolling to get out of bed. PNF patterns can assist with decreasing rigidity and increasing movement (O'Sullivan, 2001a). Verbal cues, such as "left arm," "right arm," can assist with dressing, and bathing. Music with a consistent tempo can provide an auditory cue that can help the individual maintain a rhythm during movement (Morris, 2000; Newman et al., 1995).

Individuals with PD also have increased difficulty executing complex motor sequences within the context of functional tasks. Breaking the task into small units leads to improved ability to perform the individual unit versus the complex task. During upper extremity movements, the ability to reach, grasp, and manipulate is impaired, as discussed previously. The following intervention suggestions to improve upper extremity function are adapted from Meg Morris (2000):

- Mentally rehearse the action sequence before it is performed with your patient/client and then have him or her incorporate this practice into daily activities.
- Look at the object being grasped before and during movement. This visual cue may help with planning and accuracy of the movement.
- Break fine motor tasks into individual parts and concentrate on each part separately.
- Verbally cue the task, such as "go" to move the arm for reach and "release" to let go of an object.
- Avoid environmental distractions or trying to do more than one task at a time.

Finally, adaptive equipment and techniques can

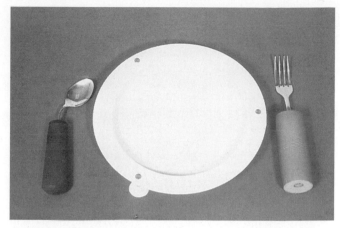

Figure 9–17. Scoop dish and utensils with enlarged handles.

assist with impaired upper extremity function during daily activities. Some suggestions include the following:

- Loose-fitting clothing, Velcro closures, elastic laces, and a reacher can assist with dressing.
- Enlarged utensil handles, plate guards, and scoop dishes can assist with feeding (Fig. 9–17).
- A raised toilet seat, tub bench, grab bars, and nonslip pads can assist in the bathroom.

Case Studies

The following case studies illustrate a therapist's approach to working with a patient with upper extremity dysfunction. The importance of the whole person and all areas of function are stressed in the case studies, as is the involvement of family members.

Case Study: Child
Michael: Child Born Prematurely

History

Michael is an 8 1/2 month old, adjusted age 4 1/2 months, who is referred for Early Intervention services. Michael's birth history is significant for premature birth at 24 weeks' gestation, birth weight of 1 pound, 4 ounces, grade III and IV intraventricular hemorrhages, retinopathy of prematurity (ROP), and bronchopulmonary dysplasia. He spent 4 months in the neonatal intensive care and underwent surgery for his ROP. Michael required ventilation and nasogastric (NG) feeding. He is currently on oxygen. He has not yet passed a hearing test. The family is involved in his overall care and concerned that he may have some longstanding impairments due to the hemorrhages he sustained.

Because Michael is under 3 years of age, he is eligible for Early Intervention services as provided through the Individuals with Disabilities Education Act (IDEA) Part C (Stephens & Tauber, 2001). These services are an entitlement, meaning that everyone who meets the eligibility criteria is entitled to services. Eligibility for services includes the following (Stephens & Tauber, 2001):

- If the child is an established risk due to a diagnosis such as Down syndrome
- If the child demonstrates a developmental delay on an appropriate evaluation tool
- If the child is at risk due to environmental risk factors such as low birth weight

Michael is eligible for services in two categories, his low birth weight and his developmental delay found on evaluation. For the state in which Michael resides, he must be delayed by 25 percent in one or more developmental areas to receive services. Early Intervention services for the birth to 3 population are family focused and occur in the natural environment, which means in the natural settings in which the child typically resides, such as home or day care.

Evaluation Findings

Michael was evaluated using the Battelle Developmental Inventory (BDI), observation, and parent interview. (Michael was evaluated based on his corrected age of 4 1/2 months.) The evaluation was completed with the mother, therapist, and Early Intervention service coordinator present. Mom expressed concern over Michael's left arm, which she felt moved less than the right. She also has some concerns over Michael's feeding.

Michael was alert and visually engaging. He visually tracked a red ring and his mom's face. He smiled and cooed at his mother and had increased movement when he saw either her or an interesting toy. He did not consistently respond to the sound of a bell, but his mother feels that he does turn, at times, to loud sounds. In supine, Michael tends to keep his head turned to the right and often held an ATNR posture (Fig. 9–18). When tracking an object, he was able to bring his head to midline and briefly to the left. His mom states that she notices that he tends to keep his head turned to the right. When in supine with his head in midline, Michael brings his hands together occasionally and will bring his right hand to his mouth. He is starting to actively bat at toys held overhead with the right hand greater than the left. He spontaneously opens both hands and will hold a placed rattle briefly in both hands. Lower extremities spontaneously kick. In supine, the center of gravity is in the midtorso area. When observed in supine, Michael's head eventually turns to the right and an ATNR is again seen.

In prone, Michael is irritable and has increased effort in breathing. He can lift his head but shoulders are elevated and retracted (left arm more so than right). In side lying, Michael's hands are together briefly, with left arm more flexed with scapular adduction. In pull to sit, Michael still demonstrates a head lag and in sitting is forwardly flexed and requires full support. During physical handling, Michael's muscle tone was noted to be slightly increased in his extremities, with the left upper extremity being slightly greater than the right. Clonus is present in both lower extremities, with the left greater than the right. During bottle feeding, Michael tended to gulp the formula and used a rather primitive suck. He displayed poor lip seal and took a long time to take 4 ounces of formula.

Intervention

Following the evaluation, an Individualized Family Service Plan (IFSP) was devised in which input from the family and team members was used to generate family-driven outcomes and objectives. The main outcome written by the family was that Michael would use his arms and legs to roll, sit, and crawl and would interact with his surroundings. The therapist was authorized to see Michael one time per week in his home for 60 minutes. The following intervention plan was devised.

Outcome: Michael will use his arms and legs to roll, sit, and crawl and will interact with his surroundings.

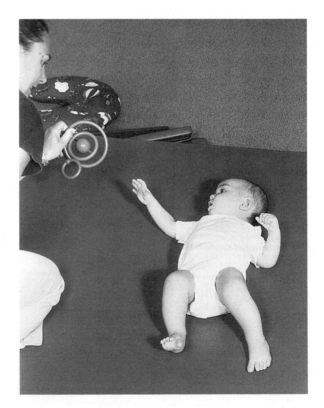

Figure 9–18. ATNR posture.

Methods and Materials   Family Training

Objective: Michael will maintain his head and hands in midline and bring his hands to his mouth in supine.

- Position Michael in a Boppy cushion (Fig. 9–19) or use rolls on his sides to help facilitate midline orientation.

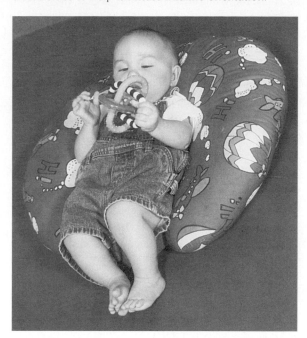

Figure 9–19. Positioning in the Boppy cushion to facilitate midline play.

- Have Michael visually regard objects brought to midline. Use objects that are visually stimulating because of possible hearing loss.
- In supine, gently facilitate head in midline with chin tuck and midline orientation of upper extremities in good alignment, without shoulder elevation or scapular adduction.
- Gradually facilitate pelvis elevation by gently flexing hips and tilting pelvis. Lower extremities can be visually regarded, and Michael can begin to bring hands to thighs and knees (Fig. 9–21).

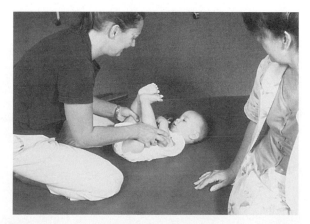

Figure 9–21. Therapist facilitating hands to knees in supine.

- Teach the family proper positioning options that promote midline orientation. Encourage use of a "jungle gym" toy in which toys are suspended above Michael to encourage batting at toys (Fig. 9–20).

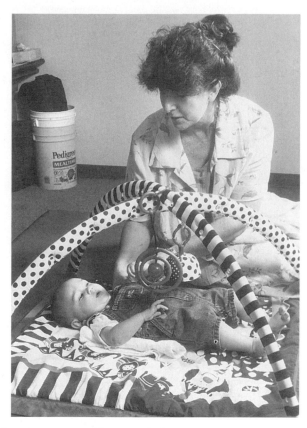

Figure 9–20. Use of suspended toys to encourage batting at toys.

- Have the family position visually stimulating objects in midline and left-hand side of crib to decrease right head turn preference.
- Teach family ways to hold Michael that incorporate hands and head in midline when carrying him and during feeding, diapering, and playing.

(Continued on the following page)

Methods and Materials	Family Training

Objective: Michael will tolerate the prone position for 2 minutes, holding head up and bearing weight on propped upper extremities.

- Place Michael in prone position with visually stimulating toys for him to visually regard. Facilitate elongation of the trunk and weight shift toward the hips to help assist with upper extremity weight bearing (Fig. 9–22).

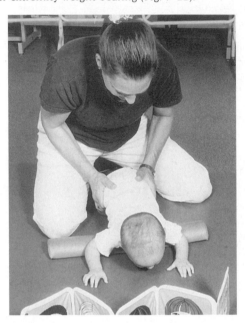

Figure 9–22. Therapist facilitating trunk elongation and upper extremity weight bearing.

- Position Michael prone over a small roll for support and introduce subtle lateral weight shifts.
- If Michael's hands are fisted, facilitate weight bearing on open hands or exploration of different toys with different textures or shape while in prone (Fig. 9–24).

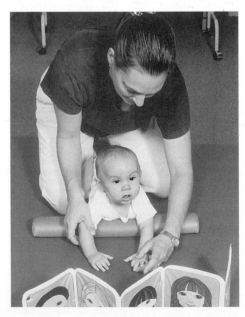

Figure 9–24. Weight bearing on upper extremities with hand open.

- Demonstrate to family prone positions that Michael will tolerate and how to use supports, such as a small roll under the chest (Fig. 9–23).

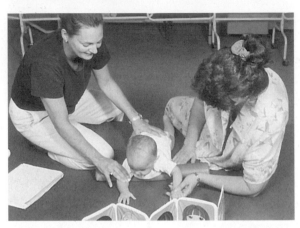

Figure 9–23. Therapist instructing family in prone positioning.

- Show family how to gently open Michael's hand if fisted and massage hand and introduce different textured and shaped toys for exploration (Fig. 9–25).

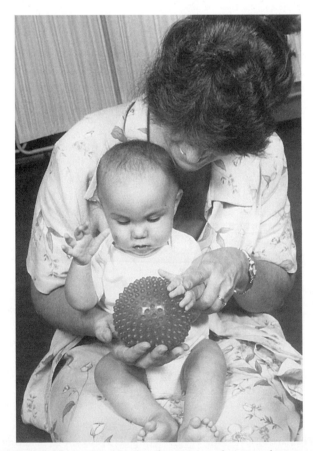

Figure 9–25. Instructing family on use of textured toys to encourage exploration of toys with his left hand.

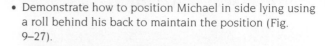

Methods and Materials	**Family Training**

Objective: Michael will bat at toys with both arms in a side-lying position and begin to roll toward prone and bear weight on arms in supported sitting.

- Roll Michael into side lying from supine on left and right sides. Facilitate elongation of the weight-bearing side (Fig. 9–26).

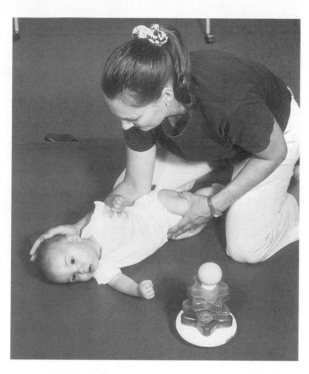

Figure 9–26. Facilitation of elongation of the weight-bearing side in side-lying position.

- Demonstrate how to position Michael in side lying using a roll behind his back to maintain the position (Fig. 9–27).

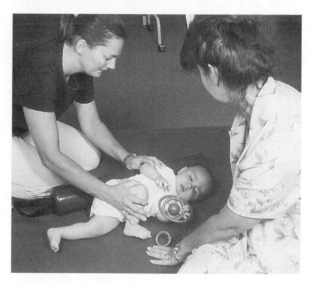

Figure 9–27. Family teaching of side-lying positioning with roll at back for support.

- Explain the importance of interaction with toys that engage Michael's visual and tactile systems to help compensate for decreased hearing.
- Demonstrate how to position Michael in supported sit with his arms propping in front or at sides.

- Once in side lying, encourage activities in which Michael is bringing hands together and visually attending to a toy held in his hand.
- Facilitate Michael's lower extremity into a weight-bearing position while in side lying (see Fig. 9–27).
- Shift weight onto left arm support in sitting on large therapy ball (Fig. 9–28).

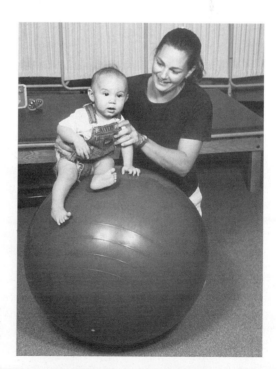

Figure 9–28. Therapist facilitating left upper extremity weight bearing on therapy ball.

Case Study: Adult

Elizabeth: Adult with Right Cerebrovascular Accident

History

Elizabeth is a right-handed 72-year-old woman with a diagnosis of a right cerebrovascular accident with left hemiparesis, which occurred 4 weeks ago. Her premorbid history is significant for mild arthritis in both hands and knees and hypertension. She is currently living with her daughter and has been referred to occupational therapy and physical therapy for outpatient services. Before her CVA, Elizabeth lived alone in a one-story home with her two cats and was independent in all her daily living skills. She has two other daughters who live in the area and are involved in her care, as well as members of her church who are assisting the family.

Evaluation Findings

Elizabeth is able to follow commands and is oriented to person, place, and time. She does exhibit some decreased attention and impulsivity but responds well to verbal cues. She demonstrates decreased perceptual abilities and moderate left neglect. Sensation is decreased to light touch, stereognosis, and localization.

Elizabeth exhibits flaccid muscle tone on the left side, greater in the upper extremity than the lower. Active movement in the left upper extremity is minimal, with the exception of some muscle tone in the pectoralis and levator scapulae and upper trapezius. Left upper extremity assumes the position of internal rotation, with the scapula downwardly rotated. The humerus is adducted, with the elbow in extension, forearm pronated, and wrist in slight flexion. A one-finger inferior subluxation is present, with complaints of some pain with PROM. Edema is present throughout the hand and wrist. Elizabeth exhibits decreased trunk control with lateral flexion to the left. Currently she is able to transfer with verbal cues for safety and impulsivity and ambulates with minimal assistance using a hemiwalker for short distances. The majority of the time is spent in a wheelchair, in which she is laterally flexed to the left. Elizabeth is able to use her right hand for grooming and eating but requires verbal cues due to left neglect and some assistance for activities requiring two hands. She requires minimal assistance for dressing due to neglect and decreased balance.

Intervention Goals

Intervention goals for Elizabeth include the following:

1. Improve postural control and alignment to help facilitate upper extremity function
2. Improve left upper extremity alignment and scapular mobility
3. Decrease left hand edema and increase pain-free ROM
4. Increase independence in ADLs
5. Educate patient and family on proper position techniques, edema management, and adaptive equipment to ensure good carryover

Intervention Strategies

Intervention strategies for Elizabeth include the following:

1. *Improve postural control and alignment to help facilitate upper extremity function*
   a. Using neurodevelopmental techniques in sitting, begin to work on subtle weight shifts and facilitation techniques to encourage trunk elongation on the left and improved upright trunk posture. Verbal and visual cues such as a mirror may also be helpful (Fig. 9–29).

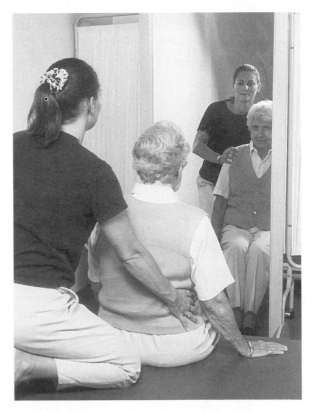

Figure 9–29. Therapist working on weight shifts in sitting in front of a mirror.

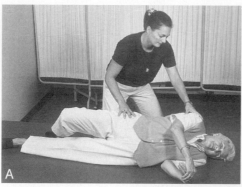
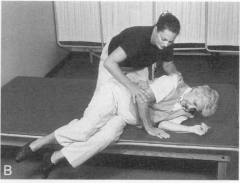
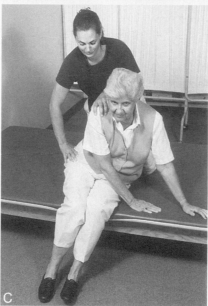

Figure 9–30. Instructing in a proper technique for rolling. Figure depicts initiation of trunk rotation (A), transition through side lying (B), and completion of movement into sitting (C).

b. Stressing symmetry, the therapist can work on functional skills, such as rolling and supine-to-sit transitions. The patient should be educated on how to roll and come to a sitting position from both sides. Cues to include the hemiplegic side may be needed due to neglect. Clasping hands together and pushing off with the lower extremity is a common technique for rolling (Fig. 9–30).

c. Improved positioning in the wheelchair is necessary. Left upper extremity should be supported with a lap tray. A left lateral support may be necessary to assist with proper trunk alignment and to bring the left upper extremity into the visual field (Fig. 9–31).

II. *Improve left upper extremity alignment and scapular mobility*

a. In sitting, the therapist begins with trunk in alignment and both upper extremities in forearm weight-bearing positions on a low table (Fig. 9–32).

b. Therapist facilitates scapular mobility and gentle approximation of the head of the humerus into the glenoid fossa.

c. Therapist provides a saddle-sling for ambulation. (Remember that a sling is only to maintain alignment achieved in therapy. It should be used with caution.) A resting hand splint is provided for nighttime use to prevent distal contracture (Fig. 9–33). A low-temperature thermoplastic wrist cock-up splint with thumb web space support is provided for use during the day.

III. *Decrease left hand edema and increase pain-free ROM*

a. Therapist uses manual pumping techniques to push fluid proximally so that it can be drained by the venous and lymphatic system. Compressive wraps, isometric contractions, and elastic gloves are other methods to decrease edema with mixed success.

b. Therapist should educate the patient and family/caretakers in pain-free ROM tech-

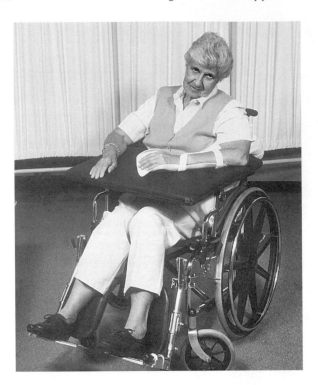

Figure 9–31. A lap tray and lateral support assist in helping achieve proper alignment in a wheelchair.

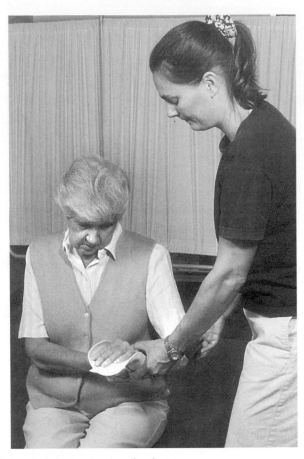

Figure 9–33. Resting hand splint.

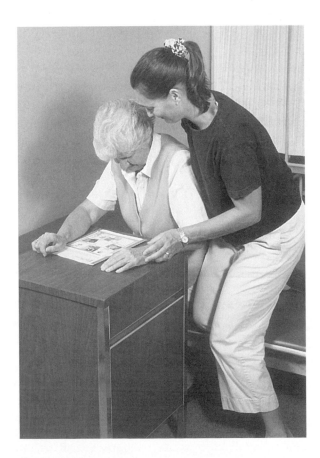

Figure 9–32. Upper extremity weight bearing at a low table.

niques. Self-ROM techniques (excerpted from O'Sullivan, 2001b, p. 551, with permission) are as follows:

1. Shoulder ROM to 90 degrees using an arm cradle position in which the unaffected upper extremity cradles the affected arm.
2. "Tabletop polishing"—the effected extremity is positioned in humeral flexion with scapular protraction and elbow extension, hand open and positioned on the table; the nonaffected hand guides the movement forward and back.
3. Tabletop positioning of the affected extremity with the trunk moving forward and back and rotating.
4. Sitting with hands clasped together and reaching towards the floor.

c. Therapist should educate the family/caretakers on strategies to decrease neglect of involved side. Elizabeth needs to be educated on positioning her left arm and not letting it fall to the side or behind her back for prolonged periods.

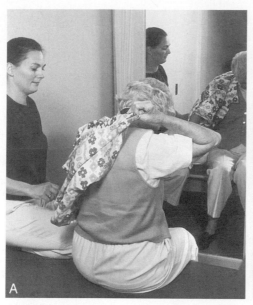
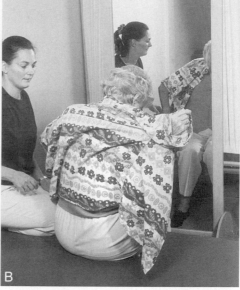

Figure 9–34. Practicing proper one-handed technique to don a shirt. Task requires reach across midline (A) and successfully moving the arm through the shirt opening (B).

IV. *Increase independence in ADLs*
a. Elizabeth should be taught one-handed techniques for grooming and dressing until she has better control of her left upper extremity. A technique for upper extremity dressing is to use loose clothing and place the hemiplegic arm in the sleeve first, bring the shirt across the back, and then place the nonaffected arm in the other sleeve (Fig. 9–34).
b. Adaptive equipment for dressing, bathing, and eating should be issued, and training on the use of the equipment should occur with Elizabeth and her family/caretakers. Some equipment recommendations include the following:
   Dressing: button hook for one-handed buttoning, long-handled shoe horn, sock aid to assist with putting on sock one handed, elastic laces, reacher (Fig. 9–35).
   Bathing: nonslip pad, grab bars, tub bench, wash mitt to slip soap into for one-handed washing.
   Eating: rocker knife for one-handed cutting, scoop dish or plate guard.
V. *Educate patient and family on proper position techniques, edema management, and adaptive equipment to ensure good carryover*
a. Techniques described earlier should all be taught to Elizabeth and her family to ensure good carryover. If possible, therapists should

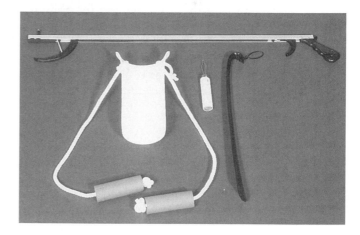

Figure 9–35. Adaptive equipment: reacher, sock-aide, button hook, long-handled shoe horn.

try to schedule family teaching sessions and meetings to discuss current goals and intervention strategies. Elizabeth should be a part of these meetings to empower her to increase her independence.

The therapist should also recommend at this time that a home visit be performed to make recommendations regarding adaptations to the home and adaptive equipment that may assist Elizabeth in being more independent.

Summary

This chapter has given a glimpse of the many systems that work together to allow individuals to use their arms and hands to interact with the environment. The sensory systems, such as vision, proprioception, and tactile, are vital in assisting the individual to reach, helping to adapt to changes in the environment, and refining the delicate in-hand manipulation skills that we often perform without much thought.

Through the development of proximal stability in weight-bearing positions as an infant and sensory exploration of objects in the environment, the individual gains the freedom to eventually engage in dynamic interactions with the environment using his or her upper extremities. These interaction can be as simple as brushing one's teeth or as complex as playing Mozart's Violin Concerto No. 4 (Fig. 9–36).

The upper extremity functions of regard, reach, grasp and manipulation, and release cannot be achieved without coordination of multiple body systems and the volition of the individual. Context, the role of the environment, and the actual tasks that are being performed have a great impact on the outcome and the ability to reach. It is through the knowledge of these intricate systems and the constraints of the environment and task that the therapist is able to assist individuals with neurological impairment in their ability to improve functional use of their upper extremity.

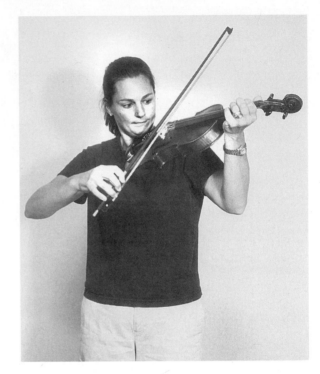

Figure 9–36. Movements of the upper extremity allow us to engage in an abundance of activities, from the most simple to the very complex.

References

Alexander, R., Boehme, R., & Cupps, B. (1993). *Normal development of functional motor skills: The first year of life.* Tucson, AZ: Therapy Skill Builders.

Amundson, S. J. (2001). Prewriting and handwriting skills. In J. Case-Smith (Ed.), *Occupational therapy for children* (4th ed., pp. 545–568). St. Louis, MO: Mosby.

Ayres, A. J. (1987). *Sensory integration and the child.* Los Angles: WPS.

Benbow, M. (1990). *Loops and other groups.* Tucson, AZ: Therapy Skill Builders.

Benbow, M. (1995). Principles and practice of teaching handwriting. In A. Henderson & C. Pehoski (Eds.), *Hand function in the child: Foundations for remediation* (pp. 255–281). St. Louis, MO: Mosby.

Bennett, S. E., & Karnes, J. L. (1998). *Neurological disabilities: Assessment and treatment.* Philadelphia: J. B. Lippincott.

Boehme, R. (1988). *Improving upper extremity control.* San Antonio, TX: Therapy Skill Builders.

Burton, A. W., & Dancisak, M. J. (2000). Grip form and graphomotor control in preschool children. *American Journal of Occupational Therapy, 54,* 9–17.

Byrne, D., & Ridgeway, M. (1998). Considering the whole body in treatment of the hemiplegic upper extremity. *Topics in Stroke Rehabilitation, 4,* 14–34.

Case-Smith, J. (1995). Object manipulation in infants and children. In A. Henderson & C. Pehoski (Eds.), *Hand function in the child:*

Foundations for remediation (pp. 136–153). St. Louis, MO: Mosby.

Case-Smith, J., Bigsby, R., & Clutter, J. (1998). Perceptual-motor coupling in the development of grasp. *Journal of Occupational Therapy, 52,* 102–110.

Cech, D., & Martin, S. (1995). *Functional movement development across the life span.* Philadelphia: W. B. Saunders.

Chaikin, L. E. (2001). Disorders of vision and visual-perceptual dysfunction. In D. A. Umphred (Ed.), *Neurological rehabilitation* (4th ed., pp. 821–854). St. Louis, MO: Mosby.

Cope, S. M., & Trombly, C. A. (1998). Grasping in children with and without cerebral palsy: A kinematic analysis. *Scandinavian Journal of Occupational Therapy, 5,* 59–68.

Danella, E., & Vogtle, L. (1992). Neurodevelopmental treatment for the young child with cerebral palsy. In J. Case-Smith & C. Pehoski, *Development of hand skills in the child* (pp. 91–110). Bethesda, MD: American Occupational Therapy Association.

Downing-Baum, S. (1995). Exercises in pediatric vision therapy. *Occupational Therapy Week, 9,* 20–22.

Duff, S. V. (1995). Prehension. In D. Chec & S. Martin, *Functional movement development across the life span* (pp. 313–354). Philadelphia: W. B. Saunders.

Duff, S. V. (2002). Prehension. In D. Chec & S. Martin, *Functional movement development across the life span* (2nd ed., pp. 428–465). Philadelphia: W. B. Saunders.

Eliasson, A. (1995). Sensorimotor integration of normal and impaired development of precision movement of the hand. In A. Henderson & C. Pehoski (Eds.), *Hand function in the child: Foundations for remediation* (pp. 40–54). St. Louis, MO: Mosby.

Erhardt, R. P. (1992). Eye-hand coordination. In J. Case-Smith & C. Pehoski (Eds.), *Development of hand skills in the child* (pp. 13–34). Bethesda, MD: American Occupational Therapy Association.

Exner, C. E. (1992). In-hand manipulation. In J. Case-Smith & C. Pehoski (Eds.), *Development of hand skills in the child* (pp. 35–46). Bethesda, MD: American Occupational Therapy Association.

Exner, C. E. (2001). Development of hand skills. In J. Case-Smith (Ed.), *Occupational therapy for children* (4th ed., pp. 289–328). St. Louis, MO: Mosby.

Fetters, L., & Kluzik, J. (1996). The effects of neurodevelopmental treatment versus practice on the reaching of children with spastic cerebral palsy. *Physical Therapy, 76,* 346–358.

Gillen, G. (1998). Upper extremity function and management. In G. Gillen & A. Burkhardt, *Stroke rehabilitation: A function based approach* (pp. 109–151). St. Louis, MO: Mosby.

Hay, L. (1990). Developmental changes in eye-hand coordination. In C. Bard, M. Fleury, & L. Hay (Eds.), *Development of eye-hand coordination across the life span* (pp. 217–244). Columbia, SC: University of South Carolina Press.

Gibson, J. J. (1966). *The senses considered as perceptual systems.* Boston: Houghton Mifflin.

Kaufman, T. (1994). Mobility. In B. R. Bonder & M. B. Wagner, *Functional performance in older adults* (pp. 42–61). Philadelphia: F. A. Davis.

Levine, K. J. (1991). *Fine motor dysfunction: Therapeutic strategies in the classroom.* Tucson, AZ: Therapy Skill Builders.

Leonard, C. T. (1998). *The neuroscience of human movement.* St. Louis, MO: Mosby.

Ma, H., & Trombly, C.A.(2001). The comparison of motor performance between part and whole tasks in elderly persons. *American Journal of Occupational Therapy, 55,* 62–67.

McCale, K., & Cermak, S. (1992). Fine motor activities in elementary school: Preliminary findings and provisional implications for children with fine motor problems. *American Journal of Occupational Therapy, 46,* 898–903.

Mcgill, R. (2001) *Motor learning concepts and applications* (5th ed.). Madison, WI: Brown and Benchmark.

Menken, C., Cermak, S. A., & Fisher, A.G. (1987). Evaluating the visual perceptual skills of children with cerebral palsy. *American Journal of Occupational Therapy, 41,* 646–651.

Montgomery, E. B. (1995). Bradykinesia and akinesia of parkinsonism: Implications for physical therapy. *Neurology Report: Neurology Section of APTA, 19,* 23–29.

Morris, M. E. (2000). Movement disorders in people with Parkinson's disease: A model for physical therapy. *Physical Therapy, 80,* 578–596.

Myers, C. A. (1992). Therapeutic fine-motor activities for preschoolers. In J. Case-Smith & C. Pehoski (Eds.), *Development of hand skills in the child* (pp. 47–62). Bethesda, MD: American Occupational Therapy Association.

Napier, J. R. (1956). The prehensile movement of the human hand. *Journal of Bone and Joint Surgery, 38,* 902–913.

Nelson, C. C. (2001). Cerebral palsy. In D. A. Umphred (Ed.), *Neurological rehabilitation* (4th ed., pp. 259–286). St. Louis, MO: Mosby.

Niemeier, P. P., Cifu, D. X., & Kishore, R. (2001). The lighthouse strategy: Improving the functional status of patients with unilateral neglect after stroke and brain injury using a visual imagery intervention. *Topics in Stroke Rehabilitation, 8,* 10–18.

Newman, E. M., Echevarria, M. E., & Digman, G. (1995). Degenerative diseases. In C.A. Trombly (Ed.), *Occupational therapy for physical dysfunction* (4th ed., pp. 735–752). Baltimore: Williams & Wilkins.

O'Sullivan, S. B. (2001a). Parkinson's disease. In S. B. O'Sullivan & T. J. Schmitz (Eds.), *Physical rehabilitation: Assessment and treatment* (4th ed., pp. 747–782). Philadelphia: F. A. Davis.

O'Sullivan, S. B. (2001b). Stroke. In S. B. O'Sullivan & T. J. Schmitz (Eds.), *Physical rehabilitation: Assessment and treatment* (4th ed., pp. 519–582). Philadelphia: F. A. Davis.

Pehoski, C. (1995). Cortical control of skilled movements of the hand. In A. Henderson & C. Pehoski (Eds.), *Hand function in the child: Foundations for remediation* (pp. 3–15). St. Louis, MO: Mosby.

Pehoski, C. (1995). Object manipulation in infants and children. In A. Henderson & C. Pehoski (Eds.), *Hand function in the child: Foundations for remediation* (pp. 136–153). St. Louis, MO: Mosby.

Pellegrino, L. (1997). Cerebral palsy. In M. L. Batshaw (Ed.), *Children with disabilities* (pp. 499–525). Baltimore: Paul H. Brookes.

Reily, M. (1962). The Elenor Clarke Slagle lecture: Occupational therapy can be one of the great ideas of 20th century medicine. *American Journal of Occupational Therapy, 16,* 1–9.

Rogers, S. L., Gordon, C. Y., Schanzenbacher, K. E., & Case-Smith, J. (2001). Common diagnoses in pediatric occupational therapy. In J. Case-Smith (Ed.), *Occupational therapy for children* (4th ed., pp. 136–189). St. Louis MO: Mosby.

Roth, E. J., & Olson, D. A. (Eds.). (2001). Introduction. *Topics in Stroke Rehabilitation, 8,* 1.

Ryerson, S. (2001). Hemiplegia. In D. A. Umphred (Ed.), *Neurological rehabilitation* (4th ed., pp. 741–789). St. Louis, MO: Mosby.

Ryerson, S., & Levit, K. (1997). *Functional movement reeducation: A contemporary model for stroke rehabilitation.* New York: Churchill Livingstone.

Scheiman, M. (1997). *Understanding and managing visual deficits: A guide for occupational therapists.* Thorofare, NJ: Slack.

Scherzer, A. L., & Tscharnuter, I. (1982). *Early diagnosis and therapy in cerebral palsy.* New York: Marcel Dekker.

Schneck, C. M. (2001). Visual perception. In J. Case-Smith (Ed.), *Occupational therapy for children* (4th ed., pp. 382–412). St. Louis, MO: Mosby.

Schneck, C. M., & Henderson, A. (1990). Descriptive analysis of the developmental progression of grip position for pencil and crayon control in nondysfunctional children. *American Journal of Occupational Therapy, 44,* 893–900.

Schumway-Cook, A., & Woollacott, M. H. (2001). *Motor control: Therapy and practical applications* (2nd ed.). Philadelphia: Lippincott Williams & Wilkins.

Shiffman, L. M. (1992). Effects of aging on adult hand function. *American Journal of Occupational Therapy, 46,* 785–792.

Stephens, L. C., & Tauber, S. K. (2001). Early intervention. In J. Case-Smith (Ed.), *Occupational therapy for children* (4th ed., pp. 708–730). St. Louis, MO: Mosby.

Stillwell, J. M., & Cermak, S. A. (1995). Perceptual functions of the hand. In A. Henderson & C. Pehoski (Eds.), *Hand function in the child: Foundations for remediation.* (pp. 55–80). St. Louis, MO: Mosby.

Strickland, J. W. (1995). Anatomy and kinesiology of the hand. In A. Henderson & C. Pehoski (Eds.), *Hand function in the child: foundations for remediation* (pp. 16–39). St. Louis, MO: Mosby.

Starkes, J. L. (1990). Eye-hand coordination in experts: From athletes to microsurgeons. In C. Bard, M. Fleury, & L. Hay (Eds.), *Development of eye-hand coordination across the life span* (pp. 309–326). Columbia, SC: University of South Carolina Press.

Sugden, D. A. (1990). Role of proprioception in eye-hand coordination. In C. Bard, M. Fleury, & L. Hay (Eds.), *Development of eye-hand coordination across the life span* (pp. 133–156). Columbia, SC: University of South Carolina Press.

Trombly, C. A., & Wu, C. (1999). Effects of rehabilitation tasks on organization of movement after stroke. *American Journal of Occupational Therapy, 53,* 333–344.

Unsworth, C., & Warburg, C. L. (2001). Assessment and intervention strategies for cognitive and perceptual dysfunction. In S. B.

O'Sullivan & T. J. Schmitz (Eds.), *Physical rehabilitation: Assessment and treatment* (4th ed., pp. 961–997). Philadelphia: F. A. Davis.

Yasukawa, A. (1992). Upper extremity casting. In J. Case-Smith & C. Pehoski (Eds.), *Development of hand skills in the child* (pp. 111–123). Bethesda, MD: American Occupational Therapy Association.

Zoltan, B. (1996). *Vision, perception and cognition: A manual for the evaluation and treatment of the neurologically impaired adult* (3rd ed.). Thorofare, NJ: Slack.

Zorowitz, R.D. (2001). Recovery patterns of shoulder subluxation after stroke: A six-month follow-up study. *Topics in Stroke Rehabilitation, 8,* 1–9.

10

Management of Impaired Lower Extremity Function

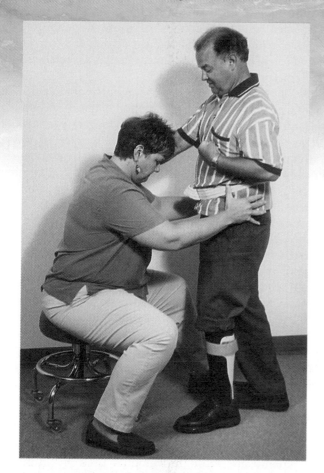

With hope, each step leads forward.
Author Unknown

This final chapter is dedicated to all the aspiring therapists and assistants of the future. Never underestimate the blessings that come from giving to others.

- Neuromuscular impairments resulting in impaired lower extremity function

- Functional limitations in gait: a task-oriented approach

  - Weight acceptance, single limb support, limb advancement

  - Effect of an assistive or orthotic device on the functional task of walking

- Lower extremity control problems associated with common neurological disorders: clinical management

Cornerstone Concepts

- Functional tasks of the lower extremity

- Locomotion: rolling, crawling and creeping, walking, and transfer tasks

  - Functional tasks of gait

  - Gait through the life span lens

- Abnormal lower extremity function and impaired locomotion

  - Implications for therapeutic intervention

Introduction

This is the final chapter on management of the common clinical dilemmas faced by individuals with movement dysfunction due to neurological disorders. This chapter will focus on the lower extremity by discussing the functional tasks of the lower extremity, describing the main locomotor or mobility tasks so important for functional retraining, and describing clinical management of common lower extremity functional limitations encountered at different ages and accompanying common neurological disorders.

Functional Tasks of the Lower Extremity

Function, as defined in this text (see Chapter 4), is the act of carrying out or performing an activity, referring to a specific role or occupation. Functional movements are the movement patterns that are used for or adapted to a function or group of similar functions (Ryerson & Levit, 1997). As such, functional movement is made up of coordinated movements of the trunk, upper extremities, and lower extremities. Functional movement is able to develop and be maintained as long as several key elements are present: adequate mobility and range of motion, appropriate muscle tone and strength, evidence of variability and isolation of movements, postural stability and central control, antigravity control, proximal stability, mature weight-bearing and weight-shifting capabilities, and the ability to make postural adjustments.

Functional movements of the extremities rely on the specific task-related movements required, often divided into two broad categories: weight-bearing or closed-chain activities and non–weight-bearing or open-chain activities. Skillful use of both the upper and lower extremities requires the ability to be functional in both weight-bearing and non–weight-bearing positions.

Lower extremity control includes the ability to support body weight on both legs, to transfer weight from one to the other, to bear weight on one leg and then move the other, and to constantly adapt to movements of the trunk and upper extremities. Human beings use lower extremity control with trunk control for safety and balance within a wide variety of position options. Lower extremity capabilities allow for all of the functions of moving the body through space, including all of the locomotor skills of rolling, crawling and creeping, walking, running, skipping, and hopping. Functionally, the main task of the lower extremities is more often concerned with weight bearing, stability, and mobility, including all the gross motor activities that accomplish the task of locomotion through space: rolling, crawling and creeping, and walking. However, lower extremity function in non–weight bearing is also important for full independent function. The author acknowledges the excellent work of Ryerson and Levit (1997, adapted with permission from Elsevier) used as a guideline to help organize portions of this chapter.

Non–Weight Bearing

Non–weight-bearing activities of the extremities are movements of the extremity in space, often referred to as **open-chain activities.** In the open chain, the distal end of the extremity is not fixed on the supporting surface and the extremity is free to move through space. Non–weight-bearing movements are used functionally to position the extremity for task performance, to execute the movement patterns required by the task, and to return the extremity from this functional position to a position of rest against the body. Non–weight-bearing movements are usually related directly to task performance (Ryerson & Levit, 1997). Open-chain movements have a great deal more variability than closed-chain weight-bearing movements. Most functional use of the upper extremity (UE) is associated with movement in the open chain.

Non–weight-bearing movements of the lower extremity have important functional uses. The swing phase of gait or flexion of the leg to go up a step or engage in a dressing activity are examples of lower extremity non–weight-bearing functional movements. Because a relatively small number of movement patterns are used to perform many similar functions, it is possible to identify the patterns of lower extremity movement that are most critical for functional performance. These generalized lower extremity patterns are movement patterns that involve predictable sequences of joint movement and patterns of muscle activation. These sequences of joint movement and muscle activation can be used with many variations to perform many similar activities. For example, unilateral stance with flexion of the opposite leg is used for the following similar but different tasks: stepping up, bring the foot up to the hand (as for dressing), or moving an object out of the way (Ryerson & Levit, 1997).

Non–weight-bearing movements of the lower extremities are vitally important in many positions, including the functional positions of sitting and standing. In sitting, non–weight-bearing lower extremity movements are those movements used in sitting to change body position or to engage in activities of daily living (Fig. 10–1). One of the most important prerequisites for non–weight-bearing movements of the leg in sitting is adequate trunk control. The trunk must be active and stable in sitting to provide stability for the leg as it lifts up. As one leg lifts off the supporting surface, the base of support (BOS) for the trunk becomes smaller. Additional trunk control is needed to adapt and adjust to the demands of the moving leg. According to Ryerson and Levit (1997), the following are the main movement components of the lower extremity required for non–weight-bearing functional performance in sitting:

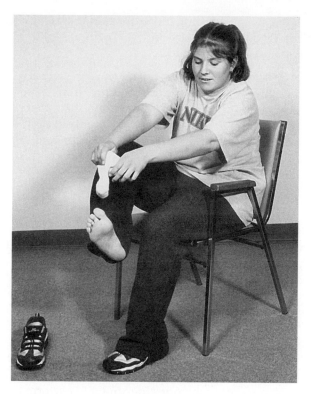

Figure 10–1. An example of a non–weight-bearing movement of the lower extremity is moving the limb into flexion to bring the foot to the hand for dressing.

- Hip flexion
- Abduction and adduction
- Knee flexion and extension
- Ankle dorsiflexion and plantar flexion

Any limitation in these movements secondary to immobility, weakness, or interference from abnormal muscle tone may result in a functional limitation.

In standing, to move the non–weight-bearing leg forward, alignment and control of the trunk, trunk and pelvic stability, and sequenced muscle activation patterns all allow the leg to move forward. In non–weight-bearing movements of the leg, the spine, pelvis, and femur move together in complex patterns that increase in complexity when balance is challenged or as the task becomes more difficult. According to Ryerson and Levit (1997), the following are the main movement components of the lower extremity required for non–weight-bearing functional performance in standing:

- Hip flexion with knee flexion
- Hip extension with knee extension
- Hip extension with knee flexion
- Hip abduction with knee extension
- Ankle plantar flexion and dorsiflexion

Any limitation in these movements secondary to immobility, weakness, or interference from abnormal

muscle tone may result in a functional limitation. Functional goals for the lower extremity during non–weight-bearing movements in standing are to move the affected leg in standing for comfort, to position the leg, to perform functional activities, and to use the leg as part of a balance response (Fig. 10–2).

Weight Bearing

The lower extremity is commonly associated with the function of weight bearing. **Weight bearing** occurs when the extremity or extremities are stabilized against a surface in a position where they support body weight and form part of the body's base of support. A weight-bearing pattern is also referred to as **closed-chain activity,** where the distal end of the body segment is fixed on the supporting surface and the proximal ends are free to move. During weight bearing, extremity muscles are active to maintain a stable contact with the supporting surface, to maintain good alignment over distal segments, and to lift and support the weight of the body against the force of gravity. Because the weight-bearing extremity is fixed on the supporting surface, any move-

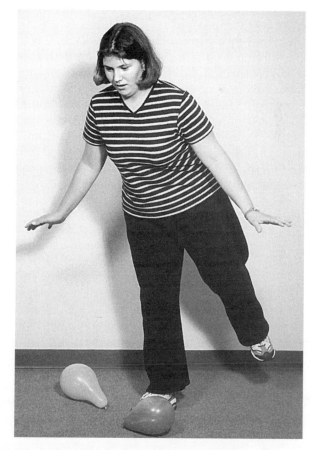

Figure 10–2. Movement of the lower extremity in non–weight-bearing as part of a balance response.

ment of the body over its distal BOS results in a change in the position of the joints of the weight-bearing extremity and a change in weight distribution over the portion of the weight-bearing extremity in contact with the support.

Clinical Connection:

Closed-chain activities are important for the development of mature upper and lower extremity patterns. In the young child, the upper extremity is often in a weight-bearing position during development in the prone position. As the young child pushes up in prone onto extended upper extremities, weight is shifted over the surface of the open hand while the baby engages in a functional activity such as reaching. This weight shifting over the weight-bearing hand serves to open the hand, activate fine motor muscles, elongate the finger flexors, increase tactile and kinesthetic sense, and ultimately prepare the hand for later precise function in non–weight-bearing activities, including precision handling. The same phenomenon occurs with the lower extremity where early stance allows for a great deal of weight shifting over the foot, allowing for the development of mature lower extremity function. ▪

As body weight is shifted around the weight-bearing extremity, the patterns of muscle activation in the weight-bearing limb change. This allows the limb to remain stable while supporting the new distribution of weight. These changes in muscle activity are important postural adaptations in the weight-bearing extremity. The part of the leg that is supporting weight and the amount and type of muscle activation used during weight support will vary according to body position and functional activity (Ryerson & Levit, 1997).

Clinical Connection:

For example, in sitting, weight bearing over the lower extremities (LEs) is between the ischial tuberosities, the posterior thigh on the supporting surface, and the feet on the supporting surface. Active weight shifting of the trunk results in movement of the hip joints, changes in weight distribution, and consequent muscle activation around all the component parts. As the trunk moves, the movement changes the amount and distribution of the weight placed on the legs, changing the demand on the lower extremity muscles and altering the state of muscle activation. ▪

According to Ryerson and Levit (1997), common components of lower extremity weight-bearing patterns in sitting are as follows:

- Pelvic weight shifting (anteroposterior and lateral)
- Hip flexion and extension
- Hip abduction and adduction

Any limitation in these movements secondary to immobility, weakness, or interference from abnormal muscle tone may result in a functional limitation. The most common lower extremity weight-bearing task, however, is that required for stance control and ambulation.

▪ Stance Control

Lower extremity function in standing is based on the ability to coordinate control between the LEs and the trunk. Lower extremity strength and coordination are necessary for both task performance and support of the body. Trunk control in standing supplies the ability to remain upright and aligned as body weight is shifted between the feet, to respond to movements of the LE so that the body remains balanced, and to initiate and respond to upper extremity movements. Trunk control is a prerequisite for unimpaired stance control. Trunk control in standing includes the ability to perform trunk movements; to control the upper trunk over the lower trunk; to produce small changes in trunk posture that are used as postural adjustments to LE movements; to coordinate trunk and LE movements in functional sequences; and for complex movement patterns, power production, speed, and balance. Lower extremity control is the ability to support weight on both LEs, to transfer weight from one LE to the other, and to adapt to movements of the trunk and arms (Ryerson & Levit, 1997).

Recordings of **postural sway** have demonstrated that quiet stance is not totally stationary. There is a slow but continual shifting of body weight between the two limbs (Murray & Peterson, 1973; Perry, 1992). During stance, the lower extremity needs to respond both to weight shifts initiated by the LEs and to those initiated by the trunk. In both instances, the muscles of the lower extremity are activated to maintain stability and balance. Independent, safe standing is an important functional goal for most patients/clients. For individuals with neurological dysfunction, the ability to control the LEs and trunk in standing is a difficult and complex task. It requires lower extremity strength, alignment, muscle firing, and sequencing patterns, but also requires postural control for movement initiation, balance, and adaptation during functional performance.

The precise interaction between trunk and leg components allows for the mobility, balance, and postural control needed for walking, running, and moving in these upright positions independently, safely, and efficiently. Lower extremity control and trunk control are important for balance and safety in standing, during upper extremity tasks, and while walking (Ryerson & Levit, 1997). O'Sullivan and Schmitz (2001) offer the following descriptive guidelines as important characteristics of functional upright postural control in stance. An understanding of these stance characteristics can serve as a set of practical guidelines to help pinpoint problems seen in therapeutic assessment and intervention. If the therapeutic goal is to establish or reestablish stance control, clinicians should strive to help the patient/client meet the following descriptive prerequisites, which indicate controlled stance:

1. The BOS is small and the center of gravity (COG) is high.
2. The **limits of stability (LOS)** are determined by the distance between the feet and the length of the feet, as well as by the height and weight of the individual (usually 12 degrees anteroposterior and 16 degrees medial/lateral for adults).
3. There is minimal postural sway.
4. Postural stability is maintained by normal postural alignment (see basic biomechanics and kinesiology texts) (see Figs. 8–1 and 10–3).
5. Postural stability is maintained by minimal but important muscular activity: in the antigravity paraspinal extensor muscles of the trunk, abdominals, gluteus maximus, hamstrings, and soleus muscles. Hip abductors are important for lateral stability.
6. Vertical postural orientation is maintained through the integration of various sensory inputs: *vestibular* by stabilizing gaze, providing inputs to the labyrinths, and regulating postural tone; *somatosensory* by providing tactile and proprioceptive information; and *visual* by responding to visual cues.
7. Several postural strategies are available for maintaining upright balance: *ankle strategy* involving small shifts of the center of mass causing ankle muscle activation; *hip strategy* whereby larger shifts in the center of mass produce flexion or extension at the hips; or a *stepping strategy* where realignment is achieved by taking a series of rapid, small steps (see Chapter 8, Figs. 8–2 through 8–4).
8. Postural control has four dimensions: *static* for maintenance of upright posture; *dynamic* for controlling functional movements while in the posture (reaching, weight shifting); *reactive* for adjusting in response to changes in the center of mass or support surface; and *anticipatory*, which allows for preparation in advance of movement execution (O'Sullivan & Schmitz, 2001).

These eight characteristics are important components for unimpaired stance control. Therapists and assistants can use these guidelines to direct intervention

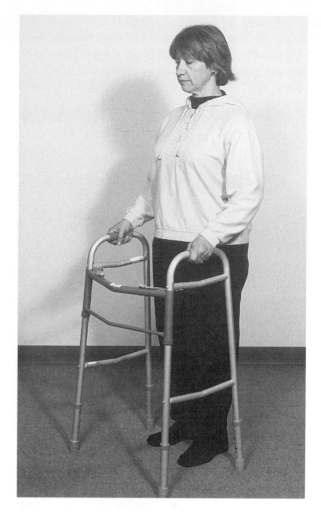

Figure 10–3. Normal alignment in stance. The figure also depicts the increase in BOS gained by the use of an assistive device.

efforts in establishing or re-establishing stance control in patients with neurological dysfunction.

Locomotion Defined

The term **locomotion** is defined as the process of moving from one place to another. Exactly how that is accomplished depends on several factors: the exact task to be done, the interaction of all the body subsystems that will perform the task, and the environment in which the task will take place (Cech & Martin, 1995, 2002). Locomotion solves a basic need of the individual: to transport the body from one location to another. Locomotion is a *variable* skill in that the movement form will differ depending on the goal and the particular movement solution needed to meet that particular goal. Locomotion, or this task of moving through space, includes many forms of movement, such as rolling, crawling and creeping, walking, running, galloping, skipping, and hopping. Locomotion is a skill that involves not only functional use of the lower extremities but also of the arm and hand complex. The arm-hand complex is often used in support of the locomotor act or can be a vital component of the movement (Craik & Oatis, 1995). Generally, however, the functional skill of locomotion is often associated mainly with lower extremity function.

Clinical Connection:

The environmental situation and the task goal will largely determine the type of locomotion that is appropriate. For example, if the goal is to get under the bed to retrieve a lost sock, and the space under the bed does not allow for upright posture or even a quadruped posture, a belly crawl may be the obvious solution to this movement dilemma. The size of the space under the bed and the parameters of the task allow for crawling and not creeping, rolling, or walking. Individuals with unimpaired locomotor abilities can exercise any number of choices from among locomotor patterns to arrive at a movement solution to accomplish a specific task. Individuals with disabilities or constraints in flexibility, strength, and fitness (to name only a few) may be limited in their options. ■

Control of the lower extremity is typically associated with locomotor abilities. The three major requirements for successful locomotion are **progression,** defined as the ability to generate a basic pattern that can move the body in the desired direction; **stability,** defined as the ability to support and control the body against gravity; and **adaptability,** defined as the ability to adapt the locomotion to meet the individual's goals and the demands of the environment (Shumway-Cook & Woollacott, 2001). This chapter will discuss the main locomotor patterns used in functional training or retraining of the individual with a neurological impairment, including rolling, crawling and creeping, transferring, and walking.

Rolling

Rolling is the earliest pattern used for locomotion, and it remains an important mobility skill throughout an individual's lifetime. As described in Chapter 4, **rolling** is defined as moving from supine to prone, or from prone to supine, usually involving some amount of rotation. Rolling has actually been described as a righting reaction because as the head rotates, the rest of the body rotates to become realigned with the head.

McGraw (1945) is credited with providing the most detailed account of how rolling progresses from infancy to the toddler stage. VanSant and colleagues (1990;

Richter, VanSant, & Newton, 1989) have done most of the observations and descriptions of rolling patterns as they change over the course of adulthood. A life span description of rolling is outlined in Table 10–1. The most significant differences in childhood versus adult rolling patterns is that during infancy, the development of a mature rolling pattern closely follows the emergence and development of functional movement components (see Chapter 4). Rolling patterns develop, change, and mature as the infant exhibits increasing mastery in antigravity extensor and flexor muscle strength, increasing dissociation both of the extremities from each other and the head and trunk from the extremities, and the emergence of smooth rotational patterns during movement. As an infant masters these fundamental movement skills, rolling progresses from being a spontaneous to a voluntary motion, and from an activity largely initiated by the head and neck and executed nonsegmentally (see Figs. 4–11 and 4–20) to a fluid segmental movement pattern with the body parts dissociated from each other (see Fig. 4–21). During adulthood, rotation and dissociation continue to be evident, but the pattern used by the adult may differ depending on upper body strength versus lower body strength, abdominal and trunk strength, and whether the individual has any limitation in flexibility (Fig. 10–4). Because segmental rolling requires dissociation between the pelvis and shoulders, an age-related change that may accompany degenerative joint changes with consequent pain and inflexibility is a return to a nonsegmental rolling pattern. Variations in the initiation of rolling patterns allow an individual to perform functionally meaningful activities, such as moving to answer the phone or retrieve a glass of water from a bedside table, or to provide automatic adjustments for comfort. The ability to roll allows an individual to change position and is a step in moving to sitting on the edge of the bed.

Throughout the life span, rolling is a meaningful and functional locomotor skill. For the retraining of rolling, Ryerson and Levit (1997) offer a very user-friendly breakdown of movement components as described in Table 10–2.

Crawling and Creeping

Crawling is defined as progression in the prone position where the belly is in contact with the supporting surface and the extremities are used in a reciprocal fashion to propel the body forward or backward. **Creeping** is defined as progression in quadruped where the belly is lifted off the supporting surface and the extremities move reciprocally to propel the body forward or backward (Cech & Martin, 1995). Developmentally, crawling typically precedes creeping and creeping requires more postural control than crawling because the belly is off the floor. Both methods require strength and are demon-

TABLE 10–1

Rolling as a Locomotor Pattern

Age	Description	Comments
Newborn	Spontaneous, involuntary	Because the newborn is in a predominantly flexed posture and because the infant does not yet have strength to overcome the force of gravity, any rolling other than accidental is not possible.
1–2 mo	Spinal extension	The emerging extension of the neck and upper spine permits rolling from side lying to supine.
4–5 mo	Log rolling	Movement is performed without segmental rotation where the body moves as a unit; permits rolling side lying to prone and prone to supine.
6–8 mo	Automatic rolling	Rolling is initiated usually by UEs, followed by trunk and LEs, although the reverse pattern may occur; a very deliberate action permitting successful movement from prone to supine and supine to prone.
8 mo	Segmental rolling	Movement is performed with deliberation, antigravity control, and segmentation, allowing rolling from supine to prone.
Adult rolling: a variety of patterns related to flexibility and muscle strength of the individual; two common patterns	Adult rolling pattern 1	From supine, movement is initiated by both upper extremities crossing to the side, followed by neck and then trunk flexion, trunk rotation, and lower extremity dissociation.
	Adult rolling pattern 2	From supine, one UE crosses over the trunk while the other pushes down into the surface; one LE pushes off the surface, followed by trunk rotation.

Sources: Adapted from McGraw, M. B. (1945). *The neuromuscular maturation of the human infant.* New York: Hafner Press; and adapted from Richter, R. R., VanSant, A. F., & Newton, R. A. (1989). Description of adult rolling movements and hypothesis of developmental sequences. *Physical Therapy, 69,* 63–71, with permission of the American Physical Therapy Association.

Figure 10–4. Adult rolling pattern where adult does not have any limitation in strength or flexibility—prone to supine (A) and supine to prone (B).

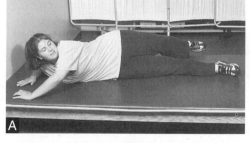 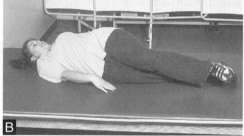

TABLE 10–2

Retraining Rolling

Functional Task: Rolling from supine to side lying, requiring a movement of the center of gravity from supine to side lying

Movement Initiation Possibilities	Transitional Movement Choices	Extremity Activity
Upper trunk flexion and rotation	Upper trunk initiation and lower trunk rotates to meet upper trunk	Upper trunk initiation and UE moves with trunk to assist
Lower trunk extension and rotation	Lower trunk initiation and upper trunk rotates to meet lower trunk	Lower trunk initiation and LE assists trunk movement
Nonsegmental pattern with spine in neutral	Nonsegmental initiation whereby upper and lower trunk move together	Nonsegmental initiation requiring that the trunk and extremities move together

Source: Excerpted from Ryerson, S., & Levit, K. (1996). *Functional movement reeducation,* with permission from Elsevier.

strated according to the demands of the environment and task. Crawling is often characterized by an actual propulsion of the body forward, accomplished by pushing off of the surface with a lower extremity and usually some degree of pulling or pushing with the upper extremity (see Fig. 4–22).

Newborn patterns of crawling and creeping have been studied extensively by McGraw (1945). Although adult patterns of prone and quadruped progression have not been studied extensively, the literature indicates that the reciprocal quadruped creeping pattern used in early childhood is the adult pattern of this movement behavior. It is safe to say that crawling and creeping are not commonly employed methods of locomotion after independent walking is achieved. The ability to creep or crawl is certainly retained throughout adulthood, retrievable if the environment or task requires it, as long as biomechanical factors such as strength and flexibility allow. Clinicians working with adults rarely concern themselves with practicing crawling or creeping. Rolling, on the other hand, is an important early locomotor pattern to be preserved and practiced at any life stage because of its obvious relevance to functional bed mobility.

Walking

Locomotion in the upright **bipedal** form demonstrated by humans occurs along a continuum from standing to walking to running and includes starting, stopping, changing direction, and altering speed (DeLisa, 1998). Gait is the means of achieving upright locomotion in the particular manner of moving on foot, which may be a walk, a jog, or a run. Walking is a particular form of gait, the most common of locomotion patterns. During walking, more than 1000 muscles are synchronized to move more than 200 bones around 100 moveable joints (Clark, 1995).

Gait Terminology

Because the task of human walking has so many components, clinicians and students must use a universal language to communicate with each other and with patients/clients about gait. For the basics of gait terminology, refer to other texts. The assumption is made in this text that the reader has a familiarity with the basic concepts and terminology related to the study of human gait. For the purposes of this text, and specifically this chapter, emphasis will be placed on the functional aspects of human upright locomotion, or gait.

Gait is studied and therefore discussed by using one or both of two description methodologies: kinematics or kinetics. **Kinematics** is the term used to describe move-

ment patterns without regard for the forces involved in producing the movement (Craik & Oatis, 1985). Information such as direction of movement or joint angles is included in a kinematic description of movement. **Kinetics,** on the other hand, is the term used to describe the forces involved in a movement. Kinetic descriptions typically include details about the muscular actions required to produce a given movement. When this chapter describes a range of motion requirement to accomplish a given gait task, a kinematic requirement is being described. Descriptions of muscular actions during gait are considered kinetic information. Therapists and assistants need to be concerned about both aspects because each contributes important requirements for efficient walking. Impairments in either may produce functional limitation or disability.

Functional Tasks of Gait

It is assumed that the readers of this text have a basic knowledge of the kinetics and kinematics of human gait. Consistent with the emphasis on functionality in this text, it is imperative that clinicians have an appreciation of the function of each of the eight subphases of gait so that observation, analysis, and intervention can be as accurate and meaningful as possible. A functional study of an individual's gait is performed by carefully assessing each phase of gait and the ability of the individual to meet the main three functional gait subtasks of limb loading, weight transfer, and limb advancement. Careful analysis of one joint at a time and one motion at a time will lead to a determination of contributing impairments and a practical clinical management plan.

Clinical Connection:

Amazingly, an entire gait cycle is completed in a little more than one second. Because gait occurs so quickly, with the subphases occurring in rapid succession, it is important that observers of gait (students and clinicians) have a method to guide observational gait analysis. The following guidelines are offered:

1. Observe the individual walking in a well-lit area devoid of obstacles, either in bare feet or wearing comfortable shoes and using an assistive device, if prescribed.

2. Observation should be of several strides, a distance of several meters with the observer standing at the middle of this distance in order to focus on typical walking and not on either the acceleration or deceleration portions of the walk.

3. Observe from a sagittal view and a frontal view, right and left sides, anterior and posterior.

4. Observe in a systematic fashion starting at the head and neck, and moving to the trunk, UEs, pelvis, hip, knee, and ankle/foot.

An active learning experience in the companion workbook includes a series of questions to be used to guide an observational gait analysis. ▪

The major requirements for successful walking are the production of a basic locomotor rhythm; support and propulsion of the body in the intended direction; dynamic control of the human body; and the ability to adapt the movement to changing environmental demands and goals (Forssberg, 1982). The literature is full of articles on gait and its analysis, with most authors agreeing upon the following as the three fundamental functional tasks associated with human gait: weight acceptance, single limb support, and limb advancement (Craik & Oatis, 1995; Pathokinesiology Department Ranchos Los Amigos, 1989).

The gait cycle, which includes an entire stride, is divided into two phases, stance and swing. These two phases are further subdivided into smaller components, or subphases, which largely describe their unique functional contribution to the overall task of walking. **Stance phase** comprises initial contact, loading, midstance, terminal stance, and preswing. **Swing phase** has three subphases: initial swing, midswing, and terminal swing. Figure 10–5 illustrates the eight subphases of gait and their functional contributions to the task of walking.

Of the three basic fundamental locomotor tasks,

stance phase is concerned with the fulfillment of all three basic tasks: weight acceptance, single limb support, and limb advancement. The subphases of stance phase all contribute to accomplishing these tasks, in varying degrees, as the lower limb functions to accomplish the principal goals of support, balance, propulsion, and the absorption of energy (Carr & Shepherd, 1998). The support function is met by the ability of the lower limb to accept weight, load weight onto it, and support the upper body. Initial contact and loading are the two subphases primarily responsible for these functions. Balance is functionally achieved through the maintenance of upright posture over the base of support, most challenged at the middle of stance (midstance) when a single limb supports the body's mass. Propulsion, as a task, involves the generation of mechanical energy to enable forward motion of the body through space and beginning limb advancement, these tasks met effectively at the terminal phases of stance, during the subphases of terminal stance and preswing. All of stance is concerned with the effective absorption and use of energy.

Of the three basic fundamental locomotor tasks, swing phase is concerned primarily with the fulfillment of mainly one of the three basic tasks: limb advancement. During swing, the lower limb's main function is to clear the foot from the ground, gain an adequate limb advancement, and prepare the foot for its landing again at initial contact. All three subphases of swing are subservient to this main functional task. During initial swing and midswing, the limb is flexed to functionally shorten the limb to clear the floor. Terminal swing is characterized by a rapid extension at the knee, effectively lengthening the limb to accomplish advancement and to form a rigid lever in preparation for landing.

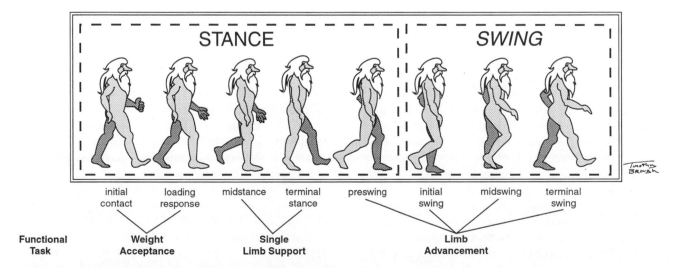

Figure 10–5. The gait cycle consists of two main phases, stance and swing, each further subdivided into five and three subphases, respectively. Specific main functional tasks are associated with each of these subphases. In this figure, the right limb (lighter shading) is the reference limb depicting the specific subphase.

It is important to remember that pelvic movement is a key component of normal gait and is often impaired in individuals with neurological disorders. The pelvis moves forward (protracts) on the swing side 4 degrees and backward (retracts) on the stance side another 4 degrees; producing an overall 8 degrees of pelvic movement in the transverse plane. The pelvis also tilts laterally about 5 degrees. These contributory motions of the pelvis are crucially important in minimizing the movement of the body's COG, thereby maximizing efficiency and contributing to a smooth forward and backward movement of the lower limb.

The muscular activation patterns recruited during human gait are a beautiful fluid pattern of activation, firing, and quieting, creating a sequence that is remarkably smooth and efficient. The major role of muscular forces during natural quiet walking is to provide the appropriate burst of power at the appropriate time in the gait cycle. Muscles act to initiate the movement, which is then carried through by the body's momentum, and then act again to brake the movement or momentum. Additional muscular force is required when walking fast and when climbing over uneven terrain, a slope, or up stairs. Muscular function during quiet walking requires a rather small amount of total force, when compared with what one would imagine is needed to accomplish the task of propelling a body mass forward. Muscles actually act over a relatively short period. During large intervals in the gait cycle, the limb is actually carried forward by its own inertia (Winter, 1985). The following sections describe the *main* muscular functional requirements during stance and swing phase (Craik & Oatis, 1985; Pathokinesiology Department Physical Therapy Department, 1989; Perry, 1992).

Throughout stance phase, the primary functional muscular requirements are subservient to the main functions of this phase: weight acceptance, loading and stabilization of the limb, energy absorption, and propulsion of the limb into swing phase. During initial contact, the limb must be positioned to accept weight. The anterior tibialis muscle maintains a stable antigravity ankle position and the hip is stabilized by activity of the gluteus medius and maximus muscles, even though the hip is positioned in flexion. All four knee extensor muscles are now firing eccentrically, having been activated during the end of swing phase, now decelerated by synergistic firing of the hamstring muscles to slow down the limb for landing. Loading of the limb is smoothed by eccentric power of the anterior tibialis muscle, lowering the foot to the floor. Shock is absorbed by eccentric control of the quadriceps muscle group, allowing weight to be accepted onto a LE with a slightly flexed knee. Activity in the gluteus maximus muscle increases as this large hip stabilizer meets the task of loading weight onto the limb. Midstance is the most precarious subphase of stance, requiring significant

restraint force supplied by the gastrocnemius and soleus muscles so that the ankle is maintained in a stable upright position, and the gluteal muscles (maximus and medius) work in concert with the entire hip abductor group to stabilize the limb in unilateral support. The quadriceps muscles are actually fairly inactive by midstance. Muscular power to the knee at this phase is largely supplied by the gastrocnemius, serving to restrain forward movement of the tibia in this closed chain, contributing to a stable stance. Terminal stance marks the beginning of the requirement to generate force for forward limb propulsion, and this power is effectively supplied by the gastrocnemius muscle, now stabilizing the knee and plantar flexing the ankle as the heel rises off the floor. Force for propulsion continues to be generated at the end of stance during preswing, from the gastrocnemius muscle, with an onset of activity in the hip adductors and rectus femoris muscle to create a burst of the limb forward into swing.

Throughout swing phase, the primary functional muscular requirements are subservient to the main functions of this phase: control of the momentum, limb advancement, and preparation again for stance. The muscular requirement for the main task of shortening the limb (to clear the floor) during initial and midswing subphases is met by the iliopsoas and anterior tibialis muscles with minimal assistance from the hamstring muscles. Maximum knee flexion must be accomplished by midswing to effectively clear the limb from the floor, but this is largely accomplished through pendular momentum rather than by active muscular contraction. Forward acceleration of the leg during initial swing is associated with a brief period of concentric quadriceps muscle force. By midswing, the quadriceps muscles are inactive, with forward acceleration being completed through pendular momentum of this swinging limb. A tremendous burst of momentum is largely responsible for supplying power from midswing into terminal swing, taking the LE from a position of maximum flexion to extension to advance the limb. The hip extensors (gluteus maximus and hamstrings) fire eccentrically to decelerate the rapidly advancing limb. The quadriceps muscles begin to fire again, now eccentrically, because initial contact will be made onto a flexed knee (for shock absorption). The anterior tibialis muscle maintains a stable ankle position in preparation for floor contact.

The joint range of motion and prime muscular force requirements needed to accomplish the functional requirements of gait at each of the eight subphases are important details for treating clinicians to know. Constraints in joint mobility or muscular force production will pose a dilemma for patients/clients trying to meet these main task requirements. If a clinician has a practical understanding of how the main functional tasks are accomplished, the clinician can then problem solve any encountered difficulties with gait as presented by a patient/client. Table 10–3 summarizes these functional requirements of gait, phase by phase (Craik & Oatis, 1985, 1995; Pathokinesiology Department Physical Therapy Department, 1989; Perry, 1992; Winter, 1985, 1987).

Gait, therefore, is made up of a series of subtasks very important to the patient and clinician. These subtasks of gait include the ability to demonstrate stable stance, unilateral LE limb loading, unweighting and advancement of an LE, effective shortening of the limb for floor clearance, effective propulsion of the limb from stance into swing, and transfer of weight to the forward advanced limb. To summarize, the following main guidelines are offered as an overview of the primary minimal muscular force requirements needed to accomplish these crucial subtasks of gait.

- Stable stance: bilateral gluteus maximus, gluteus medius, and gastrocnemius muscles
- Unilateral LE limb loading: gluteus maximus, gluteus medius, and gastrocnemius muscles on the stance side
- Effective propulsion of the limb from stance into swing: gastrocnemius muscle on the stance side
- Effective shortening of limb for floor clearance: iliopsoas, hamstrings, and anterior tibialis muscles on swing side
- Unweighting and advancing the unweighted lower extremity: hip extensors (eccentric), quadriceps and anterior tibialis muscles on the swing side
- Transfer of weight to forward advanced limb with LE stability and alignment: gluteus maximus and quadriceps muscles.

TABLE 10–3
A Practical Guide to the Functional Requirements of Gait

Subphase	Functional Task	Joint Angle Requirement	Prime Muscular Force
Initial contact	Weight acceptance Shock absorption	Ankle: 90 degrees Knee: 3–5 degrees flexion Hip: 30 degrees flexion	Tibialis anterior Quadriceps and hamstrings Gluteus maximus and medius
Loading	Weight acceptance Shock absorption	Ankle: 15 degrees plantar flexion Knee: up to 15 degrees flexion Hip: 30 degrees flexion	Tibialis anterior Quadriceps Gluteus maximus
Midstance	Single limb support	Ankle: from 15 degrees plantar flexion to 15 degrees dorsiflexion Knee: 5 degrees flexion Hip: full extension	Gastrocnemius and soleus Gluteus maximus, medius, and minimus Tensor fascia lata
Terminal stance	Single limb support Propulsion	Ankle: 15 degrees dorsiflexion to 20 degrees plantar flexion Knee: moves into full extension Hip: 10 degrees extension	Gastrocnemius
Preswing	Propulsion	Ankle: 20 degrees plantar flexion Knee: 40 degrees flexion Hip: 10 degrees extension	Gastrocnemius Hip adductors Rectus femoris
Initial swing	Limb shortening for foot clearance	Ankle: to neutral dorsiflexion Knee: 40–60 degrees flexion Hip: from extension to 30 degrees flexion	Tibialis anterior Quadriceps (controlling) Iliopsoas
Midswing	Limb shortening for foot clearance Generation of momentum	Ankle: neutral Knee: 60 degrees flexion Hip: 30 degrees flexion	Tibialis anterior Iliopsoas
Terminal swing	Limb advancement Preparation for initial contact Deceleration	Ankle: neutral Knee: to full extension Hip: 30 degrees flexion	Tibialis anterior Gluteus maximus and hamstrings

Sources: Information compiled from Craik, R. L., & Oatis, C. A. (1995). *Gait analysis: Theory and application.* St. Louis, MO: Mosby; Perry, J. (1992). *Gait analysis: Normal and pathological function.* Thorofare, NJ: Slack Inc.; Pathokinesiology Department Physical Therapy Department. (1989). *Observational gait analysis handbook.* Downey, CA: The Professional Staff Association of Rancho Los Amigos Medical Center; Winter, D. A. (1985). Concerning the scientific basis for the diagnosis of pathological gait and for rehabilitation protocols. *Physiotherapy Canada,*37, 245–252; and Winter, D. A. (1987). *The biomechanics and motor control of human gait.* Waterloo, Ontario: University of Waterloo Press.

Clinical Connection:

An appreciation of the functional contribution of different muscle groups to walking tasks offers an immediate translation into assessing and interrening with the clinical dilemmas encountered by patients with an impairment affecting those muscles or that functional task. Functionally, the muscular contributions can be summarized as follows:

Function	Muscles	Gait Phase
Shock absorbers	Quadriceps Dorsiflexors (anterior tibialis)	Initial contact Loading
Stabilizers	Gluteus maximus, medius, and minimus Tensor fascia lata Erector spinae	Stance
Propulsion	Gastrocnemius Toe flexors and ankle everters Soleus Tibialis posterior	Terminal stance Preswing
Accelerators	Adductor longus and magnus Sartorius Iliopsoas	Preswing Initial swing
Foot control	Anterior tibialis	Swing
Decelerators	Hamstrings	Terminal swing to initial contact

Source: Compiled from multiple sources.

Mastery of these concepts will form part of the basis for clinical management of gait problems demonstrated by patients/clients and discussed later in this chapter. ■

Gait Through the Life Span Lens

Immature Gait

The gait pattern of children is very different from a mature adult pattern of walking. Children have a wide-based gait, with stepping initiated primarily at the hips while keeping the knees fairly stiff. Steps are short, with increased periods of **double support** compared with adults. In children, the upper extremities are essential for balance during early walking. An understanding of the development of gait, the characteristics of immature versus mature gait, and the determinants of gait offer the clinician a framework for understanding and evaluating or assessing gait dysfunction in children. In all children through age 3, an immature gait pattern is typically characterized by the following (Burnett & Johnson, 1971):

1. Uneven **step length**
2. Swing phase characteristics: excessive hip and knee flexion, hip abduction, and external rotation
3. Stance phase characteristics: initial contact with foot flat rather than with heel contact, knee hyperextension throughout stance, loading and midstance weight bearing onto a pronated foot
4. Base of support wider than the lateral dimensions of the trunk
5. Upper extremities in a high-, medium-, and then low-guard position (see Fig. 4–42); transition from high **on-guard position** to beginning **reciprocal arm swing** normally occurs 4 to 5 months after the onset of walking
6. Lack of pelvic mobility such as tilt or rotation

Stride length is reduced and **cadence** is increased. To increase speed as needed, a child must increase cadence, because stride length is limited by leg length. Motions at the joints resemble the adult pattern by about age 3. By the age of 7, mature patterns are well established. Table 10–4 highlights the main functional gait changes that occur during childhood (Sutherland, Olshen, Cooper, & Woo, 1980).

Mature Gait

Mature, normal walking has five major attributes (Gage, 1991):

1. Stability in stance
2. Sufficient foot clearance in swing
3. Appropriate prepositioning of the foot during swing for initial contact
4. Adequate step length
5. Efficient use of energy

It is important to appreciate that these mature attributes do not magically appear, but rather develop over the course of several years, beginning with the first movements in infancy, through the early toddler years, and finally culminating in the demonstration of a mature adult walking pattern typically by age 7. The development of mature gait and the eventual emergence of these attributes are very dependent on first having the prerequisites for normal gait: adequate motor control and central nervous system (CNS) maturation (which implies an intact neurological system), adequate range of motion (ROM), strength, appropriate bone structure and composition, and intact sensation. Mature gait, usually achieved by the age of 7, is charac-

TABLE 10-4
Gait Changes over the Life Span

Age	Gait Changes
18 mo	Heel strike as point of initial contact Reciprocal arm swing emerging Usually can voluntarily increase walking speed for functional goal
2 y	Knee flexion more consistently present during stance
3 y	Gait pattern maturing: all adult components present except for increased cadence, and decreased step length still evident Running (with a nonsupport phase) is emerging
42 mo	BOS equal to or less than pelvic span
4 y	Reciprocal arm swing firmly established
6–7 y	Mature gait pattern Stride length increases as function of increasing leg length
Mature adult gait	Pelvic tilt and rotation Initial contact with a heel strike Knee flexion at midstance Mature relationship among mechanisms at the hip, knee, and ankle Mature base of support Reciprocal arm swing Refined muscle activation patterns Optimal energy efficiency
Older adulthood	Decreased velocity and slower cadence Decreased step and stride length Increased stride width and BOS Increased time in stance phase and in double support Decreased arm swing Decreased hip, knee, and ankle flexion Increased incidence of foot flat on initial contact Decreased dynamic stability during stance Re-emergence of muscular co-activation patterns

Sources: Data from Burnett, C. N., & Johnson, E. Q. (1971). Development of gait in childhood, parts 1 and 2. *Developmental Medicine and Child Neurology*, 13, 196–215; Gage, J. R. (1991). *Gait analysis in cerebral palsy*. London: MacKeith Press; Prince, F., Corriveau, H., Herbert, R., & Winter, D. A. (1997). Review article: Gait in the elderly. *Gait and Posture*, 5, 128–135; Shumway-Cook, A., & Woollacott, M. H. (2001). *Motor control: Theory and practical application* (2nd ed.). Philadelphia: Lippincott Williams & Wilkins; Sutherland, D. H., Olshen, R., Cooper, L., & Woo, S. L-Y. (1980). The development of mature gait. *Journal of Bone and Joint Surgery*, 62A, 336–353; and Wilder, P. A. (1992). Developmental changes in the gait patterns of women: A search for control parameters. PhD Thesis, Madison: University of Wisconsin.

terized by several key recognizable components (Burnett & Johnson, 1971):

1. Pelvic tilt and rotation
2. Initial contact with a heel strike
3. Knee flexion at midstance
4. A mature relationship between mechanisms at the hip, knee, and ankle
5. A mature base of support
6. Reciprocal arm swing

Free walking **velocity** increases with age until adolescence, then plateaus until senescence. With maturity, muscle activation patterns become more refined and energy efficiency improves. Table 10–4 also summarizes the characteristics of a mature adult gait pattern.

Gait Changes in the Older Adult

Balance ability, leg muscle strength, decreases in flexibility and range of motion, and changes in the availability of sensory information influence changes in the characteristics of gait in older adults. Cognitive factors may also be an important contributor. Healthy adults have reduced walking speed, shorter strides, and shorter steps than young adults. Proactive locomotor abilities also change with age, as older adults take more time to monitor the visual environment and to alter upcoming steps to avoid an obstacle by using strategies such as slowing of approach (Shumway-Cook & Woollacott, 2001).

It has been suggested that some of the gait changes in the elderly are related to the reemergence of immature walking patterns, as seen in young infants. The gait characteristics of the very young and the very old have several similarities. Both show a shorter duration of single-limb stance and an increase in double support time. In both groups, this has been interpreted as an indication of decreased balance abilities (Bril & Breniere, 1993; Gabell & Nayak, 1984; Sutherland et al., 1980). The gait of young walkers has a wide base of support as required for balance, a characteristic of the elderly as well. The muscular activation patterns in young children and older adults show co-activation of agonist and antagonist muscle groups during gait. This may be an adaptive mechanism for increasing muscle stiffness, which helps with balance control (Woollacott, 1986). It may be entirely possible that the reason for these similarities is a functional one: The two age groups, for different reasons, have difficulties with the balance system, but use similar strategies to compensate for those difficulties.

Gait characteristics common to older adults include a wider base of support, decreased reciprocal arm swing, and slower cadence. Stride length decreases and time in double support increases. These gait changes are due to a combination of musculoskeletal age-related changes, as well as to a decline in the sensory systems. Gait adaptation seen in the older adult may be associated with a general decrease in muscle strength due to loss of motor neurons, muscle fibers, and aerobic capacity (Bendall, Bassey, & Pearson, 1989; Prince, Corriveau, Hebert, & Winter, 1997). Most research indicates that the changes seen in locomotor patterns of aging adults are due to a decline in muscular strength, reflected most commonly by a decreased step length and increased time spent in double support (Wilder, 1992). The strength declines apparently most responsible for these changes in gait characteristics are losses in strength at the hip and ankle. In older adults, there is also evidence of a return to agonist and antagonist co-activation patterns, as originally seen in the toddler. This co-activation pattern may be an adaptive strategy to compensate for decreased postural control and balance deficits (Woollacott, 1989). Walking requires more energy for most older adults.

According to Shumway-Cook and Woollacott (2001), gait changes in the older adult can be summarized as follows:

1. Temporal (related to time) characteristics
   - Decreased velocity
   - Increased time in stance phase
   - Increased time in double support
   - Decreased time in swing phase
2. Spatial (pertaining to space) characteristics
   - Decreased step length
   - Decreased stride length
   - Increased stride width
3. Kinematic changes
   - Decreased vertical movement of the center of gravity
   - Decreased arm swing
   - Decreased hip, knee, and ankle flexion
   - Increased incidence of foot flat on initial contact
   - Decreased dynamic stability during stance

Table 10–4 highlights the gait changes seen in older adults.

Transfer Tasks

Because the term *locomotion* is defined as the process of moving from one place to another, the act of transferring should be discussed as a form of locomotion. A **transfer** refers to movement from one surface to another and may be accomplished independently, with assistance, or dependently. For the purposes of this text, dependent transfers will not be included in this discussion because individuals requiring total assistance

contribute varying and limited measures of independent movement to that transfer, and therefore within that context, that transfer is not considered a form of locomotion. There are many different types of transfer tasks, all using the preserved capabilities of the individual, supplemented by assistance from another person or a piece of equipment. If the patient/client is unable to bear weight through the lower extremities, an assisted or independent sliding board transfer is taught. In this case, the upper extremities and trunk muscles perform the task execution. When the lower extremities are able to accept weight bearing, several methods are available whereby the individual pushes up with his or her upper extremities to assume a stance position and a pivoting motion or series of small steps is performed to complete the transfer task.

The movement goal of a transfer is to change the center of gravity of the body from sitting on one surface to standing or sitting on another surface (Ryerson & Levit, 1997). As a model, the sit-to-stand transfer tasks will be described in this chapter because of their relevance to lower extremity functional control.

To stand up from a sitting position, the individual must have trunk control, lower extremity control, and dynamic balance. Critical components of this task include the following:

- The ability to control the upper trunk over the lower trunk during anterior/posterior weight shifts
- The ability to maintain both feet in contact with the floor
- The ability to produce extension power in the legs

The ability to stand up is one of the most demanding everyday tasks that an individual performs regularly (Berger, Riley, & Mann, 1988). Lack of independence in this task has been reported to be one of the most likely factors associated with risk of institutionalization (Branch & Meyers, 1987). For many persons, this ability to stand up from a sitting position marks the beginning of movement and function in the upright position. From standing, an individual can transfer to other chairs or seats, begin to walk, and subsequently interact more effectively with the environment.

The movement task of sit to stand is to change the center of gravity from an area defined by the hips, thighs, and feet, to one defined only by the feet. The critical components of the task are to move the body mass from over a large BOS (thighs and feet) to a small BOS, and to then extend the joints of the LEs to raise the body mass over the feet. The actual sit-to-stand task has been divided into two, three, or four phases, depending on the source. These phases are presented in Table 10–5, offering a practical guide to the clinician for retraining of this important functional task

(Schenkman et al, 1990; Shumway-Cook & Woollacott, 2001). The ability to stand from sitting occurs as a result of force generation in many muscles spanning the LE joints, as well as trunk stabilizers. EMG analyses of muscle activation during this task shows the following, presented in order of activation (Kelley, Dainis, & Wood, 1976; Millington, Myklebust, & Shambes, 1992; Richards, 1985):

1. Tibialis anterior muscle: for preparatory placement of foot backward and tibial stabilization
2. Simultaneous onset of activity in gluteus maximus, biceps femoris (hip extensors) and rectus femoris, vastus lateralis and medialis muscles (knee extensors); activity of extensors peaks at time thighs are lifted off seat
3. Varying degrees of roles of gastrocnemius and soleus muscles for postural control

Although there seems to be an assumption in the literature that sitting from standing and moving from sit to stand are fundamentally the same task in reverse, this is an erroneous assumption. The joint excursions at the hip, knee, and ankle are very similar, but in sitting from standing the muscles of the LEs are acting eccentrically, a contraction type that requires a great deal of force and control. The same muscles as listed in the sit to stand transfer are firing, but in this task (sitting from standing) these extensor muscles are creating eccentric force while the joints they cross are flexing. There is some evidence that the trunk is of less importance in this task, but the demands especially on the knee are tremendous (Carr & Shepherd, 1998).

Clinical Connection:

Age-related changes to the execution of this task often accompany the normal aging changes seen in the musculoskeletal system. Arthritis in the weight-bearing joints or the vertebral column or weakness in the lower extremity or back extensor muscles will require that the older adult develop an adaptive strategy for transferring between sitting and standing. ■

The teaching of transfers is used in neurorehabilitation to establish postural control in the trunk and strengthen movement patterns in the LEs, as well as to accomplish the actual functional movement goal itself. Transfer training can also be effectively used to build progressions that are based on the individual's needs and strengths. The therapist or assistant can slowly increase the demands of the task according to the individual's level of movement control. Intervention can focus on any number of selected goals during the activity: trunk symmetry, muscle activity in the LEs during the weight-bearing or loading phase, the ability to demonstrate postural control in stance, the ability to engage in a functional activity or rotate within the stance position, and practicing balance control to achieve patterns of movement that will then relate to standing and walking (Ryerson & Levit, 1997).

TABLE 10–5
The Sit-to-Stand Transfer

Functional Task: Moving from sitting with a wide base of support and low center of gravity to standing with a small base of support and high center of gravity. Starting position is one of sitting, upper trunk controlled over lower trunk, hips and knees in flexion, and ankles in slight dorsiflexion.

Phase	Task	Requirements of Task
1. Weight shift phase	Generation of forward momentum of upper body through forward flexion of the trunk	Activation of erector spinae muscles, contracting eccentrically Body fairly stable
2. Beginning of rise (buttocks off the chair)	Transferring of momentum from upper body to total body, allowing a lift of the body	Co-activation of hip and knee extensor muscles Stability requirement greatest during this phase
3. Lift or extension phase	Extension at hips and knees, resulting in vertical movement of body	Hip and knee extension, trunk extension, ankle postural control needed Stability requirement less than in previous phase
4. Stabilization phase	Attaining of postural stability in new upright position	Task-dependent motion complete Body stability in vertical achieved

Sources: Adapted from Schenkman, M. A., Berger, R. A., Riley, P. O., Mann, R. W., & Hodge, W. A. (1990). Whole body movements during rising to standing from sitting. *Physical Therapy*, 10, 638–651, with permission of the American Physical Therapy Association; and Shumway-Cook, A., & Wollacott, M. J. (2001). *Motor control: Theory and practical applications* (2nd ed.). Baltimore: Lippincott Williams & Wilkins.

Abnormal Lower Extremity Function and Impaired Locomotion

Impaired lower extremity function with consequent impaired mobility and locomotion is one of the most characteristic features of a variety of neurological disorders. Mobility is a critical part of attaining and maintaining independence and is an essential attribute of quality of life (Patla & Shumway-Cook, 1999). When impairments in mobility restrict the ability of the individual to move about the community or perform necessary activities of daily living (ADLs), disability results.

Although abnormal mobility is characteristic of many neurological disorders, the constellation of underlying problems contributing to mobility impairment can be varied. Some commonalities are clinically evident. Once again, to understand the nature of the patient's/client's problem so that effective clinical management can occur, one needs some kind of classification system. The most common framework seen in rehabilitation literature for understanding and classifying mobility disorders, including gait, is based on the neurological diagnosis itself. One can find a wealth of information available describing the common impairments and clinical management strategies found useful for individuals with the common disorders of cerebrovascular accident (CVA), Parkinson's disease, and cerebral palsy (CP). Because this classification approach is so common, and also because the information therein *can* be generalized to a set of common problems, this chapter will eventually describe the main mobility problems and strategies used when discussing those commonly encountered neurological disorders.

However, in a broader sense and consistent with the functional practical approach presented in this text, this chapter will first present abnormal mobility as resulting from any combination of three main functional impairments that contribute to mobility problems in individuals with neurological dysfunction:

1. Abnormal force production or weakness
2. Abnormal muscle tone
3. Coordination problems, including difficulties with muscle sequencing, timing, or interference from involuntary movements

For practical application, this chapter will then describe the main functional limitations associated with abnormal gait, because gait is the primary locomotor disorder requiring clinical attention. Regardless of the pathological cause, abnormal gait is inefficient and ineffective.

Implications for Therapeutic Intervention: Functional Costs of Pathological Gait

A skill such as walking is not an LE pattern alone, but rather it is a total body response generated by the individual who is actively solving a specific motor problem. Effective walking does not just require the control of a particular joint or body segment, but how the critical features of the movement affect and determine the overall accomplishment of functional, purposeful movement control. Gait solutions emerge that are appropriate for the individual's current condition and in relation to the task (Marshall & Jennings, 1990).

Clinical Connection:

The individual without any limiting constraints or impairments has an unlimited repertoire of movement solutions at his or her disposal. You, perhaps, can generate any number of gait styles appropriate for any presented task: picking your way over a cobbled creek bed; walking over a newly waxed, wet floor; or walking over the soft floor mat found in the therapy gym. Individuals with musculoskeletal or neurological constraints will also generate their own best movement solutions for the presented task. Clinically, sometimes these solutions were ill regarded as not being consistent with "normal" or typical movement—in this case, gait. Current approaches, however, are respectful of the individuals' right to problem solve and generate their own, perhaps atypical movement solutions, within the constraints of their own combination of abilities and challenges, as long as the movement pattern is safe and will not contribute to secondary impairments or new problems. Patients with movement challenges often present with an adaptive, perhaps atypical solution to a movement dilemma. As long as this atypical movement is not maladaptive, contributing to a lack of safety or a secondary impairment, it should be considered as effective and functional. This contemporary view is consistent with an orientation toward enablement and the current state of knowledge in motor control, motor learning, and a task-oriented approach to intervention. ▪

Regardless of the contributing factors, pathological gait is less functional and efficient than normal gait. Pathological gait is often characterized by the following functional deficits:

• Loss of stability in stance
• Insufficient foot clearance during swing

- Inappropriate prepositioning of the foot during swing for initial contact
- Inadequate step length
- Inefficient and poorly conserved energy

Although the kinematics of normal gait remain relatively stable between subjects, the kinetics, or patterns of muscle use, may vary, not only from subject to subject but also with speed and fatigue within a single subject. Research has demonstrated that there is considerable redundancy in the motor/muscular system such that if a particular muscle cannot be used, another muscle or group of muscles may take over the function (Whittle, 1991; Winter, 1987). For example, the knee during stance is under the control of at least four different muscles, and perhaps one could be recruited more so than another if circumstances required. This fact has fascinating clinical implications, offering considerable hope for successful retraining in the face of musculoskeletal impairment.

The gait patterns of individuals with neurological dysfunction are influenced primarily by deficits in force production, abnormalities of muscle tone, incoordination affecting the timing and sequencing of muscular activation patterns, and interference from involuntary movements. Functionally, these impairments may contribute to weakness, disordered motor control, immature or ineffective movement patterns, and inefficiency.

Neuromuscular Impairments Resulting in Impaired Lower Extremity Function

■ Weakness

Weakness results in the inability to generate sufficient force to meet the demands of lower extremity control, including all the locomotor skills described in this chapter. Interestingly, during normal walking, studies have demonstrated that most muscles function at a muscle grade level of fair+ or 3+ (Perry, 1992; Perry, Hoffer, Giovan, Antonelli, & Greenberg, 1986). This effort averages about 25 percent of normal strength, with no endurance or reserve. The functional limitations caused by muscle weakness depend on what muscles are weak, the extent of the weakness, and the capacity for other muscles to substitute for the weak muscles in meeting the requirements of the task. As an example, walking normally does not tax the various lower extremity muscles to their full capacity (Patla, 1995; Shumway-Cook & Woollacott, 2001). The only muscle that comes even close to maximum output during gait is the

gastrocnemius muscle, providing a major source of propulsive power. Therapists and assistants are urged to study the muscular force requirements of common locomotor tasks as presented in this chapter (Tables 10–1 to 10–3 and 10–5). Weakness in a given muscle may produce a predictable functional limitation or may require an adapted or compensatory strategy from the mover. Common functional limitations caused by key muscle weaknesses affecting locomotion are listed in Table 10–6. Clinical management includes strengthening in task-specific movements as detailed in previous chapters and later in this text.

■ Abnormalities of Muscle Tone

Abnormally low muscle tone will clinically present itself with the same functional limitations as caused by weakness. Abnormally high muscle tone, especially spasticity, results in several functional deficits that then impair locomotor abilities, especially gait. Spasticity impairs mobility in any one or any combination of five different ways:

1. Overreaction to stretch and velocity-dependent movements
2. Impaired selective control
3. Inappropriate activation, sequencing, and muscle phasing patterns
4. Increasingly apparent abnormal movement patterns
5. Altered proprioception

A discussion of how spasticity can impact gait illustrates the effects of these changes (Carr & Shepherd, 1998; Perry, 1992; Shumway-Cook & Woollacott, 2001). Spasticity results in the inappropriate activation of muscles during movements, including the gait cycle. This is especially problematic when muscles are undergoing lengthening during the movement task. Spasticity obstructs the yielding quality of an eccentric muscle contraction. A quick stretch can produce clonus. Spasticity in a given muscle group will contribute to a persistent firing pattern instead of an efficient burst of force, followed by a smooth decrease in activation. Note the importance of eccentric muscle control during the stand-to-sit transfer and during the gait cycle. During gait, the quadriceps muscle group lengthens twice, in early stance as the limb is loaded, and again when the knee flexes during propulsion at preswing. The hamstring muscles lengthen once during late swing in preparation for initial contact. The tibialis anterior muscle lengthens during loading. These times coincide with times when spasticity could interfere with fulfillment of the functional tasks associated with those muscle lengthenings (Carr & Shepherd, 1998; Perry,

TABLE 10–6

Functional Limitations in Locomotor Skills Associated with Weakness Patterns Encountered by Individuals with Neurological Dysfunction

Weak Muscle Group	Locomotor Limitation
Trunk or abdominal weakness	Impaired ability to generate force to initiate sit-to-stand transfer Impaired ability to roll Little effect on gait unless weakness is significant
Hip extensor weakness	Difficulty in lift phase of sit-to-stand transfer Difficulty with eccentric control in stand-to-sit transfer Compensation of backward trunk lean during gait to compensate for instability, especially during loading and single limb support
Hip abductor weakness	Difficulty in any component of a task requiring unilateral stance or period of single limb support: midstance of gait and stair climbing Results in a **Trendelenburg gait**, drop of pelvis on swing side opposite of the weak abductor on stance side
Hip flexor weakness	Difficulty with initiation of rolling pattern with LEs Difficulty with creeping Inadequate functional limb shortening during swing, often resulting in limb circumduction Ineffective limb advancement and prepositioning of LE for beginning of stance
Knee extensor weakness	Difficulty in lift phase of sit-to-stand transfer Difficulty with eccentric control in stand-to-sit transfer Difficulty controlling knee flexion during loading Difficulty stabilizing the knee during midstance, often resulting in knee hyperextension, knee buckling, or compensatory forward lean of the trunk
Plantar flexion weakness	Difficulty stabilizing the lower leg during stance, resulting in flexed knee (crouched) gait and ankle dorsiflexion Lack of heel rise during terminal stance Inadequate propulsion force generated at terminal stance and preswing, resulting in ineffective swing, including inadequate knee flexion during swing
Dorsiflexion weakness	Poor eccentric control during loading, resulting in foot slap Inadequate foot clearance during swing

Source: Information compiled from multiple sources. See reference list and text for details.

1992; Shumway-Cook & Woollacott, 2001). Spasticity also alters the mechanical properties of a muscle, producing increased stiffness, which then in turn affects the freedom of body segments to move rapidly. This alters the smooth relationship of limb segments to one another and limits the transfer of momentum during movement (including rolling, transfers, and gait), ultimately altering the components of the task.

As a clinical problem, spasticity is typically distributed in the following key muscles that affect locomotion, specifically gait: plantar flexors, quadriceps, hamstrings, and hip adductors. Spasticity in the plantar flexor muscles can contribute to problems in both the stance and the swing phases of gait. During stance, plantar flexion spasticity affects foot position at initial contact, creating instability, and can limit smooth dorsiflexion preventing a heel strike (Fig. 10–6). Spasticity in the plantar flexor muscles also results in inadequate propulsion during preswing. Patients often compensate

for plantar flexion spasticity by hyperextending the knee or leaning the trunk forward. During swing, spasticity in the plantar flexor muscles will lead to prolonged firing, interfering with dorsiflexion activation, resulting in an inability for the foot to clear the floor (Fig. 10–7). Spastic plantar flexor muscles also prohibit the foot from being adequately prepositioned for a stable initial contact. Quadriceps muscle spasticity can result in excessive knee extension during the stance phase of gait, limiting knee flexor control, with subsequently impaired stability of the weight-bearing limb. Hamstring muscle spasticity results in excessive knee flexion throughout stance or swing, resulting in both instability during stance and a shortened step length from an inadequately advanced limb (Fig. 10–8). Spasticity in the hip adductor muscles can result in a scissors gait, characterized by excessive adduction, and consequently a decreased BOS and instability (Fig. 10–9).

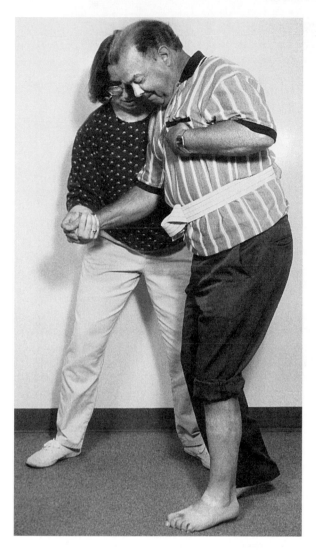

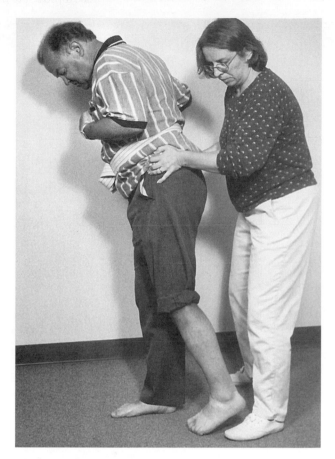

Figure 10–7. Plantar flexion spasticity preventing foot clearance during swing.

Figure 10–6. Plantar flexor spasticity will prevent smooth initial contact onto the heel, resulting in an unstable onset of stance phase. Patient compensates for instability by leaning the trunk forward.

▪ Coordination Problems

Incoordination in lower extremity function can result from pathology in a variety of neural structures, including the motor cortex, basal ganglia, and cerebellum. According to Chapter 7, coordination problems include several different movement dysfunctions, such as movement decomposition, dysmetria, inappropriate co-activation patterns, and timing problems. **Ataxia** is a common manifestation of uncoordinated control of the lower extremities. Ataxia is a problem in executing coordinated movements, characterized by dysmetria, movement decomposition, dysdiadochokinesia, and abnormal timing of multijoint movements. One of the case studies at the end of this chapter will describe the

clinical management of a patient with ataxia. **Movement decomposition** is characterized by a breakdown of movements between multiple joints, resulting in movement of individual segments rather than movement as a fluid, coordinated unit. **Dysmetria** is characterized by overshooting, underreaching, or reaching inaccurately toward the target, sometimes referred to as past-pointing. **Incoordination** occurs when the firing rates of muscles are disrupted, resulting in loss of smooth reciprocal movement, or when the CNS loses its ability to direct movement activity that requires accuracy (O'Sullivan & Schmitz, 2001; Shumway-Cook & Woollacott, 2001).

Deficits in coordination will interfere with the smooth execution of any locomotor pattern, with varying degrees of severity and functional limitation. The persistence of abnormal synergies will result in a limited ability to isolate voluntary muscle control and demonstrate smooth muscular sequencing. Inappropriate activation and sequencing will be manifested as an inability to effectively recruit a muscle, increased activation of that muscle, or inability to modulate that muscle's activity throughout the movement. Co-

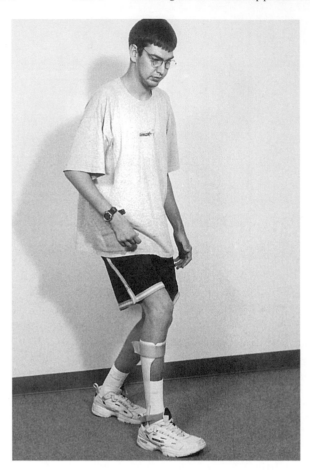

Figure 10–8. Hamstring spasticity will prevent an adequate limb advancement of the swing limb in preparation for initial contact and will also result in a shortened step length. This figure also demonstrates prevalence of pattern-only motor control pattern characterized by strong, predominant flexion of both lower extremities throughout both gait phases.

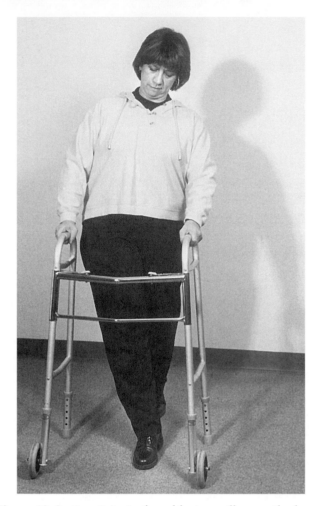

Figure 10–9. Spasticity in the adductors will cause the lower extremity to "scissor" across midline, resulting in an ineffective BOS and instability.

activation of agonist and antagonist muscle groups contributes to significant incoordination in individuals with neurological dysfunction, especially in patients post-CVA or with CP. This abnormal co-activation is thought to be due to pathologically disorganized central control programs, the need for additional postural support activity, or compensatory strategies (Knutsson, 1994; Crenna, 1998).

▪ Musculoskeletal Constraints

Although this text is emphasizing the effect of neuromuscular impairments on movement in individuals with neurological dysfunction, it would be remiss not to mention the effects of secondary impairments and deficits in other systems on functional movement performance. The primary impairments detailed previously are typical consequences of the disease or pathological processes. A secondary impairment is not always typical, may be preventable, but nonetheless can have a significant impact on functional performance and rehabilitation outcome. Neurological pathology can lead to a wide range of secondary problems, including muscular atrophy and deconditioning, joint contractures, degenerative joint disease or joint instability, and osteoporosis. Immobilization decreases the flexibility of the connective tissue and increases that tissue's resistance to stretch (Woo et al., 1975). Paralysis and subsequent immobilization can result in disuse atrophy and an actual reduction in sarcomere numbers (Duncan & Badke, 1987). Loss of flexibility, abnormal range of motion (hypomobility, as well as hypermobility), malalignment, and muscle imbalances can result. Pain can accompany any one of these musculoskeletal impairments. Contributory interferences from any of these secondary impairments, as well as deficits in cognitive processing or perceptual abilities, must be assimilated into the therapist's assessment of the composite functional picture of the patient. These areas are not a focus of this particular text, but their lack of inclusion does not minimize their relevance or importance.

Functional Limitations in Gait: a Task-Oriented Approach

Whether the underlying impairment is weakness, abnormally high muscle tone, difficulties with coordination, pain, or immobility, the resultant impact on functional performance is what is of utmost concern to both the clinician and the patient/client. Regardless of underlying pathology, age, or constellation of impairments, the individual engaged in gait training is focused on establishing or re-establishing any one of the three main functional tasks of gait, which are: weight acceptance, single limb support, and limb advancement. Intervention can be directed at training the patient to meet the basic task requirements of gait. Because human walking is a series of interconnected phases in which muscular sequencing and momentum are such crucial elements, it *is* artificial to break this whole task into component parts. In the clinical arena, both whole and part training are used, depending on the individual patient's unique needs. If part training is used to emphasize a specific functional task, it is recommended that opportunity be offered to integrate and practice the part as a portion of the whole gait task whenever and as soon as possible.

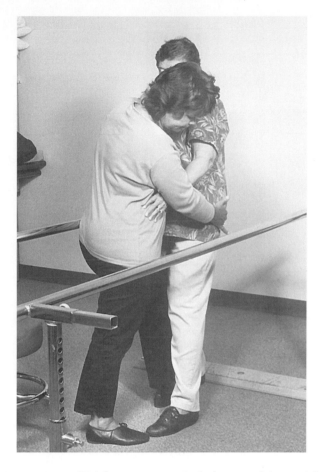

Figure 10–10. Weight acceptance includes practicing weight shifting in bilateral stance to the right and left, as well as forward and backward.

Weight Acceptance

Intervention to improve the effectiveness of meeting the functional task goal of weight acceptance is related to activities to increase stability and strength in the key muscular groups and improving postural control of the trunk in this upright position. To effectively accept weight, the lower extremity must be able to achieve a position of hip extension, slight adduction and external rotation, and knee extension, with the ankle/foot in contact with the floor. Mild deviations from these minimal requirement are permitted, but with a consequential cost to the effectiveness of the weight-bearing stance.

Intervention techniques are typically done in the upright position, with attention directed to the individual's stability, strength, and control at the trunk, pelvis, knee, and ankle. Effective intervention ideas are implemented from the intervention approaches discussed in Chapters 6 and 7. Intervention is directed at activities to increase proximal stability at the trunk and pelvis, co-

contraction strength, and control of the musculature around the hip, knee, and ankle. Weight acceptance occurs certainly at the initiation of gait as the patient/client assumes stance. Standing activities include practicing weight shifting in bilateral stance to the right and left, as well as forward and backward, within the patient's limits of stability (Fig. 10–10). During the gait cycle, weight acceptance occurs as the individual makes contact and loads onto one limb as weight is shifted from the opposite limb.

Effective techniques include sensorimotor techniques (approximation and tapping and quick stretch to activate muscle activation), rhythmic stabilization to increase co-contraction and isometric control, and techniques described by neurodevelopmental treatment (NDT) to encourage weight bearing and weight shifting through skillful physical guidance from the therapist or assistant. Figures 10–10 and 10–11 demonstrate intervention techniques useful for meeting the functional goal of weight acceptance in stance. Note the therapist's manual contact with the patient's pelvis as a key point of control.

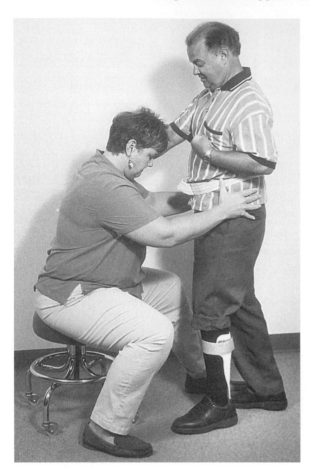

Figure 10–11. Weight acceptance is practiced as the individual makes contact and loads onto one limb as weight is shifted from the opposite limb.

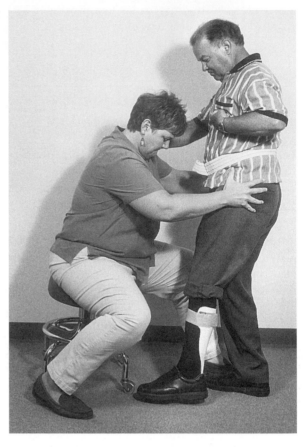

Figure 10–12. The right LE is assisted in supporting weight in single limb support as the left lower extremity advances during swing, assisted manually by the therapist's hands on the patient's pelvis.

Single Limb Support

Work on the functional task of single limb support entails practicing postural control of the trunk above a single limb, as well as stabilizing the limb when the center of mass is at its highest. Techniques to increase proximal stability, co-contraction, and strength are practiced within this functional position as described previously. Figure 10–12 demonstrates intervention techniques useful for meeting the functional goal of single limb support.

Limb Advancement

The task of limb advancement requires the generation of sufficient propulsion force from the stance leg, followed by an effective execution of swing. Once again, intervention is directed at the specific subphases of gait at which time this function is met, at the time of terminal stance through preswing on the stance limb as it

pushes into plantar flexion with the hip in hyperextension. As depicted in Figures 10–6 and 10–7, this position of plantar flexion of the ankle is an unstable position for many patients with impaired balance. Practice time can be spent in attaining an appropriate heel rise, moving the trunk forward over the stance limb, and generating force to push off. Techniques that may be effective for this task include plantar flexion strengthening exercises and movement of the trunk forward over the plantar flexed limb. Effective limb advancement requires adequate knee extensor range of motion, as well as the ability for the individual to control the momentum force generated by push-off. For effective limb advancement, the pelvis must rotate forward (protract) to place the limb for the most effective step length. Techniques to assist with active pelvic protraction include manual guidance, using the pelvis as a key point of control during the physically guided limb advancement (Figs. 10–11 to 10–13), or quick stretch at the beginning of swing to recruit activation of the pelvic protractors (Fig. 10–14). Because propulsion and momentum force are such vital components of this task, it is recommended

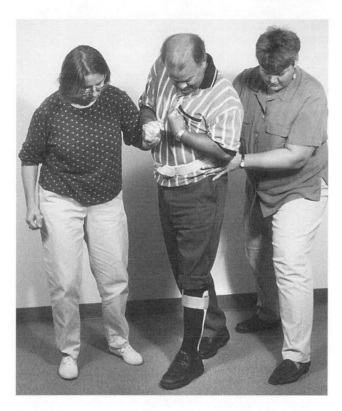

Figure 10–13. The left LE is guided into protraction during swing phase in preparation for initial contact.

that this subtask be practiced as a whole task whenever possible.

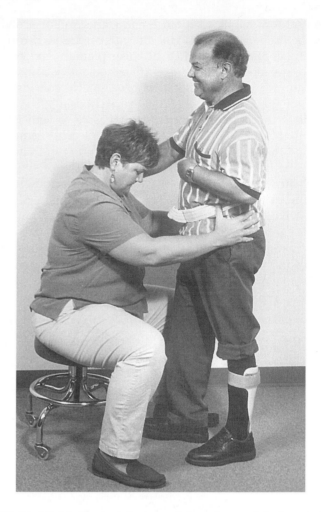

Figure 10–14. Therapist uses pelvis as key point of control during initiation of swing.

Effect of an Assistive or Orthotic Device on the Functional Task of Walking

Without a doubt, the addition of an assistive device or a lower extremity orthoses changes the nature of the walking task. When an individual uses an assistive device, the upper extremities function differently during gait than during unaided walking. The upper extremities are no longer able to engage in a reciprocal arm swing, the demands on the trunk consequently change, the ability of the trunk to freely rotate decreases, and the arms, pushing through an assistive device, are now a part of the actual gait cycle. With the exception of a rapid, swing-through gait, as demonstrated by the most proficient crutch ambulators, walking with an assistive device is slower and requires more energy (Foley, Prax, Crowell, & Boone, 1996; Franks, Palisano, & Darbee, 1991). Energy is consumed by the engagement of the upper extremities in this closed-chain activity. The use of an assistive device has also been demonstrated to impose additional attentional demands on the user, which may have an impact on

execution of the walking task itself (Wright & Kemp, 1992). An assistive device is appropriately prescribed to enhance stability in upright, widen the base of support, and allow for functional mobility in the face of significant limitations or constraints.

When an orthoses is prescribed, it is used to remediate a specific functional limitation in gait. The most common reason for the prescription of an orthoses for the individual with a neurological impairment is to correct for foot and ankle position and to aid in achievement of a stable, neutral ankle position during stance. As such, many orthoses are effective in improving lower limb stability during stance, positioning the foot adequately for weight acceptance, and therefore assisting the wearer to meet the functional tasks of stance phase (Fig. 10–15), as well as to clear the foot throughout swing (Fig. 10–16). As an artificial appliance, the benefits of an orthoses will always have an associated cost. For example, whereas a solid ankle-foot orthoses or a standard ankle-foot orthoses may correct for a dynamic drop foot deformity and position the foot in neutral for weight acceptance and stance, rollover and momentum generation will be compromised during the final phases of stance because plantar flexion is being prevented. The clinical management decision to use an orthoses is made based on a careful consideration of the costs and benefits and choosing the use of an orthoses to facilitate optimal, safe, or efficient ambulatory function. Research has clearly demonstrated the efficacy of orthotic use for improving stance stability, improving joint position for stance or swing, and increasing the overall quality of performance during gait (Embrey, Yates, & Mott, 1990; Radtka, Skinner, Dixon, & Johanson, 1997; O'Sullivan & Schmitz, 2001; Umphred, 2001).

Therapists and assistants are reminded that the gait of an individual using an orthotic or assistive device will have different characteristics than that of an unimpaired "typical" mature adult gait cycle. Nevertheless,

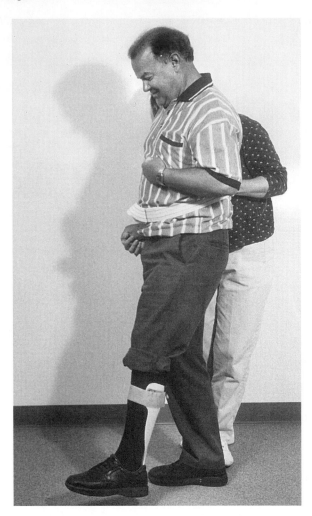

Figure 10–16. The use of an orthotic device improves performance during swing.

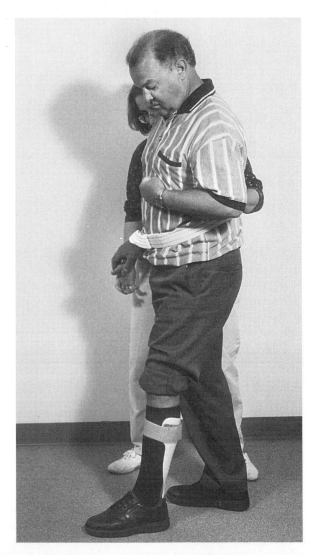

Figure 10–15. The use of an orthotic device improves performance upon stance.

meeting the functional task demands of the gait cycle and the functional subtasks of gait is still the clinical goal, aided or unaided.

Lower Extremity Control Problems Associated with Common Neurological Disorders

It is crucially important to recognize that although locomotor activities are typically associated with lower extremity function and control, locomotion, including gait, is a whole body, actually a *whole person*, activity. Human beings are not an isolated set of legs that robotically move the body through space. Rather, the lower extremities are under the control and influence of multiple systems, affected by and affecting the complementary movements of the head, arms, and trunk, moving in a concerted effort to attain a functional goal. This overly simplified but keystone idea cannot be forgotten. This cornerstone concept needs to pervade and direct the clinical management of the presenting lower extremity functional impairment of any individual, at any age, with any neurological diagnosis. Keeping this in mind, the following section will present a practical, clinical management approach to the locomotor problems associated with the most commonly encountered neurological disorders. The key management concepts can be expanded upon and applied to similar disorders with similar impairments.

Cerebral Palsy

Approximately 70 percent of children with CP are eventually able to ambulate, with the ambulatory capacity directly related to the degree of neurological involvement (Damiano & Abel, 1996; Johnson, Abel, & Damiano, 1996). Generally, all children with hemiplegia or diplegia are able to ambulate, with less success seen in children with quadriplegia or athetosis. For all children with CP, the acquisition of walking is delayed.

Children with CP often display several pathokinematic differences in gait, as verified by electromyography (EMG). These EMG studies demonstrate decreases in amplitude (which indicates strength of muscle activity on EMG) and abnormalities in timing and phasing of muscular activity. Documented differences in the gait of children with CP are as follows:

1. Amplitude on EMG is lower, which is indicative of muscular weakness. Weakness is often seen in the gluteus maximus, gluteus medius, quadriceps, gastrocnemius, and anterior tibialis muscles.
2. Movement, including gait, is characterized by co-activation or reciprocal excitation of muscle groups rather than by reciprocal inhibition and smooth muscle phasing (Cowan, Stilling, Naumann, & Colborne, 1998; Mykebust, 1990).
3. There are also mechanical changes in spastic muscle fibers. For example, the increase in tension occurring quickly after initial contact, which clinically produces a strong plantar flexion response often seen in children with CP, appears to be due to the mechanical stretching of the short gastrocnemius muscle itself rather than only to overactivity of the muscle itself (Berger, Quintern, & Deitz, 1982) (Fig. 10–17).
4. Many researchers contend that the defect in the normal function of the gastrocnemius muscle is one of the most important mechanical deficiencies in the gait of children with CP. Inadequate force production is apparent as muscle weakness with resultant stance instability and ineffective propul-

sion forward from terminal stance through preswing.
5. Lack of dorsiflexion often impairs the smooth movement of the tibia over the talus and may act as a brake on the forward movement of the trunk. This may cause knee hyperextension or cause the child to go up onto the toes with a flexed hip and knee (Fig. 10–18).
6. Sagittal plane motion of the knee is also abnormal. Initial contact is often made with the knee in significant flexion and then either extension or excessive knee flexion throughout stance. In mildly involved children, the knee flexion phase during midstance is present but reduced in size (Olney, 1989).
7. Hip joint motion is likely to be impaired in more severely involved children (Olney, 1989).
8. Examination of joint motion patterns during gait shows more hip adduction, flexion, and internal rotation, exaggerated knee flexion during stance, and a forefoot strike pattern (Fig. 10–19).

Clinically, four common characteristic gait patterns are often observed in children with CP: a crouch gait, a gait characterized by genu recurvatum, a stiff leg gait, or a gait typical of hemiplegia (O'Byrne, Jenkinson, & O'Brien, 1998; Perry, 1992). The most common, *crouch gait*, is a bilateral impairment characterized by excessive hip and knee flexion, dorsiflexion, and usually an anterior tilt of the pelvis (see Figs. 10–17 and 10–18). Excessive hip and knee flexion is probably caused by a combination of overactivity of hip and knee flexors with weakness of antigravity hip and knee extensors. Increased excitement or gait speed may contribute to an exaggeration of undesirable movement patterns (Fig. 10–20). Poor control of the gastrocnemius muscle is thought to be the main impairment in a crouch gait. The weak gastrocnemius muscle does not effectively restrain the forward movement of the tibia in stance, causing the knee to remain flexed. Weakness of the quadriceps muscle is not considered to be a main contributing factor in stance control in a crouch gait, but rather contributes more to an ineffective step length by not extending the limb sufficiently at terminal swing. *Genu recurvatum* presents the opposite clinical picture. The knee assumes a position of hyperextension during stance and the ankle often goes into excessive plantar flexion (Fig. 10–21). The hip may still continue to demonstrate excessive flexion, as the trunk moves forward to compensate (Perry, 1992). A *stiff leg gait* is characterized by extension at the trunk, posterior tilt of the pelvis, and excessive hip and knee extension, usually in combination with internal rotation and adduction of the hips. The ankles are typically plantar flexed (Cowan et al., 1998). The gait of a child with *hemiplegic* CP is characterized by asymmetry, uneven

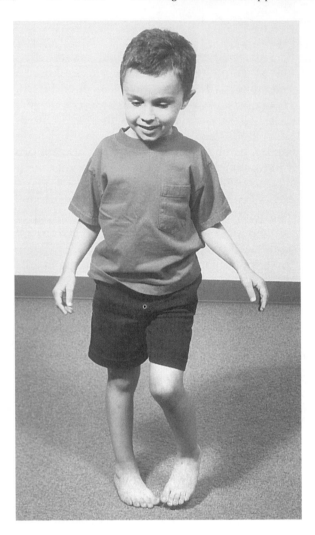

Figure 10–17. Strong plantar flexion response moving into initial contact, often seen in children with CP, may be due in part to mechanical stretching and limited range of a short gastrocnemius muscle.

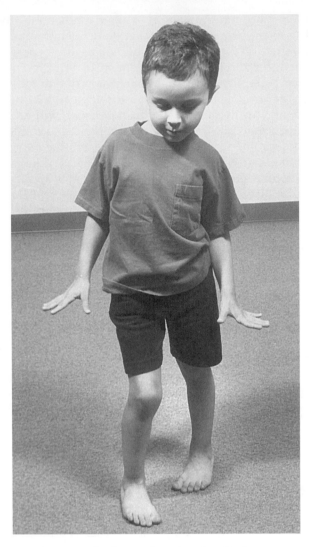

Figure 10–18. Lack of smooth active dorsiflexion may cause the child to go up onto his forefoot (R) with a flexed knee and compensate by hyperextending the knee (L) of the trailing limb.

weight bearing and step length, hip retraction, knee flexion, and ineffective heel strike, usually with a plantar flexed ankle.

The energy cost of ambulation for children with CP is higher than for children without impairment (Olney, 1989; Olney, Costigan, & Hedden, 1987; Olney, MacPhail, Hedden, & Boyce, 1987; Rose, Gamble, Medeiros, Burgos, & Haskell, 1989). Generally, children with CP ambulate at about half the speed of children without CP, with an energy demand estimated to be triple the demand for healthy children (Campbell & Ball, 1978; Mossberg, Linton, & Fricke, 1990). Energy cost is high due to the following factors: unnecessary levels of muscle activity that do not result in movement, erratic activation and firing patterns, and the inability to efficiently transfer weight to the accepting limb (Olney et al., 1987). Both heart rate and oxygen cost are reliable measures of energy cost (Rose et al., 1989).

▪ Clinical Management

Intervention with the child with CP is focused specifically on reducing impairments, preventing secondary impairments, and decreasing functional limitations, in an effort to promote optimal development and independent function. Interventions attempt to promote optimal postural alignment and train the child to develop movements that are conducive to musculoskeletal development, neurophysiological control, and improved function, through exercise, positioning, and adaptive equipment. Intervention includes activities to improve force generation and functional strength, management of abnormal muscle tone, and task-specific training to reduce functional limitations and promote independent mobility. Reducing the effects of multisystem impairments and improving

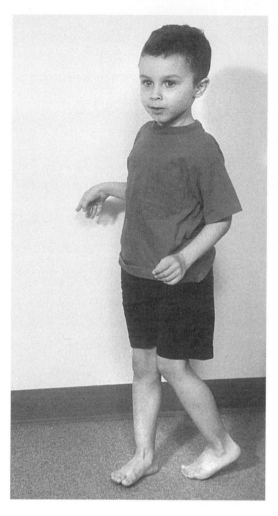

Figure 10–19. Joint patterns during gait often show more hip adduction, flexion, and internal rotation; exaggerated knee flexion; and a forefoot strike pattern.

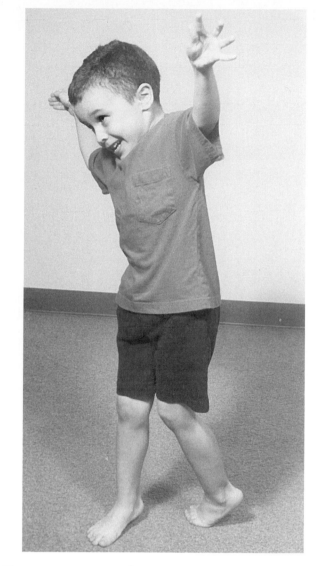

Figure 10–20. Increased excitement may contribute to exaggeration of undesirable movement patterns.

selective control, anticipatory regulation, and learning of effective and efficient movement facilitate improvements in functional control (Olney & Wright, 2000).

Ambulation is a major concern of therapists and assistants working with young children with CP. Intervention emphasis is on prewalking skills, such as attaining effective and well-aligned weight bearing, promoting dissociation and weight shift, and improving balance. In children with developmental disabilities, impaired attainment of key functional movement components such as dissociation and rotation (see Chapter 4), often hinders control of the reciprocal limb movements required by all the locomotor functions of rolling, crawling, creeping, and walking. Refer to the information presented in Chapters 4, 6, and 7 for intervention suggestions appropriate for training of motor control and motor development in children with CP.

This section will discuss only suggestions specific to the clinical management of gait disorders.

Specific intervention strategies include activities to promote the acquisition of key functional movement components, such as antigravity flexion and extension strength, stable weight bearing and smooth weight shifting, upright postural control, dissociation, and rotation. Many children have difficulty specifically with adequate force production, lack of lower extremity dissociation, decreased single limb support, and evidence of limited postural reactions during weight shifting. For example, children with spastic diplegia often have difficulty dissociating one LE from the other and dissociating LE movements from the trunk (see Figs. 10–20 and 10–22). Intervention could emphasize practicing coming to stand or stabilization of the LE weight-bearing position so that the child can work on

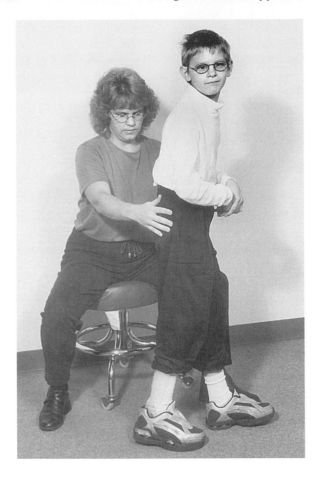

Figure 10–21. Genu recurvatum, seen in the child with a right hemiplegic CP, prevents the right lower extremity from offering a stable and effective contribution to upright mobility. The limb is often literally left behind, unengaged and not integrated into functional gait.

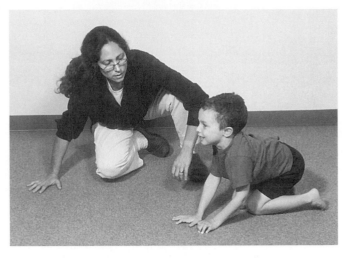

Figure 10–22. Children with spastic diplegic CP often have difficulty dissociating one LE from the other, impairing the ability to demonstrate independent transitional movements.

LE strengthening and weight bearing (Fig. 10–23). Practicing lateral trunk postural reactions may assist with the emergence of LE dissociation, in response to weight shifting (Fig. 10–24). Intervention for commonly encountered gait difficulties in children with CP requires facilitation of smooth, useable functional movement components and integration of functional movement patterns into both preambulatory and gait activities. Typically, therapy will focus on work in stance, coming to stand, weight shifting while in stance, forward progression, and limb advancement. Orthoses and assistive devices are prescribed as needed to assist in the attainment of safe ambulation. At the end of this chapter, a case study is presented that details an example of a gait training program for a child with CP.

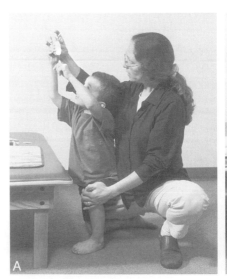
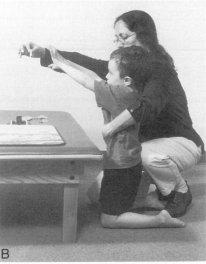

Figure 10–23. Functional strengthening can be done in half kneel while reaching, targeting increased hip strengthening and LE dissociation (A). Play in kneeling challenges the hip and abdominal muscles bilaterally to control a stable pelvic position (B).

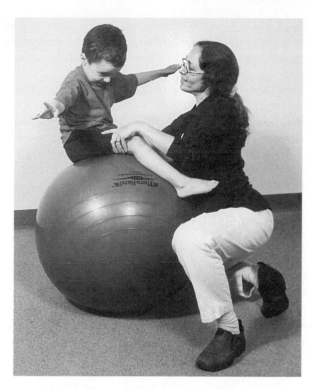

Figure 10–24. Practicing lateral trunk postural reactions.

Clinical Connection:

Key concepts in maximizing an efficient gait for children with CP include attention to the following.

Attempts should be made to achieve smoothness of both speed and joint position during gait. Decrease the tendency to hip hike, circumduct, exhibit excessive trunk displacement, or scissor the LEs, because these deviations create a high-energy demand.

Self-selected velocity is usually the most efficient. Attempt to achieve normal, smooth levels of speed so that gait is not jerky. ▪

Cerebrovascular Accident and Adult Hemiplegia

It is safe to say that *all* students and clinicians in physical and occupational therapy will have the opportunity to treat a patient/client who has had a stroke. It is entirely possible that some students and clinicians will not have the opportunity to treat a child with CP or an adult with a spinal cord injury; but this is not so for stroke. Appropriately, a great deal of academic preparation in physical therapy and occupational therapy programs discusses the CVA and clinical presentation of patients after a CVA.

Assessment and clinical management of locomotor deficits experienced by individuals who have had a stroke has been studied and documented extensively in physical and occupational therapy literature. Brunnstrom (1970) and the Bobaths (1970) have extensively published and taught intervention approaches specifically for individuals with adult hemiplegia, with clinical updates evident in the literature, as practice has changed (Lennon, 2001; Sawner & LaVigne, 1992). Proprioceptive neuromuscular facilitation (PNF) offers many suggestions for retraining and strengthening the movements of the pelvis to improve hemiplegic gait (Trueblood, Walker, Perry, & Gronley, 1989; Wang, 1994). Carr and Shepherd (1987) have detailed a Motor Retraining Programme (MRP), specifically designed to address the movement and motor control issues of stroke patients. A common thread to all intervention approaches is the attention directed to the trunk, and the importance of trunk control and strength on the ability of the individual to move from place to place. Because Chapter 8 of this text has discussed postural control, including trunk control and balance in great detail and Chapter 9 discusses the upper extremity, those concepts or techniques will not be repeated here, but the reader is reminded to integrate those concepts into a holistic management approach. This section will focus on the clinical management of gait disturbances as a main locomotor problem of patients/clients with hemiplegia.

The gait of persons with hemiplegia has several common characteristics. Velocity is decreased. Individuals who have had a stroke walk more than 50 percent slower than their healthy counterparts (Waters, Hislop, Perry, & Antonelli, 1978). Their gait is also characterized by increased double support time, reflecting increased time on the involved limb. Although the energy expenditure in a selected period is not higher, the energy demand overall is higher because it takes longer to cover the same distance (Gersten & Orr, 1971; Perry, 1992). Step length is shorter with the involved leg. Kinetic data show a loss of the normal phasing and modulation of muscle activity during the gait cycle. Although there are individual variations, three fairly distinct patterns have been identified:

1. A tendency for the flexor muscles to be active primarily during swing and the extensor muscles to be active primarily during stance in patients who demonstrate pattern-only motor control (see Figs. 10–8 and 10–25) (Perry, Giovan, Harris, Montgomery, & Azaria, 1978)
2. A tendency for premature and continued activity of the stance muscles (Fig. 10–25)
3. A tendency for co-contraction and co-activation patterns (Montgomery, 1987)

The causes of gait dysfunction in patients with

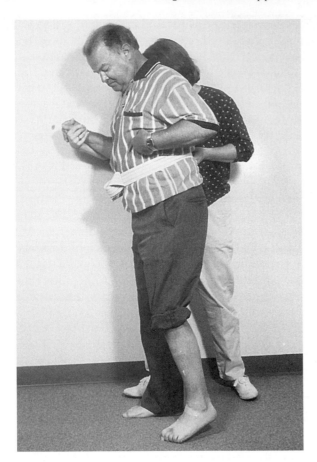

Figure 10–25. Example of pattern-only motor control—in this case, excessive extension persisting into the onset of swing phase. Continued activity of stance muscles interferes with an effective push-off and smooth transition into swing phase.

hemiplegia are due to disordered motor control, a lack of voluntary muscle control and weakness, interference from abnormal muscle tone and muscle stiffness, and a disorganized postural control mechanism. Table 10–7 summarizes the common gait deviations and possible causes and offers some intervention suggestions for the gait problems commonly observed in patients/clients following a stroke. The following summarizes some specific intervention guidelines for retraining of gait in individuals following a stroke.

▪ Clinical Management

Clinical management of the walking difficulties encountered by patients/clients with a stroke requires an analysis and intervention for the whole body as it cooperates during the gait cycle. Specific impairments such as decreased joint range of motion or muscle weakness need to be addressed. Gait training, along with all other functional mobility training, is optimally initiated early. Specific activities include activities to improve upright balance, the ability to demonstrate effective stance control, the ability to shift weight over the supporting limb, sufficient limb stability, and the ability to advance each limb. Intervention emphasis is on preambulation activities, as well as during the actual task of gait training. During gait training, the individual is offered opportunity to practice functional, task-specific locomotor skills: walking forward, walking backward, stepping sideways, and practice of elevation activities such as stepping over a step, clearing obstacles, negotiating

TABLE 10-7			
Common Gait Deviations Seen in Stroke: Possible Causes and Intervention Suggestions			
Deviation	**Gait Phase**	**Possible Cause**	**Intervention Suggestion**
Forward trunk lean	Throughout stance	Unawareness of affected side, poor proprioception Weak hip extensor strength or presence of hip flexion contracture Knee instability Plantar flexion spasticity	Increase awareness and movement control of affected body side. Strengthen voluntary hip extension. Stretch contracture, if present. Activate active dorsiflexion and dampen plantar flexion spasticity.
Pelvic retraction	Throughout gait cycle, most apparent during swing	Spasticity Weak voluntary protraction and pelvic control Weak abdominal muscles Shortening of pelvic retractors	Quick stretch to protractors before initial swing. Make manual contact and use pelvis as key point of control. Strengthen abdominal muscles for increased pelvic control. Stretch shortened pelvic retractors.
Hip hiking	Throughout swing	Inadequate hip or knee flexion Inadequate dorsiflexion Spasticity	Increase active antigravity range of motion into flexion: hip, knee, or ankle. Use orthotic device to compensate for foot drop. Use motor retraining to eliminate synergistic pattern.

TABLE 10-7

Common Gait Deviations Seen in Stroke: Possible Causes and Intervention Suggestions

Deviation	Gait Phase	Possible Cause	Intervention Suggestion
Circumduction	Throughout swing	Extensor spasticity Inadequate hip or knee flexion, dorsiflexion Plantar flexion contracture	Increase active antigravity range of motion in flexion: hip, knee, or ankle. Use orthotic device to compensate for foot drop. Use motor retraining to eliminate synergistic pattern.
Inadequate hip flexion	Throughout swing	Extensor spasticity, especially in quadriceps muscles Weakness or abnormally low LE muscle tone Inadequate hip flexion	Increase active antigravity control and range of motion in antigravity flexion.
Trendelenburg gait	Observed as pelvic drop on swing side or compensated by lateral trunk lean over stance limb	Weak hip abductor muscles	Strengthen hip abductor muscles in unilateral stance, especially to control contralateral pelvic position.
Scissoring	Throughout stance and swing	Spasticity in hip adductor muscles	Strengthen active hip abduction with strengthening of voluntary adductor control.
Excessive knee flexion during stance	Throughout stance, but especially at initial contact and loading	LE weakness or abnormally low muscle tone Increased flexor muscle tone or presence of LE flexor synergy Flexion contracture Poor proprioception	Increase voluntary strength of LE muscles, especially eccentric extensor cortical, during weight acceptance task. Stretch contracture, if present. Increase sensory awareness or augment for loss.
Knee hyperextension	Stance, especially at loading and midstance	LE muscle weakness, especially inadequate co-contraction control of hamstrings and quadriceps, hip extension weakness Pelvic retraction Quadriceps spasticity, increased extensor muscle tone in LE Plantar flexion contracture	Strengthen voluntary LE antigravity muscles and hamstring/quadriceps muscle control during weight-bearing tasks. Use motor retraining to increase active pelvic protraction, pelvic control during gait, and quadriceps muscle control. Stretch plantar flexion contracture and increase ankle dorsiflexion to at least neutral.
Inadequate knee flexion	Swing, especially midswing	Inadequate antigravity flexion Spastic quadriceps muscles	Increase active antigravity hip and knee flexion control.
Foot slap	Stance, at initial contact and loading	Inadequate dorsiflexor muscle strength, especially poor eccentric control Equinus gait or plantar flexion contracture	Increase voluntary dorsiflexor control, especially eccentric control. Stretch plantar flexion contracture and increase dorsiflexion. Use orthotic assistance.
Foot drop	Throughout swing and from terminal stance through preswing	Inadequate dorsiflexor muscle strength, especially antigravity control Muscle weakness Spasticity	Increase voluntary dorsiflexor control. Use orthotic assistance.

Source: Information compiled from multiple sources. See reference list and text for details.

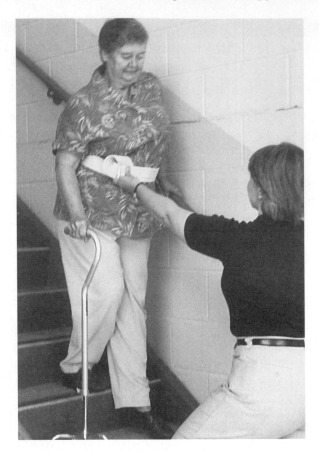

Figure 10–26. Stair use is an important functional locomotor skill.

uneven terrain or inclines, and using stairs (Fig. 10–26; see Figs. 7–16 and 7–17).

For an overall understanding of the movement difficulties of patients following a stroke, Ryerson and Levit (1997) offer a practical approach to organizing the functional retraining of gait in hemiplegia by dividing the main functional limitations into three areas: trunk impairments, impairments encountered in stance, and impaired swing. This model will be used to direct the clinical suggestions described next. This same organizational model so effectively promoted by Ryerson and Levit (1997) for the clinical management of clients with stroke can be expanded and applied to intervention with clients with other disorders, including ataxia and Parkinson's disease.

▪ Trunk Impairments

It is important to assist in the re-establishment of trunk alignment and control during the functional task of walking. Intervention with the trunk also cannot be separated from intervention directed to intervention with the individual's involved upper extremity (see Chapter 9). If the trunk becomes asymmetrical, control of the pelvis is compromised. Asymmetrical posture has

been identified as a common movement problem in patients with hemiplegia (Wu, Huang, Lin, & Chen, 1996). The therapist or assistant can use manual guidance, key points of control, balance activities, and strengthening activities to aid the individual first in gaining symmetrical midline trunk control over a stable upright base of support (Fig. 10–27). As forward progression begins, attention is then directed to re-educating the individual to shift weight through the lower extremities while retaining control of the trunk, allowing for smooth movement between the upper trunk over the lower trunk as the gait cycle proceeds (Fig. 10–28).

▪ Stance Impairments

Lower extremity intervention must establish compatible proximal and distal movement control. The proximal goals focus on increasing hip extension in conjunction with trunk extension control to maintain alignment over the pelvis. Distal intervention goals are then sequenced and combined with proximal goals during movement throughout stance. The therapist or

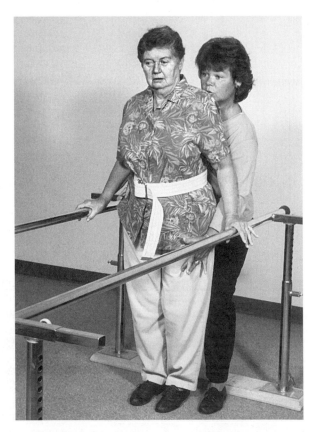

Figure 10–27. While facing a mirror, therapist uses verbal, visual, and manual guidance to cue patient for correct trunk, pelvic, and LE position. Patient is challenged to work on attaining/maintaining midline trunk control over a stable, upright BOS.

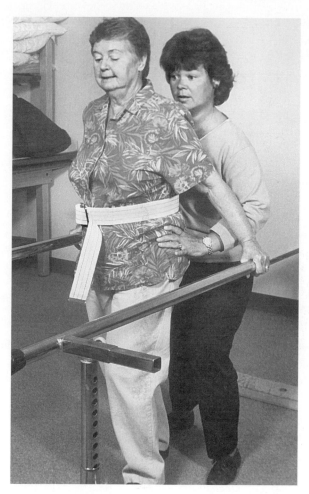

Figure 10–28. Therapist cues patient to initiate weight shift of lower extremity in a forward direction while maintaining control of the upper trunk as the lower trunk begins to rotate forward.

assistant intervenes to correct and cue for correct trunk and pelvic position (see Fig. 10–27), initiate the weight shift from the lower extremity in a forward direction (see Fig. 10–28), and re-establish ankle, knee, and hip control. During single limb support, individuals with hemiplegia often experience the greatest risk of instability, because the center of gravity is at its highest point in midstance. At the hip, intervention is directed to shift and move forward without excessive lateral movement. At the knee, intervention is directed to retrain and strengthen the musculature around the knee, including retraining for isometric, concentric, and eccentric control. At the ankle, intervention is directed at increasing effective dorsiflexor control, concentrically and eccentrically as appropriate.

▪ Swing Impairments

During swing, atypical muscle firing, inappropriate initiation patterns, and the inability to sustain appro-

priate firing are more noticeable. Forward momentum is often lost, resulting in a choppy, inefficient gait. If the pelvis is retracted, initiation of swing phase often occurs with pelvic elevation and shortening of the trunk. The clinician's first attention needs to be at the trunk and pelvis, assisting with trunk control and active pelvic protraction so that the LE can be advanced effectively (Fig. 10–29). The use of PNF and NDT techniques focusing on strengthening pelvic mobility and protraction have been demonstrated to be clinically successful, contributing to improvement not only in pelvic stability but mobility, resulting in an improved swing and longer step length (Trueblood et al., 1989). In intervention, problems with muscle firing and timing are retrained with the stance limb forward to replicate the demands of the swing cycle. The use of orthoses or functional electrical stimulation is known to be effective in assisting with foot clearance during swing (Bertoti, 2000; Pease, 1998) (see Fig. 7–3). Carryover into walking will not occur unless opportunity for practice is offered within the whole naturally occurring task of walking. Practice is offered to move smoothly from preswing into a controlled flexion and advancement of the hemiplegic limb.

Ataxia

By clinical definition, ataxia is a problem of defective muscular coordination especially manifested when voluntary movement is attempted (*Taber's,* 2001). Evidence of dysmetria, movement decomposition, dysdiadochokinesia, and abnormal timing of multijoint movements often characterize ataxia. As a symptom of disordered motor control, ataxia can accompany many neurological disorders, including multiple sclerosis; cerebellar, midbrain, or spinal disease; Friedreich's ataxia; chronic alcoholism; and some types of CP. The common denominator is that the movement disorder of ataxia is caused by neurological damage that interferes with normal spinocerebellar functioning, thus resulting in defective coordination of movement. As such, it is a classic sign of cerebellar disease. Ataxia is common in multiple sclerosis (MS). Because this particular symptom presents with a unique array of management dilemmas for rehabilitation professionals, this section will discuss the movement problems associated with the symptom of ataxia, regardless of the causative pathophysiology. Clinical management of ataxia as it interferes with lower extremity function and locomotion will not only be described here but will be the focus of a case study at the end of this chapter.

Ataxia may be manifested in the trunk, extremities, head, mouth, or tongue. As implied by its presentation as a coordination disorder, multijoint motions and patterns of movement are more affected than single

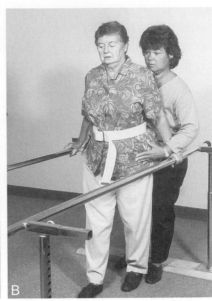
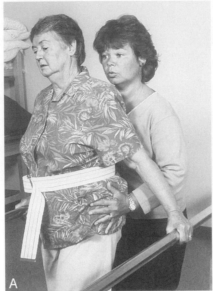

Figure 10–29. At the hip, intervention is directed at cueing pelvic control without excessive lateral movement. Therapist cues and guides the patient by assisting at the pelvis at the end of swing (A), as well as at the initiation of swing (B).

joint movements. The patient/client with ataxia typically presents with incoordination, tremor, and disturbances of posture, balance, and gait. Therapy is directed at promoting postural stability, accuracy of limb movements, and functional balance and gait (O'Sullivan, 2001a). Ataxia is most often associated with problems with reaching or difficulties with gait. Ataxic gait is one in which there is uneven step length, width is irregular, rhythm is absent, and the feet are often lifted too high (Figs. 10–30 and 10–31). The normal relationship between stance and swing phases of gait is altered. Arm swing is typically absent (Melnick & Oremland, 2001). Movement is typically wide-based with evidence of

poor proximal stability at the shoulders and pelvis (Fig. 10–32). Movement is also disturbed secondary to incorrect force generation, timing abnormalities, and inability to regulate posture.

Clinical Connection:

Unfortunately, many of us have seen the slurred speech, impaired balance, and uncoordinated gait pattern of someone who is drunk. Those symptoms present themselves, although temporarily, because of

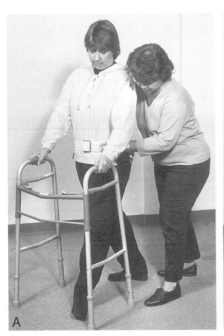
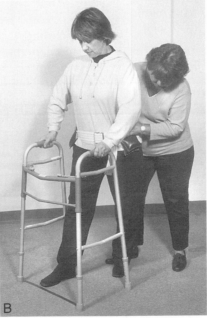

Figure 10–30. Gait of a person with ataxia is often irregular and jerky, resulting in poor foot placement and an ineffective BOS.

the effect of alcohol consumption on spinocerebellar neural connections and pathways, among others. Alcohol intoxication causes temporary ataxic symptomatology. ▪

Lesions or diseases affecting the cerebellum can also produce a condition of generalized weakness, known as **asthenia.** It has been hypothesized that asthenia is caused by a loss of cerebellar facilitation to the motor cortex, which in turn can reduce the activity of spinal motor neurons during voluntary movement (Bremer, 1935; Melnick & Oremland, 2001). The result is that posture is poorly maintained, and patients complain of a feeling of heaviness, excessive effort required for simple tasks, and early onset of fatigue during conscious effort (Holmes, 1939). Hypotonia also often accompanies cerebellar dysfunction. All these difficulties will decrease the smoothness and efficiency of lower extremity functioning, mobility, and gait.

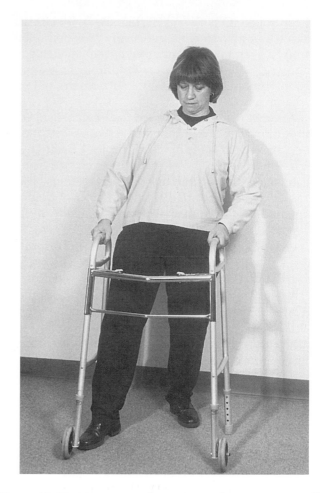

Figure 10–32. Movement of a patient wth ataxia is typically wide based, with evidence of poor stability at shoulders, trunk, and pelvis.

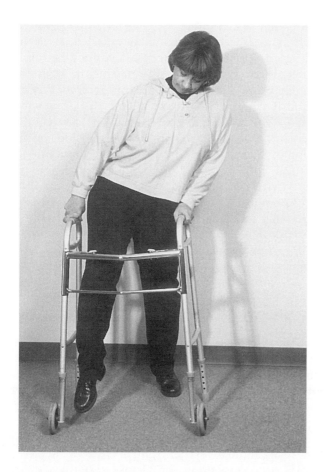

Figure 10–31. Gait of a person with ataxia can be characterized by excessive hip and knee flexion (high steppage), with the ankle poorly prepositioned in plantar flexion for initial contact.

▪ Clinical Management

Intervention will certainly be multifaceted, directed at improving postural control; decreasing the interfering effects of instability; improving functional locomotor skills, including transfers and gait; and improving accuracy of limb movement during functional activities. Activities to improve postural stability and balance are described in Chapter 8 of this text. This section will focus on activities to improve lower extremity control and locomotion.

Postural stability and strength can be improved by focusing on static control in a variety of different weight-bearing postures, such as prone on elbows, sitting, quadruped, kneeling, and standing. Refer to Table 4–2 for a summary of the use of developmental positions as strengthening exercises. Progression can include training in a series of postures that increase postural demands by varying the BOS, and increasing the number of body segments that must be coordinated and controlled (O'Sullivan, 2001a, 2001c). Specific techniques to improve stability, especially proximal stability around the shoulders and pelvis, are effective (see Chapter 6). Techniques that are helpful include approximation, rhythmic stabilization, and isometrics at varying points within the range.

Dynamic postural responses can be challenged by incorporating controlled mobility activities (see Chapter 6) into functional retraining. Examples of activities in which controlled mobility is utilized include weight-shifting activities and movement transitions. Movements are typically started as small and then gradually progressed into larger increments of range. Assistance and guidance are given judiciously, with encouraged active movement and voluntary control from the patient/client. Functional activities such as bridging and transitioning between sitting and standing are effective ways to integrate controlled mobility into an individual's movement repertoire. PNF is effective to establish and strengthen the agonist-antagonist relationship during movement. Any of the appropriate facilitation techniques used with PNF can be selected (see Table 6–2). Frenkel's exercises are useful in the remediation of the dysmetria so often seen in patients/clients with uncoordinated movement (Frenkel, 1902).

Clinical Connection:

Proximal stability may improve, contributing to a decrease in ataxia, through the judicious use of light weights. Weights can be used proximally or distally, both uses attempting to increase proprioceptive awareness of the limb. Placement of weight proximally, such as through use of a weighted belt or putting rolled coins into a patient's pockets, may serve as a joint approximation input, contributing to increased proximal stability around the pelvic/hip area. The same method would be appropriate for improving UE stability and awareness though the use of light weights over the shoulder, sewn into a vest or shoulder pads. Alternately, the use of distal weights around the ankles or wrists has met with clinical success in increasing proprioceptive awareness and aiding in effective upper or lower limb placement. Therapists and assistants are encouraged to try both methods and to assess the patient's response. If it is effective, continue; if not, discontinue. ■

Functional training focuses on the development of problem-solving skills and appropriate compensatory strategies to ensure that ADL tasks can be performed safely and with maximum independence. Training includes practice of all mobility skills, including rolling, bed mobility, transfer training, and ambulation. Consistent with the style of this chapter, the following gait training strategies are suggested as organized to assist the individual with ataxia to successfully execute the main tasks of gait (Ryerson & Levit, 1997).

■ Trunk Impairments

Exercises and activities to improve static and dynamic postural control and balance can be incorporated into preambulation activities and gait training. Standing and walking activities should stress adequate weight transfer with trunk rotation and retraining to re-establish a reciprocal arm swing, however limited. Trunk-strengthening exercises, rhythmic stabilization, and biofeedback are all effective techniques. PNF patterns that emphasize trunk rotation are useful.

■ Stance Impairments

Stance function can be impaired by interference from a constellation of constraints, as discussed previously in this chapter: weakness, especially in the hip and knee extensors; contracture; sensory impairment; and interference from abnormally low muscle tone or uncoordinated movement. Suggestions for the clinical management of all these impairments have been detailed elsewhere. Lower extremity intervention must establish compatible proximal and distal movement control. The proximal goals focus on increasing hip extension in conjunction with trunk extension control to maintain alignment over the pelvis, with adequate postural control. Distal intervention goals are then sequenced and combined with proximal goals during movement throughout stance. The therapist or assistant intervenes to correct and cue for correct trunk and pelvic position and initiation of the weight shift from the lower extremity in a forward direction and to help re-establish ankle, knee, and hip control.

■ Swing Impairments

During swing, atypical muscle firing, inappropriate initiation patterns, and the inability to sustain appropriate firing are more noticeable. Forward advancement of the limb is often demonstrated as a wide-based, abducted advancement of the limb, with evidence of dysmetria resulting in poor limb prepositioning for stance placement (see Fig. 10–30). Momentum is often lost, resulting in a very jerky, ineffective swing (see Fig. 10–31). In intervention, problems with muscle firing and timing are retrained with the stance limb forward to replicate the demands of the swing cycle. The use of proximal or distal weights may help in decreasing the ataxic movement, assisting with accuracy of swing. Remember, however, that carryover into walking may not occur unless opportunity is given for practice within the whole naturally occurring task of walking. Practice is offered to move smoothly from preswing into a controlled flexion and advancement of the moving limb.

Parkinson's Disease

The main motor impairments associated with Parkinson's disease include muscular rigidity, resting tremor, bradykinesia, and akinesia, all of which have been described elsewhere in this text. Specifically for this chapter, a discussion of the lower extremity functional challenges encountered by individuals with Parkinson's disease offers another opportunity to problem solve the clinical management of gait disturbances encountered by these patients/clients.

For clarification, it is important to contrast and compare the two symptoms of akinesia and bradykinesia. **Akinesia** refers to difficulty *initiating* movement. Akinesia will create difficulty for the individual to initiate the weight shift to begin a gait cycle or to shift the trunk forward to initiate a sit-to-stand transfer. **Bradykinesia,** in contrast, refers to slowness or difficulty *maintaining* movement once initiated. Patients with Parkinson's disease may present with both akinesia and bradykinesia in varying degrees. Recent studies have demonstrated that difficulties in movement initiation experienced by individuals with Parkinson's disease are more limiting than difficulties with initiation experienced by older counterparts without the disease and that these difficulties become more pronounced in older patients with Parkinson's disease than in their younger counterparts (Halliday, Winter, Frank, Patla, & Prince, 1998; Martin et al., 2002).

The impairment of rigidity and voluntary muscle weakness will also have effects on functional use of the lower extremities and locomotor skills. Patients will demonstrate loss of flexibility, abnormal co-activation patterns, and contracture development secondary to lack of movement. In the lower extremities, contractures commonly develop in the hip and knee flexors, hip adductors, and plantar flexors. These positional changes will have a negative effect on the ability to effectively load the lower extremity, a position requiring hip extension, knee control, and an ankle position of at least neutral. A forward flexed trunk leads commonly to a kyphotic deformity, which compromises trunk mobility and antigravity strength of both flexor and extensor muscle groups (see Fig. 7–17A). Rolling becomes less segmental, and a more rigid pattern is typically seen. Sit-to-stand will be characterized by difficulty with not only the initiation phase of the transfer, but also the

trunk extension and execution phase (see Table 10–5 and Figs. 7–38 and 7–39).

The gait pattern of a patient with Parkinson's disease has several unique clinical characteristics. As mentioned previously, difficulties with initiation (akinesia) and momentum (bradykinesia) will prevail. Hip, knee, and ankle motions are reduced, with a generalized lack of extension at the hip and knee and dorsiflexion at the ankle. Trunk and pelvic motions are diminished, resulting in lack of reciprocal arm swing, limited rotation and dissociation, and inability of pelvic motion to contribute effectively to the gait cycle, limiting rotation, momentum, and limb advancement. Stride length is decreased, and the patient is observed to walk with small, shuffling steps (see Fig. 7–17). The abnormally stooped posture contributes to the development of a **festinating gait,** characterized by a progressive increase in speed with a shortening in stride length (O'Sullivan, 2001b). The gait can then take on an accelerating quality, called a **propulsive gait,** sometimes requiring that the patient/client come in contact with an object or a wall in order to stop. Patients with Parkinson's disease have great difficulty turning and changing direction while walking. Overall velocity may be decreased, but cadence is increased, contributing to inefficiency. Heel strike is lost on initial contact, with either a flatfooted or toe-heel progression seen. This flatfooted gait will decrease the ability of the individual to step over obstacles or walk on carpeted surfaces. The gait and postural difficulties experienced by patients with Parkinson's disease are the two impairments that can cause the greatest handicap to these individuals. This section will focus on clinical management of the gait disturbance. See Chapter 8 for a discussion of postural control.

▪ *Clinical Management*

For the sake of consistency, it is helpful to discuss the clinical management of common gait disturbances experienced by individuals with Parkinson's disease by applying the same model to guide discussion as used previously in this chapter. A familiarity with the symptoms and impairments as described previously readily demonstrates that individuals with Parkinson's disease will encounter difficulty with all three subtasks of gait: weight acceptance, single limb support, and limb advancement. These functional limitations will be caused by the constellation of impairments and symptoms that trouble the patient with Parkinson's disease: weakness, rigidity, abnormal muscular activation and sequencing, loss in flexibility, deformity and contracture formation, and impaired movement coordination. As presented in the other pathologies within this chapter, this section will discuss clinical management suggestions for the gait difficulties experienced by patients with Parkinson's disease by examining how these gait subtasks can be the focus of intervention, framed within a discussion of intervention directed at the trunk impairment or impairments seen during stance or swing phase (Ryerson & Levit, 1997).

Because of the nature of the disorder of Parkinson's disease, it is important to emphasize the importance of varying the practice of movement skills within and across varying environmental contexts. Patients with Parkinsonism will perform better if the environment is familiar and if cognitive attention to the actual movement task is shifted from the movement to the actual familiar task. Embedding an exercise program, including a locomotor training program, within a meaningful environment or activity is much more effective than rote exercise or part practice. Random practice may enable the patient/client to learn the correct schema or rule by which to regulate the speed and direction of functional movement, such as moving around in a living space. Gait training needs to include walking in crowds, through doorways, and on different surfaces. Practice in walking at different speeds and with differing stride lengths is also functionally important (see Fig. 7–17*B*). Task-specific training has been demonstrated to be optimally effective in the rehabilitation of individuals with Parkinson's disease (Morris, 2001).

▪ Trunk Impairments

The trunk of a patient with Parkinson's disease may be stooped, flexed, and rigidly limited in rotation (see Fig. 7–17*A*). Patients with Parkinson's disease often do not demonstrate a reciprocal arm swing, consistent with inflexibility and lack of trunk rotation. To increase trunk rotation, PNF patterns (see Fig. 8–17), NDT techniques using key points of control and manual guidance (see Figs. 7–38 and 8–19), and exercise to practice active trunk rotation have all been shown to be effective. It may be easier to practice these techniques first in sitting, where postural control is not as challenged, and then integrate the reciprocal movement patterns into upright standing and then during gait. Because bilateral symmetrical movement patterns are easier than reciprocal patterns, they can be tried first, followed by diagonal movements (Melnick, 2001). Clinical studies have demonstrated that the use of rhythm and auditory cues facilitates movement very effectively for individuals with Parkinson's disease. Dancing incorporates rotation, movement, and coordination in a familiar and rhythmic manner. Trunk strengthening programs are important to focus on strengthening of the spinal extensors for improvement in posture and postural control and increasing spinal flexibility. Relaxation exercises

have also been found to be beneficial in improving mobility, effective ventilation, and reducing stress (Schenkman et al., 1989).

▪ Stance Impairments

Rhythm, especially as in a marching motion, seems to enable the individual to move continuously with the required alternating flexion and extension without being hindered by akinetic "freezing" (see Chapter 5). Rhythmic exercise has been shown to decrease rigidity and bradykinesia and to improve gait over time (Gauthier, 1987; McIntosh, 1997). Functional strength training can be effectively used to increase strength, especially of the muscles so vitally important for stance control: pelvic stabilizers, hip extensors, knee extensors, and eccentric control of the anterior tibialis and gastrocnemius muscles. Traditional stretching techniques can be used to elongate shortened muscles, especially the hip and knee flexors and plantar flexors. Weight-shifting activities offer multiple opportunities for integrating functional strength and postural responses into a movement pattern (see Figs. 7–38 and 7–39). Work in stance can include activities to encourage heel strike at initial contact, effective weight acceptance over a stable and extended lower extremity, and weight shifting over the leg, as well as to the other extremity. Attention to gait initiation should occur during smooth practice of both stance and swing phase, to take advantage of the natural momentum that occurs during the gait cycle (Halliday et al., 1998).

▪ Swing Impairments

Activities that encourage smooth control of the momentum force generated at the end of stance will offer the patient/client opportunity to control the advancing limb. Increasing active hip flexion and knee extension will correlate with a more effectively advanced limb and a longer stride. Once again, the use of rhythm or auditory cues can be very effective. Functional task training that includes clearing obstacles, negotiating uneven terrain, and changing speeds can be practiced in varying environments. Individuals with Parkinsonism may require a focus on eccentric strength training so that increased voluntary control can be channeled into the deceleration tasks of the muscles that naturally elongate during gait: hip extensors, hamstrings and quadriceps, and both ankle compartments.

Spinal Cord Injury

Although spinal cord injury (SCI) is not emphasized in any previous chapter in this text, it is important to mention this disorder here because this chapter deals specifically with lower extremity function, the main locus of impairment for the individual with a SCI. First, it is important to differentiate between the types of CNS symptoms seen in patients with spinal cord injury compared with the symptomatology associated with patients with disorders affecting the areas of the CNS superior to the spinal cord. This is often an area of confusion for students, so a brief and rather simple explanation is offered.

The spasticity seen in spinal upper motor neuron (UMN) lesions differs from that seen in cerebral UMN lesions. **Spinal spasticity,** resulting from a noncongenital SCI, can be quite extreme, with a characteristic distribution in the extensor muscles of the lower extremities, often with severe episodes of muscle spasm (Pedretti, 1996; Preston & Hecht, 1999). Research suggests that this increased muscle tone is the result of residual influence of supraspinal centers, such as the cortex, on the spinal cord and ineffective modulation of spinal pathways (Craik, 1991). **Cerebral spasticity** is the type described throughout this text, as often seen in patients with CP, traumatic brain injury, brain tumor, or after CVA. In this clinical presentation, the degree of hypertonicity often fluctuates as a result of a change in the patient's position, and the antigravity muscles are predominantly affected (flexors in the UEs and extensors in the LEs) (Young, 1994). In MS, the spasticity stems from both spinal and cerebral disease (Blumenkopf, 1997). It is important to mention these differences because the clinical manifestation may appear different to the clinician or student, although the universal fact in *all* instances is that in spasticity, voluntary muscle control and activation is deficient, muscular weakness prevails, and the abnormally high muscle tone is a pathological sign of disordered motor control. Regardless of the underlying pathophysiology, the therapeutic intervention strategies are more similar than dissimilar.

It is also important to at least briefly acknowledge the difference between a congenital spinal cord injury and one that occurs after birth. A congenital spinal cord injury is associated with the most severe form of spina bifida, a condition known as myelomeningocele, in which the spinal cord and meninges of a developing fetus are contained in a sac external to the vertebral column (Fig. 10–33). Within this sac, the spinal cord and associated neural tissue show extensive abnormalities. Incomplete closure of the neural tube, abnormal growth of the spinal cord, and a tortuous pathway of neural elements make the transmission of nervous impulses abnormal (Schneider & Krosschell, 2001). The clinical result is a sensory and motor impairment at the level of the lesion and below, presenting as a flaccid paralysis (Stark, 1977). The most common site of myelomeningocele is the lumbosacral spine. The resulting physical

Myelomeningocele

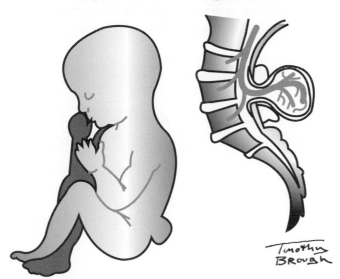

Figure 10–33. Myelomeningocele: a neural tube defect whereby the spinal cord and spinal nerves are exterior to the vertebral column, with subsequent sensory and motor impairment.

impairments are numerous, including paralysis and denervation of the musculature in the lower extremities to an extent dependent on the level of the lesion. On the other hand, spinal cord injury of postnatal onset interrupts the connection between the spinal cord and the rest of the CNS, but the neural connections and tissue had originally been normally formed. The clinical result in this instance is flaccidity at the exact level of the lesion and spasticity below the level of the lesion.

■ Clinical Management

It is not the intent of this text or this chapter to discuss in any detail the clinical management of either a child with myelomeningocele or an individual with a spinal cord injury. Management strategies are unique to those disorders and covered in depth in other sources. However, this section of this chapter would be remiss if these disorders were not at least mentioned. Locomotor management typically includes orthotic and assistive device prescription as required to compensate for the loss of movement in the muscles affected by the spinal lesion. Programs to establish or restore mobility include strengthening of key musculature; selective stretching; and functional training in all mobility skills, including rolling, floor or mat mobility, transfers, standing, ambulation, and wheelchair training. The techniques that have proven useful in the rehabilitation of patients with spinal cord injury are a unique set of clinical management strategies, based on the strengthening of preserved musculature and functional abilities and the augmenting of those capabilities with assistive technology and adaptive equipment. Refer to other sources for an in-depth discussion (Campbell, 2000; Cech & Martin, 2000; O'Sullivan, 2001c; Pedretti, 1996; Trombly, 1995; Umphred, 2001).

Case Studies

The following case studies will describe the clinical management of locomotor difficulties with a child with CP and an adult with cerebellar ataxia.

Case Study: Child

Amanda: Child with Spastic Diplegic CP

History

Amanda was born at 27 weeks gestation with a birth weight of 2 pounds, 5 ounces. Delivery was via an emergency Cesarean section precipitated by maternal eclampsia. She was in the NICU for 10 weeks; her neonatal course was complicated by pneumothoraces, renal failure, cardiopulmonary arrest, and several episodes of apnea. Amanda has a mild visual deficit, requiring eyeglasses. She has undergone successful surgery for strabismus. History is negative for medications or seizures. Diagnosis of cerebral palsy, spastic diplegia, was made at 10 months of age. Developmental milestones were delayed; mother reports that Amanda did not sit until after 1 year of age and that she began pulling to stand at furniture at 3 years and ambulating with an assistive device at age 4. She is now 6 years old and is attending the first grade in a local classroom. She uses a posterior walker and wears bilateral molded ankle foot orthoses (MAFOs). She has had no orthopedic surgical procedures. This evaluation is conducted at the request of the school district to specifically address issues surrounding functional mobility and independence while at school.

Evaluation

Transitional movements that lack rotation and dissociation characterize functional mobility on the floor during play and floor-to-stand transfer. Antigravity flexion and extension strength appear to be adequate. Sitting positions and transitions show limited choices. Amanda moves out of floor sitting by assuming a quadruped position; she is not able to transition with rotation to side sitting or half kneel. Movement on the floor is characterized by scooting forward using her

arms and flexed lower extremities to propel herself forward, rather than reciprocally creeping. Amanda pulls to stand at support, including a posterior walker that she has used independently for the past 3 years. She pulls to stand by using her upper extremities; the lower extremities remain flexed, passively coming underneath her (Fig. 10–34). Stance posture is characterized by capital extension, a forward flexed trunk, anterior pelvic tilt, hips in flexion and adduction, knees flexed, and ankles in plantar flexion. The left knee is more flexed than the right throughout stance, with weight typically shifted forward onto the arms and then onto the walker, with limited weight borne through the LEs (Fig. 10–35).

Muscle tone is high throughout both lower extremities, with muscular weakness in all isolated voluntary movements. In the lower extremities, increased muscle tone is distributed primarily to the hip extensors, hip adductors, hamstrings, and plantar flexors, with a few beats of unsustained clonus noted at the left ankle. There is a Babinski sign bilaterally. Muscle tone is low in the trunk, with very poor abdominal tone. Muscle tone in the LEs and the trunk appears to increase with excitement and newly introduced activities. Amanda has limited voluntary muscle control of any isolated action in the lower extremities. There is very little dissociation of one lower extremity from the other.

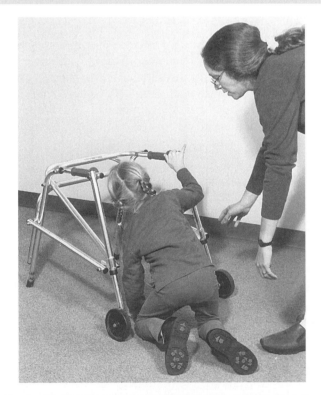

Figure 10–34. Transition from floor to stand at support characterized by flexed LEs and poor dissociation between the LEs, preventing smooth weight shift. Because of the weak LEs, reliance on UEs to pull up is evident.

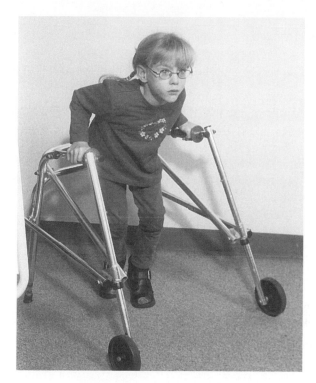

Figure 10–35. Stance posture demonstrating increased reliance on UEs bearing weight onto the assistive device, a forward-flexed, unstable trunk posture and ineffective weight bearing through the LEs.

Motor control is characterized by movement patterns of predominantly full flexion or extension with little dissociation or rotation. Movements are stereotypical, with little variety. Position and gravity exert an influence on body posture and muscle tone. Posturing is often asymmetrical, with increased muscle tone, especially on the left body side. Observations of movements are consistent with lack of sophisticated motor control and a predominance of some tonic automatic responses, including postural reflexes, continuing to influence movement and posture. Isolated voluntary motor control with varying movement combinations is not evident. Rather, Amanda demonstrates a limited repertoire of movement patterns and the presence of some apparent compensatory strategies, which may prove to be undesirable. Challenging Amanda's balance results in increased muscle tone in both lower extremities and an increased extension posturing of her trunk. Mature balance reactions are delayed and weak. Functional independence in an upright position is limited.

A functional assessment of strength reveals weakness of hip extension, hip abduction, knee extension, and limited stabilization of the weight-bearing foot. There is also evidence of poor abdominal strength and lack of pelvic control. Amanda encounters difficulty attempting to isolate and demonstrate hip extension

and knee extension strength through the available range against gravity. Spasticity is quite strong, assessed at a score of 4 on the modified Ashworth Scale. Spasticity does interfere with and mask voluntary isolated movement. Amanda is not able to perform upright kneeling, shift into half kneel, or stand mid-floor without manual assistance or support. Amanda presents with a crouched stance posture with forward flexed trunk, anterior pelvic tilt, hips in flexion and adduction, knees flexed, and ankles in plantar flexion. On both sides, the gait cycle is characterized by consistent hip and knee flexion, limited hip abduction, and initial contact onto the ball of the foot. There is limited rollover and no push-off, with very little stability throughout stance. Limited limb advancement is evident with lack of full knee extension at terminal swing. Initial contact occurs onto a plantar flexed ankle, hip and knee flexed. During midstance, both knees remain flexed, with evidence of limited stance stability. Generally, gait dysfunction is noted with overactivity of the knee flexors and weakness of the gastrocnemius, quadriceps, and hip extensor and abductor muscles (Fig. 10–36). Stance phase function is characterized by instability and an impaired ability to accept weight for adequate limb support. Swing phase function is impaired by difficulty advancing the limb in preparation for weight transfer. Functionally, Amanda is independent in the use of a posterior walker, which presently limits her to level surfaces and use of an elevator between floors at school. She is currently wearing bilateral molded ankle-foot orthoses, which fit her well.

Upper extremity range of motion is within normal limits. Hips appear to be clinically stable. Goniometric assessment of the lower extremities reveals minimal hip flexion contractures (hip flexion 5 to 120 degrees on left; lack of complete hip extension on left; full range on right) and a 15-degree flexion contracture at the left knee. None of these limitations are significant enough to require orthopedic surgical intervention. These data suggest muscle weakness and significant spasticity rather than range-of-motion limitations as the main impairment contributing to Amanda's movement dysfunction.

Present Movement Problem

Amanda is an active, well-adjusted, happy 6-year-old girl with spastic diplegic CP, who is currently expressing frustration about her limited upright mobility and discomfort secondary to spasticity. Muscle tone is severely high in both lower extremities, left more so than right. Spasticity is most evident in the hamstring and adductor muscles, contributing to a crouch position throughout stance and gait. Her movement disorder is characterized by muscle weakness, abnormal

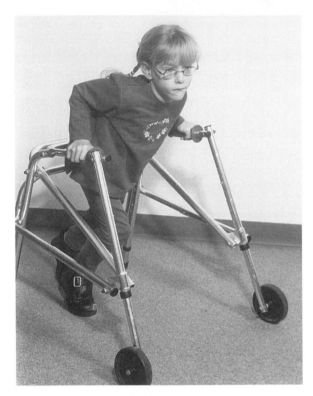

Figure 10–36. Gait is characterized by predominant hip and knee flexion, initial contact onto the ball of the foot, apparent instability, and ineffective weight acceptance.

muscle tone, limited motor control, predominance of immature postural patterns that influence voluntary activity, stereotypical movement patterns, and decreased evidence of mature postural control mechanisms. Movement is characterized by poor rotation and dissociation and limited antigravity control. Weakness is a predominant feature of the lower extremities, especially in hip extension, knee extension, and stance control at the ankle. Spasticity interferes with function, and Amanda complains of painful spasms, especially after a long day at school. There is some evidence of secondary musculoskeletal impairments, including minimal to moderate limitations in range of motion. Amanda is currently using a posterior walker and bilateral orthoses, both of which fit well and continue to be appropriate.

Intervention

The physical and occupational therapist met with Amanda, her parents, and Amanda's teacher to discuss findings of the assessment and plan an intervention strategy. Amanda's primary goal was stated as a desire to be more independently mobile so that she could "stand taller" and walk a "little better, to keep up with my friends." After meeting with the family, Amanda,

and Amanda's physician, a decision was made to schedule Amanda for placement of a baclofen pump so that spasticity could be ameliorated and a strengthening program could be directed to all the functional muscle groups of the LEs. An increase in voluntary, isolated antigravity muscle strength is anticipated with exercise in combination with a decrease in the symptom of spasticity in both lower extremities. The effects of the baclofen injection are expected to assist the therapists and assistants in helping Amanda to make selective strength gains and ensure translation of these anticipated strength gains into the attainment of improved functional skills (see Chapter 6). Figure 10–37 shows the placement of the pump under Amanda's skin, delivering a prescribed dose of baclofen to the intrathecal spinal space.

The following summarizes some of the intervention activities, carried out at school, at an outpatient rehabilitation center during weekly appointments, and at home. Intervention will take on an eclectic, integrated approach, utilizing techniques from NDT, PNF, a therapeutic exercise approach, task-oriented training, dynamic systems approach to motor control, and motor learning. All members of the therapy team from PT and OT participate in treating Amanda. The therapy goals and sample activities to meet these objectives are outlined next, accompanied by figures depicting the intervention. Goals and activities focus on the following:

1. Increase strength. Strengthening efforts will be focused on key lower extremity muscles and the trunk.
   - Amanda will demonstrate increased strength in gluteus maximus, quadriceps, hamstrings, and gastrocnemius muscles bilaterally.
     1. Gluteus maximus: active hip extension in functional positions such as kneeling and stance. Strengthen hip extension during functional tasks including: stability in kneeling, half kneeling, and stance (Figs. 10–38 and 10–39). Progress to unilateral limb loading with adequate hip extension. Activities including partial squat for eccentric work and walking backward may be attempted. Integrate activities into play and functional tasks.
     2. Quadriceps: Strengthen the quadriceps muscles for eccentric control during appropriate subphases of gait, such as initial contact and loading, concentrically during terminal swing, and isometrically for stance control. Activities such as squat to stand are effective for eccentric strengthening of the quadriceps, as well as the gluteus maximus muscles.

3. Hamstring muscles: Strengthen the hamstring muscles to be activated effectively during isometric knee stabilization in stance and semi-squat activities. Activate the hamstring muscle group to work eccentrically to decelerate the advancing limb during the swing phase of gait.

4. Gastrocnemius: Strengthen the gastrocnemius muscles to stabilize the hindfoot and act on the knee in the closed chain to stabilize stance. Work toward co-contraction and balance around the ankle.

2. Increase range of motion. Amanda, her teachers, and her family will learn to remind Amanda about her positioning choices so that Amanda is encouraged to attempt alternative and varied sitting positions, such as side sitting or sitting against furniture for support. Positioning in prone for some period will be encouraged at home, perhaps for television time or sleep.

3. Improve quality of movement. Therapy will focus on guiding Amanda in mastering movement options that encourage the development of postural control. Therapy will facilitate the carryover of rotation and dissociation into transitional movement and will decrease stereotypical patterns.

• Amanda will incorporate rotation and dissociation into transitional movements during adaptive physical education and while moving at home.

1. Facilitate and practice floor mobility with rotation incorporated into the movement, such as supine to and from sit, sitting to and from quadruped, and prone to and from sitting.

2. Transfer to and from upright with rotation incorporated into functional transitional movements: kneel to and from half kneel, half kneel to and from stance (see Fig. 10–38).

• Amanda will demonstrate increased variety of movement options.

1. Explore and practice various movement choices.

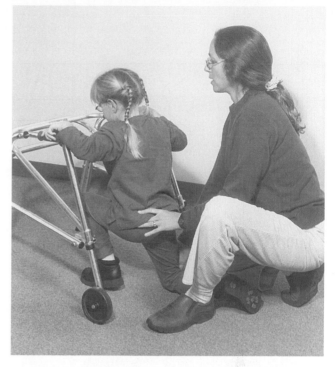

Figure 10–38. Work in half kneeling to strengthen isolated hip extension (R) and to promote development of dissociated movement patterns during a functional task.

2. Examine possible barriers to these movement choices and explore new possibilities. For example, Amanda's family room and classroom can be modified to ensure that bookcase and table heights allow Amanda to practice her newly learned mobility skills and retrieve items such as books independently. She will also be encouraged to help her mother at the kitchen table, standing at support.

4. Increase mobility. Encourage Amanda to explore different opportunities for independent mobility, such as transfers; practice in stance for selected daily activities, such as standing at the sink, toilet, or drinking fountain; and correct use of the walker.

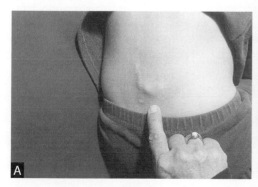
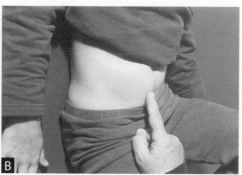

Figure 10–37. Placement of baclofen pump: posterior view (A); anterior view (B).

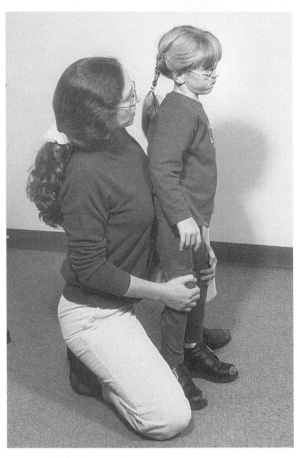

Figure 10–39. Work on bilateral strengthening and control of gluteus maximus, quadriceps, and gastrocnemius muscles to effectively maintain functional upright stance control.

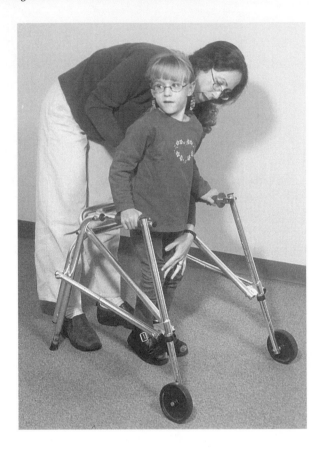

Figure 10–40. Child encouraged to practice stance with erect trunk, neutral pelvis, hip and knee extension, and a plantigrade foot.

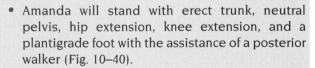

- Amanda will stand with erect trunk, neutral pelvis, hip extension, knee extension, and a plantigrade foot with the assistance of a posterior walker (Fig. 10–40).
  1. Muscles targeted for strengthening are the bilateral gluteus maximus, gluteus medius, and gastrocnemius in stance.
- Amanda will ambulate 25 feet with training focusing on several functional subtasks.
  1. Unilaterally load one lower extremity while simultaneously unweighting and advancing the contralateral lower extremity. *Effective unilateral limb loading* is described as a stable pelvic position, hip and knee extended to accept/maintain upright weight bearing, and heel on the floor. Muscles targeted to strengthen include the gluteus maximus, gluteus medius, and gastrocnemius on the weight-bearing side.
  2. *Effective limb advancement* is described as forward translation of the lower extremity through space with hip flexion and knee flexion followed by knee extension to advance the limb with adequate step length. The foot clears the floor throughout swing so that the limb is appropriately positioned in preparation for the next floor contact (Fig. 10–41). Muscles targeted for strengthening may include rectus femoris, hamstrings, quadriceps, and anterior tibialis.
  3. The next task is to transfer weight to the forward advanced limb with appropriate stability and lower extremity alignment. The lower extremity accepting the weight transfer must have a level pelvic position, hip moving into extension, knee extended with the heel in contact with the floor (see Fig. 10–41). Muscles targeted for strengthening include the iliopsoas, gluteus maximus, hamstrings, and quadriceps.
  4. Practice gait cycles with smooth limb loading, limb advancement, and weight transfer (Fig. 10–42) (Bertoti, 2000).

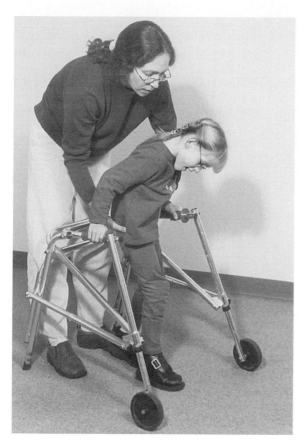

Figure 10–41. Effective limb advancement with improved knee extension at terminal swing and floor contact onto a stable foot.

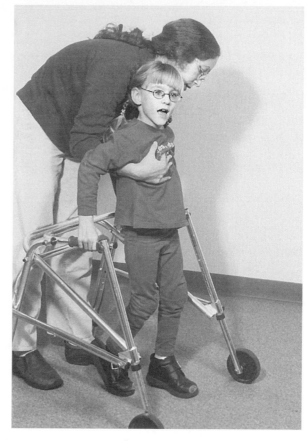

Figure 10–42. Practice of successive gait cycles and emphasis on the functional subtasks of each phase.

Case Study: Adult

Anna: Adult with Ataxic MS

History

Anna is a 47-year-old woman, diagnosed with multiple sclerosis 5 years ago. She is the married mother of an only son, now grown and attending college. She has a busy but attentive husband, who is a full-time teacher. Anna and her husband live in a small town home, spending summers in a cottage at the seashore. Anna is presently admitted for a brief inpatient rehabilitation visit, having experienced an exacerbation of her MS symptoms and a change in functional abilities. Anna is cooperative and talkative, actually somewhat euphoric and inappropriate at times, although very pleasant to work with.

Evaluation

Anna presents in a wheelchair, which she has used over the past 2 years for long distances and when tired. She had used a walker in the past but is currently experi-encing difficulty in accurate and safe use of this as an assistive device. Anna is willing to begin using a different device but wishes to remain ambulatory, however limited, so that she can access the small stores on the oceanfront boardwalk and walk around her small backyard bird sanctuary. Anna is independent in all mobility with the use of a wheelchair. Transfers in and out of the chair are executed safely and consistently. Ambulation safety and efficiency with the walker are of great concern.

Muscle tone is low throughout the trunk and extremities, with hypotonia more pronounced in the proximal muscle groups as compared with the distal groups. Anna has generalized weakness throughout, and she complains of a feeling of limb heaviness, clumsiness, and frequent fatigue. Sensation is mildly diminished to sharp and light touch, intact to dull and firm touch. Proprioceptive sense is decreased, especially in the distal lower extremities. Following this exacerbation, Anna now presents with a foot drop bilaterally, often interfering with functional placement and control of the lower extremities during upright activities. Range of motion is within functional limits.

Present Movement Problem

Anna is able to enjoy most independent mobility when using a wheelchair as an assistive device for long distances and when tired. Increasing fatigue, weakness in the trunk and extremities, ataxic movements of the lower extremities, and a bilateral foot drop compromise functional ambulation. The therapists and assistants in the rehabilitation facility met with Anna to discuss her goals and intervention. Table 6–8 and the questions posed in the Clinical Connection on page 206 of Chapter 6 were used to guide the discussion and arrive at functional goals for Anna. Anna would like to retain some limited ambulation ability. The therapy team has concurred that the amount of generalized weakness and fatigue, proximal instability, and drop foot were the main impairments contributing to Anna's present movement problem and functional limitations.

Intervention

Intervention was planned to include both physical and occupational therapy while in the rehabilitation center, with follow-up home visits upon discharge. The team referred Anna immediately for fitting with bilateral ankle foot orthoses to stabilize the position of the foot and prevent the foot drop, stabilizing the ankle at neutral and preventing plantar flexion. Anna and the team decided that training in gait and functional activities with the assistance of a rolling walker would most appropriately meet Anna's functional goals.

The following summarize some of the intervention activities. The therapy goals and sample activities to meet these objectives are outlined next, accompanied by figures depicting the intervention. From these suggestions, as each individual task is used to assist Anna in the development of gait skills required to access activities of daily living, the therapist analyzed each movement attempt at each task and the movement dilemma, as described in Tables 6–6 and 6–8. All movement skills are practiced within the context of functional activity.

1. Anna will demonstrate increased static postural stability of the trunk while in upright during the performance of functional activity. Activities include a trunk strengthening program, the use of rhythmic stabilization and isometric exercise while in sitting, and standing at a support (see Fig. 6–16).
2. Anna will demonstrate increased dynamic postural stability of the trunk while engaged in a locomotor activity. Activities will include practice of trunk stabilization during the execution of a sit-to-stand and return-to-sit transfer (Fig. 10–43), reaching across midline while maintaining stability in stance (Fig. 10–44), and gait activities that require direction change and trunk movement (Fig. 10–45).
3. Anna will demonstrate increased stance control as demonstrated by an average BOS and erect trunk, hip, and knee extension. Activities will include strengthening activities in stance within the base of the rolling walker as integrated into a functional use of the walker. Activities will occur at stance upon completion of the sit-to-stand transfer, while performing an activity such as answering the phone in stance, within the base of the walker at the kitchen or bathroom sink, or while standing to use the microwave oven (see Fig. 10–44A). Activities will include retraining and practice in lower extremity control in the ability to support weight on both legs (Fig. 10–46), to transfer weight from one leg to the other (Fig. 10–47), and to adapt to movements of the trunk and arms while in stance. The intervention suggestions and guidelines described in this chapter are all appropriate. Strengthening activities will be directed to the antigravity paraspinal extensor muscles of the trunk, abdominals, gluteus maximus, pelvic stabilizers, quadriceps, gastrocnemius (closed chain), and soleus muscles.
4. Anna will demonstrate increased control in the accurate transfer of weight from one LE to the other during walking. Activities will include practice during the subphases of gait, especially preswing to initial contact on the opposite limb. The therapist or assistant will use manual guidance, biofeedback, visual and verbal feedback, and training within the gait cycle to focus on this skill.
5. Anna will demonstrate more accurate foot position during gait as assisted by an orthotic device. Practice will occur to familiarize Anna with the new proprioceptive experience of weight bearing and foot clearance, as aided by an ankle-foot orthosis. Activities will be done to establish stable initial contact and to train Anna in loading onto an ankle fixed at neutral.
6. Anna will demonstrate more accurate control of swing phase and more accurate limb advancement. Activities will include the use of approximation and manual guidance to increase proprioception and proximal stability at the pelvis girdle. Light weights will be added to a belt to enhance this augmented input. Reinforcement and feedback will include use of bright tape on the floor and a mirror to draw Anna's attention to placement of the advanced limb (Fig. 10–47).

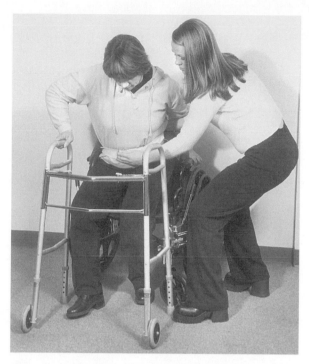

Figure 10–43. Practicing sit-to-stand transfers offers an opportunity to improve functional postural control of the trunk and strength and stability of all four extremities.

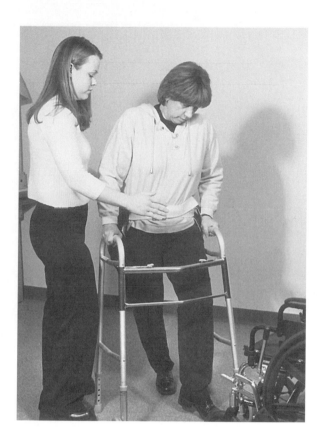

Figure 10–45. Effective functional training includes practicing the task of walking while changing directions and negotiating a turn.

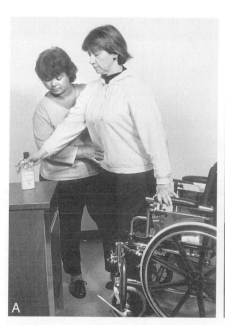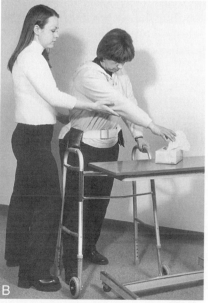

Figure 10–44. An activity useful for practicing trunk stabilization is executing a sit-to-stand transfer and then performing a functional task from that position (A). Reaching across midline in stance effectively strengthens trunk stabilizers and offers a task-embedded opportunity for practicing postural control of the trunk and stance control of the LEs (B).

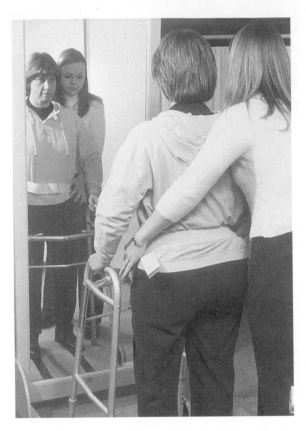

Figure 10–46. Use of a mirror, verbal instruction, manual cues, and weights on the pelvis to increase kinesthetic awareness of effective stance posture.

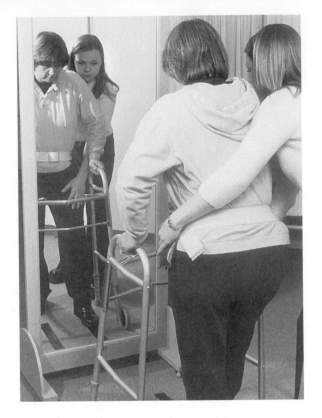

Figure 10–47. Retraining in the gait subtask of transferring weight to the advanced limb. Therapist uses manual guidance, tape on floor, weights on patient's pelvis, mirror, and verbal instruction all as teaching aides to assist in practicing an effective, accurate, and safe lower limb advancement.

Summary

This chapter has presented a practical approach to guide the student and clinician in understanding the functional tasks of the lower extremity, describing how those tasks may be impacted in individuals with neurological dysfunction. The tasks of the lower extremity were first classified as weight-bearing or non–weight-bearing functional movement tasks, then further described through a discussion of stance control and the locomotor functions of human beings: rolling, crawling and creeping, transfer tasks, and gait. An analysis of the movements required for successful execution of these common locomotor tasks can aid the clinician in problem solving for patients/clients experiencing difficulties with these tasks and subsequently designing and carrying out an effective intervention strategy. A task-oriented approach useful for the training or retraining of rolling, sit-to-stand transfer, stance control, and gait was presented.

To assist with the intervention of gait disturbances in the individual who is neurologically impaired, a model for task analysis was presented so that clinicians and students can discern with which part of the task during gait the patient/client is having difficulty: weight acceptance, single limb support, or limb advancement. This analysis can then be used to aid in clinical decision making as the clinician seeks to answer the following clinical questions:

- Why is the patient having trouble with that functional subtask?
- What constraints or impairments are contributing to a particular functional limitation for that patient for that task?
- Of these, what constraints or impairments are removable or remediable, and if so, how?

For example, patients with CP or who have had a CVA will encounter difficulties with all three functional subtasks of gait, although patients with Parkinson's disease may have more difficulty with limb advancement than with weight acceptance or single limb support.

This is the final chapter in this text. This text has attempted to offer therapists and assistants a practical theoretical framework from which to understand movement problems encountered by patients/clients with neurological impairments. The author has attempted to immediately translate the theoretical background underlying these movement problems into application of intervention strategies.

References

Bendall, M. J., Bassey, E. J., & Pearson, M. B. (1989). Factors affecting walking speed of elderly people. *Age and Ageing, 18,* 327–332.

Berger, W., Quintern, J., & Deitz, V. (1982). Pathophysiology of gait in children with cerebral palsy. *Electroencephalography and Clinical Neurophysiology, 53,* 538–548.

Berger, R. A., Riley, P. O., & Mann, R. W. (1988). Total body dynamics in ascending stairs and rising from a chair following total knee arthroscopy. In *Proceedings of the 34th Annual Meeting of the Orthopedic Research Society.* Atlanta, GA: Orthopedic Research Society.

Bertoti, D. B. (2000a). Cerebral palsy: Lifespan management. In *Orthopaedic interventions for the pediatric patient, orthopaedic section home study course.* Alexandria, VA: American Physical Therapy Association.

Bertoti, D. B. (2000b). Electrical stimulation: A reflection on current clinical practices. *Research and Engineering Society of North America, special issue: Assistive Technology, 12,* 21–32.

Blumenkopf, B. (1997). Intrathecal baclofen for spasticity. In P. D. Charles, *Treatment advances in spasticity.* Nashville, TN: Symposium at Vanderbilt University Medical Center.

Bobath, B. (1970). *Adult hemiplegia: Evaluation and treatment.* London: William Heinemann Medical Books.

Branch, L. G., & Meyers, A. R. (1987). Assessing physical function in the elderly. *Clinical Geriatric Medicine, 3,* 29–51.

Bremer, F. (1935). Le cervelet. In G. H. Roger & L. Binet (Eds.), *Traite de physiologie normale et pathologique, 10,* Paris: Masson.

Bril, B., & Breniere, Y. (1993). Posture and independent locomotion in childhood: Learning to walk or learning dynamic postural control? In G. J. P. Savelsbergh (Ed.), *The development of coordination in infancy.* Amsterdam: North Holland.

Brucker, J. (1998). *The gait workbook: A practical guide to clinical gait analysis.* Thorofare, NJ: Slack.

Brunnstrom, S. (1970). *Movement therapy in hemiplegia: A neurophysiological approach.* New York: Harper & Row.

Burnett C. N., & Johnson, E. Q. (1971). Development of gait in childhood, Parts 1 and 2. *Developmental Medicine and Medical Child Neurology, 13,* 196–215.

Campbell J., & Ball, J. (1978). Energetics of walking in cerebral palsy. *Orthopedic Clinics of North America, 9,* 374–377.

Campbell, S. K., Vander Linden, D. W., & Palisano, R. J. (Eds.). *Physical therapy for children.* Philadelphia: W. B. Saunders.

Carr, J., & Shepherd, R. (1987). *A motor relearning programme for stroke.* Rockville, MD: Aspen Publishers.

Carr, J., & Shepherd, R. (1998). *Neurological rehabilitation: Optimizing motor performance.* Oxford: Butterworth Heinemann.

Cech, D., & Martin, S. (1995). *Functional movement development across the life span.* Philadelphia: W. B. Saunders.

Cech, D., & Martin, S. (2002). Functional movement development across the life span (2nd ed.). Philadelphia: W. B. Saunders.

Clark, J. E. (1995). Dynamical systems perspective on gait. In R. B. Craik & C. A. Oatis (Eds.), *Gait analysis: Theory and application* (pp. 79–86). St. Louis, MO: Mosby.

Cowan, M. M., Stilling, D. S., Naumann, S., & Colborne, G. R. (1998). Quantification of antagonist muscle coactivation in children with spastic diplegia. *Clincal Anatomy, 11,* 314–319.

Craik, R. L. (1991). Abnormalities of motor behavior. In M. J. Lister (Ed.), *Contemporary management of motor control problems: Proceedings of the II-Step Conference.* Alexandria, VA: Foundation for Physical Therapy.

Craik, R. L., & Oatis, C.A. (1985). Gait assessment in the clinic: Issues and approaches. In J. M. Rothstein (Ed.), *Measurement in physical therapy.* London: Churchill Livingstone.

Craik, R. L., & Oatis, C.A. (1995). *Gait analysis: Theory and application.* St. Louis, MO: Mosby.

Crenna, P. (1998). Spasticity and "spastic" gait in children with cerebral palsy. *Neuroscience and Biobehavioral Reviews, 22,* 571–578.

Damiano, D. L., & Abel, M. F. (1996). Relationship of gait parameters and gross motor function in spastic cerebral palsy. *Developmental and Medical Child Neurology, 38,* 389–396.

DeLisa, J. A. (1998). *Gait analysis in the science of rehabilitation.* Baltimore: Department of Veterans Affairs, Veterans Health Administration.

Duncan, P., & Badke, M. B. (1987). *Stroke rehabilitation: The recovery of motor control.* Chicago: Year Book.

Embrey, D. G., Yates, L., & Mott, D. H. (1990). Effects of neurodevelopmental treatment and orthoses on knee flexion during gait: A single-subject design. *Physical Therapy, 70, 10,* 626–637.

Foley, M. P., Prax, B., Crowell, R., & Boone, T. (1996). Effects of assistive devices on cardiorespiratory demands in older adults. *Physical Therapy, 76, 12,* 1313–1319.

Forssberg, H. (1982). Spinal locomotor functions and descending control. In B. Sjolund & A. Bjorklund (Eds.), *Brain stem control of spinal mechanisms.* New York: Elsevier Biomedical Press.

Franks, C. A., Palisano, R. J., & Darbee, J. C. (1991). The effect of walking with an assistive device and using a wheelchair on school performance in students with myelomeningocele. *Physical Therapy, 71,* 570–577.

Frenkel, H. S. (1902). *The treatment of tabetic ataxis by means of systematic exercise.* Philadelphia: Blakiston.

Gabell, A., & Nayak, U. S. L. (1984). The effect of age on variability in gait. *Journal of Gerontology, 39,* 662–666.

Gage, J. R. (1991). *Gait analysis in cerebral palsy.* London: MacKeith Press.

Gauthier, L., Dalziel, S., & Gauthier, S. (1987). The benefits of group occupational therapy for patients with Parkinson's disease. *American Journal of Occupational Therapy, 41,* 360–365.

Gersten, J. W., & Orr, W. (1971). External work of walking in hemiparetic patients. *Scandinavian Journal of Rehabilitation Medicine, 3,* 85–88.

Halliday, S. E., Winter, D. A., Frank, J. S., Patla, A. E., & Prince, F. (1998). The initiation of gait in young, elderly, and Parkinson's disease subjects. *Gait and Posture, 8,* 8–14.

Holmes, G. (1939). The cerebellum of man. *Brain, 62,* 1.

Johnson, D., Abel, M. F., & Damiano, D. D. (1996). Evolution of gait in cerebral palsy. *Journal of Pediatric Orthopaedics, 17,* 392–396.

Kelley, D. L., Dainis, A., & Wood, G. K. (1976). Mechanics and muscular dynamics of rising from a seated position. In P. V. Komi (Ed.), *Biomechanics.* Baltimore: University Park Press.

Knutsson, E. (1994). Can gait analysis improve gait training in stroke patients? *Scandinavian Journal of Rehabilitation Medicine Supplement, 30,* 73–80.

Lennon, S. (2001). Gait re-education based on the Bobath concept in two patients with hemiplegia following stroke. *Physical Therapy, 81, 3,* 924–935.

Marshall, R. N., & Jennings, L. S. (1990). Performance objectives in the stance phase of human pathological walking. *Human Movement Science, 9,* 599–611.

Martin, M., Shinberg, M., Kuchibhatla, M., Ray, L., Carollo, J. J., & Schenkman, M. L. (2002). Gait initiation in community-dwelling adults with Parkinson disease: Comparison with older and younger adults without the disease. *Physical Therapy, 82,* 566–577.

McGraw, M. B. (1945). *The neuromuscular maturation of the human infant.* New York: Hafner Press.

McIntosh, G. C., Brown, S. H., Rice, R. R., & Thaut, M. H. (1997). Rhythmic auditory-motor facilitation of gait patterns in patients with Parkinson's disease. *Journal of Neurology, Neurosurgery and Psychiatry, 62,* 22–26.

Melnick, M. E. (2001). Basal ganglia disorders: Metabolic, hereditary, and genetic disorders in adults. In D. A. Umphred (Ed.), *Neurological rehabilitation* (4th ed.). St. Louis: Mosby.

Melnick, M. E., & Oremland, B. (2001). Movement dysfunction associated with cerebellar problems. In D.A. Umphred (Ed.), *Neurological rehabilitation* (4th ed.). St. Louis: Mosby.

Millington, P. J., Myklebust, B. M., & Shambes, G. M. (1992). Biomechanical analysis of the sit-to-stand motion in elderly persons. *Archives of Physical and Medical Rehabilitation, 73,* 609–617.

Montgomery, J. (1987). Assessment and treatment of locomotor deficits in stroke. In P. Duncan & M. B. Badke, *Stroke rehabilitation: The recovery of motor control.* Chicago: Year Book.

Morris, M. E. (2000). Movement disorders in people with Parkinson disease: A model for physical therapy. *Physical Therapy, 80,* 578–597.

Mossberg, K. A., Linton, K. A., & Fricke, K. (1990). Ankle-foot orthoses: Effect on energy expenditure of gait in spastic diplegic children. *Archives of Physical and Medical Rehabilitation, 71,* 490–494.

Murray, M. P., & Peterson, R. M. (1973). Weight distribution and weight-shifting activity during normal standing posture. *Physical Therapy, 53, 7,* 741–748.

Mykebust, B. M. (1990). A review of myotatic reflexes and the development of motor control and gait in infants and children: A special communication. *Physical Therapy, 70,* 188–203.

O'Byrne, J. M., Jenkinson, A., & O'Brien, T. M. (1998). Quantitative analysis and classification of gait patterns in cerebral palsy using a three-dimensional motion analyzer. *Journal of Child Neurology, 3,* 101–108.

Olney, S. J. (1989). New developments in the biomechanics of gait in children with cerebral palsy. In *Topics in pediatrics: Lesson 1.* Alexandria, VA: American Physical Therapy Association.

Olney, S. J., Costigan, P.A., & Hedden, D. M. (1987). Mechanical energy patterns in gait of cerebral palsied children with hemiplegia. *Physical Therapy, 67,* 1348–1354.

Olney, S. J., MacPhail, H. E. A., Hedden, D. M., & Boyce, W. F. (1987). Work and power in hemiplegic cerebral palsy gait. *Physical Therapy, 67,* 1348–1354.

Olney, S. J., & Wright, M. J. (2000). Cerebral palsy. In S. K. Campbell, D. W. Vander Linden, & R. J. Palisano (Eds.), *Physical therapy for children.* Philadelphia: W. B. Saunders.

O'Sullivan, S. B. (2001a). Multiple sclerosis. In S. B. O'Sullivan & T. J. Schmitz (Eds.), *Physical rehabilitation: Assessment and treatment* (4th ed.). Philadelphia: F. A. Davis.

O'Sullivan, S. B. (2001b). Parkinson's disease. In S. B. O'Sullivan & T. J. Schmitz (Eds.), *Physical rehabilitation: Assessment and treatment* (4th ed.). Philadelphia: F. A. Davis.

O'Sullivan, S. B. (2001c). Strategies to improve motor control and motor learning. In S. B. O'Sullivan & T. J. Schmitz (Eds.), *Physical rehabilitation: Assessment and treatment* (4th ed.). Philadelphia: F. A. Davis.

O'Sullivan, S. B., & Schmitz, T. J. (2001). *Physical rehabilitation laboratory manual: Focus on functional training.* Philadelphia: F A. Davis.

Pathokinesiology Department Physical Therapy Department. (1989). *Observational gait analysis handbook.* Downey, CA: The Professional Staff Association of Rancho Los Amigos Medical Center.

Patla, A. E. (1995). A framework for understanding mobility problems in the elderly. In R. L. Craik & C. A. Oatis (Eds.), *Gait analysis: Theory and application.* St. Louis, MO: Mosby.

Patla, A. E., & Shumway-Cook, A. (1999). Dimensions of mobility: defining the complexity and difficulty associated with community mobility. *Journal of Aging and Physical Activity, 7,* 7–19.

Pease, W. S. (1998). Therapeutic electrical stimulation for spasticity: quantitative gait analysis. *American Journal of Physical Medicine and Rehabilitation, 77,* 351–355.

Pedretti, L. W. (1996). *Occupational therapy: Practice skills for physical dysfunction* (4th ed.). St. Louis, MO: Mosby.

Perry, J. (1992). *Gait Analysis: Normal and Pathological Function.* Thorofare, NJ: Slack.

Perry, J., Giovan, P., Harris, L. J., Montgomery, J., & Azaria, M. (1978). The determinants of muscle action in the hemiparetic lower extremity (and their effect on the examination procedure). *Clinical Orthopedics, 131,* 71–89.

Perry, J., Hoffer, M. M., Giovan, P., Antonelli, P., & Greenberg, R. (1986). Predictive value of manual muscle testing and gait analysis in normal ankles by dynamic electromyography. *Foot and Ankle, 6,* 254–259.

Preston, L. A., & Hecht, J. S. (1999). *Spasticity management rehabilitation strategies.* Bethesda, MD: American Occupational Therapy Association.

Prince, F., Corriveau, H., Hebert, R., & Winter, D. A. (1997). Review article: Gait in the elderly. *Gait and Posture, 5,* 128–135.

Radtka, S. A., Skinner, S. R., Dixon, D. M., & Johanson, M. E. (1997). A comparison of gait with solid, dynamic, and no ankle-foot orthoses in children with spastic cerebral palsy. *Physical Therapy, 77,* 395–409.

Richards, C. L. (1985). EMG activity level comparisons in quadriceps and hamstrings in five dynamic activities. In D. A. Winter, R. P. Norman, & R. P. Wells (Eds.), *International series on biomechanics IX-A.* Champaign, IL: Human Kinetics Publishers.

Richter, R. R., VanSant, A. F., & Newton, R. A. (1989). Description of adult rolling movements and hypothesis of developmental sequences. *Physical Therapy, 69,* 63–71.

Rose, J., Gamble, J. G., Medeiros, J., Burgos, A., & Haskell, W. L. (1989). Energy cost of walking in normal children and in those with cerebral palsy: Comparison of heart rate and oxygen uptake. *Journal of Pediatric Orthopedics, 9,* 276–279.

Ryerson, S., & Levit, K. (1997). *Functional movement reeducation.* Philadelphia: Churchill Livingstone.

Sawner, K., & LaVigne, J. (1992). *Brunnstrom's movement therapy in hemiplegia* (2nd ed.). New York: J. B. Lippincott.

Schenkman, M. A., Berger, R. A., Riley, P. O., Mann, R. W., & Hodge, W. A. (1990). Whole-body movements during rising to standing from sitting. *Physical Therapy, 10,* 638–651.

Schenkman, M. A., Donovan, J, Tsubota, J., Kluss, M., Stebbins, P., & Butler, R. B. (1989). Management of individuals with Parkinson's disease: Rational and case studies. *Physical Therapy, 69,* 944–955.

Schneider, J. W., & Krosschell, K. J. (2001). Congenital spinal cord injury. In D. A. Umphred (Ed.), *Neurological rehabilitation* (4th ed.). St. Louis, MO: Mosby.

Shumway-Cook A., & Woollacott, M. H. (2001). *Motor control: Theory and practical application* (2nd ed.). Philadelphia: Lippincott Williams & Wilkins.

Stark, G. D. (1977). *Spina bifida: Problems and management.* Boston: Blackwell Scientific.

Sutherland, D. H., Olshen, R., Cooper, L., & Woo, S. L-Y. (1980). The development of mature gait. *Journal of Bone and Joint Surgery, 62A,* 336–353.

Trombly, C. A., & Radomski, M. V. (2001). *Occupational therapy for physical dysfunction* (5th ed.). Hagerstown, MD: Lippincott Williams & Wilkins.

Trueblood, P. R., Walker, J. M., Perry J., & Gronley, J. K. (1989). Pelvic exercise and gait in hemiplegia. *Physical Therapy, 69,* 32–40.

Umphred, D. A. (2001). *Neurological rehabilitation* (4th ed.). St. Louis, MO: Mosby.

Taber's cyclopedic medical dictionary. (2001). Philadelphia: F. A. Davis.

Wang, R. (1994). Effect of proprioceptive neuromuscular facilitation on the gait of patients with hemiplegia of long and short duration. *Physical Therapy, 74,* 12, 1108–1115.

Waters, R. L., Hislop, H. J., Perry, J., & Antonelli, D. (1978). Energetics: Application to the study and management of locomotor abilities. Energy cost of normal and pathologic gait. *Clinical Orthopedics, 131,* 54–63.

Whittle, M. W. (1991). *Gait analysis: An introduction.* Oxford, UK: Butterworth Heinemann.

Wilder, P. A. (1992). Developmental changes in the gait patterns of women: A search for control parameters. PhD Thesis, Madison: University of Wisconsin.

Winter, D. A. (1985). Concerning the scientific basis for the diagnosis of pathological gait and for rehabilitation protocols. *Physiotherapy Canada, 37,* 245–252.

Winter, D. A. (1987). *The biomechanics and motor control of human gait.* Waterloo, Ontario: University of Waterloo Press.

Woo, S. L. V., Matthews, J. V., Akerson, W. H., Amiel, D., & Convery, F. R. (1975). Connective tissue response to immobility. *Arthritis and Rheumatism, 18,* 257–264.

Woollacott, M. (1986). Gait and postural control in the aging adult. In W. Bles & T. Brandt (Eds.), *Disorders of posture and gait.* Amsterdam: Elsevier.

Wright, D. L., & Kemp, T. L. (1992). The dual-task methodology and assessing the attentional demands of ambulation with walking devices. *Physical Therapy, 72,* 306–315.

Wu, S., Huang, H., Lin, C., & Chen, M. (1996). Effects of a program on symmetrical posture in patients with hemiplegia: A single-subject design. *American Journal of Occupational Therapy, 50,* 1, 17–23.

Young, R. R. (1994). Spasticity: A review. *Neurology, 44,* S12–S20.

Glossary

absolute refractory period: brief period immediately after the action potential when the membrane cannot respond to any stimulus, regardless of how strong (Chapter 2).

accessory optic tract: projections from the optic tract to the olivary nucleus in the pons (Chapter 8).

accommodation: ability to focus on a near object and then a far object (Chapter 9).

action potential: temporary reversal of the resting membrane potential in response to a chemical, electrical, or sensory stimulus that is then sufficient enough to be propagated as an electrochemical signal along the length of the axon (Chapter 2).

activities of daily living (ADL): includes the self-care tasks of sleeping/resting, eating, grooming, bed mobility, dressing, toileting, functional mobility, bathing, and sexual activity required for independence in everyday living (basic activities of daily living or BADLs); often also includes community mobility, home management, care of others and pets, and communication devices (instrumental activities of daily living or IADLs). ADL requires basic skills whereas instrumental ADL requires more advanced problem-solving and social skills (Chapter 1).

activity limitation: denotes that activity performance of the individual is limited due to a functional limitation, dependent not only on the person's body structure/body function, but also secondary to the way a task is designed or how the environment may support or constrain performance (Chapter 1).

adaptability: one of the three major requirements for successful mobility, defined as the ability to adapt the mobility to meet the individual's goals and the demands of the environment (Chapter 10).

adaptation: occurs secondary to stimuli placed upon the system, such as the modeling that occurs within bone secondary to muscle pull (Chapter 4).

afferent: a neuron whose function is to respond to or convey a sensory signal (Chapter 2).

aging: refers to the changes in physical, sensory, and psychosocial performance that occur to some degree in all elderly persons with the passage of time. Although aging can occur at different rates, the structural and functional consequences are surprisingly consistent across the different physiological systems, with profound behavioral consequences (Chapter 3).

agnosia: inability to recognize common objects with the senses (Chapter 2).

agraphia: difficulty with writing (Chapter 2).

akinesia: slowness in initiating movements, often accompanying basal gangliar damage (Chapter 2). Symptom referring to difficulty initiating movement, creating difficulty for the individual to initiate the weight shift to begin a gait cycle or to shift the trunk forward in order to initiate a sit-to-stand transfer (Chapters 2, 3, and 10).

alexia: difficulty with reading (Chapter 2).

alpha motor neuron: a specific type of anterior horn cell, named for its large size, that innervates skeletal muscle (Chapter 2).

ambient vision: describes the "field of view" function of vision; the "Where is it?" or big picture function, as contrasted with focal vision (Chapter 8).

andragogy: the field of study concerned with understanding the instructional processes for adults (Chapter 5).

ankle strategy: postural control that is initiated from the ankles and feet (Chapter 8).

anomia: inability to name an object (Chapter 2).

anterior horn cell: a large neuron located in the gray matter of the spinal cord that sends out axons through the anterior or ventral spinal root, eventually giving rise to peripheral nerves that innervate muscle fibers (Chapter 2).

anterior spinothalamic tract: one of the two main sensory or afferent tracts, carrying information about pain and temperature. The fibers of this tract enter the dorsal horn, synapse, and cross to the other side of the spinal cord within three segments (Chapter 2).

anticipatory control: preparations for movement that relate to the task and the environment as it currently exists (Chapter 8). The programming of action based on mental representation of an object's properties that has developed through prior experience (Chapter 9).

antigravity extension: the voluntary, active movement, first of the neck and then of the trunk, against the force of gravity, first evident in prone with head lifting and then extension of the trunk (Chapter 4).

antigravity flexion: develops as a baby combats the force of gravity, first in the supine and side-lying positions, evidenced by head lifting, foot play in supine, beginning bridging, and successful voluntary movement out of supine (Chapter 4).

aphasia: language and communication disorder caused by brain damage (Chapter 2).

appropriate compensations: use of movement patterns that resemble normal movements, incorporate the involved and uninvolved body segments into the movement pattern, and promote the integration of the individual's active movement patterns into functional performance (Chapter 6).

apraxia: difficulty with planning a movement where the individual's movements are typically slow and clumsy, with mild proximal weakness and loss of coordination around the proximal joints (Chapter 2).

areflexia: a clinical sign of hypotonia where the stretch reflexes are absent (Chapter 7).

arousal: the overall level of alertness or excitement of the cerebral cortex (Chapter 5). State of alertness to the environment (Chapter 8).

associated movements: characterized by involuntary movement of one body part during the voluntary movement of another body part, often seen in the presence of abnormal muscle tone, especially spasticity. They are probably seen as the result of lost supraspinal inhibitory mechanisms that normally suppress the coupling of movements between limbs (Chapter 2).

associated reactions: movements of a body part that occur involuntarily in accompaniment to another movement (Chapter 4).

associative learning: involves the association of ideas to help the learner to detect and establish causal relationships in the environment; two events or stimuli are temporarily paired, allowing for conclusions to be drawn about causal relationships in the environment and relationships to be predicted (Chapter 5).

astasia: literally means "without stance," describing a normal period at around 2 months of age when no weight bearing is accepted through the lower extremities when placed on feet (Chapter 4).

asthenia: a condition of generalized weakness, often accompanying cerebellar disease (Chapter 10).

astrocytes: nonexcitable neuroglial cells found mostly in the gray matter of the central nervous system, directly in contact with blood vessels; involved in the exchange of substances in the bloodstream, thereby serving an important role in the maintenance of the blood-brain barrier (Chapter 2).

asymmetry: position or posture characterized by a lack of correspondence of body parts on one side of the body compared with the opposite side (Chapter 4).

ataxia: wide-based movements, often accompanying cerebellar damage (Chapter 2). A problem in executing coordinated movements, characterized by dysmetria, movement decomposition, dysdiadochokinesia, and abnormal timing of multijoint movements (Chapter 10).

athetoid movements: a type of dystonic movement characterized as slow involuntary writhing or twisting, usually involving the upper extremities more than the lower extremities (Chapter 2).

athetosis: dystonic movement disturbance characterized by slow, involuntary writhing or twisting, usually involving the upper extremities more than the lower extremities, whereby muscle tone appears to fluctuate in an unpredictable manner from low to high; most commonly manifested as a type of cerebral palsy (Chapter 7).

attention: the capacity of the brain to process information from the environment or retrieve information from long-term memory (Chapter 5). Directing cognitive processes to a significant feature in the environment (Chapter 8).

attractor states: a complex set of biomechanical, neuromotor, cognitive, and environmental variables governing transition from one stage of development to the next, allowing for the perception of a state of readiness for developmental change. This state describes the coming together of all the vital variables allowing a transition to occur (Chapter 4).

autogenic inhibition: also called nonreciprocal inhibition, mediated by the Golgi tendon organ proprioceptors; refers to an inhibitory input to an agonist muscle (the prime mover) and an excitatory message to the antagonist (opposing) muscle (Chapter 2).

automatic movements: those movements that occur in response to a given stimulus, often without conscious, voluntary effort, including reflexes, postural reactions such as righting, equilibrium and protective reactions, and associated reactions (Chapter 4).

autonomic dysreflexia: a potentially life-threatening accompanying impairment to spinal cord injury occurs because the autonomic nervous system is no longer under effective central nervous system control and a state of disarray, or dysreflexia, can result from otherwise minimal disturbances perceived by the body; can be caused by overdistention of the bladder, a urinary tract infection, a pinched catheter tube, or even monthly menstrual cramps (Chapter 2).

Babinski sign: extension of the great toe with fanning of the other toes into abduction upon stimulation of the lateral sole of the foot; a classic diagnostic sign of spasticity (Chapter 7).

balance: the ability to move into and change weight-bearing positions while resisting gravity and remaining in an upright posture (Chapter 8).

ballistic style of reach: corrections in the reaching trajectory made at the end of the movement instead of during the movement (Chapter 9).

base of support: the plane defined by the weight-bearing points of the body (Chapter 8).

basic activities of daily living (BADL): the self-care tasks of sleeping/resting, eating, grooming, bed mobility, dressing, toileting, functional mobility, bathing, and sexual activity required for independence in everyday living (Chapter 1).

binocular vision: vision from both eyes, allowing for depth perception and the ability to judge distance (Chapter 3).

bipedal: on two feet (Chapter 10).

body image: the mental representation of the emotions and thoughts associated with your body (Chapter 8).

body righting: movement of the body to realign the body with the head (Chapter 8).

body scheme: an understanding of the position of the whole body and the relationship of the body parts to each other and to the whole (Chapter 8).

body sway: movement of the body during quiet stance (Chapters 3 and 8).

bottom-up approach: a more traditional approach to assessment and intervention, which focuses on the deficits of components of function, such as strength, range of motion, and balance, believed to be prerequisites to successful occupational and functional performance (Chapter 6).

bradykinesia: symptom referring to slowness of movement or difficulty maintaining movement once initiated, often accompanying basal ganglia damage (Chapters 2 and 10).

cadence: number of steps per unit of time (steps/minute) (Chapter 10).

cataracts: an age-related decrease in the transparency of the lens of the eye (Chapter 3).

center of mass (COM): point in which all mass is centered in relation to gravity (Chapter 8).

central vestibular disorders: disorder arising from the pathology within the projection fibers and/or tracts of the vestibular system (Chapter 8).

cephalocaudal: a directional term, denoting developmental change in a head-to-toe direction (Chapters 2 and 4).

cerebral shock: time of profound depression of motor function in which all muscles of the affected body segments are involved; used to describe the temporary flaccid state in the muscles of the person following a brain injury when the nervous system is in a state of shock after a lesion of acute onset (Chapter 7).

cerebral spasticity: the type of spasticity described as often seen in patients/clients with cerebral palsy, traumatic brain injury, brain tumor, or after a cerebrovascular accident, whereby the degree of hypertonicity often fluctuates as a result of a change in the person's position, and the antigravity muscles are predominantly affected (flexors in the UEs and extensors in the LEs) (Chapter 10).

cerebrospinal fluid (CSF): fluid that cushions the nervous system, circulating around the brain and spinal cord within the subarachnoid space of the meninges, offering support, transportation of nutrients, and removal of metabolic wastes (Chapter 2).

cerebrovascular accident (CVA): commonly called a stroke; caused by either a hemorrhage or occlusion in any of the cerebral blood vessels (Chapter 2).

choreiform movement: a type of dystonic movement characterized as involuntary, quick, jerky, rapid, and irregular whereby muscle tone appears to fluctuate in an unpredictable manner from low to high (Chapter 2).

circle of Willis: circular arrangement of cerebral arteries interconnected at the base of the brain, arising from the carotid arteries and the vertebral arteries and then including the anterior cerebral artery, posterior cerebral arteries, and middle cerebral arteries (Chapter 2).

classical conditioning: type of associative learning involving learning to pair stimuli; the process whereby an initially weak stimulus becomes highly effective in producing a response when it is paired with another stronger stimulus (Chapter 5).

clinical reasoning: the process of generating hypotheses, seeking answers, and making decisions on possible solutions for a clinical dilemma (Chapter 1).

clonus: spasmodic alternations of muscle contractions between antagonistic muscle groups, caused by hyperactive stretch reflexes; indicative of an upper motor neuron lesion, a common clinical sign of spasticity (Chapter 7).

closed-chain activity: a weight-bearing extremity pattern, where the distal end of the body segment is fixed on the supporting surface and the proximal ends are free to move (Chapter 10).

closed-loop motor control theory: based on the reflex theories on motor control, which viewed movement as the summation of sensory input to the central nervous system. This theory proposed that errors in motor performance were compared with an internal reference of correction, which in turn could influence subsequent movement (Chapter 3).

closed skills: skills that, according to Gentile's classification, require "fixation," meaning that the learner works toward developing the capability to perform the pattern automatically and efficiently; the learner is given the opportunity to "fixate" the required movement coordination pattern so that it can be performed consistently with little variety introduced into the task (Chapter 5).

cogwheel rigidity: a type of rigidity characterized by alternate episodes of resistance and relaxation; often associated with lesions of the basal ganglia, such as in Parkinson's disease (Chapter 2).

collateral sprouting: regenerative or additional neuronal sprouts that arise in an area of injury from nearby undamaged neurons, occurring within five days of the injury (Chapter 2).

compensation: a behaviorial substitution where alternative behavioral strategies are adopted to accomplish a task whereby function is achieved through alternative processes. Function returns, but not in its original premorbid form (Chapter 6).

compensatory strategies: alternative movement strategies that replace typical movement patterns when age-related changes or impairment prevent the use of the typical pattern of coordination; developed by the individual in an attempt to control all the elements that are free to vary and use the remaining systems to compensate to achieve functional goals (Chapter 6).

conjugate: joined or paired (Chapter 3).

constant practice: organizing practice sessions so that the same task is practiced repeatedly during the session (Chapter 5).

constraints: limitation or restriction imposed on the movement such that the movement manifested by a patient/client is the end result of all the possibilities, as well as the limitations, offered by all the contributing systems (Chapter 3).

context: the setting within which an activity or task is placed or the circumstances that surround an event (Chapter 5).

contextual interference: a practice situation where performance of one task results in a performance detriment of another task (Chapter 5).

controlled mobility: the ability to move while maintaining a stable upright posture; often referred to as dynamic stability (Chapter 6).

corticospinal tract: The main motor or descending tract, also called the pyramidal tract. This tract originates in the frontal lobe, crosses to the opposite side in the brainstem, and continues through many interconnections and synapses to the ventral horn of the spinal cord onto the anterior horn cell (Chapter 2).

crawling: progression in prone where the belly remains on the floor as the arms and legs move reciprocally to propel the body either forward or backward (Chapters 4 and 10).

creeping: progression in quadruped where the belly is off of the floor as the arms and legs move reciprocally to propel the body either forward or backward (Chapters 4 and 10).

critical periods: times when axons are competing for synaptic sites and pathways are organizing, so that damage to the central nervous system will have different behavioral effects depending on whether the damage occurs before or after a certain time. Various central nervous system structures have different critical periods (Chapter 3).

cross-modality processing: the assimilation of information from more than one sensory modality into a composite sensory picture (Chapter 3).

cruising: walking sideways while holding onto a supporting surface (Chapter 4).

decerebrate rigidity: refers to a state of sustained contraction of the trunk and all four limbs into extension, usually indicative of a brainstem lesion (Chapter 7).

decision making: selecting from an array of possible solutions (Chapter 8).

declarative learning: type of associative learning that results in knowledge that can be continuously recalled, thus requiring awareness and attention. A skill learned in this way can be demonstrated in other contexts than that within which it was learned (Chapter 5).

decorticate rigidity: refers to a state of sustained contraction and posturing of the trunk and lower limbs in extension, and the upper limbs in flexion, usually indicative of a corticospinal tract lesion at the level of the diencephalon, above the superior colliculus (Chapter 7).

decussates: crosses (Chapter 3).

degrees of freedom: the variety of potential movement combinations that can occur at a specific joint and then cumulatively within the human body (Chapter 3).

dendrites: cell processes that carry impulses toward the cell body (Chapter 2).

dendritic arborization: term used to describe the proliferative growth, thickening, and branching of dendrites secondary to neuronal use (Chapter 2).

depolarization: a decrease in membrane potential, making it more positive and more likely to reach action potential threshold, thereby having an excitatory or facilitatory effect (Chapter 2).

development: a continuous process of adaptive change toward competence, aptly implying that development is a lifelong process. This term is also often used in the more limited sense of describing the beginning growth and organization of each system (Chapter 3). A change in form and function, where form and function are intertwined. Development is not simply growth; rather, developmental changes occur through the processes of growth, maturation, adaptation, and learning (Chapter 4).

diffuse lesion: affecting bilaterally symmetrical structures but not crossing midline as a single lesion (Chapter 2).

diplegia: motor weakness or paralysis, mainly in the lower extremities and trunk, usually also accompanied by abnormal muscle tone; associated with some types of cerebral palsy (Chapter 2).

diplopia: double vision (Chapter 2).

directionality: sense of position relative to the self; that is, the position of an object in the environment is described using directional language with the self as reference (Chapter 8).

disability: the inability to perform actions, tasks, or activities usually expected in specific social roles that are customary for the individual, within a specific sociocultural context and physical environment; includes required roles such as self-care, home management, work (job/school/play), and community/leisure (Chapter 1).

disablement: the typical consequences of disease or pathological processes; further defined as the loss or abnormality of physiological, psychological, or anatomical structure or function (Chapter 1).

dissociation: breaking up of mass movement patterns, characterized by the ability to separate movement in one body part from associated movement in another (Chapter 4).

distributed practice: defined as organizing the practice so that rest periods either equal or exceed the practice periods (Chapter 5).

divided attention: the ability to perform several tasks at the same time (Chapter 5).

dodging: the rapid deceleration and redirection of movement (Chapter 8).

dorsal horn: area in the posterior region of the spinal cord where all sensory afferents enter the central nervous system (Chapter 2).

double support: period of the gait cycle when both LEs are in contact with floor; approximately 22 percent of a given gait cycle (Chapter 10).

dynamic action system: any system that demonstrates change over time. Change may be required as a response to growth, maturation, aging, disease, or the requirements of the environment or the task (Chapter 3).

dynamic balance: refers to the ability to maintain equilibrium when moving from point to point (Chapter 3). Ability to move without falling even to the extremes of the base of support (Chapter 8).

dynamic tripod grasp: a grasp pattern in which the pencil is controlled between the thumb and index finger (Chapter 9).

dysarthria: speech difficulties associated with coordination of phonation, respiration, and articulation (Chapter 2).

dyscalculia: difficulty with doing math (Chapter 2).

dysdiadochokinesia: the inability to perform rapid alternating movements (Chapter 7).

dyskinesia: involuntary movements (Chapter 3).

dysmetria: inability to gauge distance in reaching or stepping; often accompanies cerebellar damage (Chapter 2). Movement dysfunction characterized by overshooting or reaching beyond the target; sometimes referred to as past-pointing (Chapters 7 and 10).

dyspraxia: a processing and sensory integration disorder resulting in the inability to plan and execute a movement appropriate for a given task (Chapter 3).

dystonia: a syndrome dominated by sustained muscle contractions and disordered muscle tone, often causing abnormal postures, twisting or writhing movements, and repetitive abnormal postures; often associated with basal ganglia disturbances; disorder of muscle tone and postural control (Chapters 2 and 3).

early development: in this text, refers to the changes that occur during prenatal growth and organization (Chapter 3).

edema: swelling. A localized condition in which body tissues contain an excessive amount of tissue fluid (Chapter 9).

efferent: neuron that will respond to and convey a motor or action signal (Chapter 2).

electromotive force: created by the differences in permeability and potential across an excitable cell membrane, giving rise to an electric current (Chapter 2).

emotional lability: unstable emotional state; mood changes (Chapter 2).

endolymph: fluid contained within the semicircular canals of the vestibular apparatus (Chapter 8).

equilibrium: the act of re-establishing balance once one's balance is disturbed (Chapter 4). Adjustments made to posture in order to maintain a position (Chapter 8).

equilibrium reactions: adjusted according to a change in the body's orientation in space, comprised of righting responses of the head and trunk and protective extension responses of the extremities (Chapter 4). Movements made to restore balance after it is lost (Chapter 8).

excitatory postsynaptic potential (EPSP): a small, local, and nontransmitted or nonpropagated depolarization in the postsynaptic neuron resulting from the stimulation of a single presynaptic excitatory neuron (Chapter 2).

explicit learning: a process that develops an initial mapping between the performer's body and environmental conditions, requiring active processing of information and effort during practice (Chapter 5).

exteroceptors: sensory receptors that give the central nervous system information about the external world, such as touch (Chapter 2).

extrinsic feedback: augmented or amplified information about movement provided to the mover from an external source (Chapter 5).

eye-hand coordination: Skillful use of the hand and arm via integration of visual perceptual information (Chapter 9).

facilitation: the promotion of any natural process; specifically, the effect produced in nerve tissue by the passage of an impulse (Chapter 6).

facilitatory: depolarization effect on a neuron, making it more likely to reach action potential threshold, often called excitatory (Chapter 2). Term used to describe the use of stimulation to activate or increase the likelihood of a specific response (Chapter 6).

feedback: the use of sensory information for the control of action in the process of skill acquisition (Chapter 5).

feed-forward input: the ability to anticipate movement (Chapter 9).

festinating gait: gait characterized by a progressive increase in speed with a shortening in stride length; seen in individuals with Parkinson's disease (Chapter 10).

fine movements: developmental term used to describe more refined, precise movements (Chapter 4).

first-order neuron: extends from the sensory receptor and enters the central nervous system, with the cell body located in the dorsal root ganglion (Chapter 3).

flaccidity: muscle weakness or paresis, typically seen following a period of initial brain damage, where muscle tone is absent (Chapter 2). State of abnormally low muscle tone, characterized as the complete loss of muscle tone (Chapter 7).

focal lesion: lesion limited to a single location (Chapter 2).

focal vision: the ability to recognize and identify objects in the environment (Chapter 8).

frames of reference (FOR): set of interrelated internally consistent concepts and principles that provide a systematic basis for a practitioner's interaction with patients/clients (Chapter 9).

function: the purpose or role of something; term used to describe the functioning of the body, as well as the functioning of the individual in activities within specific environments necessary for particpation in society (Chapter 1). The act of carrying out or performing an activity, referring to a specific role or occupation (Chapter 4).

functional goals: goals based on the needs and desires of the individual and on the functional impairments that have been identified by the therapist during evaluation, representing a desired significant change in the patient's/client's level of independence and reflecting a practical improvement in a specific functional limitation (Chapter 6).

functional limitation: restriction of the ability to perform—at the level of the whole person—a physical action, activity, or task in an efficient, typically expected, or competent manner (Chapters 1 and 6).

functional movement: those movements used to meet basic needs, perform daily tasks, accomplish goals and engage in purposeful activity and occupations. Functional movements are the movement patterns that are used for or adapted to a function or group of similar functions (Chapter 4).

functional reach: the distance a person can reach forward beyond arm's length while keeping a fixed base of support in the standing position (Chapter 8).

functional training: a method of retraining the movement system using repetitive practice of functional tasks in an attempt to establish or reestablish the individual's ability to perform activities of daily living (Chapter 6).

gamma motor neurons: smaller motor neurons located within the ventral or anterior horn of the spinal cord that innervate the intrafusal muscle fibers within the muscle spindle (Chapter 2).

ganglia (singular: ganglion): grouping of nerve cells outside the central nervous system with common function, form, and connections (Chapter 2).

generativity: assuming responsible adult roles in community; being worthwhile; looking beyond oneself and embracing future generations (Chapter 4).

generator potential: a local, unpropagated potential in the terminal part of the sensory nerve axon, which is then graded and additive if summation occurs (Chapter 2).

gestational age: age of a fetus expressed in weeks, 40 weeks being full term for humans (Chapter 3).

Golgi tendon organ (GTO): a type of proprioceptor located at the musculotendinous junction of skeletal muscle; arranged perpendicular to the pull of the muscle, allowing the GTO to constantly monitor tension and detect fatigue, as a muscle contracts and pulls on its tendon (Chapter 2).

grasp: the voluntary closing of the hand onto an object (Chapters 4 and 9).

grasp reflex: automatic response where strong finger flexion accompanies tactile stimulation to the palm of the hand, especially the ulnar side (Chapter 4).

gross movements: developmental term used to describe large, undefined, or mass movements (Chapter 4).

growth: an increase in size and weight; changes in the physical dimensions of the body (Chapter 4).

gyri (singular: gyrus): ridges in the surface of the cerebrum, serving to increase the surface area without affecting the size of the brain (Chapter 2).

habituation: type of nonassociative learning involving a decrease in a behavior due to repeated exposure to a nonpainful stimulus (Chapter 5).

handling: term used in neurodevelopmental treatment (NDT) to describe manual guidance given to facilitate automatic postural movements and to encourage the activation and emergence of typical movement components (Chapter 6).

haptic perception: recognition of objects and object properties by the hand without the use of vision (Chapter 9).

head control: the ability of the head to maintain a stable position (co-contraction) and move automatically (righting) or voluntarily (concentrically or eccentrically), vital for offering a stable base of support for the visual and vestibular systems (Chapter 4). The ability to keep the head in an upright position despite changing body positions (Chapter 8).

head lag: demonstrated by lack of or insufficient flexion antigravity control of the neck muscles, so that the head lags behind the trunk on passive pull to sit (Chapter 4).

hemifield: half of one eye's visual field (Chapter 3).

hemiparesis or hemiplegia: motor weakness or paralysis on one side of the body (Chapter 2).

heterarchy: where the contributing systems are not arranged in a hierarchy; rather, all the contributing systems work parallel to each other (Chapter 3).

heteroarchical: Organization involving the interaction of many subsystems, collectively contributing to the unified whole, where the parts of the system cooperate together and not in a fixed or centrally instructed way (Chapter 6).

heterotopia: displaced gray matter in the cerebral cortex, which results from abnormal neuronal cell migration during prenatal development, often causing a seizure disorder (Chapter 3).

hierarchical: "top-down" organization, where the lowest level is overseen by a higher level, all superseded by a highest level of control (Chapter 6).

hierarchy: when contributing systems are arranged in a linear fashion, where one is more important than another (Chapter 3).

high on-guard position: positioning of the arms in abduction and external rotation; seen when a new upright position of either sitting or standing is attempted (Chapter 4).

hip strategy: control of posture that comes from the pelvis and trunk (Chapter 8).

homolateral limb synkinesis: a term used to describe the dependency that often is observed between hemiplegic limbs, such as when flexion of the upper extremity elicits flexion of the lower extremity on the hemiplegic side (Chapter 2).

homonymous hemianopsia: loss of contralateral half of each visual field, the nasal half of one eye and the temporal half of the other, corresponding to the hemiplegic side in a patient with a stroke (Chapter 2).

hydrocephalus: obstruction in the flow of cerebrospinal fluid, producing enlargement of the ventricles (Chapter 2).

hyperpolarization: an increase in resting membrane potential, making it more negative, making a neuron less likely to reach an action potential threshold, thereby having an inhibitory effect (Chapter 2).

hyperreflexia: a clinical sign of hypertonia where the stretch reflexes are exaggerated and overly reactive (Chapter 7).

hypokinesis: decreased activity, often seen in the older adult (Chapter 3).

hyporeflexia: a clinical sign of hypotonia where the stretch reflexes are diminished (Chapter 7).

hypotonia: a reduction in muscle stiffness, often seen in spinocerebellar lesions and in developmental disorders, such as a type of cerebral palsy or Down syndrome (Chapter 2). State of abnormally low muscle tone characterized by a reduction in muscle stiffness, low muscle tone, weak neck and trunk control, poor muscular co-contraction, and limited stability (Chapter 7).

impairments: the typical consequences of disease or pathological processes; further defined as the loss or abnormality of physiological, psychological, or anatomical structure or function. Impairments occur at the tissue, organ, and system level, and signs and symptoms indicate them (Chapter 1).

implicit learning: occurs with repeated practice as the learner attempts to anticipate more precisely what is needed to be more efficient; this type of learning involves predicting the impact of forces, such as the effects of gravity and momentum, as well as active muscular force, on the emergent and intended movement, the learner learns how to estimate movement characteristics and anticipate the appropriate force requirements (Chapter 5).

incoordination: occurs when the firing rates of muscles are disrupted, resulting in loss of smooth reciprocal movement, or when the central nervous system loses its ability to direct movement activity that requires accuracy (Chapters 7 and 10).

in-hand manipulation skills: the ability to move an object within the hand after grasp (Chapter 9).

inhibitory: hyperpolarization effect on a neuron, making it less likely to reach an action potential threshold (Chapter 2). Term used to describe the use of stimulation to suppress or decrease the likelihood of a specific response (Chapter 6).

inhibitory postsynaptic potential (IPSP): a small, local, and nontransmitted or nonpropagated hyperpolarization in the postsynaptic neuron resulting from the stimulation of a single presynaptic inhibitory neuron (Chapter 2).

instrumental activities of daily living (IADL): activities of daily living such as shopping, community living skills, home management, or using public transportation to go to work (Chapter 1).

intention tremor: tremor accompanying purposeful movement, often associated with cerebellar pathology (Chapter 2). Sometimes called an action tremor, a tremor evidenced upon purposeful movement of the body part, typically seen during reaching with the upper extremity or stepping with the lower extremity; a symptom commonly seen in patients with cerebellar lesions (Chapter 7).

interactive reasoning: takes place during any face-to-face encounter between the treating professional and the patient/client, including body orientation, activity, eye contact, eye movement, nonverbal behavior, and direct verbal cues including voice elements (Chapter 1).

internal representations: mental representations of an object's properties that are developed through prior experience (Chapter 9).

interoceptors: sensory receptors that give the central nervous system information about the viscera and inside of the body (Chapter 2).

intrinsic feedback: sensory information from within one's body that comes from the proprioceptors and skin, visual, vestibular, and auditory receptors either during or following movement production (Chapter 5).

joint receptors: proprioceptors located within the structure of the joint and its ligaments, including Ruffini-type endings or spray endings, Paciniform endings, ligament receptors, and free nerve endings, all distributed throughout various portions of the joint capsule. These receptors signal joint position, detect the end of a joint range, and give very accurate information to the central nervous system about even the minute fractionation of joint range of motion (Chapter 2).

judgment: discerning the appropriateness of a particular set of circumstances (Chapter 8).

key points of control: parts of the body, usually the pelvis or shoulder, chosen by the therapist or assistant as optimal to be used to physically guide a person's movement (Chapter 6).

kinematics: the terms used to describe movement patterns, such as direction of movement or joint angles, without regard for the forces involved in producing the movement (Chapter 10).

kinetics: the term used to describe the forces involved in a movement, such as muscular forces (Chapter 10).

knowledge of performance (KP): a type of extrinsic feedback that provides information about the nature of the movement pattern underlying the goal outcome (Chapter 5).

knowledge of results (KR): a type of extrinsic feedback relating to the outcome or result of an action with respect to the attempted goal (Chapter 5).

labyrinthine righting: movement of the body or head in response to receptors in the vestibular apparatus of the inner ear (Chapter 8).

Landau reaction: extension of the neck and trunk when held in horizontal suspension; made possible by the development of sufficient antigravity extensor control and strength (Chapter 4).

lateral geniculate nucleus of the thalamus: a subcortical nucleus that receives input from the optic tract and sends secondary neurons to the visual cortex (Chapter 8).

laterality: awareness of the two sides of the body (Chapter 8).

lateral tripod grasp: pencil grasp in which the pencil is stabilized against the side of the middle finger, with the index pad on the pencil and the thumb adducted with the thumb pad against the side of the index finger (Chapter 9).

lead pipe rigidity: a type of rigidity characterized by a constant resistance to movement throughout the range. Rigidity often accompanies basal ganglia damage (Chapter 2).

learning: can be considered as a type of adaptation, resulting in a relatively permanent change in behavior, usually as a result of practice (Chapters 4 and 5).

learning style: refers to how information is processed, which is unique to an individual (Chapter 5).

lesion: an area of damage or dysfunction (Chapter 2).

limits of stability (LOS): determined by the distance between the feet and the length of the feet, as well as by the height and weight of the individual (usually 12 degrees anteroposterior and 16 degrees medial/lateral for adults) (Chapter 10).

locomotion: the process of moving from one place to another, accomplished using any one of a number of motor patterns: rolling, crawling, creeping, walking, running, galloping, hopping, and skipping (Chapters 4 and 10).

long-term memory: memories that are actually stored in the brain and available for later retrieval; the process initially reflects functional changes in the efficiency of brain synapses and in later stages is accompanied by actual structural changes in these synaptic connections (Chapter 5).

long-term potentiation (LTP): strengthening of a synapse that occurs following repetitive stimulation and activity (Chapter 2).

lower motor neuron (LMN) lesions: lesions that affect the anterior horn cell or the peripheral nerve, producing decreased or absent muscle tone along with associated symptoms of paralysis, signs of muscle denervation, and atrophy (Chapter 7).

lower motor neurons (LMNs): neurons that arise from the spinal cord and cranial nerve motor nuclei. They innervate skeletal muscles directly and are considered peripheral nerves (Chapter 2).

macular degeneration: an age-related pigmentary change in the retina, causing cloudy vision or a "blind spot"; very common in older adulthood (Chapter 3).

manipulation: includes all the actions of reach, grasp, and release; the movement of the object while it is being held; adjustments to the object (Chapter 4).

manipulatives: objects that are manipulated in the hands to encourage fine motor skills (Chapter 9).

massed practice: consists of a sequence of practice and rest times in which the rest time is much less than the practice time (Chapter 5).

maturation: refers to the qualitative changes that enable one to progress to a higher level of functioning, characterized by fairly fixed order of progression that may vary in pace and sequence between individuals (Chapter 3). Increase in complexity within body systems, allowing for more sophisticated functioning, including such processes as the myelination of nerves (Chapter 4).

maturity: implies a period of relative developmental stability, with most changes driven by individual responses to environmental or task demands (Chapter 3).

meaning: refers to the sense that is made or the personal implications that are drawn; existing at multiple levels, from the immediate and superficial to the enduring and fundamental. Meaning arises from a combination of social, personal, and cultural factors, but it is also dynamic and can change over time or even within a single encounter (Chapter 5).

memory: learning and recalling information (Chapter 8).

meninges: membranes that surround the spinal cord, offering protection from infection and contusion; made up of the pia mater, arachnoid mater, and dura mater (Chapter 2).

mental practice: the cognitive rehearsal of a motor task without any overt movement (Chapter 5).

microglia: nonexcitable neuroglial phagocytic cells (a clean-up crew) that form part of the nervous system's defense against infection and injury (Chapter 2).

micrographia: abnormally small handwriting (Chapter 9).

mobility: movement function whereby moving is the main task goal (Chapter 4). Characterized by the ability to move into a posture (Chapter 6).

model: a schematic representation of a theory; useful for conceptualizing ideas (Chapter 3).

modulate: ability to refine or change; made possible within the human nervous system through many processes, including convergence (Chapter 3).

monocular vision: vision from one eye (Chapter 3).

motility: eye movement (Chapter 8).

motivation: the internal state that tends to direct or energize a system toward a goal (Chapter 5).

motor control: a field of study directed at the study of movement as the result of a complex set of neurological, physical, and behavioral processes. Motor control is the ability of the individual to maintain and change posture and movement based on an interaction among the individual, task, and environment (Chapters 3 and 5).

motor cortex: the frontal lobe, further subdivided into the primary motor cortex, the premotor cortex, and the supplementary motor area (Chapter 2).

motor development: the process of change in motor behavior that is related to the age of the individual (Chapter 4).

motor learning: a set of internal processes that brings about a relatively permanent change in the capacity for motor performance as a result of experience or practice. Motor learning involves both the acquisition of new skills and the retention of and transfer of skills to novel situations (Chapter 5).

motor program: a generalized prestructured plan that can then be modified according to the specific task demands; an abstract structure in memory that is prepared in advance of the movement so that when it is executed, the result causes movement to occur without the involvement of feedback (Chapter 5).

motor unit: the alpha motor neuron and all the muscle fibers it innervates (Chapter 2).

movement decomposition: movement dysfunction characterized by a breakdown of movements between multiple joints, resulting in movement of individual segments, rather than movement as a fluid, coordinated unit (Chapters 7 and 10).

movement equivalence: an important concept describing the many-to-one relationship among the three levels of task analysis, such that between movement patterns and the action goal there can be many appropriate and preferred combinations (Chapter 6).

movement system: the functional interaction of several subsystems and structures that contribute to the act of moving (Chapter 3).

movement time: the time taken to execute a task-specific movement, once it has been initiated (Chapter 7).

multifocal lesion: lesion limited to several, nonsymmetrical locations (Chapter 2).

muscle spindle: a unique type of proprioceptor, located between the fibers of skeletal muscle, which has both sensory and motor properties. It detects length change and velocity of length change in skeletal muscle (Chapter 2).

muscle tone: a state of readiness of skeletal muscle so that the muscular system is in a state of arousal, prepared for the task demands to be placed on it; determined by the level of excitability of the entire pool of motor neurons controlling a muscle, the intrinsic stiffness of the muscle itself, the absence of neuropathology, and the level of sensitivity of many different reflexes (Chapter 2).

narrative reasoning: a clinical reasoning approach that involves learning about the patient's story, in which the therapist then can discern the role that occupational performance has played in the person's life (Chapter 1).

neck righting: movements made by the neck to realign the head in reference to the body (Chapter 8).

negative features: signs due to a loss in or deficit of motor behavior, such as weakness, slowness of movement, loss of dexterity or coordination, and fatigability (Chapter 7).

neurodevelopmental treatment (NDT): intervention approach originally developed by Drs. Karl and Berta Bobath (Chapter 6).

neurofacilitation approach: also known as a neurophysiological or sensorimotor approach; first proposed for intervention with the neurologically impaired, growing out of the reflex and hierarchical models (Chapter 6).

neuroglia: nonexcitable support cells of the nervous system, each with specific support functions, such as formation of myelin, guidance of developing neurons, maintenance of extracellular ion levels, and reuptake of chemical transmitters following neuronal activity. Includes astrocytes, microglia, oligodendrocytes, and Schwann cells (Chapter 2).

neuromodulators: a substance that can change or alter the properties or qualities of a neuron, making neurons more or less responsive to incoming stimuli (Chapter 2).

neuromuscular facilitation techniques: a group of approaches used to retrain muscle responses after central nervous system injury (Chapter 8).

neuron: an excitable cell that receives and sends signals to other excitable cells composed of a cell body, or soma (containing the cell nucleus), dendrites, and an axon (Chapter 2).

neuro-occupation: a new term seen in the occupational therapy literature, reflective of the inexorable link being drawn among the neurosciences, an individual's nervous system, and the way in which that individual engages in occupation (Chapter 6).

neurophysiological approach: a sensorimotor approach based originally on the work of Margaret Rood (Chapter 6).

neuroplasticity: a term used to describe the ability of the nervous system to change in response to experience, changing conditions (including injury), and repeated stimuli (Chapter 2).

neurorehabilitation: the application of neuroscience to the rehabilitation of individuals with brain injury (Chapter 1).

neuroscience: study of the functioning of the nervous system (Chapter 1).

neurotransmitter: an excitatory or inhibitory chemical released into the synaptic cleft (Chapter 2).

nodes of Ranvier: anatomical locations in an axon where there are breaks in the myelin, allowing current to conduct quickly, jumping efficiently from node to node (Chapter 2).

nonassociative learning: occurs when a single stimulus is given repeatedly, so that the nervous system learns about the characteristics of the stimulus (Chapter 5).

nonregulatory conditions: characteristics of the performance environment that are irrelevant and do not influence the movement characteristics of the skill (Chapter 5).

non–weight-bearing activities: activities of the extremities where the extremity is free to move in space; often referred to as open-chain activities (Chapter 10).

normal muscle tone: constant resting state of readiness so that skeletal muscle is literally on a steady state of alert or arousal for the task demands to be placed on it. It is determined by the level of excitability of the entire pool of motor neurons controlling a muscle, the intrinsic stiffness of the muscle itself, the absence of neuropathology, and the level of sensitivity of many different reflexes (Chapter 2).

nuclei (singular: nucleus): grouping of nerve cells inside the central nervous system serving a common function, often with a common target (Chapter 2).

nystagmus: a normal consequence of head movement, characterized by alternating slow movement of the eyes in the direction opposite to head movement and then the rapid resetting of the eyes in the direction of the head movement (Chapter 3). An involuntary, rhythmic oscillation of the eye generally more to one side than the other (Chapter 8).

occupation: uniquely human task behavior that is characterized by the qualities of personal meaning and purpose used in the context of occupational therapy. Occupation is the means through which a patient/client (consumer) achieves therapeutic goals for maximum independence and life satisfaction. Successful engagement in occupation is the desired end product for intervention (Chapter 6).

occupationally embedded: a term used to describe occupations that have greater meaning and purpose to a given individual; embedding movement education or re-education into an occupation (Chapter 5).

oculomotor components: eye movements that are used for visual regard (Chapter 9).

oligodendrocytes: nonexcitable neuroglial cells that predominate in the white matter of the central nervous system, have long processes composed almost exclusively of myelin, produce the myelin for the central nervous system, and act as a support network (Chapter 2).

on-guard position: position of the upper extremities into shoulder external rotation and horizontal abduction, scapular retraction, and elbow flexion for the purpose of widening the base of support to increase stability; further classified into a position of high, medium, or low on guard, accompanying a respective increase in upright stability and balance (Chapter 10).

ontogenetic sequence: skill attainment follows in sequential fashion, with one skill building on successful completion of another (Chapter 8).

open-chain activities: a non–weight-bearing extremity pattern where the distal end of the extremity is not fixed on a supporting surface and is free to move (Chapter 10).

open-loop feedforward motor control system: based on the hierarchical or neuromaturational motor control theories, proposing that movements are selected, planned, and initiated based on a central reference that has been established by past experience (Chapter 3).

open skills: skills that, according to Gentile's classification, require "diversification" of the basic movement pattern acquired during the first stage of learning, so that the learner is required to adapt to continuously changing regulatory conditions (Chapter 5).

operant conditioning: type of associative learning involving trial and error; learning to associate a certain response, from among many that have been made, with a consequence (Chapter 5).

opisthotonus: a strong and sustained contraction of the extensor muscles so that the individual assumes a hyperextended posture; seen in severe cases of brain damage (Chapter 7).

optical righting: movement of the body or head in response to the eyes (Chapter 8).

optic chiasm: formed by fibers from the optic nerves from each eye, located at the base of the brain. At the chiasm, axons originating from the nasal portions of both retinas cross, whereas those from the temporal portions do not (Chapter 3).

orientation: maintenance of body segments in relationship to each other to allow completion of functional tasks (Chapter 8).

orienting reactions: movements by the head or body made to bring an object in the environment into clearer vision or physical reach (Chapter 8).

osteoporosis: age-related change in bone mineral density severe enough to increase vulnerability to fracture (Chapter 3).

parallel processing: refers to the way that the nervous system manages and processes all the information being conveyed by multiple sources, where similar information is conveyed by multiple sources so that the information-carrying capabilities of the nervous system are maximized. Parallel processing also allows for redundancy and, often, recovery of function (Chapter 3).

paraplegia: motor weakness or paralysis of the lower extremities (Chapter 2).

parasympathetic nervous system: a division of the autonomic nervous system responsible for maintaining homeostasis and balanced body functions (Chapter 2).

participation restriction: denotes that activity performance is restricted, creating a disability for that individual within that specific environment in the performance of a selective task, thus restricting the ability of the person to participate freely in society (Chapter 1).

pathology/pathophysiology: synonymous with disease, condition, or disorder; usually consistent with the medical diagnosis, is primarily identified at the cellular level, and can be the result of many different etiologies, such as infection, trauma, or degenerative processes. Any single disorder may disrupt normal anatomical structures or physiological processes (Chapter 1).

pattern recognition: the ability to observe a phenomenon, identify significant characteristics (cues), determine whether there is a relation among the cues, and make a comparison or decision; it requires that a comparison can be made to an expectation or a familiar pattern (Chapter 1).

pedagogy: field of study concerned with understanding the instructional processes for children as learners (Chapter 5).

perception: adding meaning to sensory impulses; integration of multiple sensory input modalities by the cortex (Chapter 8).

perceptual learning: a more complex form of nonassociative learning involving the formation of sensory memories that can then serve as a spontaneous rehearsal mechanism for that action or occurrence (Chapter 5).

performance: a temporary change in behavior readily observable during practice sessions, often resulting from short-term training (Chapter 5).

peripheral neuropathy: age-related change in the somatosensory system whereby nerve conduction velocities are decreased and sensation is diminished (Chapter 3).

peripheral vestibular disorders: disorders that affect the structures of the vestibular system located within the inner ear (Chapter 8).

perseveration: persistence of a single thought, utterance, or movement (Chapter 2).

phase shift: transition from one preferred pattern of coordination to another, a key principle in a dynamic-systems view on motor development; during this phase shift, the system is in a relative state of instability until a new preferred pattern is established (Chapter 4).

phasic stimuli: term used by the neurophysiological approach to intervention to describe a stimulus used to facilitate a mobility response, such as quick stretch and quick ice, employed to stimulate the initiation of a movement or the activation of a muscular response (Chapter 6).

physical practice: type of practice that allows the learner to gain direct experience, crucial for the shaping of a motor program (Chapter 5).

physiological flexion: a term used to describe the predominate flexed posture of full-term babies, precipitated by the posture assumed secondary to the confines of the womb as the baby grew in size during the last prenatal weeks (Chapter 4).

plexus: a network of nerves, bundled and subdivided so that the branching allows for a rich representation of spinal nerve origin in the peripheral nerve terminal (Chapter 2).

positive features: abnormal behavior due directly to the central nervous system lesion, including the presence of abnormal movement patterns such as pathological reflex responses (e.g., Babinski reflex) or hyperactive reflex responses such as a hyperreactive stretch reflex. Positive features or signs are all really exaggerations of normal phenomena, considered to be due to the pathological involvement in the brain (Chapter 7).

posterior (or dorsal) white columns: one of the two main sensory or ascending tracts carrying information about position sense (proprioception), vibration, two-point discrimination, and deep touch. The fibers of this tract enter the spinal cord in the dorsal horn, ascend the spinal cord, and then cross to the other side of the brain at the level of the brainstem (Chapter 2).

postrotatory nystagmus: a reversal in the normal eye movement occurring when the spinning stops, used often as a clinical assessment tool to evaluate the intactness of the vestibular system (Chapter 3).

postural accompaniments: adjustments made to the motor plan simultaneously to its execution, allows sensory feedback to influence movement (Chapter 8).

postural alignment: keeping the body centered about the vertical midline (Chapter 8).

postural control: mature movement control, demonstrating a functioning relationship between stability (holding a posture) and mobility (moving) (Chapters 4 and 8).

postural control of the trunk: the task whereby the trunk, as the center of the body mass, must maintain the body in a balanced, erect position against gravity, and it must adapt to the moving extremities (Chapter 4).

postural preparations: adjustments made to the motor plan before execution of the movement plan (Chapter 8).

postural reactions: adjustments made to the motor plan after it has been executed; allows for response to unanticipated environmental conditions (Chapter 8).

postural sway: a slow but continual shifting of body weight between the two lower limbs during quiet stance (Chapter 10).

postural tone: activation of specific anti-gravity muscles to stabilize the weight-bearing joints and the trunk (Chapter 8).

postural tremor: a type of tremor that can be observed when the individual bears weight through the limb or encounters resistance to movement of the limbs, head, trunk, or neck (Chapter 7).

power grasp: grasping in which the whole hand is used with the thumb held close to the other digits, such as in the grasp used to pick up a large object (Chapter 9).

practice: the continuous and repeated effort to become proficient at a skill (Chapter 5).

practice order: the sequence in which the tasks are practiced; can be blocked, serial, or random (Chapter 5).

praxis: knowledge of where the body is in space and the sequence of movements that must be planned to perform a motor task, based on the interaction of tactile, vestibular, and proprioceptive information (Chapter 3).

precision grasp: a grasp in which the thumb is held in opposition and is often used to grasp small or medium objects (Chapter 9).

preferred pattern of movement: movement pattern

that emerges as a coordinated interaction of all the contributing subsystems, within the strengths and constraints of the contributing systems at a given developmental time (Chapter 4).

prehensile: adapted for grasping or holding (Chapter 9).

premorbid: before the development of the disease (Chapter 3).

presbyopia: farsightedness; a normal age-related change that occurs because the lens of the eye loses some of its elasticity, so that the lens is unable to adjust its curvature to focus on objects on the very near points of vision (Chapter 3).

problem solving: requires clinical flexibility, so that input strategies can be constantly modified to meet the dynamic needs of the patient/client; is developed based on experience, a thorough knowledge of the area, sensitivity to the total environment, and the ability to integrate all three and respond optimally (Chapter 1).

procedural learning: type of associative learning involving mastering a task through repetition over many trials, so that the rules for that movement develop, allowing for the automatic performance of that task (Chapter 5).

procedural reasoning: the type of knowledge used when a practitioner applies learned professional or academic knowledge to a clinical problem, generating sets of hypotheses about possible clinical situations and possible results (Chapter 1).

progression: one of the three major requirements for successful locomotion, defined as the ability to generate a basic pattern that can move the body in the desired direction (Chapter 10).

proprioceptive neuromuscular facilitation (PNF): intervention approach developed in the 1950s describing methods of promoting or hastening the response of the neuromuscular mechanism through stimulation of the proprioceptors (Chapter 6).

proprioceptors: sensory receptors that give the central nervous system information about the state and position of the musculoskeletal system; includes muscle spindles, joint receptors, and Golgi tendon organs (Chapter 2).

propulsive gait: gait characteristic sometimes seen in individuals with Parkinson's disease, where the gait takes on an accelerating quality sometimes requiring that the patient/client come in contact with an object or a wall in order to stop (Chapter 10).

protective extension: extension motion of the upper or lower extremities toward the supporting surface, elicited in preparation for catching oneself from a fall (Chapter 4).

proximal stability: a term used to describe the required co-contraction around shoulder and pelvic girdles required for successful, coordinated use of the upper or lower extremities, respectively (Chapter 4).

purposeful activity: goal-directed behaviors or tasks that comprise occupations whereby the activity is *purposeful* if the individual is an active, voluntary participant and if the activity is directed toward a goal that the individual considers meaningful (Chapter 5).

pursuits: smooth eye movements following a target throughout the visual field (Chapter 8).

quadriplegia: motor weakness or paralysis of all four extremities, neck, and trunk (Chapter 2).

quadruped: all-fours position; belly off the floor and arms extended (Chapter 4).

Ralmiste's phenomenon: an example of an associated reaction where resistance applied to a movement on the uninvolved side of the body will cause a similar response in the involved lower extremity (Chapter 2).

reach: the directing or adjusting of the hand as it approaches an object (Chapter 4). The ability to move the hand toward an object within the constraints of time and space (Chapter 9).

reaction time: the time between the person's decision to move and the actual initiation of the movement (Chapter 7).

reactive control: movement adjustments made in response to ongoing feedback (Chapter 8).

reafference: the ability of the cerebellum to receive sensory feedback from the receptors about the movements as the movement is occurring (Chapters 2 and 3).

receptor field: a particular area from which it is possible to excite a receptor; variance in field size and the density of receptors within a given area of skin determine the degree of touch discrimination (Chapter 2).

receptor potential: a local change in potential at the receptor site, converting the stimulus into electrical energy so it can be transmitted throughout the nervous system (Chapter 2).

reciprocal: alternate flexion and extension of opposite extremities (Chapter 4).

reciprocal arm swing: rhythmic swinging of the upper extremities during walking so that as one lower extremity advances during swing phase, the opposite upper extremity swings forward (Chapter 10).

reciprocal innervation: when an agonist muscle is signaled to contract, its antagonist is signaled to relax (Chapter 2).

reciprocal interweaving: term used to describe the spiraling process of development, made up of periods that alternate between states of equilibrium and disequilibrium; the process of coordinated and progressive intricate interweaving of opposing muscle groups into an increasingly mature relationship, proposed by Gesell as a characteristic of motor development of children (Chapter 4).

recovery: the achievement of function through original processes (Chapter 6).

reflex: a largely automatic, somewhat stereotypical, consistent, and predictable motor response to a specific stimulus, usually sensory (Chapter 4).

reflexogenic zones: stimulus area that elicits a reflex response (Chapter 3).

refractoriness: term describing the period when an excitable membrane (nerve or muscle) is resistant to stimulation (Chapter 2).

regenerative sprouts: grow from the distal end of the cut axon, near the injury site, sometimes traveling over great distances in attempting to reconnect to their target (Chapter 2).

regulatory conditions: characteristics of the performance environment that influence (regulate) the characteristics of the movement used to perform the skill (Chapter 5).

relative refractory period: period during repolarization of an excitable membrane, when membrane excitability is depressed but a response can be triggered with repeated or intensified stimuli (Chapter 2).

release: the method by which an object leaves the hand (Chapters 4 and 9).

repolarization: period of the action potential following depolarization, where the Na$^+$ gates close and gates allowing movement of K$^+$ open, resulting in a movement of K$^+$ outward (Chapter 2).

resting membrane potential: the functional implication of the resting potential is that it creates an environment of readiness to respond to change (–70 to –90 mV for nerves, up to –90 mV inside a muscle fiber), which is why scientists characterize only nerves and muscles as possessing this property of a cell membrane described as excitable (Chapter 2).

resting tremor: a tremor occurring in a body part that is not being voluntarily activated and is supported against gravity, ceasing once movement is initiated; a symptom of a basal ganglia disorder, especially Parkinson's disease (then called a "pill-rolling" tremor) (Chapter 2).

righting: a postural response of the head or trunk elicited secondary to displacement or movement, ensuring the realignment of the head or trunk with each other or with regard to an outside stimulus (Chapter 4).

righting reactions: movements made to realign the body in reference to a stimulus in the environment (Chapter 8).

rigidity: a form of hypertonicity, characterized by a heightened resistance to passive movement but independent of the velocity of that stretch or movement. There are two types of rigidity, lead pipe and cogwheel. Rigidity is often associated with lesions of the basal ganglia, commonly seen in Parkinson's disease (Chapter 2).

rolling: considered a form of locomotion, defined as moving from supine to prone or from prone to supine, involving some degree of body rotation (Chapter 4). Earliest pattern used for locomotion, defined as moving from supine to prone or from prone to supine, usually involving some amount of rotation (Chapter 10).

rotation: can be demonstrated because of a balanced control of both flexors and extensors and dissociation between body segments (Chapter 4). Rolling an object or rotating an object 180 to 360 degrees, along the fingertips (Chapter 9).

saccades: precise eye movements from target to target within the visual field (Chapter 8).

schema: an abstract memory construct that represents a rule or a generalization about a motor action, perception, or event, proposed by Schmidt (Chapters 3 and 5).

schwann cells: nonexcitable neuroglial cell found in the peripheral nervous system (PNS) having a similar function there as the oligodendrocytes do in the central nervous system (Chapter 2).

second-order neuron: transports somatosensory information to the thalamus, usually crossing in the brainstem or spinal cord where its cell body lies (Chapter 3).

selective attention: the ability to focus on a specific stimulus while screening out extraneous stimuli (Chapter 5).

senile muscular atrophy: muscular wasting associated with the aging process (Chapter 3).

sensitive periods: times when the individual is more sensitive to certain kinds of stimulation (Chapter 4).

sensitization: type of nonassociative learning involving increased responsiveness to a threatening or noxious stimulus (Chapter 5).

sensorimotor approach: also known as a neurophysiological or neurofacilitation approach; first proposed for intervention with the person with a neurological impairment; growing out of the reflex and hierarchical models (Chapter 6).

sensory cortex: where incoming sensory information is processed and given meaning; primarily located in the parietal lobe (Chapter 2).

sensory integration (SI): the neurological process whereby the spatial and temporal aspects of inputs from different sensory modalities are integrated, associated, and unified. The brain processes sensory information and then is able to select, enhance, inhibit, compare, and associate the information for use in a flexible, constantly changing pattern

(Chapter 3). A sensorimotor intervention approach, based on the work of Jean Ayres, whereby controlled sensory input may be used to help individuals to experience sensation, explore the environment, and process the sensations within a movement or learning task. Sensory stimulation activities emphasize active exploration and processing of tactile, proprioceptive, and vestibular stimulation within a context of purposeful movement (Chapter 6).

shaping: a term borrowed from the education field, referring to a gradual process whereby a behavior is changed from an initial status to a desired terminal outcome (Chapter 5).

shift: moving of an object or adjusting an object on the fingertips (Chapter 9).

short-term memory: working memory, which lasts only for a few minutes. We use short-term memory to remember a series of numbers, such as a phone number, for a brief period (Chapter 5).

shoulder-hand syndrome: a chronic pain syndrome often seen in individuals following a CVA, which begins with hand edema and shoulder pain (Chapter 9).

skill: a level of functional motor mastery that enables the individual to produce highly coordinated movement; characterized by precision in timing and direction (Chapter 6).

somatosensation: sensory information about the body (soma), therefore including the cutaneous sensations of touch and the proprioceptive sensations from ligaments, muscles, joints, and tendons (Chapter 3).

somatosensory: sensations from or awareness of the body (Chapter 2).

somatosensory system: includes all those structures involved in the reception of signals from the periphery to the integration and interpretation of those signals related to all the simultaneous incoming information (Chapter 3).

Souques' phenomenon: associated reaction often seen in patients with hemiplegia whereby elevation of the hemiplegic upper extremity with the elbow extended above the horizontal may elicit an extension and abduction response of the fingers (Chapter 2).

spasticity: sign of upper motor neuron damage, demonstrated as a velocity-dependent increase in resistance of a muscle to passive stretch; associated with a wide range of abnormal motor behaviors including hyperactive stretch reflexes, abnormal posturing of the limbs, excessive co-activation of the antagonist muscles, associated movements, clonus, and stereotypical movement synergies (Chapter 2).

spatial summation: integration of multiple postsynaptic potentials that arrive simultaneously but at different locations on the postsynaptic membrane (Chapter 2).

spinal reflexes: earliest synaptic connections, at the spinal cord level, allowing for the pairing of sensory inputs and motor responses. Many of these spinal reflexes are permanent, "hard-wiring" the developing human quite early, equipping the fetus with survival capabilities such as the ability to suck and gag (Chapter 3).

spinal shock: time of profound depression of motor function in which all muscles of the affected body segments are involved; used to describe the temporary flaccid state in the person with a spinal cord injury when the nervous system is in a state of shock after a lesion of acute onset (Chapter 7).

spinal spasticity: increased muscle tone hypothesized to be the result of residual influence of supraspinal centers, such as the cortex, on the spinal cord and ineffective modulation of spinal pathways, often resulting from a noncongenital spinal cord injury. It can be quite extreme, with a characteristic distribution in the extensor muscles of the lower extremities, often with severe episodes of muscle spasm (Chapter 10).

splinter skills: skills that cannot be generalized to other environments or to variations of the same task (Chapter 6).

stability: movement function whereby the holding of a posture is the main task goal (Chapter 4). Static postural control, characterized by the ability to maintain a stable posture, attained through muscular co-contraction ensuring the maintenance of upright posture (Chapter 6). One of the three major requirements for successful locomotion, defined as the ability to support and control the body against gravity (Chapter 10).

stance phase: the phase of the gait cycle when the lower extremity is in contact with the floor, comprising the five subphases of initial contact, loading, midstance, terminal stance, and preswing (Chapter 10).

static balance: the ability of the body to maintain equilibrium while in a stationary position (Chapter 3). See *stability* (Chapter 8).

step length: spatial distance from initial contact of one foot to initial contact of the opposite foot (Chapter 10).

stiffness: a change in the viscoelastic physical properties of the muscle accompanying hypertonicity, which contributes to the increased resistance to passive stretch (Chapter 7).

strategy: refers not only to a description of the movement pattern used to accomplish the task, but also includes how an individual appears to organize motor, sensory, and perceptual information necessary to performing a task in different environments (Chapter 6).

stretch reflex: a monosynaptic, simple reflex arc mediated at the spinal cord level (Chapter 2).

stride length: spatial distance from initial contact of one foot to initial contact of the same foot again (Chapter 10).

sulci (singular: sulcus): depressions in the surface area of the cerebrum, serving to increase the surface area without affecting the size of the brain (Chapter 2).

superior colliculus: an area in the dorsal midbrain that acts as the integrative and relay center for visuospatial information to the skeletal muscles (Chapter 8).

sustained attention: requires the ability to maintain attention for a task-appropriate length of time (Chapter 5).

sway: slight anteroposterior or lateral movements in space representing the postural adjustments being constantly made to keep us in an upright position (Chapter 8).

swing phase: the phase of the gait cycle when the lower extremity is not in contact with the floor, comprising the three subphases of initial swing, midswing, and terminal swing (Chapter 10).

symmetry: position or posture characterized by correspondence in relative position of parts on opposite sides of the body (Chapter 4).

sympathetic nervous system: part of the autonomic nervous system commonly known as responsible for "fight-or-flight" responses, because it assists in responding to stressful situations; composed of fibers that arise from the thoracic and lumbar portions of the spinal cord (Chapter 2).

synapse: a specialized zone where neurons communicate with each other, classified as either electrical or chemical, occurring between two axons (axoaxonic), between the cell body and axon (axosomatic), or between dendrites and axons (axodendritic) (Chapter 2).

synaptic cleft: space (about 200 Å wide) between the presynaptic terminal of one end of a synapse and postsynaptic element terminal at another (Chapter 2).

synergies: stereotypical patterns of movement that don't change or adapt to environmental or task demands. Abnormal synergies reflect an inability to move a single joint without simultaneously generating movement in other joints, and movement out of the fixed pattern is often difficult if not impossible. There is a flexion and extension synergy of both the upper and the lower extremity (Chapter 2). Patterned, recognizable flexion or extension movements of the entire limb, evoked by attempts to move or by sensory stimuli, characteristically seen during the period of recovery following a neurolog-

ical incident such as a cerebrovascular accident (Chapter 6). Groups of muscles that work together, often as a bound unit, to produce a movement (Chapter 3).

systems approach: a functional approach of viewing the nervous system as subservient to functional purpose, where structures may contribute to more than one function and thereby be a part of more than one system (Chapter 2).

tandem: toe-to-heel foot placement while walking in a straight line (Chapter 8).

temporal summation: additional excitatory postsynaptic potentials arriving at the same location on the postsynaptic membrane quickly enough so that the potentials can add to each other (Chapter 2).

tetraplegia: motor weakness or impairment of all four extremities (Chapter 2).

theory: a statement of relationships among important concepts (Chapter 1).

therapeutic use of self: term used by the occupational therapy profession in reference to interactive reasoning as a major component of clinical reasoning and goal setting with patients/clients (Chapter 1).

third-order neuron: arises from a cell body in the thalamus and projects to the sensory cortex (Chapter 3).

threshold: a critical voltage level that must be reached before depolarization of a cell membrane can occur (Chapter 2).

tonic stimuli: term used by the neurophysiological approach to intervention to describe a stimulus used to facilitate a stability response, such as approximation or resistance, employed to assist in the development of control in a chosen stability activity such as holding in a sitting position (Chapter 6).

top-down approach: the contemporary view on assessment and intervention that is so patient/client centered that it starts with an inquiry into how functional the individual is, whether there is adequate role competency for that individual in his or her own environment, and whether the role and ability to function is meaningful for that person. (Chapter 6).

tract: a group of nerve fibers that are similar in origin, destination, and function that carry impulses to and from various areas within the nervous system, sometimes traveling on one side (ipsilateral) and sometimes crossing (contralateral) (Chapter 2).

training: occurs when the performer is provided with solutions to problems, often resulting in short-term or limited performance capabilities (Chapter 5).

transfer: refers to movement from one surface to another and, as such, can be considered as a type of locomotion or mobility skill (Chapter 10).

transfer of learning: refers to the gain or loss of task performance as a result of practice or experience on some other task; the positive influence that a previously practiced skill has on the learning of a new skill or performing the same skill in a new environmental context (Chapter 5).

transition: change from one position to another (Chapter 4).

translation: when an object is moved from the fingertips to the palm or palm to fingertips (Chapter 9).

tremor: a rhythmic, involuntary, oscillatory movement of a body part, demonstrated as a result of damage to the central nervous system (Chapter 2).

two-point discrimination: the ability to detect that the skin is being touched by two points or objects at once, a function made possible through the inhibitory surround mechanism within the parietal lobe (Chapter 2).

undesirable compensations: compensations that do not utilize the individual's available movement patterns and work in opposition to the overall goal of optimal independent functional movement, by promoting asymmetries and poor alignment in the trunk and limbs; decreased weight acceptance, leading to inefficient or unsafe movement production; and/or the development of secondary impairments (Chapter 6).

upper motor neuron (UMN): neuron that arises from the cortex (Chapter 2).

upper motor neuron (UMN) lesions: affect the central nervous system, anywhere from the spinal cord superiorly, producing signs of UMN syndrome; typically associated with hypertonicity or hypotonicity, depending on the site of the lesion and the time of onset (acute versus chronic) (Chapter 7).

variable practice: organizing practice sessions so several variations of the same or similar tasks can be performed during the same session (Chapter 5).

velocity: temporal characteristic of movement, defined as distance covered over time (Chapter 10).

ventral horn: area in the front or anterior region of the spinal cord (Chapter 2).

vergence: the ability to regard a single object clearly whether it is near or far in the visual field (Chapter 9).

vertigo: a false sense of motion, typically accompanying a vestibular disorder (Chapter 3). A sensation of movement in the absence of actual physical movement (Chapter 8).

vestibulo-ocular reflex (VOR): regulation of eye position in the orbit to ensure that a steady image is held on the retina during movement, so that the eyes remain fixed on an object when the head or the body is moving (Chapters 3 and 8).

visual cognition: the ability to mentally manipulate visual information and synthesize it with other sensory information to solve problems, formulate plans, and make decisions (Chapter 9).

visual discrimination: the ability to detect features of an object in order to recognize it, match it, or categorize it (Chapter 9).

visual field: the extent of space within which you can see an object, projected onto the opposite side of the retina (Chapter 3).

visual fixation: the ability to sustain gaze on an object when looking at a stationary target (Chapter 9).

visual inattention: decreased visual scanning and regard (Chapter 9).

visual memory: receiving, storing, and retrieving visual information within the central nervous system (Chapter 9).

visual-motor control: the process by which a person uses visual information to perform smooth and precise movements (Chapter 9).

visual neglect: see *visual inattention* (Chapter 9).

visual perception: the ability to make meaning of what is seen (Chapter 9).

visual recall: the ability to recall visual information (Chapter 9).

volar: the palmar surface of the hand (Chapter 9).

volition: the will or desire to make a choice or decision (Chapter 9).

voluntary grasp: conscious control of grasp (Chapter 9).

weakness: an inability to generate normal levels of muscular force; a major impairment of motor function in patients/clients with nervous system damage (Chapter 7).

weight bearing: permitted by effective co-contraction and stability in postures, which further reinforces the ability to assume more weight (Chapter 4). Occurs when the extremity or extremities are stabilized against a surface in a position where they support body weight and form part of the body's base of support; also referred to as a closed-chain activity (Chapter 10).

weight shifting: a characteristic of mature movement control, occurring as one body part stabilizes simultaneously with the other body part being unweighted enough to move (Chapter 4).

Index

Entries with page numbers followed by b, f, and t indicate boxes, figures, and tables, respectively.